Basic Mechanisms
and Clinical Treatment
of Tumor Metastasis

Academic Press Rapid Manuscript Reproduction

Proceedings of an international symposium held at Fukuoka, Japan,
6–8 December 1982

Basic Mechanisms and Clinical Treatment of Tumor Metastasis

Edited by

MOTOMICHI TORISU

Kyushu University School of Medicine
Fukuoka, Japan

TAKESHI YOSHIDA

The University of Connecticut Health Center
Farmington, Connecticut

1985

ACADEMIC PRESS, INC.

(Harcourt Brace Jovanovich, Publishers)

Orlando   San Diego   New York   London
Toronto   Montreal   Sydney   Tokyo

ACADEMIC PRESS, INC.
Orlando, Florida 32887

United Kingdom Edition published by
ACADEMIC PRESS INC. (LONDON) LTD.
24/28 Oval Road, London NW1 7DX

Library of Congress Cataloging in Publication Data

Main entry under title:

Basic mechanisms and clinical treatment of tumor
   metastasis.

   Proceedings of the International Symposium on Basic
Mechanisms and Clinical Treatments of Tumor Metastasis,
held at Fukuoka, Japan, Dec. 6-8, 1982.
   Bibliography: p.
   Includes index.
   1. Metastasis--Congresses. I. Torisu, Motomichi.
II. Yoshida, Takeshi. III. International Symposium on
Basic Mechanisms and Clinical Treatments of Tumor
Metastasis (1982 : Fukuoka-shi, Japan) [DNLM:
1. Neoplasm metastasis--Physiopathology--Congresses.
2. Neoplasm metastasis--Therapy--Congresses. QZ 202 B311
1983]
RC269.B27 1985   616.99'4   83-21463
ISBN 0-12-695680-4 (alk. paper)

PRINTED IN THE UNITED STATES OF AMERICA

85 86 87 88   9 8 7 6 5 4 3 2 1

CONTENTS

PART I
Cellular Behavior of Metastatic Tumors
Chairpersons:
Gloria H. Heppner and Hiroshi Kobayashi

1. ROLE OF CELLULAR HETEROGENEITY IN TUMOR BEHAVIOR
    Gloria H. Heppner, Scott E. Loveless, Fred. R. Miller, Keith H. Mahoney, and Amy M. Fulton

2. THE QUANTITATION OF SOME ASPECTS OF INVASION *IN VIVO* AND *IN VITRO*
    Leonard Weiss and Okhee W. Suh

3. SPONTANEOUS REGRESSION OF XENOGENIZED TUMOR METASTASIS IN RATS
    Hiroshi Kobayashi

v

4. **EXPERIMENTAL STUDIES OF OPERATIVE STRESS
    ON TUMOR GROWTH IN RATS**

*Takao Hattori, Tetsuya Toge, Wataru Takiyama, Toshihiro Hirai,
and Toshiyuki Ikeda*

PART IIA
Regulations of Metastatic Tumor Cells
Chairpersons:
George Poste and Kokichi Kikuchi

5. **TUMOR CELL HETEROGENEITY AND THE PATHOGENESIS
    OF CANCER METASTASIS**

George Poste

6. **MOLECULAR MECHANISM OF ADHESIVENESS
    AND DISSOCIATION OF CANCER CELLS**

Hideo Hayashi, Yasuji Ishimaru, Ryuichi Hattori, and Shinya Kurano

7. **SYSTEMIC AND LOCAL REGULATION OF HUMAN NATURAL
    KILLER CYTOTOXICITY**

*Sidney H. Golub, Peter M. Moy, J. Dixon Gray, Linda M. Karavodin,
Norihiko Kawate, Masayuki Niitsuma, and Martyn W. Burk*

8. SIGNIFICANCE OF LOCAL T CELL RESPONSE TO HUMAN CANCER

Kokichi Kikuchi, Kiyoshi Kasai, Hiroyoshi Hiratsuka, Tomoaki Usui, Hirofumi Kamiya, and Izuru Shimokawara

9. NATURAL AND INDUCED RESISTANCE TO METASTASIS FROM MOUSE MAMMARY CARCINOMAS

Jan Vaage

PART IIB

Chairpersons:
Takeshi Yoshida and Hideo Hayashi

10. THE CELL SURFACE MARKERS OF TUMORICIDAL MACROPHAGES

Tohru Tokunaga, Kiyoko S. Akagawa, and Tadayoshi Taniyama

PART III
The Effects of Soluble Mediators
on Tumor Cell Metastasis

Chairpersons:
Stanley Cohen and Takeru Ishikawa

15. NONCYTOTOXIC EFFECTS OF LYMPHOKINES ON TUMOR CELLS

Stanley Cohen, William Munger, Marion C. Cohen, and Takeshi Yoshida

16. *IN VIVO* EFFECTS OF LYMPHOKINES ON TUMOR CELLS

Takeshi Yoshida, Helen D'Silva, Marion C. Cohen, Mark Donskoy, and Stanley Cohen

17. INDUCTION OF HUMAN SPECIFIC KILLER T CELL AGAINST AUTOLOGOUS CANCER CELLS AND ITS PROPAGATION BY T CELL GROWTH FACTOR

Takeru Ishikawa, Tsutomu Ikawa, Yukinori Ichino, and Mikio Toya

18. PROSTAGLANDINS IN TUMOR CELL METASTASIS

Kenneth V. Honn and Bonnie F. Sloane

PART IV
Immunological Aspects of Metastatic Tumors
Chairpersons:
Reiko F. Irie and Takehiko Tachibana

19. CLINICOPATHOLOGICAL AND IMMUNOLOGICAL ASPECTS OF METASTATIC MALIGNANT MELANOMA IN MAN

Alistair J. Cochran and Duan-Ren Wen

20. THE PRIMARY IMMUNOREGULATORY ROLE OF REGIONAL LYMPH NODES ON THE DEVELOPMENT OF LOCAL TUMOR AND LYMPHATIC METASTASIS

Kikuyoshi Yoshida and Takehiko Tachibana

21. ANTIBODIES TO TUMOR-ASSOCIATED GANGLIOSIDES (GM2 AND GD2): POTENTIAL FOR SUPPRESSION OF MELANOMA RECURRENCE

Reiko F. Irie, Tadashi Tai, and Donald L. Morton

22. A STUDY OF IMMUNE COMPLEX OF GLOMERULI IN CANCER PATIENTS, ASSOCIATED WITH IgG–RHEUMATOID FACTOR AND ANTINUCLEAR ANTIBODY

Tetsuzo Sugisaki, Hiroaki Nakajima, Takanori Shibata, and Hisashi Kawasumi

23. ANTIBODY THERAPY OF METASTATIC PROLIFERATION OF HUMAN NEOPLASTIC CELLS HETEROTRANSPLANTED INTO IMMUNODEFICIENT MICE

Emilio A. Machado, Bismarck B. Lozzio, Carmen B. Lozzio, David A. Gerard, James R. Mitchell, Carl J. Wust, and Elena G. Bamberger

PART VA
Clinical and Experimental New Approaches to Cancer Treatment
Chairpersons:
G. Mathé and Motoharu Kondo

PART VB

Chairpersons:
M. J. Embleton and Kikuo Nomoto

28. EXPERIMENTAL IMMUNOTHERAPY OF HUMAN MELANOMA WITH HUMAN MONOCLONAL ANTIBODY TO A TUMOR ANTIGEN (OFA-I-2) USING ATHYMIC NUDE MICE

Mitsuo Katano and Reiko F. Irie

29. POSTOPERATIVE LONG-TERM IMMUNOSTIMULATORY PROTEIN-BOUND POYSACCHARIDE KUREHA (PSK) THERAPY FOR ADVANCED GASTRIC CANCER

Ryunosuke Kumashiro, Youichiro Hiramoto, Takeshi Okamura, Tadashi Kano, Chiaki Sano, and Kiyoshi Inokuchi

30. THE ANTITUMOR AND TUMOR METASTASIS-INHIBITORY ACTIVITIES OF LENTINAN IN PRECLINICAL ANIMAL MODELS AND ITS POSSIBLE IMMUNE MECHANISMS

Goro Chihara

PART VC

Chairpersons:
Donald L. Morton and Motomichi Torisu

CONTRIBUTORS AND PARTICIPANTS

Numbers in parentheses indicate the pages on which the authors' contributions begin.

*KIYOKO S. AKAGAWA (193), Department of Tuberculosis, National Institute of Health, Tokyo 141, Japan

TADAHIRO AMAYA, Department of Clinical Research, Fujisawa Pharmaceutical Corp., Ltd., Osaka, Japan

HATSUO AOKI, Department of Cell Biology, Fujisawa Research Laboratory, Osaka, Japan

*ICHIRO AZUMA (449), Institute of Immunological Science, Hokkaido University, Sapporo 060, Japan

*R. W. BALDWIN (485), Cancer Research Campaign Laboratories, University of Nottingham, Nottingham NG7 2RD, England

*ELENA G. BAMBERGER (405), Laboratory of Experimental Hematology and Oncology, University of Tennessee Memorial Research Center, Knoxville, Tennessee 37920

*D. BELPOMME (477), Institut de Cancérologie et d'Immunogénétique (INSERM, CNRS), et Service des Maladies Sanguines et Tumorales, Groupe Hospitalier Paul-Brousse, 94804 Villejuif, France

*MARTYN W. BURK (123), Division of Surgical Oncology, John Wayne Clinic, Jonsson Comprehensive Cancer Center, University of California at Los Angeles School of Medicine, Los Angeles, California 90024

*GORO CHIHARA (535), National Cancer Center Research Institute, Tokyo 104, Japan

*ALISTAIR J. COCHRAN (338), Division of Surgical Oncology, John Wayne Clinic and Armand Hammer Laboratory, Departments of Pathology and Surgery, University of California at Los Angeles School of Medicine, Center for the Health Sciences, Los Angeles, California 90024

*MARION C. COHEN (273, 285), Department of Pathology, University of Connecticut Health Center, Farmington, Connecticut 06032

*STANLEY COHEN (273, 285), Department of Pathology, University of Connecticut Health Center, Farmington, Connecticut 06032

*HELEN D'SILVA (285), Department of Pathology, University of Connecticut Health Center, Farmington, Connecticut 06032

*M. DELGADO (477, 617), Institut de Cancérologie et d'Immunogénéti-

que (INSERM, CNRS), et Service des Maladies Sanguines et Tumorales, Groupe Hospitalier Paul-Brousse, 94804 Villejuif, France

*F. DE VASSAL (617), Institut de Cancérologie et d'Immunogénétique (INSERM, CNRS), et Service des Maladies Sanguines et Tumorales, Groupe Hospitalier Paul-Brousse, 94804 Villejuif, France

*MARK DONSKOY[1] (285), Department of Pathology, University of Connecticut Health Center, Farmington, Connecticut 06032

*M. J. EMBLETON (485), Cancer Research Campaign Laboratories, University of Nottingham, Nottingham NG7 2RD, England

*MASAZUMI ERIGUCHI[2] (223), Department of Surgery, Institute of Medical Science, University of Tokyo, Toyko 108, Japan

*GENSHICHIRO FUJII (223), Department of Clinical Oncology, Institute of Medical Science, University of Tokyo, Tokyo 108, Japan

*TAKASHI FUJIMURA (593), Department of Surgery, Kyushu University School of Medicine, Fukuoka 812, Japan

*AMY M. FULTON (3), Department of Immunology, Michigan Cancer Foundation, Detroit, Michigan 48201

*P. FUMOLEAU (477), Institut de Cancérologie et d'Immunogénétique (INSERM, CNRS), et Service des Maladies Sanguines et Tumorales, Groupe Hospitalier Paul-Brousse, 94804 Villejuif, France

*DAVID A. GERARD (405), Laboratory of Experimental and Comparative Pathology, Department of Medical Biology, Memorial Research Center, University of Tennessee College of Medicine, Knoxville, Tennessee 37920

*SIDNEY H. GOLUB (123), Division of Oncology, Department of Surgery, University of California at Los Angeles School of Medicine, Los Angeles, California 90024

*J. DIXON GRAY (123), Division of Oncology, Department of Surgery, University of California at Los Angeles School of Medicine, Los Angeles, California 90024

*J. GUERRIN (477, 617), Institut de Cancérologie et d'Immunogénétique (INSERM, CNRS), et Service des Maladies Sanguines et Tumorales, Groupe Hospitalier Paul-Brousse, 94804 Villejuif, France

*RISHAB K. GUPTA (561), Division of Surgical Oncology, John Wayne Clinic and Armand Hammer Laboratories, Jonsson Comprehensive Cancer Center, University of California at Los Angeles School of Medicine, Los Angeles, California 90024

*OSAMU HASHIMOTO (239), Department of Surgery, Okayama University Medical School, Okayama 700, Japan

[1]Present address: Department of Pathology, Hahnemann University Hospital, Philadelphia, Pennsylvania 19102.

[2]Present address: Institut de Cancérologie et d'Immunogénétique, Hôpital Paul-Brousse, 94804 Villejuif, France.

*AKIKAZU HATOSAKI (239), Department of Surgery, Okayama University Medical School, Okayama 700, Japan

HIROAKI HATTORI, Dai Nippon Pharmaceutical Corp., Ltd., Osaka, Japan

*RYUICHI HATTORI (101), Department of Pathology, Kumamoto University Medical School, Kumamoto 860, Japan

*TAKAO HATTORI (53), Department of Surgery, Research Institute for Nuclear Medicine and Biology, Hiroshima University, Hiroshima 734, Japan

*HIDEO HAYASHI (101), Department of Pathology, Kumamoto University Medical School, Kumamoto 860, Japan

*GLORIA H. HEPPNER (3), Department of Immunology, Michigan Cancer Foundation, Detroit, Michigan 48201

*TOSHIHIRO HIRAI (53), Department of Surgery, Research Institute for Nuclear Medicine and Biology, Hiroshima University, Hiroshima 734, Japan

*YOUICHIRO HIRAMOTO (523), Second Department of Surgery, Kyushu University School of Medicine, Fukuoka 812, Japan

*HIROYOSHI HIRATSUKA (143), Department of Pathology, Sapporo Medical College, Sapporo 060, Japan

*KENNETH V. HONN (311), Departments of Radiology, Radiation Oncology, and Biological Sciences, Wayne State University, Detroit, Michigan 48202

*TAKASHI HOSHINO (573), Department of Immunology, Fukui Medical School, Fukui 910-11 Japan

MASAO HOSOKAWA, Laboratory of Pathology, Cancer Institute, Hokkaido University School of Medicine, Sapporo, Japan

*JAMES F. HUTH (561), Division of Surgical Oncology, John Wayne Clinic and Armand Hammer Laboratories, Jonsson Comprehensive Cancer Center, University of California at Los Angeles School of Medicine, Los Angeles, California 90024

*YUKINORI ICHINO (293), Department of Otolaryngology, Kumamoto University School of Medicine, Kumamoto, Japan

*TSUTOMO IKAWA (293), Department of Otolaryngology, Kumamoto University School of Medicine, Kumamoto, Japan

*TOSHIYUKI IKEDA (53), Department of Surgery, Research Institute for Nuclear Medicine and Biology, Hiroshima University, Hiroshima 734, Japan

*KIYOSHI INOKUCHI (449, 523), Department of Surgery, Kyushu University School of Medicine, Fukuoka 812, Japan

TAKEO INOUE, Department of Gynecology, Aichi Cancer Center Hospital, Nagoya 464, Japan

*REIKO F. IRIE (371, 511), Division of Surgical Oncology, University of

California at Los Angeles School of Medicine, Los Angeles, California 90024

*TAKERU ISHIKAWA (293), Department of Otolaryngology, Kumamoto University School of Medicine, Kumamoto 860, Japan

*YASUJI ISHIMARU (101), Department of Pathology, Kumamoto University Medical School, Kumamoto 860, Japan

*HIDEAKI ITOH (593), Department of Surgery, Kyushu University School of Medicine, Fukuoka 812, Japan

TAKESHI IWAMURA, Department of Surgery, Miyazaki Medical College, Miyazaki 889, Japan

KAZUNORI IWASAKI, Department of Surgery, Kyushu University School of Medicine, Fukuoka 812, Japan

*C. JEANNE (617), Institut de Cancérologie et d'Immunogénétique (INSERM, CNRS), et Service des Maladies Sanguines et Tumorales, Groupe Hospitalier Paul-Brousse, 94804 Villejuif, France

*HIROFUMI KAMIYA (143), Department of Pathology, Sapporo Medical College, Sapporo 060, Japan

*TADASHI KANO (523), Second Department of Surgery, Kyushu University School of Medicine, Fukuoka 812, Japan

TAMOTSU KANO, Biochemical Research Laboratory, Kureha Chemical Industrial Corp., Ltd., Tokyo, Japan

*LINDA M. KARAVODIN (123), Division of Oncology, Department of Surgery, University of California at Los Angeles School of Medicine, Los Angeles, California 90024

*KIYOSHI KASAI (143), Department of Pathology, Sapporo Medical College, Sapporo 060, Japan

*MITSUO KATANO[3] (511, 593), Division of Surgical Oncology, University of California at Los Angeles School of Medicine, Los Angeles, California 90024

HARUKI KATO, Department of Medicine, Kyoto Prefectural University School of Medicine, Kyoto 700, Japan

*HISASHI KAWASUMI (385), Department of Internal Medicine, Showa University School of Medicine, Tokyo 142, Japan

*NORIHIKO KAWATE (123), Department of Surgery, Tokyo Medical College, Tokyo 160, Japan

*KOKICHI KIKUCHI (143), Department of Pathology, Sapporo Medical College, Sapporo 060, Japan

*YUTAKA KIMURA (593), Kimura Surgical Hospital, Fukuoka 812, Japan

*HIROSHI KOBAYASHI (41), Laboratory of Pathology, Cancer Institute, Hokkaido University School of Medicine, Sapporo 060, Japan

MASAO KOBAYASHI, Department of Surgery, Kyoto Prefectural University School of Medicine, Kyoto 700, Japan

[3]Present address: Department of Surgery, Saga Medical School, Saga 840-01, Japan.

*MOTOHARU KONDO (623), Department of Medicine, Kyoto Prefectural University of Medicine, Kyoto 602, Japan

*RYUNOSUKE KUMASHIRO (523), Second Department of Surgery, Kyushu University School of Medicine, Fukuoka 812, Japan

*SHINYA KURANO (101), Department of Pathology, Kumamoto University Medical School, Kumamoto 860, Japan

*B. LE MEVEL[4] (617), Institut de Cancérologie et d'Immunogénétique (INSERM, CNRS), et Service des Maladies Sanguines et Tumorales, Groupe Hospitalier Paul-Brousse, 94804 Villejuif, France

*LANCE A. LIOTTA (209), Laboratory of Pathology, National Cancer Institute, National Institutes of Health, Bethesda, Maryland 20205

*S. E. LOVELESS[5] (3), Department of Immunology, Michigan Cancer Foundation, Detroit, Michigan 48201

*BISMARCK B. LOZZIO[6] (405), Laboratory of Experimental Hematology and Oncology, University of Tennessee Memorial Research Center, Knoxville, Tennessee 37920

*CARMEN B. LOZZIO (405), Laboratory of Experimental Hematology and Oncology, and Laboratory of Medical Genetics, Department of Medical Biology, Center for the Health Sciences, University of Tennessee Memorial Research Center, Knoxville, Tennessee 37920

*EMILIO A. MACHADO (405), Laboratory of Experimental and Comparative Pathology, Department of Medical Biology, Memorial Research Center, University of Tennessee College of Medicine, Knoxville, Tennessee 37920

SHUZO MAEDA, New Product Evaluation Overseas Group, Fujisawa Pharmaceutical Corp., Ltd., Osaka, Japan

*KEITH H. MAHONEY (3), Department of Immunology, Michigan Cancer Foundation, Detroit, Michigan 48201

*G. MATHÉ (477, 617), Institut de Cancérologie et d'Immunogénétique (INSERM, CNRS), et Service des Maladies Sanguines et Tumorales, Groupe Hospitalier Paul-Brousse, 94804 Villejuif, France

*R. METZ (477, 617), Institut de Cancérologie et d'Immunogénétique (INSERM, CNRS), et Service des Maladies Sanguines et Tumorales, Groupe Hospitalier Paul-Brousse, 94804 Villejuif, France

*FRED R. MILLER (3), Department of Immunology, Michigan Cancer Foundation, Detroit, Michigan 48201

*J. L. MISSET (477, 617), Institut de Cancérologie et d'Immunogénétique (INSERM, CNRS), et Service des Maladies Sanguines et Tumorales, Groupe Hospitalier Paul-Brousse, 94804 Villejuif, France

*JAMES R. MITCHELL (405), Laboratory of Experimental Hematology and Oncology, University of Tennessee Memorial Research Center, Knoxville, Tennessee 37920

[4]Present address: Centre René Gauducheau, 44000 Nantes, France.
[5]Present address: E. I. DuPont de Nemours, Wilmington, Delaware 19898.
[6]Deceased.

*HIROAKI MIWA (239), Department of Surgery, Okayama University Medical School, Okayama 700, Japan

*YOJU MIYAMOTO (223), Department of Clinical Oncology, Institute of Medical Science, University of Tokyo, Tokyo 108, Japan

TADANORI MIYATA, Department of Surgery, Kyushu University School of Medicine, Fukuoka 812, Japan

*V. MORICE (617), Institut de Cancérologie et d'Immunogénétique (INSERM, CNRS), et Service des Maladies Sanguines et Tumorales, Groupe Hospitalier Paul-Brousse, 94804 Villejuif, France

NAOTO MORIYA, Department of Surgery, Okayama University Medical School, Okayama, Japan

*DONALD L. MORTON (371, 561), Division of Surgical Oncology, John Wayne Clinic and Armand Hammer Laboratories, Jonsson Comprehensive Cancer Center, University of California at Los Angeles School of Medicine, Los Angeles, California 90024, and Surgical Services, Veterans Administration Medical Center, Sepulveda, California 91343

*PETER M. MOY (123), Division of Oncology, Department of Surgery, University of California at Los Angeles School of Medicine, Los Angeles, California 90024

*WILLIAM MUNGER (273), Department of Pathology, University of Connecticut Health Center, Farmington, Connecticut 06032

KAZUYO NAITO, Department of Surgery, Kyoto Prefectural University School of Medicine, Kyoto 700, Japan

*HIROAKI NAKAJIMA (385), Department of Internal Medicine, Showa University School of Medicine, Tokyo 142, Japan

HIDEKI NAKANO, Chugai Pharmaceutical Corp., Ltd., Tokyo, Japan

*MASAYUKI NIITSUMA (123), Department of Surgery, Tokyo Medical College, Tokyo 160, Japan

*KIKUO NOMOTO (449), Department of Immunology, Institute for Bioregulation, Kyushu University, Fukuoka 812, Japan

*TAKENORI OCHIAI (465), Second Department of Surgery, Chiba University School of Medicine, Chiba 280, Japan

*HIDECHIKA OKADA[7] (255), National Cancer Research Institute, Tokyo 104, Japan

*NORIKO OKADA[7] (255), Department of Bacteriology, The Kitasato Institute, Tokyo 108, Japan

*TAKESHI OKAMURA (523), Second Department of Surgery, Kyushu University School of Medicine, Fukuoka 812, Japan

*KUNZO ORITA (239), Department of Surgery, Okayama University Medical School, Okayama 700, Japan

*M. V. PIMM (485), Cancer Research Campaign Laboratories, University of Nottingham, Nottingham NG7 2RD, England

[7]Present address: Department of Microbiology, Fukuoka University School of Medicine, Fukuoka 814-01, Japan.

*R. PLAGNE (477, 617), Institut de Cancérologie et d'Immunogénétique (INSERM, CNRS), et Service des Maladies Sanguines et Tumorales, Groupe Hospitalier Paul-Brousse, 94804 Villejuif, France

*GEORGE POSTE (79), Smith Kline and French Laboratories, Philadelphia, Pennsylvania 19101, and Department of Pathology and Laboratory Medicine, University of Pennsylvania Medical School, Philadelphia, Pennsylvania 19104

*RAYMONDO G. RUSSO (209), Laboratory of Pathology, National Cancer Institute, National Institutes of Health, Bethesda, Maryland 20205

*MASAKI SAKATA (593), Department of Surgery, Kyushu University School of Medicine, Fukuoka 812, Japan

*CHIAKI SANO (523), Second Department of Surgery, Kyushu University School of Medicine, Fukuoka 812, Japan

*HIROSHI SATO (465), Second Department of Surgery, Chiba University School of Medicine, Chiba 280, Japan

*M. SCHNEIDER[8] (617), Institut de Cancérologie et d'Immunogénétique (INSERM, CNRS), et Service des Maladies Sanguines et Tumorales, Groupe Hospitalier Paul-Brousse, 94804 Villejuif, France

*MORIMASA SEKIGUCHI (223), Department of Clinical Oncology, Institute of Medical Science, University of Tokyo, Tokyo 108, Japan

*B. SERROU[9] (617), Institut de Cancérologie et d'Immunogénétique (INSERM, CNRS), et Service des Maladies Sanguines et Tumorales, Groupe Hospitalier Paul-Brousse, 94804 Villejuif, France

*TAKANORI SHIBATA (385), Department of Internal Medicine, Showa University School of Medicine, Tokyo 142, Japan

*IZURU SHIMOKAWARA (143), Department of Pathology, Sapporo Medical College, Sapporo 060, Japan

*BONNIE F. SLOANE (311), Departments of Pharmacology and Radiation Oncology, Wayne State University School of Medicine, Detroit, Michigan 48201

*TETSUZO SUGISAKI (385), Department of Internal Medicine, Showa University School of Medicine, Tokyo 142, Japan

*OKHEE W. SUH (23), Departments of Experimental Pathology and Biomathematics, Roswell Park Memorial Institute, Buffalo, New York 14263

*TAKEHIKO TACHIBANA (355), Department of Immunology, Research Institute for Tuberculosis and Cancer, Tohoku University, Sendai 980, Japan

*TETSUO TAGUCHI (549), Department of Oncologic Surgery, The Research Institute for Microbial Diseases, Osaka University, Osaka 565, Japan

[8]Present address: Centre Antoine Lacassagne, Service d'Hématologie–Cancérologie, 06054 Nice, France.
[9]Present address: Laboratoire d'Immunopharmacologie des Tumeurs, Centre Paul Lamarque, 34-033 Montpellier, France.

*TADASHI TAI (371), Division of Surgical Oncology, University of California at Los Angeles School of Medicine, Los Angeles, California 90024

*MASAHARU TAKESUE (593), Kimura Surgical Hospital, Fukuoka 812, Japan

SHOJIRO TAKETSUKA, Department of Surgery, Okayama University Medical School, Okayama 700, Japan

*WATARU TAKIYAMA (53), Department of Surgery, Research Institute for Nuclear Medicine and Biology, Hiroshima University, Hiroshima 734, Japan

*HIROKO TANAKA (255), National Cancer Center Research Institute, Tokyo 104, Japan

*TADAYOSHI TANIYAMA (193), Department of Tuberculosis, National Institute of Health, Tokyo 141, Japan

*UNNUR P. THORGEIRSSON (209), Laboratory of Pathology, National Cancer Institute, National Institutes of Health, Bethesda, Maryland 20205

*TETSUYA TOGE (53), Department of Surgery, Research Institute for Nuclear Medicine and Biology, Hiroshima University, Hiroshima 734, Japan

*TOHRU TOKUNAGA (193), Department of Tuberculosis, National Institute of Health, Tokyo 141, Japan

HIROYUKI TOMIKURA, Chugai Pharmaceutical Corp., Ltd., Tokyo, Japan

YUJI TOMOOKA, Department of Pediatrics, Kyushu University School of Medicine, Fukuoka 812, Japan

*MOTOMICHI TORISU (593, 623), Department of Surgery, Kyushu University School of Medicine, Fukuoka 812, Japan

*MIKIO TOYA (293), Department of Otolaryngology, Kumamoto University School of Medicine, Kumamoto 860, Japan

*ATSUSHI UCHIDA[10] (573), Institute for Applied and Experimental Oncology, University of Vienna, A-1090 Vienna, Austria

*TOMOAKI USUI (143), Department of Pathology, Sapporo Medical College, Sapporo 060, Japan

*JAN VAAGE (163), Department of Experimental Pathology, Roswell Park Memorial Institute, Buffalo, New York 14263

*LEONARD WEISS (23), Department of Experimental Pathology, Roswell Park Memorial Institute, Buffalo, New York 14263

*DUAN-REN WEN (338), Division of Surgical Oncology, Department of Surgery, University of California at Los Angeles School of Medicine, Center for the Health Sciences, Los Angeles, California 90024

[10]Present address: Division of Immunology, Paterson Laboratories, Christie Hospital and Holt Radium Institute, Manchester M20 9BX, England.

*CARL J. WUST (405), Department of Microbiology, University of Tennessee, Knoxville, Tennessee 37996

HISAKAZU YAMAGISHI, Department of Surgery, Kyoto Prefectural University School of Medicine, Kyoto, Japan

*YUICHI YAMAMURA (449), Osaka University, Osaka 553, Japan

*KOSEI YASUMOTO (449), Second Department of Surgery, Kyushu University School of Medicine, Fukuoka 812, Japan

*KIKUYOSHI YOSHIDA (355), Department of Immunology, Research Institute for Tuberculosis and Cancer, Tohoku University, Sendai 980, Japan

*TAKESHI YOSHIDA[11] (273, 285, 593), Department of Pathology, University of Connecticut Health Center, Farmington, Connecticut 06032

TOSHIKAZU YOSHIKAWA, Department of Medicine, Kyoto Prefectural University School of Medicine, Kyoto, Japan

MAKOTO YOSHIMURA, Biochemical Research Laboratory, Kureha Chemical Industry Corp., Ltd., Tokyo, Japan

[11]Present address: Merck Sharp & Dohme Research Laboratories/Japan, MSD (Japan) Co., Ltd., Tokyo 107, Japan.

PREFACE

Since the early 1960s extensive basic and clinical studies on immunochemotherapy have been performed throughout the world. In Japan, for example, the clinical application of immunochemotherapy has been an important part of the treatment of various malignant neoplasms for more than a decade. Although these trials have produced both fruitful and disappointing results, we are convinced that the metastatic spread and growth of tumors can be controlled if we can successfully activate, maintain, and enhance the natural immunologic mechanisms of cancer patients. To achieve this we must determine the most appropriate form of immunotherapy for each case, based on the general immune status of the patient. Therefore, information on the basic mechanisms of cancer spreading and on the complex immune status of tumor-bearing individuals is urgently needed for clinical investigators. To address this need we have prepared this volume based on an international symposium entitled "Basic Mechanisms and Clinical Treatments of Cancer Metastasis," at which world experts in basic research on cancer metastasis and clinical investigators in immunochemotherapy of cancer gathered and discussed the direction of research needed to find the most effective immunological treatment of cancer and its metastasis.

There have been many books dealing separately with the basic mechanism of tumor metastasis or with the clinical results with immunochemotherapy of cancer. This volume is unique in that basic and clinical studies on cancer metastasis have been brought together in an attempt to stimulate both basic and clinical investigators to find the best method for the eventual control of metastasis. Another unique feature of the book is the inclusion of rather extensive studies of clinical trials of cancer immunochemotherapy by Japanese investigators who have played a pivotal role in the clinical assessment of various immunomodulating drugs. The chapters dealing with this aspect provide us with an excellent opportunity to evaluate this approach. Most of these studies provide new data or only partially published data that have not been accessible to the international scientific community.

The four chapters in the first part of this volume cover both the *in vivo* and *in vitro* behavior of metastatic tumor cells. The second part includes ten chapters that address the pathogenesis of cancer metastasis and its possible modulation by immune cells per se or by those treated with immunopotentiators in experimental animals. The third part of the book contains four chapters on the effects of various soluble immune mediators on tumor cell growth and metastasis. The five chapters in the fourth part deal with the immunobiology and immunopathology of human tumor cell metastasis. The final part of this volume discusses clinical treatments of cancer and metastasis. Most of these chapters discuss both successful and unsuccessful trials with cancer immunotherapy using various new biological and chemical compounds.

We trust that this volume will provide a better understanding of our present knowledge concerning the basic mechanisms of cancer metastasis and the current immunochemotherapeutic approaches to cancer treatment. We hope that these chapters will stimulate readers to search for new approaches in their own research. This volume should be particularly useful for active investigators in the fields of tumor biology and clinical research on cancer metastasis, and for academic clinicians in oncology.

Motomichi Torisu
Takeshi Yoshida

ACKNOWLEDGMENTS

The organizers of the International Symposium, "Basic Mechanisms and Clinical Treatments of Tumor Metastasis," express their sincere appreciation to the following for their generous financial support: Chugai Pharmaceutical Co., Ltd., Sankyo Co., Ltd., Kureha Chemical Industry Co., Ltd., Mitsui Pharmaceuticals Inc., Fujisawa Pharmaceutical Co., Ltd., Shionogi and Co., Ltd., Nipponzoki Pharmaceutical Co., Ltd., Eisai Co., ICI Pharma Ltd., Morishita Pharmaceutical Co., Ltd., Takeda Chemical Industry Co., Ltd., Green Cross Co., Ltd., Zeria Pharmaceuticals, Nippon Kayaku Co., Ltd., Ono Pharmaceutical Co., Ltd., Daiichi Seiyaku Co., Ltd., Kyowa Hakko Kogyo Co., Ltd., Bayer A.G., Mochida Pharmaceuticals Co., Inc., Funai Corp., Sumitomo Chemical Co., Ltd., Taiho Pharmaceutical Co., Ltd., Nippon Boeringer Ingelheim Co., Ltd., Torii and Co., Ltd., Nippon Roussel Co., Ltd., Kaken Pharmaceutical Co., Ltd., Sandoz Pharmaceutical Co., Ltd., and Dainippon Pharmaceutical Co., Ltd.

We also acknowledge the patronage of the Fukuoka Cancer Society. We express our sincere gratitude to Drs. Kiyoshi Inokuchi, Hideya Endo, Motoharu Kondo, Tetsuzo Sugisaki, Takeru Ishikawa, Masaki Sakata, and Kikuo Nomato, who have supported us in a variety of ways. Without such support, this publication and the symposium would not have been possible. Finally, but not least, we are extremely grateful for the excellent secretarial efforts of K. Matsui, Y. Horie, K. Yasutake, K. Yamamoto, Y. Asai, and H. Yamashita, who helped run the symposium.

PART I

Cellular Behavior of Metastatic Tumors

Chairpersons

Gloria H. Heppner
Hiroshi Kobayashi

CHAPTER 1

ROLE OF CELLULAR HETEROGENEITY
IN TUMOR BEHAVIOR

Gloria H. Heppner
Scott E. Loveless
Fred R. Miller
Keith H. Mahoney
Amy M. Fulton

Department of Immunology
Michigan Cancer Foundation
Detroit, Michigan

BASIC MECHANISMS AND CLINICAL TREATMENT
OF TUMOR METASTASIS

3

I. TUMOR CELL HETEROGENEITY OF MAMMARY TUMORS

    Over the last 5 years there has been great interest in the
basis for neoplastic variability among cancers of different individuals and within single neoplasms. Attention has been drawn
particularly to the presence of multiple tumor cell subpopulations,
either occurring simultaneously or developing over the course of
tumor progression. Clonal heterogeneity has been demonstrated in
a wide spectrum of cancers of different organ sites and histological types (reviewed in Heppner and Miller, 1982). Breast cancer
has been no exception; formal demonstration of distinct tumor subpopulations has been achieved with both mouse (Dexter et al.,
1978; Macinnes et al., 1981; Michalides et al., 1982) and rat
(Bennett et al., 1978; Neri and Nicolson, 1981; Dulbecco et al.,
1981) mammary cancers, with autochthonous (Dexter et al., 1978) as
well as transplanted (Neri and Nicolson, 1981) tumors, and with
tumors of both viral (Dexter et al., 1978) and chemical (Tseng,
1980; Neri and Nicolson, 1981) etiology. Evidence consistent with
the existence of distinct tumor cell subpopulations has also been
presented in human breast cancers (Brennan et al., 1979; Parbhoo,
1981; Weiss et al., 1981; Nuti et al., 1982). Although clonal diversity is not the only basis for intratumor heterogeneity (Weiss,
1980; Dethlefsen, 1980; Vaupel et al., 1981; Heppner and Miller,
1982), it would seem to be a major and common factor.
    The existence of multiple tumor subpopulations provides a
ready explanation for many clinical and experimental observations
in tumor biology. For example, tumor progression may arise from
sequential selection of tumor variants (Nowell, 1976). Treatment
failure can be understood as due to resistant clones already
present at the time of diagnosis, as well as those arising later
(Goldie and Coldman, 1979). Cancers thus seem to consist of multiple units, each one of which is responsible for certain characteristics of the whole neoplasm. The purpose of this presentation
is to review work of our laboratory, which is seeking to under--
stand how cellular heterogeneity affects tumor behavior. As will
be discussed, the picture is much more complex than the simple
"multiple unit" scheme would imply.

A. A Mouse Mammary Tumor Model of Tumor
    Heterogeneity

    Our work has utilized a series of tumor subpopulations that
were isolated from a single strain BALB/cfC$_3$H mouse mammary cancer
(Dexter et al., 1978; Heppner et al., 1978). Four of these subpopulations (designated 66, 67, 68H, and 168) derive from the
autochthonous parent tumor; the fifth (4.10) comes from a lung
metastasis of a subcutaneous implant of the tenth in vivo-passage
generation of the original tumor. These subpopulations are now
long-term lines that undoubtedly have undergone changes since

their original isolation. We are using them as "tools" to study the consequences of tumor heterogeneity, not as immutable members of their parent tumor. Evidence suggesting that they are, however, descendants of distinct subpopulations of one tumor has been presented elsewhere (Dexter et al., 1978).

Our five subpopulations, and certain of their clonal derivatives, differ in a wide array of characteristics: karyotype (Dexter et al., 1978), in vitro growth properties (Dexter et al., 1978), antigenicity (Dexter et al., 1978; Hager and Heppner, 1982), immunogenicity (Miller and Heppner, 1979a), drug sensitivity (Heppner et al., 1978), tumor latency period and growth rate (Dexter et al., 1978), and ability to metastasize (Miller et al., 1983). Although these subpopulations are in general stable and "breed true" after sequential in vitro—in vivo passage, 68H acts like a tumorigenic "stem cell" line and produces further variants on growth in vivo (Hager et al., 1981).

B. Tumor Subpopulation Interactions

The fact that one can isolate subpopulations of tumor cells that behave differently from their parent tumor, as well as from each other, suggests that tumor behavior is not just a simple composite of the individual characteristics of the subunits. Rather it would seem, and experimental evidence suggests (Hauschka, 1953; Klein and Klein, 1956; Jansson and Revesz, 1976; Keyner et al., 1978; Newcomb et al., 1978), that the behavior of the individual subpopulations can be modified by the presence of other subpopulations. We have demonstrated that subpopulations can "interact" to alter growth (Heppner et al., 1980; Miller et al., 1980), sensitivity to drugs (Miller et al., 1981; Heppner, 1982), and immunogenicity (Miller and Heppner, 1979b).

The results of our work support the concept of a tumor as an "ecosystem" (Heppner, 1982). The individual subpopulations are influenced by each other directly, and through each other by the host, to behave in a more homogeneous fashion than their heterogeneous characteristics might suggest. This is not to imply that their individual characteristics are not important, but to point out that they are subject to mutual regulation. For example, relatively slow-developing line 4.10 tumors can retard the growth of 168 tumors when cells of the two tumor lines are injected on opposite sides of the same mouse (Miller et al., 1980). The mechanism of this growth interaction depends on the host having an intact immune system and involves the ability of 4.10 tumors to elicit a strong immunity to themselves, and to 168 tumors, whereas 168 tumors are themselves essentially nonimmunogenic. We have also demonstrated other tumor subpopulation growth interactions that do not depend on the host and that can be seen in vitro (Heppner et al., 1980). The direction of these interactions can be either stimulatory or inhibitory to growth of particular subpopulations. In one case there is evidence for the release of a

factor from one subpopulation that can inhibit growth of other
subpopulations at a distance. There is an element of specificity
to all these growth interactions in that they are seen with certain combinations of subpopulations. The demonstration of multiple, diverse mechanisms suggests that tumor subpopulation growth
interactions are "opportunistic," that is, they do not occur
through general mechanisms but depend on the environmental circumstances of the cells and their individual characteristics. Similar conclusions can be drawn from our studies of interactions
that affect immunogenicity and sensitivity to chemotherapeutic
drugs. Knowing the immunological or drug sensitivity characteristics of the tumor subpopulations, as determined on isolated
clones, does not predict these characteristics when the subpopulations are growing together.

The characteristic that has received the greatest attention of
students of tumor heterogeneity is the ability to metastasize
(Fidler and Kripke, 1977). Many cancers, including our mammary
tumor, have yielded subpopulations that differ in invasive and
metastatic properties. Even metastasis, however, is subject to
the influence of tumor subpopulation interaction. Both experimental and clinical observations are suggestive of growth interactions between metastatic cells and other subpopulations within
primary cancers (Sugarbaker et al., 1977; Gorelik et al., 1982).
Poste (Chapter 5, this volume) discusses the role of clonal interactions in stabilization of the metastatic phenotype (Poste et
al., 1981). Data from our laboratory indicate other types of interactions affect metastasis. A brief description of this work
follows.

Line 168 tumors only rarely metastasize from primary implants
growing either subcutaneously or in the mammary fatpad. However,
intravenous (iv) injection of 168 cells, particularly at doses
greater than 10^5 cells, may result in lung "metastases." Tumors
of line 410.4 (a highly metastatic variant of 410) metastasize to
lung from both the subcutis and fatpad, as well as after iv injection (Miller et al., 1983). Strain BALB/c mice were injected
subcutaneously (sc) with 2 X 10^5 line 168 cells. The tumors were
allowed to grow to a mean diameter of 12 mm, at which time the
mice were divided randomly into three groups: One received iv saline, one received iv 168 cells, and the third received iv 410.4
cells. Five weeks later, when the mean diameter of the sc tumor
was 28 mm, the mice were sacrificed. None of the mice that had
received either saline or 168 cells iv had visible lung metastases.
About half the mice that had received 410.4 cells had lung metastases. Individual metastases were isolated and placed in monolayer culture. Lines 410.4 and 168 cells have distinctive morph-
ologies in monolayer; 410.4 cells are polygonal, whereas 168 cells
are fusiform. Interestingly, cultures from some of the metastases
contained cells morphologically identical to 168 cells, as well as
to 410.4 cells. Cells of both types could grow to form large colonies in vitro.

In a second experiment the effect of 410.4 cells on lung

TABLE I

Metastasis of "Nonmetastatic" Mammary Tumor Cells

Experiment number	Cell type (iv)	Incidence of metastasis[a]	Cell type in metastases
1[b]	Saline	0/5	—
	168 (10^4)[c]	0/7	—
	410.4 (10^4)	4/7	168 cells in 2/9 metastases[d]
			410.4 cells in 9/9 metastases
2	67 (3×10^6)	0/5	—
	410.4 (10^4)	1/5	—
	67 (3×10^6) + 410.4 (10^4)	9/10	67 cells in 7/13 metastases[e]
			410.4 cells in 9/13 metastases

[a] Number of mice with metastases/number in group.
[b] All mice bore subcutaneous line 168 tumors.
[c] Number of cells injected.
[d] Nine metastases cultured from three mice.
[e] Thirteen metastases cultured from six mice.

colony formation by another essentially nonmetastatic line, 67, was tested. In this experiment BALB/cfC$_3$H mice were injected iv with line 67 cells alone, line 410.4 cells alone, or a mixture of the two. Five weeks later the mice were sacrificed and individual metastases were cultured from the latter group. Again cultures yielded growing colonies of both types of cells. A summary of the data from both experiments is shown in Table I.

A third experiment utilized another combination of metastatic and nonmetastatic subpopulations. In this experiment, only cells of the metastatic line grew in monolayer cultures of the lung metastases, that is, there was no interaction in production of metastasis.

These data are clearly still preliminary. For experiments 1 and 2 we need more definitive evidence that the monolayer cultures contain the two tumor cell types, since cellular morphology alone is inadequate. Current efforts are directed toward introducing drug resistance markers into the various subpopulations to aid in their isolation from metastatic nodules. The results suggest, however, that tumor subpopulations may complement each other, so that cells that would not metastasize by themselves can do so with the "right" partner. Perhaps the mechanism involves the production and systemic release by one partner of some factor, such as a proteinase, which can aid the other subpopulation through an

essential step in the metastatic cascade. A tempting candidate
for such a mechanism would be enzyme-containing membrane vesicles
(Dvorak *et al.*, 1981), especially in the light of the report in
the B16 melanoma system that fusion of membrane vesicles from
metastatic cells with "nonmetastatic" cells can transfer the ability to metastasize (Poste and Nicolson, 1980). Alternatively,
an effect on the host, such as suppression of immunity, might be
an underlying mechanism for the interaction. Again the mechanisms
would depend on the characteristics of the participating subpopulations. Only those subpopulations that could compensate for the
particular factor or circumstance that prevents the nonmetastatic
population from metastasizing on its own would be expected to
"interact." Whatever the mechanism, the complex nature of the
role of cellular heterogeneity in tumor behavior is once again
evident.

The experiments in Table I are examples of subpopulation interactions that promote metastasis. Other experimental protocols
may demonstrate inhibition. In one experiment, BALB/c mice were
injected sc with a mixture of 168 cells and cells of 4501, a metastatic clone of 4.10. Control mice were injected with either
168 or 4501 cells. As expected, none of the 15 mice bearing 168
tumors alone developed metastasis, whereas 4 of 7 mice bearing
4501 tumors alone had lung metastasis 38 days after tumor injection. However, none of the 6 mice bearing both tumors had developed metastasis when the experiment was terminated at 63 days.
The mechanism of this inhibition is as yet unknown, but we have
previously demonstrated production by monolayers of 168 cells of
a factor that could inhibit growth of some tumor cells *in vitro*
(Heppner *et al.*, 1980).

II. HOST CELL HETEROGENEITY OF MAMMARY TUMORS

In addition to multiple tumor cell subpopulations, tumors consist of a variety of normal cells, including infiltrating lymphocytes and macrophages. These cells are thought to contribute to
the behavior of cancers and, indeed, much effort has been directed
toward making them more effective in controlling tumor growth and
spread. An underlying assumption in this effort is that the infiltrating cells represent a "response" of the host to neoplastic
cells. Neoplastic cells are viewed as strong or weak immunogens,
and the effectiveness of the host response is looked at in quantitative terms. Just as with the "multiple unit" scheme of tumor
heterogeneity (see earlier), this view ignores much of the subtlety
of host—tumor cell association. Some years ago we reported that
individual mouse mammary tumors contained distinctive patterns of
infiltrating macrophages and lymphocytes (Blazar and Heppner,
1978). These patterns persisted even when the tumors were passaged into new hosts. This suggested that the pattern of host

TABLE II

T Cell Content of Mammary Tumor Subpopulations

	Phenotypes				Mean recovered cells (%)			
Tumor	Mean latency period (days)	Metastatic frequency[b] (%)	Primary immunogenicity[c]	Secondary immunogenicity[d]	ALS$^+$	Thy-1.2$^+$	Lyt-1.2$^+$	Lyt-2.2$^+$
68H (13)[a]	60	0	++	—	36	24	25^e	8
168 (11)	19	3	$\pm$	—	12^e	9^e	4	8
410 (11)	24	8	++	++	39	29	8	24^e
410.4 (3)	14	82	n.d.^{f}	+	38	24	0	22
4501 (4)	14	66	n.d.	—	35	23	4	22

[a] Number of experiments in parentheses.

[b] Spontaneous metastasis from a subcutaneous implant.

[c] Based on relative growth in normal adult mice versus mice immunosuppressed by 400 rad irradiation 2 days prior to injection ± thymectomy.

[d] Based on ability to induce transplantation immunity to a secondary challenge.

[e] $p < .002$, Wilcoxon rank sum test. Indicated value compared to rest of values in the same column for tumors 68H, 168, and 410.

[f] n.d., Not determined.

"immune" response to these tumors was, in fact, determined not by
the host, but by the tumor. We have since extended this work to
see how tumor heterogeneity might contribute to the nature of the
infiltrating cells (Rios et al., 1983).

A.   Patterns of Lymphocyte Infiltration
      in Tumor Subpopulations

     Tumors were removed when at least 10 mm in diameter, the cells
were placed into suspension, and the lymphocytes were isolated by
the isokinetic gradient method of Pretlow (1971). Mean total cell
recovery for tumors of the five subpopulations studied ranged from
43 to 71%. The mean percentage of these cells recovered in fractions 4 and 5 of the gradient, where most of the lymphocytes are
found, ranged from 13 to 45%. The mean percentage of recovered
cells in fraction 10, the peak tumor cell fraction, ranged from 10
to 72%. Since our earlier work showed that BALB/cfC$_3$H mammary
tumors contain very few, if any, B cells (Blazar and Heppner,
1978), we concentrated on identifying T cells within the lymphocyte fractions. To do this we used monoclonal antisera (New England Nuclear, Boston, Massachusetts) against T cell antigens in
standard cytotoxicity assays. The tumor subpopulations were chosen on the basis of differences in their immunological and growth
characteristics. A summary of results is presented in Table II.
In this table the percentages of lymphocyte subpopulations are expressed in terms of the total number of cells recovered from the
entire gradient. Since there is a greater cell loss in the late
fractions than in the early lymphocyte-containing fractions, these
percentages do not represent the true T cell content of the tumors,
but they do provide a relative indication of the number of T cells
among the tumor subpopulations.
     As Table II shows, different mammary tumor lines contain char-
acteristic amounts and distribution of T cells and T cell subsets.
Line 168 tumors are relatively poor in lymphocytes (anti-lymphocyte serum, ALS[+]), as well as in T cells (Thy-1.2[+]) and in T cells
of the helper phenotype (Lyt-1.2[+]) and T cells of the killer-suppressor phenotype (Lyt-2.2[+]). The other lines contain comparable
numbers of ALS[+] and Thy-1.2[+] cells. However, 68H tumors contain
relatively more Lyt-1.2[+] than Lyt-2.2[+] cells. The opposite pattern is seen in all the other tumor lines. That these T cell patterns are the function of the tumor rather than the host is illustrated in Table III. Strain BALB/cfC$_3$H mice were injected on
opposite sides with 68H cells and 168 cells. Controls were injected on two sides with cells of the same lines. The T cell distribution in the tumors was characteristic for the tumor type,
irrespective of the identity of the contralateral tumor.
     As can also be seen in Table II, the number of lymphocytes and
the T cell distribution does not correlate with tumor growth, metastatic ability, or immunogenicity. Interestingly, the tumor
with the highest number and proportion of Lyt-1.2[+] is also the

TABLE III

T Cell Distribution in Bilateral Tumor Subpopulations[a]

	Control		Experiment		Control	
	Side 1	Side 2	Side 1	Side 2	Side 1	Side 2
Cell type	68H	68H	68H	168	168	168
Ratio of Lyt-1.2:Lyt-2.2	5	2.3	3.5	0.2	0.8	0.3

[a]Mean of three experiments.

tumor with the longest latency period. In contrast, a relatively high proportion of Lyt-2.2$^+$ cells was found in the four tumor lines with relatively short latency periods. Mule et al. (1981) have also presented data suggestive of a similar correlation between Lyt phenotype and tumor growth.

B. Patterns of Macrophage Infiltration
   in Tumor Subpopulations

We have also isolated and characterized the macrophage component of tumors produced by the various subpopulation lines (Loveless and Heppner, 1983; Mahoney et al., 1983). In our initial work the macrophages were isolated by adherence to plastic from enzyme digests of whole (15-mm diameter) tumors. The macrophages were identified by morphology, the presence of Fc receptors, and the ability to phagocytize latex beads. Using these methods, tumors of the four lines studied, namely 66, 67, 68H, and 410.4, were found to contain comparable percentages (20-25%) of macrophages. Thus, like other investigators, we found no correlation between macrophage content and either immunogenicity or ability to metastasize (Evans and Lawler, 1980; Talmadge et al., 1981).

Our next step was to test tumor-associated macrophages for cytotoxicity to tumor cells. Although cultured cells of all our tumor subpopulations are equally susceptible to killing by MVE-2-activated macrophages (mean cytotoxicity level at 10 macrophages: 1 tumor cell = ~50%), for these studies line 67 cells were used as a standard target. Target cells were labeled with [^{3}H]thymidine ([^{3}H]dThd) and added to varying numbers of adherent, tumor-isolated macrophages. The extent of isotope release was determined after a 48-h incubation period. As shown in Fig. 1, tumoricidal activity was consistently seen with macrophages from the metastatic tumors, 66 and 410.4 (14 of 14 experiments). Macrophages from nonmetastatic tumors, 68H and 67, were tumoricidal at a much lower frequency (6 of 15 experiments).

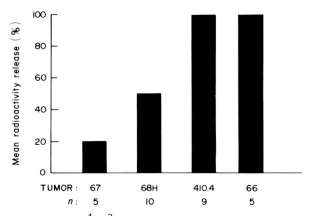

Fig. 1.   About 10^4 [^{3}H]dThd-labeled tumor cells were coincu-
bated with adherent, trypsin-resistant cells isolated from enzyme-
dissociated mammary tumors.   Two days later, supernatant material
was assayed for radioactivity.   Differences in mean radioactive
release between experimental and spontaneous release were assessed
by ANOVA with Dunnett's t-test and considered significant at the
$p < .05$ level. n, Number of individual tumors tested.

We have subsequently extended these observations in a detailed
study on the distribution of macrophage subpopulations in metastatic versus nonmetastatic mammary tumors.   Like tumor cells and
lymphocytes, macrophages are a heterogeneous population.   The existence of macrophage subpopulations has been reported on the basis
of antigenic (Sun and Lohmann-Matthes, 1982), enzymatic (Morahan
et al., 1980), and functional (Morahan et al., 1980; Campbell et
al., 1980) criteria.   We have attempted to separate macrophage
subpopulations by counterflow centrifugal elutriation (in a Beck-
man J2-21 centrifuge with JE-6B elutriation head) of whole-tumor
suspensions, followed by adherence of each fraction on plastic.
Both total cell viability (trypan blue) and cell recovery exceeded
90%.   As is indicated in Table IV, a greater proportion of macrophages from our metastatic tumors separated into the "heavier"
fractions of the elutriation gradient than did the macrophages
from the nonmetastatic tumors.   This suggests that macrophages
from the metastatic tumors consist of a higher proportion of larger and more dense, mature cell populations than do macrophages
from the nonmetastatic tumors.   This was most noticeable for tumor
66, in which 17% of the macrophages were found in fraction 4.
The macrophages in each fraction were assayed for the ectoen-
zymes leucine aminopeptidase (LAP), alkaline phosphodiesterase I
(APD), and 5'-nucleotidase (5'N).   The ectoenzyme LAP is reported
to be characteristic of activated, cytotoxic macrophages whereas
activated macrophages have low levels of the latter two ectoen-
zymes (Morahan et al., 1980).   This is consistent with our observations of low APD and 5'N levels and relatively high LAP levels,

TABLE IV

Tumor-Associated Macrophages of Metastatic
and Nonmetastatic Mammary Tumors

Tumor	Phenotype	Macrophage distribution $2:3^a$	LAP concentration[b] $2:3^a$	PGE distribution[c] $2:3^a$
66 (4)[d]	Metastatic	1.4 (75)[e]	0.6 (9.3)[f]	2.5
410.4 (3)	Metastatic	1.2 (81)	n.d.[g]	n.d.
67 (5)	Nonmetastatic	2.4 (84)	1 (2.3)	0.1
168 (3)	Nonmetastatic	2.0 (80)	1 (3.7)	0.3

[a] Ratio of elutriation fraction 2:fraction 3.
[b] LAP, Leucine aminopeptidase (nmol/min/μm^2).
[c] PGE, Prostaglandin E.
[d] Number of experiments given in parentheses.
[e] Percentage of total macrophages in fractions 2 + 3 given in parentheses.
[f] Mean LAP concentration of macrophages in fractions 2 + 3 given in parentheses.
[g] n.d., Not determined.

in tumor 66 macrophages (Table IV). Furthermore, the LAP activity
was greater in fraction 3 than in fraction 2 macrophages, again
suggesting that line 66 tumors contain relatively more mature cells
(Wachsmuth and Stoyle, 1977).

Prostaglandin E levels were also assessed in the fractions from
the various tumors as a marker for "suppressor" macrophages (Stenson and Parker, 1980). Distribution of PGE was inversely correlated
with LAP concentration.

Taken all together, these data suggest that metastatic mammary
tumor subpopulations are differentially infiltrated with more mature,
tumoricidal macrophages, as compared to macrophages of nonmetastatic
tumors, and that cytotoxic macrophages are separable physically from
suppressor macrophages. Thus, just as with the T cells, the types
of tumor-associated macrophages are determined by the tumor, not by
the host. Furthermore, since different tumor subpopulations are
associated with different infiltrating cells, tumor cell heterogeneity can influence host cell heterogeneity.

C. Macrophages and Metastatic Subpopulations

    The observation that macrophages from our metastatic tumors
are more likely to be tumoricidal *in vitro* than are macrophages
from nonmetastatic tumors appears paradoxical. Other investigators have reported, in the Maloney sarcoma system for example, that
cytotoxic macrophages are characteristic of regressing tumors
(Russell *et al.*, 1977; Taniyama and Holden, 1979). However, Weiss
(1978) has suggested that tumor-associated macrophages may aid
metastasis by secreting proteases that allow tumor cells to escape
into the circulation and lymphatic drainage. We have been in-
trigued by the reports of Weitzmann and Stossel (1981, 1982) that
human peripheral blood phagocytes are able to cause genetic muta-
tions in bacteria under the conditions of the Ames assay (Ames *et
al.*, 1975). The activity appears to be related to reactive oxygen
metabolites formed during the respiratory burst of phagocytosis.
Some of these metabolites are reported to be tumoricidal and to be
produced by activated macrophages (Nathan *et al.*, 1979). The production of mutation-causing agents by activated macrophages could
be an explanation for our observations linking macrophage tumoricidal activity with metastatic tumors, since those tumor cell populations that escape cytotoxicity *in vivo* may contain a higher
frequency of genetic variants than do tumor populations not exposed to such "endogenous" mutagens. Increasing the frequency of
variants would be expected to increase the chance of metastasis
(Nowell, 1976; Cifone and Fidler, 1981). As a preliminary effort
to test this hypothesis, we have assessed the mutagenic ability
of tumor-associated macrophages from metastatic mammary tumors.
    Whole-tumor suspensions of lines 66 and 410.4, and plastic-
adherent or nonadherent cells from them, were tested for mutagenic
activity against histidine-requiring auxotrophs of *Salmonella
typhimurium,* tester strain 98. The mammalian cells were mixed
with the bacteria and immediately plated in solidified, histidine-
deficient agar. Two days later the number of bacterial colonies
was counted and used to calculate the frequency of revertants to
histidine independence. The results in Table V show that whole-
tumor cell suspensions increased the mutation frequency almost
2.5 times above background. Other experiments (data not shown)
indicate that the degree of increase in mutagenic frequency is related to the number of tumor cells added. Adherent cells, of
which >90% were macrophages by standard criteria, removed from
suspensions of 66 and 410.4 tumors increased the mutation frequency almost 5.5-fold. Nonadherent cells (i.e., all cells left in
suspension after the macrophages were removed) were not mutagenic.
    To date, experiments with nonmetastatic tumors have been neg-
ative in the Ames assay. Much more data are necessary, however,
before firm conclusions can be made.
    Clearly, we have a great deal of work to do before we know
whether the ability of macrophages from metastatic tumors to increase bacterial mutation frequency is in any way related to metastasis. Our observations do, however, provide another mechanism

TABLE V

Mutagenicity of Macrophages Isolated
from Metastatic Mouse Mammary Tumors: Ames Assay

Preparation	Frequency of mutagenicity[a]	Revertant index[b] (mean ± SE)
Tumor suspension	7/9	2.4 ± 0.5
Nonadherent cells	0/5	1.3 ± 0.1
Adherent cells[c]	5/5	5.4 ± 2.3
2-NHA[d]	7/7	24.0 ± 3

[a] Number of positive experiments/total experiments.
[b] Number of revertants in test/number of revertants in control using TA98 *Salmonella* test strain.
[c] Characterized as macrophages by Fc receptor, latex bead phagocytosis, and morphology.
[d] 2-NHA, 2-napthohydroxymic acid—a known mutagen used as positive control.

whereby the production of tumor cell variants may be effected. Numerous mechanisms for the origin of tumor cell heterogeneity have been suggested. These include multifocal origin of cancer (Parbhoo, 1981), tumor cell genetic instability (Nowell, 1976) perhaps reflected in increased spontaneous mutation rates (Cifone and Fidler, 1981), genomic rearrangements (Sager, 1982), and gene amplification (George and Powers, 1982), as well as differentiation of neoplastic stem cells (Pierce, 1974). Attention has also been given to the possibility that somatic cell fusion and subsequent chromosomal redistribution at mitosis might produce tumor cell variants (DeBaetselser *et al.*, 1981; Kerbel *et al.*, 1982). We here suggest that host infiltrating cells might also "fuel" heterogeneity by releasing mutagens into the growing neoplasm. This hypothesis, coupled with the well-appreciated potential of infiltrating cells to select out particular subpopulations during tumor progression, places emphasis on the role of the host in tumor heterogeneity. We have shown that tumor heterogeneity can lead to heterogeneity in infiltrating lymphocytes and macrophages (see earlier). This host cell heterogeneity may then "close the circle" by contributing, directly, to production of new variants and, indirectly, to their emergence during tumor progression. The capacity of tumor cell subpopulations to interact with each other, and to provoke heterogeneous host cell responses that may both influence and be influenced by the outcome of these interactions, further underscores the concept of a tumor as a dynamic, evolving ecosystem (Heppner, 1982).

ACKNOWLEDGMENTS

    The authors wish to acknowledge the contributions of Dr.
Bonnie E. Miller to the work demonstrating tumor subpopulation
interactions and of Ms. Angie Rios to the isolation of tumor-associated lymphocytes. Our work is being supported by NIH Grants
CA-27437 and CA-27419, by a grant from Concern Foundation, by the
E. Walter Albachten bequest to the Michigan Cancer Foundation,
and by the United Foundation of greater Detroit.

REFERENCES

Ames, B. N., McCann, J., and Yamasaki, E. (1975). *Mutat. Res. 31*,
    347-364.
Bennett, D. C., Peachey, L. A., Durbin, H., and Rudland, P. S.
    (1978). *Cell 15*, 283-298.
Blazar, B. A., and Heppner, G. H. (1978). *J. Immunol. 120*,
    1881-1886.
Brennan, M. J., Donegan, W. L., and Appleby, D. E. (1979). *Am. J.
    Surg. 137*, 260-262.
Campbell, M. W., Sholley, M. M., and Miller, G. A. (1980). *Cell.
    Immunol. 50*, 153-168.
Cifone, M. A., and Fidler, I. J. (1981). *Proc. Natl. Acad. Sci.
    USA 78*, 6249-6252.
DeBaetselser, P., Gorelik, E., Eshlar, Z., Ron, Y., Katzav, S.,
    Feldman, M., and Segal, S. (1981). *J. Natl. Cancer Inst. (US)*
    67, 1079-1087.
Dethlefsen, L. (1980). *In* "Cell Biology of Breast Cancer" (C. M.
    McGrath, M. A. Rich, and M. J. Brennan, eds.), pp. 145-160.
    Academic Press, New York.
Dexter, D. L., Kowalski, H. M., Blazar, B. A., Fligiel, Z., Vogel,
    R., and Heppner, G. H. (1978). *Cancer Res. 38*, 3174-3181.
Dulbecco, R., Henahan, M., Bowman, M., Okada, S., Battifora, H.,
    and Unger, M. (1981). *Proc. Natl. Acad. Sci. USA 78*, 2345-2349.
Dvorak, H. F., Quay, S. C., Orerstein, N. S., Dvorak, A. M., Hahn,
    P., Bitzer, A. M., and Carvallo, A. C. (1981). *Science (Washing-
    ton, D.C.) 212*, 923-924.
Evans, R., and Lawler, E. M. (1980). *Int. J. Cancer 26*, 831-835.
Fidler, I. J., and Kripke, M. L. (1977). *Science (Washington,
    D.C.) 197*, 893-895.
George, D. L., and Powers, V. E. (1982) *In* "Tumor Cell Hetero-
    geneity Origins and Implications" (A. H. Owens, Jr., D. S. Coffey,
    and S. B. Baylin, eds.), pp. 399-410. Academic Press, New York.
Goldie, J. H., and Coldman, A. J. (1979). *Cancer Treat. Rep. 63*,
    1727-1733.
Gorelik, E., Segal, S., Shapiro, J., Katzav, S., Ron, Y., and
    Feldman, M. (1982) *Cancer Metastasis Rev. 1*, 83-94.

Hager, J. C., and Heppner, G. H. (1982). *Cancer Res. 42*, 4325-4329.

Hager, J., Fligiel, S., Stanley, W., Richardson, A. M., and Heppner, G. H. (1981). *Cancer Res. 41*, 1293-1300.

Hauschka, T. S. (1953). *J. Natl. Cancer Inst. (US) 14*, 723-736.

Heppner, G. H. (1982). *In* "Tumor Cell Heterogeneity Origins and Implications" (A. H. Owens, Jr., D. S. Coffey, and S. B. Baylin, eds.), pp. 225-236. Academic Press, New York.

Heppner, G. H., and Miller, B. E. (1983). *Cancer Metastasis Rev. 2*, 5-23.

Heppner, G. H., Dexter, D. L., DeNucci, T., Miller, F. R., and Calabresi, P. (1978). *Cancer Res. 38*, 3758-3763.

Heppner, G., Miller, B., Cooper, D. N., and Miller, F. R. (1980). *In* "Cell Biology of Breast Cancer" (C. M. McGrath, M. J. Brennan, and M. A. Rich, eds.), pp. 161-172. Academic Press, New York.

Jansson, B., and Revesz, L. (1976). *In* "Methods in Cancer Research" (H. Busch, ed.), Vol. 13, pp. 227-290. Academic Press, New York.

Kerbel, R. S., Dennis, J. W., Largarde, A. E., and Frost, P. (1982). *Cancer Metastasis Rev. 1*, 99-140.

Keyner, D., Christman, J., Acs, G., Silagi, S., Newcomb, E. W., and Silverstein, S. C. (1978). *J. Cell. Physiol. 95*, 159-167.

Klein, G., and Klein, E. (1956). *Ann. N.Y. Acad. Sci. 63*, 640-661.

Loveless, S. E., and Heppner, G. H. (1983). *J. Immunol. 131*, 2074-2078.

Macinnes, J. I., Chan, E. C. M., Percy, D. H., and Morris, V. L. (1981). *Virology 113*, 119-129.

Mahoney, K. H., Fulton, A. M., and Heppner, G. H. (1983). *J. Immunol. 131*, 2079-2085.

Michalides, R., Wagenaar, E., and Sluyser, M. (1982). *Cancer Res. 42*, 1154-1158.

Miller, B. E., Miller, F. R., Leith, J., and Heppner, G. H. (1980). *Cancer Res. 40*, 3977-3981.

Miller, B. E., Miller, F. R., and Heppner, G. H. (1981). *Cancer Res. 41*, 4378-4381.

Miller, F. R., and Heppner, G. H. (1979a). *J. Natl. Cancer Inst. (US) 63*, 1457-1464.

Miller, F. R., and Heppner, G. H. (1979b). *Proc. Amer. Assoc. Cancer Res. 21*, 201.

Miller, F. R., Miller, B. E., and Heppner, G. H. (1983). *Invasion and Metastasis 3*, 22-31.

Morahan, P. S., Edelson, P. J., and Gass, K. (1980). *J. Immunol. 125*, 1312-1317.

Mule, J. J., Forstrom, J. W., George, E., Hellstrom, I., and Hellstrom, K. E. (1981). *Int. J. Cancer 28*, 611-614.

Nathan, C. F., Silverstein, S. C., Brukner, L. H., and Cohn, Z. A. (1979). *J. Exp. Med. 149*, 100-113.

Neri, A., and Nicolson, G. L. (1981). *Int. J. Cancer 28*, 731-738.

Newcomb, E. W., Silverstein, S. C., and Silagi, S. (1978). *J. Cell. Physiol. 95*, 169-177.

Nowell, P. C. (1976). *Science (Washington, D.C.) 194*, 23-28.

Nuti, M., Horan Hand, P., Colcher, D., and Schlom, J. (1982). *Proc. Amer. Assoc. Cancer Res. 23*, 267.

Parbhoo, S. P. (1981). *In* "Systemic Control of Breast Cancer" (B.A. Stoll, ed.), pp. 55-77. Heinemann, London.

Pierce, G. B. (1974). *In* "World Symposium on Model Studies in Chemical Carcinogenesis" (P. O. P. T.'so and J. A. DiPaolo, eds.), pp. 463-472. Dekker, New York.

Poste, G., and Nicolson, G. (1980). *Proc. Natl. Acad. Sci. USA 77*, 399-403.

Poste, G., Doll, J., and Fidler, I. J. (1981). *Proc. Natl. Acad. Sci. USA 78*, 6626-6630.

Pretlow, T. G. (1971). *Anal. Biochem. 41*, 248-255.

Rios, A. M., Miller, F. R., and Heppner, G. H. (1983). *Cancer Immunol. Immunother. 15*, 87-91.

Russell, S. W., Gillespie, G. Y., and McIntosh, A. T. (1977). *J. Immunol. 118*, 1574-1579.

Sager, R. (1982). *In* "Tumor Cell Heterogeneity Origins and Implications" (A. H. Owens, Jr., D. S. Coffey, and S. B. Baylin, eds.), pp. 411-423. Academic Press, New York.

Stenson, W. F., and Parker, C. W. (1980). *J. Immunol. 125*, 1-5.

Sugarbaker, E. V., Thorntwaite, J., and Ketcham, A. C. (1977). *In* "Cancer Invasion and Metastasis: Biologic Mechanisms and Therapy" (S. D. Day, ed.), pp. 227-238. Raven, New York.

Sun, D., and Lohmann-Matthes, M. L. (1982). *Eur. J. Immunol. 12*, 134-140.

Talmadge, J. E., Key, M., and Fidler, I. J. (1981). *J. Immunol. 126*, 2245-2248.

Taniyama, T., and Holden, H. T. (1979). *Int. J. Cancer 24*, 151-160.

Tseng, M. T. (1980). *Cancer Res. 40*, 3112-3115.

Vaupel, P. W., Frinak, S., and Bicher, H. E. (1981). *Cancer Res. 41*, 2008-2013.

Wachsmuth, E. D., and Stoyle, J. P. (1977). *J. Reticuloendothel. Soc. 22*, 485-497.

Weiss, L. (1978). *Int. J. Cancer 22*, 196-203.

Weiss, L. (1980). *In* "Cell Biology of Breast Cancer" (C. M. McGrath, M. J. Brennan, and M. A. Rich, eds.), pp. 189-205. Academic Press, New York.

Weiss, L., Holmes, J. C., and Ward, P. M. (1983). *Brit. J. Cancer 47*, 81-89.

Weiss, M. A., Michael, J. G., Pesce, A. J., and DiPersio, L. (1981). *Lab. Invest. 45*, 46-57.

Weitzman, S. A., and Stossel, T. P. (1981). *Science (Washington, D.C.) 212*, 546-547.

Weitzman, S. A., and Stossel, T. P. (1982). *J. Immunol. 128*, 2770-2772.

DISCUSSION

MATHÉ: I would like to mention that we have, with Dr. Olsson, observed that AKR leukemia cells are, at least for antigens, detected by monoclonals of four types. To cure 50% of the mice, we have to use three monoclonals. So, I would like to ask you, if you have studied NK and suppressor cells, don't you think that the contrary hypothesis of yours, according to which the microenvironment variation may be responsible to metastasis variation.

HEPPNER: I tried to indicate that a tumor is a system of interacting cells: tumor cell subpopulations influence other tumor cell subpopulations; tumor cell heterogeneity influences host cell heterogeneity; host cells affect tumor cells and tumor cell heterogeneity. It is the principle of an ecosystem.

LIOTTA: Dr. Heppner, you showed that highly metastatic subpopulations, when mixed with nonmetastatic subpopulations, induced the nonmetastatic cells to be recovered from iv-induced lung metastasis. Did you do the same experiment with primary tumors? How were the subpopulations identified?

HEPPNER: In the first experiment, I showed the nonmetastatic cells were placed subcutaneously and the metastatic cells were injected intravenously. We could isolate both nonmetastatic and metastatic cells from metastatic foci in the lung. So far, our identification has been on the basis of morphological criteria.

GOLUB: Are the types of macrophages found in metastases the cause of the metastasis? Can you isolate macrophages from metastatic tumors that will cause nonmetastatic subpopulations to then metastasize?

HEPPNER: Basically, there are two types of mechanisms whereby more mature macrophages "become" associated with metastatic tumors: (1) mature macrophages may be differenitally attracted to or retained by metastatic tumors and (2) metastatic tumors may provide an environment in which macrophages mature. We are currently attempting to determine which mechanism is acting here. Without this information we cannot design the types of experiments you suggest.

TOKUNAGA: Could you exclude a possibility that macrophages selected some particular population of *Salmonella*?

HEPPNER: What we measure is the increased frequency of *Salmonella*
             mutants against a spontaneous mutation rate background.
             If the macrophages were simply selecting the *Salmonella*
             mutants, they could not increase the mutation rate.

WEISS: There is no question that the cancer cells in a tumor
             are heterogeneous; all cell populations show distri-
             butions in any property. For example, flow cytometry
             of "pure" cell populations shows this type of hetero-
             geneity. There is also no question that cell lines can
             be *developed* from tumors—these lines certainly have
             distinct metastasis-related properties, as shown by
             Fidler and his colleagues. The question really is
             whether "subpopulations" preexist in tumors? Are they
             really *isolated* by techniques involving many generations
             in culture (and *in vitro* mutation) or are they *generated*
             by these techniques? In the classical setting, metas-
             tasis of metastases is an essential part of the patho-
             logy of metastasis. If the "preexisting" "metastatic
             phenotype" has more than academic interest, then metas-
             tases should metastasize more than their appropriate
             primary cancer. We have been unable to demonstrate
             this (Weiss *et al.*, 1983). Finally, in answer to Pro-
             fessor Mathé's question, we have demonstrated reversible
             surface changes in cancer cells in rats and mice, de-
             pending on the organ in which they grow. This type of
             (organ) site-induced, environmental modulation of cancer
             cells occurs *after* they reach the target organs, and
             does not appear to depend on organ-specific subpopu-
             lations. The distinction is between cause and effect.

HEPPNER: Although it is difficult to prove absolutely that mam-
             mary tumor subpopulations preexisted in the parent tumor
             from which we derived our lines, that parent tumor
             was—at the time of removal from the autochthonous ani-
             mals—heterogenous in regard to morphology, karyotype,
             and expression of mammary tumor virus-associated anti-
             gens. We do not claim that our mammary tumor subpop-
             ulations are immutable descendants of clones within the
             parent tumor. We are using them as a model system to
             reconstruct tumor heterogeneity and to study its con-
             sequences. There are many reasons why metastases may
             not be more metastatic than their parent tumor. To
             begin with, there are interactions between subpopula-
             tions that affect metastasis. In my paper, I presented
             our data showing that tumor cells that would not metas-
             tasize alone may do so in the presence of metastatic
             cells. Clearly, if you isolated such a metastasis, it
             may be *less* metastatic than its primary. Poste has
             presented data showing that new clonal variants are gen-
             erated within metastasis—some of them are less metas-
             tatic than the parent tumor.

MORTON: (1) May the induction of metastatic potential of an ordinarily nonmetastatic tumor by concomitant presence of
a metastatic tumor be an induced effect due to specific
or nonspecific immunosuppression induced by metastatic
tumors? (2) May the mutagenicity of macrophages not be
an artifact of the Ames system secondary to genetic
hybridization with transfer of histidine-inducing genes
to *Salmonella* from the mouse macrophages that would
appear as mutants in the Ames assay? (3) What are the
implications of your data for cancer therapy?

HEPPNER: (1) It may be that the mechanism you suggest is correct.
Whatever the mechanism, however, "nonmetastatic" cells
are metastasizing. (2) We have no data to rule out this
possibility absolutely. The particular strain of *Salmonella* we used detects frame shifts. We are repeating
the work with another strain that detects point muta-
tions. (3) I think from the way you ask this question
that you think the implications are bad. In fact, tumor heterogeneity may aid therapy. In all our studies
on subpopulation interactions that affect drug sensitivity, the presence of a sensitive subpopulation
increases the sensitivity of a less sensitive subpopulation (Miller *et al.*, 1981).

CHAPTER 2

THE QUANTITATION OF SOME ASPECTS OF INVASION *IN VIVO* AND *IN VITRO**

Leonard Weiss

Department of Experimental Pathology
Roswell Park Memorial Institute
Buffalo, New York

Okhee W. Suh

Departments of Experimental Pathology
and Biomathematics
Roswell Park Memorial Institute
Buffalo, New York

Some of the work described here was supported by Grant #CD-21 to L. Weiss from the American Cancer Society, Inc.

I. INTRODUCTION

Any understanding of invasion of tissues by cancer cells requires consideration of the cancer cells, the tissues they invade, and other noncancerous cells with which they interact.

Invasion is essentially a local event that may culminate in metastasis, which is a distant event. By comparing certain features of squamous cell carcinomas, which invade and metastasize albeit infrequently and late, with basal cell carcinomas, which invade but only very rarely metastasize (Mikhail et al., 1977; Safai and Good, 1977), some of the essential relationships between invasion and metastasis can be identified. An early event in invasion by squamous cell carcinomas is an apparent loosening of the cancerous tissues as evidenced by a reduction in the number of desmosomes, with the formation of spaces that are then penetrated by processes from individual cancer cells (Sugár, 1968). This is followed by penetration of the host tissues through disrupted basement lamina, and on histologic examination, irregular masses of epidermal cells are seen to proliferate toward subcutaneous tissues and to invade the dermis (Hashimoto et al., 1973; Lever, 1975, p. 476). In contrast, in basal cell carcinomas, although thin processes are seen in the intercellular spaces, they do not usually penetrate the basal lamina border of the tumor (Cutler et al., 1980). In both tumors metastases most commonly involve lymph nodes, although lung metastases have been described as the most common site in one series of metastatic basal cell carcinomas (Farmer and Helwig, 1980). In neither lesion have cancer cells been described in local blood vessels, although in the absence of special staining procedures this statement is of dubious value, and initial dissemination, when it occurs, is presumably via the lymphatic system.

The metastatic process consists of a number of sequential steps, and, although cancer cells apparently leave tumors in large numbers, comparatively few overt metastases are generated by them. The term metastatic inefficiency has been introduced (Weiss et al., 1982) to account for the costliness of metastasis in terms of cancer cells--"For many are called, but few are chosen." In the examples given, part of the metastatic inefficiency is concerned with the manner in which cancer cells penetrate or fail to penetrate host tissues, and part is concerned with an apparent failure to intravasate. It is not suggested that these are the only two loci of metastatic inefficiency, since it has been known for many years that the presence of cancer cells in the bloodstream is not synonymous with metastasis (Goldmann, 1897; Iwasaki, 1915), and subsequent studies have shown that the delivery of 10^5 cancer cells to the lungs results in only approximately 10—200 tumor colonies (Weiss et al., 1982).

In this communication, we wish to discuss the development of a technique for investigating the manner in which melanoma cells invade human host tissues; we will then examine the consequences

of invasive failure of melanomas in relation to metastasis in
mice, and finally, we will comment on some differential blocks to
cell movement *in vitro*.

II. INVASION—ASSESSMENT OF THE CONTRIBUTION OF ACTIVE MOVEMENT *IN VIVO*

Invasive movements of cancer into host tissues can occur
through two basic, nonexclusive mechanisms. These are, first,
through expansion due to growth and, second, active crawling movements of cancer cells. In the former, the expansive forces (*vis
a tergo*) drive the cancer into the surrounding host tissues. The
path followed, other things being equal, will be that of least
mechanical resistance. In a mechanically homogeneous environment,
a benign tumor may expand uniformly in all directions in the form
of an encapsulated sphere. In a nonhomogeneous environment, host
tissue compliance or resistance may result in a convoluted tumor
shape, as seen, for example, when a lipoma meets a bone; however,
lipomas are benign tumors and are not usually considered as invasive. In contrast, when the discrete margins of malignant tumors
are examined microscopically, often a pseudocapsule of compressed
normal tissue is seen that is penetrated by single cancer cells
or tumor spicules. Thus, even where expansion of a cancer into
macroscopically homogeneous media is achieved by growth, penetration appears to require microscopic dissolution of the host tissues, involving destruction of host cells (Dingemans and Roos,
1982), sometimes in a tissue-specific pattern (Carr *et al.*, 1976).
    The contribution of active cell movements to invasion is not
clear, although the capability of cancer cells to move over glass
slides has been recognized for more than a century. Also well
recognized are the *in vivo* movements of cells in embryogenesis,
the movements of cancer cells into embryonic tissues *in vitro*,
extravasatory movements of cancer cells in rabbit ear chambers,
and the active movements of cancer and noncancer cells over artificial substrate *in vitro*. While there is no question that cancer
cells are capable of active movements *in vitro* where they may mimic
some phases of invasion (loss of contact inhibition; Abercrombie,
1967) when confronted by certain noncancerous cells, the problem
still remains of assessing the contributions of active cell movement to invasion under natural conditions.
    We have tried to develop a technique to reconstruct the events
in invasion by human cutaneous melanomas, from the information
contained in standard hematoxylin and eosin-stained sections of
surgical specimens. We have made the assumption that when a melanoma expands by an uncomplicated growth process, each cell divides
into two in a geometric progression, such that if the densities of
cancer cells at the tumor edge are examined in three-unit squares

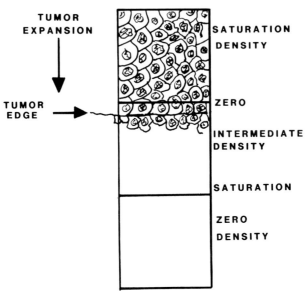

Fig. 1. In a tumor where expansion is by growth, it is expected that within a three-square microscope eyepiece grid placed at the tumor margin, the top grid would show saturation density of cancer cells, the intermediate grid would show a density between saturation and zero, and the bottom grid would contain no cancer cells. The transition from saturation to zero occurs over three squares.

of tissue section as shown in Fig. 1, the square over the tumor proper will contain cancer cells at saturation density, the square over the host tissue proper will contain no cancer cells at all, whereas the intermediate square over the cancer—host tissue interface will contain a variable number of cells progressing from zero to saturation density as the melanoma expands. In contrast to this abrupt transition in cancer cell densities expected to be associated with expansion by growth, in the presence of active cell movement the transition pattern from saturation to zero densities is expected to be more gradual, as shown in Fig. 2. This is partly because of the distribution of cell velocities seen when cells move over uniform surfaces, partly because of randomness in cell direction, and partly because of nonhomogeneity in the tissues being invaded with respect to mechanical and physicochemical properties. While there is no way that we can discriminate in a histological section between the effects of these variables on cell density patterns, apart from the unlikely possibility that they are self-canceling, it can be reasonably expected that the mark of active cancer movement through the tissues will be gradual, centrifugal diminution in cancer cell density in proceeding from the main body of the tumor in the direction of invasion.

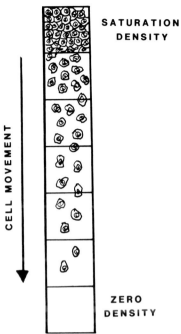

Fig. 2.   Where expansion of a cancer occurs by active cell movement, a diffusive, centrifugal cancer cell density gradient is expected, which is more gradual than that shown in Fig. 1.   In this case, the transition from saturation to zero density occurs over seven squares.

The validity of the model was tested on sections of human malignant melanomas.   Density counts were made over whole-tumor sections at known magnifications of ×205, using an eyepiece with a net micrometer grid containing 100 squares, each square being equivalent to 2210 μm^2 of tissue, respectively.   Melanoma cell density maps were constructed from these data for superficial nod- ular melanomas where growth was away from the dermis (into the air!), and where expansion had to be by growth, since there were no tissues to invade.   We also constructed density maps for mela- nomas invading the dermis and subcutaneous tissue, and data dis- cussed here are for one example of each.   In Fig. 3, the mean cell densities are shown from the advancing edges of a nodular and an invasive tumor as a function of distance expressed in number of eyepiece squares.   It can be seen that in the case of the nodular tumor, the transition from zero to saturation densities occurs over 3 eyepiece squares, whereas in the invasive tumor, the transition occurs over approximately 10 squares.   These observa- tions are in accord with our expectations for expansive growth and invasive cell movements, respectively.   Although there is a progressive centrifugal decrease in mean cancer cell densities in the invasive segment, which is compatible with a "diffusion"

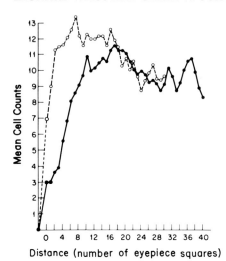

Distance (number of eyepiece squares)

Fig. 3. *Observed* density gradients in a nodular melanoma
(O---O) show the expected transition from zero to saturation over
three eyepiece squares with 50-μm sides. This transition in the
invasive tumor (●---●) occurs over 10 squares (∿400 μm).

process associated with cell locomotion, examination of the coef-
ficients of variation of these means indicates a lack of continuity
in the progression. Not surprisingly, then, the invasive movements
of the melanoma cells cannot be described in terms of an *ideal* diffusion process.

The densities of cancer cells in the individual squares of the
density maps of tumors were compared by the use of *mean moving av-
erages* (MMA), which are the predicted cell densities in individual
squares calculated from the densities in the surrounding eight
squares. Where y is the observed cell density in a square, the
differences between the observed and predicted densities.

$$W = y - \text{MMA} \tag{1}$$

and

$$\chi^2 = W^2/\text{MMA} \tag{2}$$

In cases where $\chi^2 > 3.84$, the cell density in that square is significantly different from the predicted value. ($\chi^2 = 3.84$ for
$p = .05$, with 1 degree of freedom.)

A total of 2181 and 2836 squares were used for MMA calculations
from respective sections of the nodular part of a melanoma (N), and
a part of the same melanoma (I) that was invading the dermis and
subcutaneous tissues. By the use of χ^2 tests, it was shown that in
section N, 2.8% (61) squares contained significantly higher densities of cancer cells, and 1.3% (29) contained significantly lower

densities; in section I, 3.5% (98) squares were high points and
2% (57) were low points. Neither the overall numbers of high and
low points, nor the sums of all the significantly different squares
are significantly different in the two sections. However, the patterns of high and low points are different. Thus, while nearly
all of the significantly low-density squares are located around
the *periphery* of the nodular tumor (N), they appear within the
general confines of the invasive segment (I). The higher accumulation of low-density squares in section I is accounted for both
by a distribution of low cell densities in regions near the advancing tumor edge, and low-density "troughs" in the body of the tumor
around its high points.

The high points at the peripheral regions of the invasive tumors are by definition significant discontinuities in the centrifugal density gradient of melanoma cells. We interpret this observation to indicate that the progenitors of the cancer cells at
the high points must have reached these locations by active locomotion, because the presence of surrounding *very* low-density zones
precludes their location as a result of a contiguous growth process. This reconstruction of events further suggests that a phase
of proliferation occurred after the crawling cells came to rest.
By examination of the proportion of high points in different zones,
we conclude that these proliferative regions are too frequent to
have occurred as random events. The region of centrifugal diminution in cancer cell density extends approximately 500 μm (9-10
squares) from the main tumor edge. If our interpretation of the
pathologic significance of the high-density regions is correct,
then the initial event in invasion, in the case examined at least,
is a migration of melanoma cells from their origin, for a distance
of approximately 0.5 mm in the direction of the dermis. Some of
the migrating cells then stop and proliferate. The proliferating
regions eventually merge, and the process of migration followed by
proliferation is then repeated.

It must be emphasized that our present interpretation of limited measurements is speculative. However, the technique of statistical reconstruction that we have developed makes it possible
to quantitate this aspect of invasion. This technique will be
described in detail elsewhere.

III. INVASION AND METASTASIS

In the case of hematogenous and lymphogenous metastasis, intravasation of cancer cells is a critical event. Weiss *et al.*
(1982) attempted to assess the level of control of the invasive
process on the subsequent development of metastases. Use was made
of various sublines of the B16 mouse melanoma maintained *in vitro*,
and the results of various experiments are summarized in Table I.

TABLE I

Effect of Intravenous and Intramuscular Injections of Mice
with B16 Melanoma Cells, with and without Massage[a,b]

B16 Cell type	iv Injection (10^5 cells + 21 days)		im Injection (10^5 cells + 21–23 days)		im Injection (10^5 cells + Massage + 21 days)	
	Mice with lung tumors (%)	Mean no. lung tumors (±SE)	Mice with lung metastases (%)	Mean no. lung metastases (±SE)	Mice with lung metastases (%)	Mean no. lung metastases (±SE)
BL6	12/12 (100)	227 ± 27	25/25 (100)	8 ± 2	23/23 (100)	34 ± 8
F10	45/45 (100)	110 ± 11	23/64 (34)	2 ± 0.5	13/36 (36)	1 ± 0.4
F10FA	12/12 (100)	35 ± 8	48/96 (50)	7 ± 3	n.d.[c]	n.d.
F10^{lr-6}	34/41 (83)	8 ± 4	34/68 (50)	2 ± 0.3	14/33 (42)	2 ± 0.8
Wild	28/30 (93)	9 ± 3	12/30 (40)	1 ± 0.2	25/37 (68)	2 ± 0.4

[a] Data from Weiss et al. (1982).
[b] Note: comparison of pulmonary colonization after tail-vein injections, with pulmonary metastasis after im injections, with and without massage.
[c] n.d., Not determined.

Twenty-one days after tail-vein injections of 10^5 melanoma cells, mice receiving the BL6 (Hart, 1979) and F10 lines (Fidler *et al.*, 1976) had developed means of 227 and 110 pulmonary tumors, respectively. The other four sublines generated progressively fewer tumors, down to a mean of nine in the case of the wild type. That the development of pulmonary tumors following intravenous injection is not synonymous with metastasis is demonstrated by the results of intramuscular injection of the same sublines. Although intramuscular tumors grew in all of the recipients, only means of eight and two overt pulmonary metastases (i.e., >0.2 mm diameter) developed in mice with B16B16 and B16F10 tumors, respectively, and only 40% of the mice bearing B16 wild-type tumors had pulmonary metastases at all, with a mean of only one metastasis. The B16F10 line, which exhibited a high degree of pulmonary colonization potential following intravenous injection, showed low metastatic potential, in that only 34% of animals bearing the tumor developed pulmonary metastases, and the mean number was two metastases. Thus, a metastasis-controlling block was demonstrated between lung colonization potentials and metastatic potential; if B16F10 cells could get into the venous blood going to the lungs, pulmonary colonies were formed with an efficiency of 0.1% ($110/10^5$), so the fact that a mean of only two pulmonary metastases were formed in animals bearing B16F10 tumors indicated with invasive failure, reflected in a low rate of entry of B16 cells into the venous system, was a rate-regulating step in metastasis.

As there is ample evidence that massage of primary cancers increases the incidence of metastasis, a technique was devised to massage intramuscular tumors reproducibly to determine whether this would promote the release of cancer cells into the bloodstream and restore the differential in numbers of lung tumors seen after direct intravenous injections of the different cell types. The results given in Table I show that massage enhanced metastasis in the case of the intramuscular tumors caused by B16BL6 cells, but produced only slight but significant enhancement in the case of the B16 wild type, and no enhancement at all with the F10 and F10^{1r-6} lines. This evidence is in accord with the suggestion that the failure of the F10 tumors to achieve their full lung colonization potential is due to failure to intravasate in sufficient quantities to produce metastases within the time frame of the experiments.

The group of B16 tumors thus fell into two groups, as shown in Fig. 4. First, the B16 line was selected by Hart for invasiveness and it intravasated to a small amount that was detectable by massage-enhanced metastasis. Second, by the same criteria, the F10 and F10^{1r-6} lines fell into a group in which intravasation was not detectable by massage. It therefore appears that within the constraints of the experiments, although the F10 had much greater lung *colonization* potential than the F10^{1r-6} line, this did not translate into increased *metastatic* potential because of invasive failure, manifest at the level of intravasation possibly at the level of the basement membranes of small vessels. This is compat-

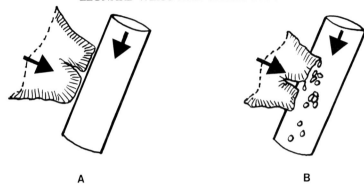

A   **B**

Fig. 4.   (A) Where tissue invasion occurs without tumor intravasation, massage will not cause the additional intravascular release of cancer cells, and will not increase pulmonary metastasis.
(B) Where both invasion and intravasation occur, massage promotes
metastasis.

ible with the hypothesis that collagen IV, which is found in the
basement membrane of blood vessels, is a major "barrier" to invasion, and with the observation of Liotta *et al.* (1980) that the
B16BL6 line cells secreted a high level of type IV collagenolytic
activity into their medium on culture.   Unfortunately, we are un-
aware of matching data for the other B16 lines used in the experiments summarized in Table I.   It must be emphasized that as all of
these tumors metastasize to some extent, invasive failure is relative with respect to *rate* and not an all-or-none phenomenon.

IV.   INVASION AND HOST TISSUE "BARRIERS"

     It is assumed that in some way, different components of the
connective tissues offer differential barriers to invasion
(Sträuli *et al.*, 1980; Kuettner and Pauli, 1981), and that invasive capacity may be accounted for by whether cancer cells possess
an adequate complement of enzymes with the capability of degrading
these barriers (Sträuli *et al.*, 1980; Recklies and Poole, 1982;
Zeidman, 1982).   This view may be oversimplistic, as there are dis-
crepancies between malignancy and normalcy with respect to enzymes;
in addition, the physicochemical nature of the stroma represents a
balance between degradation and synthesis, and "bystander" cells
involved in inflammatory and other responses may play key roles in
maintaining or disrupting the connective tissue steady state.
Also, natural tissue inhibitors of invasion have been demonstrated,
and it is probable that there is some degree of specificity in the
microscopic invasive routes followed by different cancer cells in
different host organs.   A number of these points are discussed

in detail in the book edited by Liotta and Hart (1982). A few of
these variables will be considered in relationship to work done
within our own group.

A. Necrosis and Invasion

Necrosis is a common regional feature of many human and animal tumors, as a consequence of vascular insufficiency due to a
variety of underlying causes, host defense reactions, lethal muta-
tions, and last, but by no means least, as a result of therapy.
Host cells including macrophages and polymorphs may be attracted
to necrotic tissues and play an additional role in maintaining or
extending the underlying pathologic process, and conversely, products of necrotic regions may diffuse out into the surrounding tissues (Weiss and Holmes, 1980).

The interactions in embryonic systems between living and dead
cells, and the relationship between active morphogenetic migratory
movements are well recognized. However, in the case of tumor systems the pathophysiologic consequences of necrosis, as distinct
from its causes, have been largely overlooked (Bowen and Lockshin,
1981).

In one series of studies, it was shown that saline extracts of
necrotic material from cancers affected the migration of both cancer cells and macrophages from capillary tubes *in vitro*. Necrotic
extracts from mouse lymphosarcomas and fibrosarcomas significantly
reduced the migration of both lymphosarcoma and fibrosarcoma cells
with no evidence of specificity. However, necrotic extracts from
the lymphosarcoma enhanced the migration of Walker-256 (W-256)
cells, whereas extracts from fibrosarcoma inhibited their migration.

Active cell movements depend on three components: (1) formation
of adhesions between cells and their substrata, (2) generation of
locomotor forces acting at the regions of adhesion, and (3) detachment of relative parts of cells from their substrata as movement
proceeds.

It was shown that necrotic extracts from both W-256 tumors and
lymphosarcomas increase the rates of adhesion *in vitro* of W-256
cells. Necrotic extracts from lymphosarcomas inhibit the migration
and retard the adhesion of lymphosarcoma cells; extracts from W-256
tumors have little or no effect on the migration of lymphosarcoma
cells but significantly reduce their rate of adhesion. In addition,
extracts from W-256 tumors reduce the rate of adhesion of Ehrlich
ascites tumor cells, while extracts from lymphosarcomas increase
the rate (Weiss and Holmes, 1980). These observations preclude
simple relationships between the action of necrotic extracts on
cell movement and on the rate of cell adhesion.

Some effects of necrotic extracts on cell detachment have also
been studied. In the case of W-256 tumors growing either subcutaneously or in the livers of rats, it was shown, using a standardized technique, that more viable cancer cells were shaken free

from juxtanecrotic regions of tumors than from regions distant
from the necrotic regions. When juxtanecrotic samples were exposed to necrotic extract, no enhancement of detachment was observed; in contrast, when distant cortical regions of tumor were
exposed, more cells were detached. This suggests a diffusion gradient outward, from the central necrotic region of a tumor, of
material facilitating cancer cell detachment. In addition, more
parenchymal cells were shaken free from liver samples taken adjacent to a tumor edge than from zones 0.5 and 1.0 cm from the edge.
This enhancement of parenchymal cell detachment was also mimicked
by incubation of liver samples with necrotic extracts. Thus,
material lying free within necrotic regions of a tumor and dif-
fusing outward, can not only promote detachment of cancer and liver cells, presumably by mechanically weakening intercellular material, but can in some cases increase cell migration. Necrosis
would therefore be expected to promote invasion (Weiss, 1977).

The necrotic extracts are rich in neutral proteases, acid
phosphatase, β-glucuronidase, 2-galactosidase, hexosaminidase (no
collagenolytic or fibrinolytic activities were detected). As the
labilization of lysosomes has been shown to be associated with
cell detachment (Weiss, 1965), and as detachment can also be mediated by extrinsic enzymes (Weiss, 1963), the question arises whether
the mechanism of action of the necrotic extracts is mediated by
their direct action on the intercellular material, by their indirect action in labilizing lysosomal enzymes, or by other mechanisms. It was shown that exposure of cultures of W-256 cells growing in glass-bottomed chambers to necrotic extracts, followed by
exposure to shearing pressures of 1.9 Nm^{-2} for 2 min, facilitated
their detachment. This necrotic extract-induced detachment was
reduced but not completely abrogated by prior exposure of the cells
to the lysosome stabilizer hydrocortisone hemisuccinate (Weiss,
1978). Although it is difficult to give definitive explanations
of these data, it seems likely that necrotic materials promote
cell detachment both by their direct enzymatic activity and by
labilizing lysosomes, thereby promoting nonlethal degradation of
the pericellular regions.

The effects of necrotic extracts from W-256 tumors and Gardner
lymphosarcomas have also been studied on the *in vitro,* transmem-
brane migration of W-256 and lymphosarcoma cells and rat and mouse
peritoneal macrophages (Turner and Weiss, 1980). The extracts increased the rates of migration of all cell types by their chemo-
kinetic activity; this effect was partially reduced in the presence
of aprotinin, a neutral protease inhibitor. Rat liver lysosome
preparations containing lower levels of neutral protease activity
than the necrotic extracts either inhibited or were without effect
on migration rates, and the lysosome stabilizer hydrocortisone did
not inhibit the action of the necrotic extracts. These results
indicated that the diffusion of materials from the necrotic regions
of tumors may therefore enhance the outward movement of cancer
cells and the inward "necrotactic" movement of macrophages. The
extracts appear to act partially through their neutral protease

activity, but an indirect effect on motility through lysosomal labilization was not demonstrable. Necrosis is a common enough feature of solid tumors not to be overlooked in relation to its effect on invasion.

B. Resistance to Cell Movement

    An attempt was made by Folger *et al.* (1978) to determine the effects of viscosity of the medium on the migration rates of guinea pig macrophages from capillary tubes *in vitro*. The purpose of the experiments was to develop a technique to determine at what point the viscosity of the medium balanced the locomotor forces, thereby preventing movement. A highly significant linear correlation was obtained between migration indices (determined planimetrically) and viscosity ($N.s_2m^{-2}$) over the viscosity range of 0.71 to 3.09×10^{-3} $N.s.m^{-2}$ obtained by the addition of agarose. Extrapolation of the linear regression line indicated that no migration was expected when the viscosity of the medium reached 3.30×10^{-3} $N.s.m^{-2}$, corresponding to 0.82% agarose. Additional experiments suggested that the slowing of movement with increase in viscosity was due to "vertical" resistance to contact of macrophages with the surface of the dish over which they moved, not "horizontal" viscous "drag" on the whole cells. It was therefore suggested that within defined limits, a feedback mechanism exists, enabling macrophages to increase their locomotor forces in response to increased environmental viscosity or resistance. To date, experiments of this type have not been made with cancer cells; however, this type of environmentally responsive variability in cell motility may well add to the complexity of invasion by active cell movement.

C. Individuality with Respect to "Barriers"

    The depth of migratory penetration into cellulose membranes of rat peritoneal exudate cells, W-256 cancer cells, and Gardner lymphosarcoma (GL) cells was determined *in vitro* (Turner and Weiss, 1980). In some experiments, the membranes were impregnated with either collagen I or fibrin. The monocytoid cells migrated a mean distance of 52 μm into medium-filled 3-μm diameter pores, but did not penetrate either collagen- or fibrin-impregnated pores. Over incubation periods of 4 and 8 h, W-256 cells penetrated (fluid) medium-filled, 8-μm diameter pores to mean depths of 27 and 57 μm, respectively. In the presence of collagen I, the W-256 did not penetrate the membranes at all, and in the presence of fibrin, penetration was reduced to a mean depth of 14 μm in 4 h. Gardner lymphosarcoma cells penetrated medium-filled 8-μm pores to mean depths of 43 and 91 μm after 2 and 4 h incubation, respectively, but in contrast to the W-256 cells, they penetrated collagen-impregnated pores to respective mean depths of 2 and 22 μm, and did not penetrate the fibrin-filled pores at all after incubation for periods up to 19 h. In the presence of necrotic extracts, which exhibited no demonstrable collagenolytic or fibrinolytic activities, there was faster movement of cells through pores that they had previously been shown to penetrate, but where movement was totally inhibited by fibrin or collagen impregnation, necrotic extracts had no effect (Turner and Weiss, 1982). In these experiments the necrotic extracts therefore appear to act directly on cell movement (chemokinesis) rather than on the matrices through which the cells moved.

Whether a cell moves or does not move into a matrix cannot be simply and directly correlated with whether or not it releases enzymes capable of degrading the matrix in question. Thus, the migration of W-256 tumor cells into fibrin-impregnated membrane pores was unaffected in the presence of the antifibrinolytic agent aprotinin, and GL cells migrate into collagen-impregnated pores in the presence of fetal calf serum, which has anticollagenolytic activity. In addition, Schor et al. (1980) have shown that collagenolytic activity is not required for cancer cell migration into collagen in their own *in vitro* test system.

In invasion, cells from a primary cancer must traverse a number of chemically different connective tissue "barriers," and in addition, when invasion results in hematogenous metastasis, additional "barriers" must be overcome in the processes of intravasation and extravasation. The individuality exhibited by two types of cancer cells for barriers consisting of only fibrin or collagen I, suggests that useful information relating to this one aspect of invasion could be obtained by testing a number of cancer cells of different invasive and metastatic potential against a whole spectrum of impregnated membranes. The penetrants, used singly and in combination, would include collagens I to V, elastin, laminin, and fibronectin. By use of a combination of quantitative techniques for the measurement of invasion *in vivo* described earlier, and the membrane penetration test used by us and others, these aspects of invasion could be quantitated and correlated, and the cancer cells' own contribution to enzymatic tissue degradation could be assessed.

REFERENCES

Abercrombie, M. (1967). *Nat. Cancer Inst. Monogr. 26,* 249-277.
Bowen, I. D., and Lockshin, R. A. (eds.) (1981). "Cell Death in Biology and Pathology." Chapman & Hall, London.
Carr, I., McGinty, F., and Norris, P. (1976). *J. Pathol. 118,* 91-99.
Cutler, B., Posalaky, A., and Katz, H. I. (1980). *J. Cutaneous Pathol.* 7, 310-314.
Dingemans, K. P., and Roos, E. (1982). *In* "Liver Metastasis" (L. Weiss and H. A. Gilbert, eds.), pp. 51-76. Hall, Boston.
Farmer, E. R., and Helwig, E. B. (1980). *Cancer (Philadelphia)* 46, 748-757.

Fidler, I. J., Gersten, D. M., and Budmen, M. B. (1976). *Cancer Res. 36*, 3160-3165.
Folger, R., Weiss, L., Glaves, D., Subjeck, J. R., and Harlos, J. P. (1978). *J. Cell Sci. 31*, 245-257.
Goldmann, E. E. (1897). *Bruns Beitr. Klin. Chir. 18*, 595-612.
Hart, I. R. (1979). *Am. J. Pathol. 97*, 587-600.
Hashimoto, K., Yamanishi, Y., Maeyens, E., Dabbous, M. K., and Kanzaki, T. (1973). *Cancer Res. 33*, 2790-2801.
Iwasaki, T. (1915). *J. Pathol. Bacteriol. 20*, 85-105.
Kuettner, K. E., and Pauli, B. U. (1981). *In* "Bone Metastasis" (L. Weiss and H. A. Gilbert, eds.), pp. 131-165. Hall, Boston.
Lever, W. F. (1975). "Histopathology of the Skin," 5th ed. Lippincott, Philadelphia.
Liotta, L. A., and Hart, I. R. (eds.) (1982). "Tumor Invasion and Metastasis." Nijhoff, The Hague.
Liotta, L. A., Tryggvason, K., Garbisa, S., Hart, I., Foltz, C. M., and Shafie, S. (1980). *Nature (London) 284*, 67-68.
Mikhail, G. R., Nims, L. P., Kelly, A. P., Dittmars, D., and Eyler, W. R. (1977). *Arch. Dermatol. 113*, 1261-1269.
Recklies, A. D., and Poole, A. R. (1982). *In* "Liver Metastasis" (L. Weiss and H. A. Gilbert, eds.), pp. 77-95. Hall, Boston.
Safai, B., and Good, R. A. (1977). *Arch. Pathol. Lab. Med. 101*, 327-331.
Schor, S. L., Allen, T. D., and Harrison, C. J. (1980). *J. Cell Sci. 46*, 171-186.
Sträuli, P., Barrett, J. A., and Baici, A. (eds.) (1980). "Proteinases and Tumor Invasion." Raven, New York.
Sugár, J. (1968). *Eur. J. Cancer 4*, 33-38.
Turner, G. A., and Weiss, L. (1980). *Int. J. Cancer 26*, 247-254.
Turner, G. A., and Weiss, L. (1982). *Invasion Metastasis 2*, 361-368.
Weiss, L. (1963). *Exp. Cell Res. 30*, 509-520.
Weiss, L. (1965). *Exp. Cell Res. 37*, 540-555.
Weiss, L. (1977). *Int. J. Cancer 20*, 87-92.
Weiss, L. (1978). *Int. J. Cancer 22*, 196-203.
Weiss, L., and Holmes, J. C. (1980). *In* "Proteinases and Tumor Invasion" (P. Sträuli, A. J. Barrett, and A. Baici, eds.), pp. 181-199. Raven, New York.
Weiss, L., Mayhew, E., Rapp, D. G., and Holmes, J. C. (1982). *Br. J. Cancer 45*, 44-53.
Zeidman, I. (ed.) (1982). "Role of Proteases in Metastasis (Selected Abstracts)." I.C.R.D.B. Program, N.C.I./N.I.H., Washington, D. C.

DISCUSSION

COHEN: In your maps, the high-density cells tend to be at the
           periphery and clustered. Two possible mechanisms in-
           volve either intermittent forces inducing movement or
           conversely, mechanisms that inhibit movement that are
           intermittently overcome. As you indicated, mononuclear
           infiltration is often seen in melanomas. Do you find
           an association between such inflammatory infiltrates
           and the presence of clusters of high-density cells?
           This would suggest a role of the immune system in in-
           fluencing the effects you have described.

WEISS: On the basis of our density-mapping techniques, we can-
           not answer your question, although on the basis of other
           work, including your own, it seems likely that host
           defense reactions modify both the cancer cells and the
           tissues invaded by them.

MATHÉ: Have you studied the effect of vinca alkaloids on cell
           movement? It has been observed by J. P. Levy in Paris
           that in the case of erythroblastic leukemia the erythro-
           blasts produce a growth factor to which they are sensi-
           tive. Could you search if the melanoma cell could not
           be able to secrete the tumor chemokinetic factor, which
           would explain why the local invasion stops?

WEISS: We have not to date examined sections taken from patients
           on chemotherapy. If we can obtain specimens from patient
           on vincristine, and so on, before their tumors were ex-
           cised, we will certainly examine them with your sugges-
           tion in mind; however, as far as I am aware, the vinca
           alkaloids are not used to treat melanomas. Analysis of
           density maps at best permit a reconstruction of events;
           they do not in themselves permit discrimination between
           the possible mechanisms involved. Certainly the dis-
           tance from the edge of the main body of the tumor at
           which cancer cell movement stops could be regulated by
           the rates of degradation of diffusible chemokinetic
           factors and agents affecting the mechanical strength of
           host tissues.

MACHADO: Is it not possible that isolated melanoma cells are
           actually inside lymphatic vessels? Thus, the small pro-
           liferations are perhaps satellite micrometastases.

WEISS: Some of the melanoma cells observed by us are doubtless
           in lymphatic vessels. Indeed, we suggest that active
           cell movement through the tissues is a factor weighting
           for entry into the lymphatic system. We have only

examined hematoxylin and eosin-stained material, so we
cannot estimate the proportions of intralymphatic cancer
cells. Although this location of cells is well recognized and of obvious importance, I do not think it is
frequent enough to introduce major errors in our own
work. The proliferative areas would correspond to satellite micrometastases, but we are of the opinion that
the cancer cells reached the proliferative locations by
active movement.

COCHRAN: Could your density variations be related to tumor size
and penetration of fixative into tissues? How do you
allow for content of macrophages and lymphocytes? Are
you sure that you can identify single melanoma cells
deep to the tumor and if so, how? If single cells do
exist deep to the tumor, why do they not excite and
attract collections of immunocytes?

WEISS: Our material was subject to standard formalin fixation
and histologic processing. All measurements relate to
this material, not to tissues in the fresh state. I
agree that single cancer cells always present identification problems. However, in the case of malignant
melanomas, the major problem is to distinguish between
melanophages and melanoma cells. On occasion we have
been unable to identify cells positively, and have not
included them in our density maps. However, this happens infrequently, and the potential error is not great
in our opinion. We have not enumerated immunocyte
densities.

LIOTTA: We have confirmed your results in studies on invasion in
murine tumors transplanted into muscle (*J. Theoret.
Biol.*, 1976). Fixation artifact in our studies was
controlled. Tumor cell distribution at the invasion
front behaved as a classic diffusion process, therefore,
supporting the concept that invasion is an active process not simply related to growth pressure.

WEISS: Thank you for your comments; we are aware of your own
work. Although we do not find that the *migration* pattern of melanoma cells follows a classic diffusion process, we are in general agreement with your own conclusions. The challenge was, of course, to *numerically*
evaluate the relative contributions of *vis a tergo* and
active cell movements to invasion in humans.

COCHRAN: The dermis comprises two separate and physically different zones, the *papillary dermis* and *reticular dermis*—these present different physical media for the

invading cell. How does your model relate to these factors, or are your observations concerned only with the papillary dermis?

WEISS: Our own observations to date are limited to cancer cell density gradients and statistically high- and low-density points. We have independent evidence from *in vitro* experiments that the chemical nature of the materials through which cells migrate, produces differential effects. Thus, W-256 tumor cells will migrate through membranes with fibrin-impregnated pores but not through collagen I. In contrast, Gardner lymphosarcoma cells will migrate through collagen I-impregnated pores but not through fibrin (Turner and Weiss, 1983).

LIOTTA: How would you *merge* your finding with those of Dr. W. Clark who showed that the depth of invasion and thickness correlated with prognosis?

WEISS: Our system is too time consuming to be applied to routine measurements of clinical specimens. I think that our own studies may add some perspective to Clark's classification. Although ultimately we will be seeking correlations between density patterns, clinical histories, and Clark's classification, we have not done this to date.

MORTON: (1) Have you looked at melanomas present in the skin of varying thickness? (2) Would the S-100 marker molecule described by Dr. Cochran not be useful in quantitative studies and more rapid than morphologic approach?

WEISS: Thank you for your suggestion. We will do this, and we have already planned to do similar studies of metastatic melanomas in different organs. I cannot comment on the potential usefulness of the S-100 marker, because I would guess that the reaction of melanoma cells with the marker is very variable.

POSTE: Comment: We have been doing studies on the morphometry of malignant melanoma using monoclonal antibodies and computerized image analysis methods. This is proving very difficult because of antigenic heterogeneity among the donor cells, which dictates the need to use a panel of antibodies. Even under these conditions many tumor cells fail to stain, and variations in tumor cell fluorescence (variation in epitope density?) also make it exceptionally difficult to use quantitative fluorometric measurements to define tumor—host margin in any sophisticated method using image analysis methods.

CHAPTER 3

SPONTANEOUS REGRESSION OF XENOGENIZED
TUMOR METASTASIS IN RATS

Hiroshi Kobayashi

Laboratory of Pathology
Cancer Institute
Hokkaido University School of Medicine
Sapporo, Japan

I. INTRODUCTION

There have been no reports on spontaneous regression of tumor metastasis. However, in viral xenogenization of tumor cells, primary tumors and their metastases regress after the temporary growth of tumors by an artificial infection of tumors in rats with foreign antigenic viruses.

BASIC MECHANISMS AND CLINICAL TREATMENT
OF TUMOR METASTASIS

II.   XENOGENIZATION OF TUMOR CELLS

    Figure 1 shows the growth pattern of various types of rat
tumors after infection of the tumors with Friend virus. Such
virus-infected tumors are unable to grow in syngeneic and autochthonous hosts; even if they grow for a while, they regress eventually. Most rat tumors regress in the pattern with a small amount
(<10 mm) of temporary growth of the tumors (Kobayashi *et al.*,
1969, 1970, 1977, 1978; Kuzumaki *et al.*, 1978; Kobayashi, 1979,
1982).
    The reason for the regression of tumors is that a foreign an-
tigen produced on the cell surface after an artificial infection
of tumors with such a foreign antigenic virus as Friend virus, is
foreign in the host, since the tumor cells come from rats, while
the virus is obtained from mice, the two being different species.
In other words, Friend virus is infectious to mice but not to
adult rats. However, the virus is able to infect rat tumor cells
under certain conditions. Such regression of tumors, referred to
as "viral xenogenization" of tumors, can be observed not only in
rat tumors infected with virus, but also in mouse and hamster
tumors by artificial infection with foreign antigenic nonlytic
viruses (Eiselein and Boggs, 1970; Barbieri *et al.*, 1971; Evermann
and Burnstein, 1975).

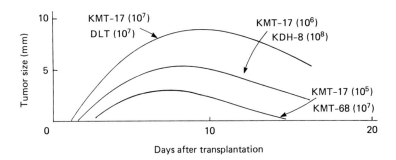

    Fig. 1. Viral xenogenization as seen in regression of rat
tumors modified by Friend virus. Numbers in parentheses indicate
numbers of tumor cells transplanted.

III. REGRESSION OF METASTASIS
      OF XENOGENIZED TUMORS

    Metastasis developed in the regional lymph nodes regresses
as well after initial enlargement of the lymph nodes if tumor cells
were previously modified or xenogenized by virus infection, while

uninfected ordinary types of tumor will grow and kill the host in
all cases (Figs. 2-11). In other words, xenogenized highly immunogenic tumor cells are also able to metastasize into lymph nodes
regardless of the high immunogenicity of xenogenized tumor cells.
It thus seems that immunogenicity is not directly related to such
processes of metastasis formation as liberation, intravasation,
and lodgement of tumor cells. Immunogenicity may be related to
the growth of tumor cells at a final stage of metastasis after
the tumor cells have reached the tissue (Kodama *et al.*, 1974a,b,
1975).

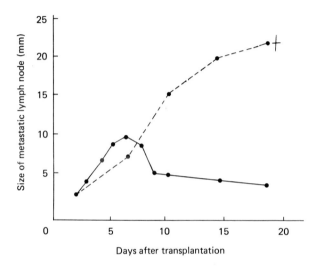

Fig. 2.   Regression of tumor metastasis in regional lymph node.
●---● KMT-17 tumor; ●——● virally modified KMT-17 tumor.

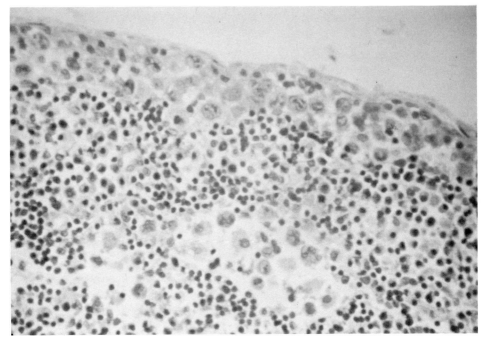

Fig. 3. An early stage of metastasis of rat tumor cells infected with Friend virus.

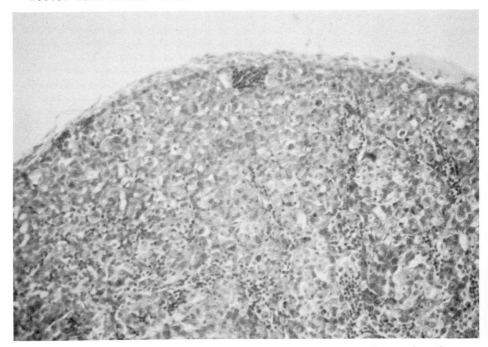

Fig. 4. An abundant number of tumor cells proliferating in a lymph node that is almost wholly occupied by tumor cells.

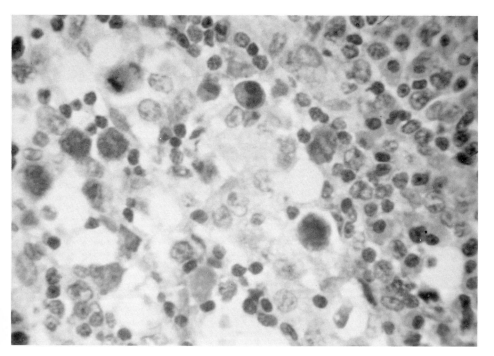

Fig. 5. High magnification of a lymph node in which virus-infected xenogenized tumor cells grow well.

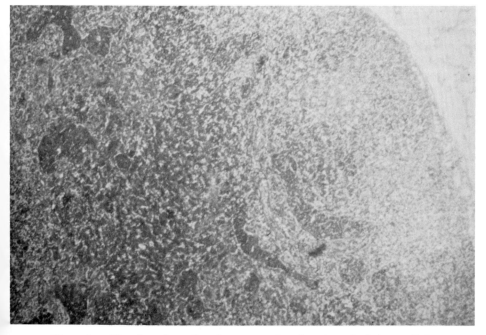

Fig. 6. The lymph node, however, begins to shrink, and tumor cells disappear gradually.

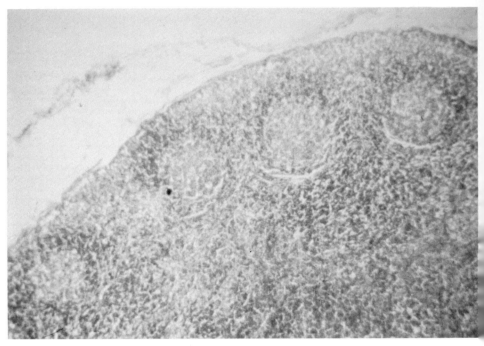

Fig. 7. Finally, the normal structure of the lymph node appears again. No perceptible signs exist that there was tumor metastasis in the lymph node.

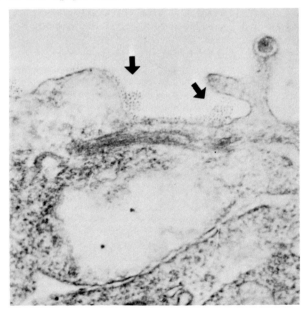

Fig. 8. A new antigen appearing on the cell surface as indicated by granules of immunoferritin. There is a virus budding, and the new foreign antigen (arrows) that is produced on the surface after xenogenization may be recognized as foreign by the host.

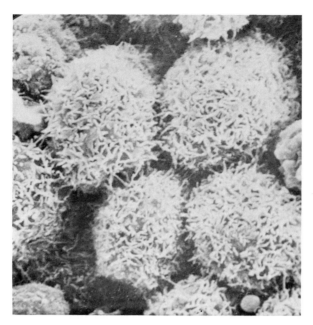

Fig. 9. A scanning electron micrograph showing tumor cells with a number of microvilli on the surface; there are fibrosarcoma cells before infection with virus.

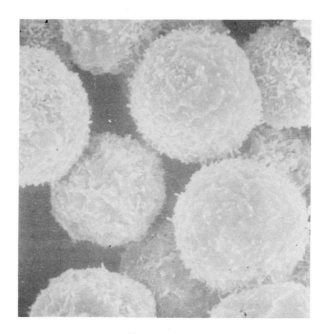

Fig. 10. After the infection of the same line of tumor cells
with Friend virus, the cell surface becomes converted to the appearance shown here; that is, a number of the microvilli seen in
Fig. 9 disappear, and the surface looks smooth, so that it appears
tumor cells may be easily liberated and intravasated.

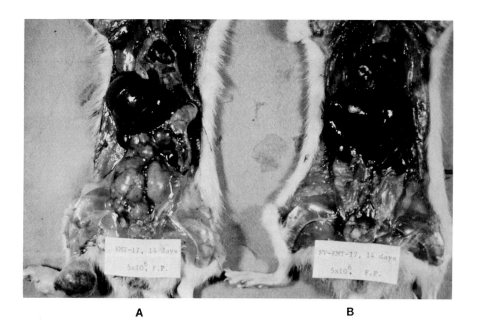

A   B

Fig. 11.   (A) An enlarged lymph node metastasized from a primary tumor.   (B) The metastasized lymph nodes regress 2 weeks after a xenogenized tumor has been transplanted into the leg.   Resistance to rechallenged tumor growth is observed in such tumor-
regressed rats.   However, when lymph nodes are removed from the
body after regression of the tumor, the resistance will be weakened.

IV. SPECIFIC IMMUNOTHERAPY TO TUMOR METASTASIS
    BY XENOGENIZED TUMOR CELLS

    In order to treat metastasis of uninfected tumors, prior im-
munization is not allowed.   The immunization must be done after
tumor development.   When an uninfected KMT-17 tumor was injected
into a footpad and the tumor was surgically removed several days
later, metastasis developed in 38 of 56 cases.   However, when
virus-infected xenogenized tumor cells were used for the immunization of the host after surgery, metastasis developed in only 28
of 65 cases.   This rate was significantly lower than that of the
control (Kobayashi et al., 1975).
    However, the difference between the two groups was not so big.
The main reason for this is the time limit required to make xenogenized tumor cells strongly immunogenic in inhibition of the

TABLE I

Immunotherapy with Viable Xenogenized Tumor Cells (KMT-17)
against the Metastasis of Original Tumor Cells

Treatment	No. of rats dead of metastasis[a]
Immunotherapy with viable xenogenized tumor cells after surgery	28/65 (43%) $p < .01$
Surgery alone	38/56 (68%)

[a]Two-month observation.

tumor metastasis, since the tumor used in this experiment grows
very rapidly and produces metastasis before immunity develops
(Table I).

REFERENCES

Barbieri, D., Belehradek, J., Jr., and Barski, G. (1971). *Int. J. Cancer 7*, 364.
Eiselein, J., and Biggs, M. W. (1970). *Cancer Res. 30*, 1953.
Evermann, J. F., and Burnstein. T. (1975). *Int. J. Cancer 16*, 861.
Kobayashi, H. (1979). *Adv. Cancer Res. 30*, 279-299.
Kobayashi, H. (1982). *In* "Immunological Approaches to Cancer Therapeutics" (E. Mihich, ed.), pp. 405-440. Wiley, New York.
Kobayashi, H., Sendo, F., Shirai, T., Kaji, H., and Saito, H. (1969). *J. Natl. Cancer Inst. (US) 42*, 413-319.
Kobayashi, H., Sendo, F., Kaji, H., Shirai, T., Saito, H., Takeichi, N., Hosokawa, M., and Kodama, T. (1970). *J. Natl. Cancer Inst. (US) 44*, 11-19.
Kobayashi, H., Gotohda, E., Hosokawa, M., and Kodama, T. (1975). *J. Natl. Cancer Inst. (US) 54*, 997-999.
Kobayashi, H., Kodama, T., and Gotohda, E. (1977). "Xenogenization of Tumor Cells," pp. 1-124. Hokkaido Univ. School of Medicine, Sapporo.
Kobayashi, H., Takeichi, N., and Kuzumaki, N. (1978). "Xenogenization of Lymphocytes, Erythroblasts, and Tumor Cells," pp. 1-174. Hokkaido Univ. School of Medicine, Sapporo.
Kodama, T., Gotohda, E., Takeichi, M., Kuzumaki, N., and Kobayashi, H. (1974a). *J. Natl. Cancer Inst. (US) 52*, 931-939.
Kodama, T., Gotohda, E., Takeichi, N., Kuzumaki, N., and Kobayashi, H. (1974b). *Abstr. Int. Cancer Congr. 11th*, pp. 639-640.

Kodama, T., Gotohda, E., Takeichi, N., Kuzumaki, N., and Kobayashi, H. (1975). *Cancer Res. 35,* 1628-1636.
Kuzumaki, N., Fenyo, E., Klein, E., and Klein, G. (1978). *Transplantation 26,* 304-307.

DISCUSSION

COHEN: It's important not to restrict the explanation of these phenomena to immunologic mechanisms. Since viruses are involved in this system, other possibilities include direct effects of interferon, as well as indirect effects indicated by Dr. Golub. Also, as we and others have shown, viruses induce *cytokines,* and some of these mediators can influence inflammatory cells.

KOBAYASHI: Even with virus-induced cytokine and some other cytotoxic factors, there have been no reports so far describing the regression of such a large number of transplanted tumor cells. As we have already described, the mechanism of regression of tumors infected with foreign antigenic virus could possibly be explained by immune competent cells such as T cells, macrophages, and humoral antibodies. This may also depend on the conditions of virus infection of cells such as the dose of virus used and the amount of surface antigen produced.

COCHRAN: What happens if you place your Friend virus-infected cells into tissue culture, rather than back into the animals? Do the xenogenized cells survive in culture?

KOBAYASHI: Yes, xenogenized tumor cells can survive in culture, as can the unxenogenized ordinary type of tumor cells, since no cytopathic effect of the virus is seen. Xenogenized tumor cells can also grow in *in vivo*-immunosuppressed hosts.

LIOTTA: The lymph node was depleted during regression of the micrometastases. This speaks against a cell-mediated immune mechanism.

KOBAYASHI: Yes, we agree. We have not studied the histology of the regressing tumors extensively. However, it is difficult to draw a conclusion, since the rejection mechanism of the tumor may vary depending on the dose of a virus and the amount of surface antigen produced. Humoral immunity is evidently involved in explaining the regression of such high-antigenic xenogenized tumors, but maybe not all.

MATHÉ: I would like to know if with xenogenization you mainly
            obtain a nonspecific immunity potentiation or a specif-
            ic virus-antigenic stimulation. Have you examined NK,
            macrophages, and cytotoxic T cells?

KOBAYASHI: Both specific and nonspecific immunity may be involved
            in explaining the rejection mechanism of virus-infected
            tumors and the subsequent production of antitumor im-
            munity following regression of the tumor.

GOLUB: Have you examined the possible involvement of NK cells
            or interferon in the viral-infected cell immunotherapy?
            Are there strain differences in mice and can these be
            correlated to NK levels?

KOBAYASHI: As far as we have tested, it seems that activated NK
            cells or interferon will not explain the entire mech-
            anism of the strong immunogenicity of tumor cells caused
            by infection with virus in rats. We have not yet ex-
            amined any mice.

MORTON: What is the histopathological character of the regres-
            sing viral-infected tumor at the primary site and in the
            regional lymph nodes?

KOBAYASHI: We have not yet studied the histology of regressing
            primary and metastatic tumor extensively.

CHAPTER 4

EXPERIMENTAL STUDIES OF OPERATIVE STRESS
ON TUMOR GROWTH IN RATS

Takao Hattori
Tetsuya Toge
Wataru Takiyama
Toshihiro Hirai
Toshiyuki Ikeda

Department of Surgery
Research Institute for Nuclear Medicine and Biology
Hiroshima University
Hiroshima, Japan

BASIC MECHANISMS AND CLINICAL TREATMENT
OF TUMOR METASTASIS

I. INTRODUCTION

It is generally accepted that surgery is the most powerful
means for the cure of cancer, as shown in the history of surgery
for gastric cancer in Japan. By escalation of operative intervention to extirpate all the lymph nodes with the stomach and
sometimes a part of neighboring tissues, the long-term survival
rate of patients with gastric cancer has increased strikingly.
In the case of gastric cancer located near the esophagocardial
junction, however, the situation differs somewhat. Resection of
esophagocardial cancer can now be carried out with a reasonably
low mortality rate via a thoracoabdominal approach, but the prognosis of patients so treated does not seem to have changed over
the last two decades. The difficulty of detecting esophagocardial
cancer in the early stage was the only excuse for its poor prognosis. Hitherto the influence of surgical stress of thoracotomy
on tumor growth has not come up for discussion. However, new
surgical techniques for esophagocardial cancer that were established by us (Hattori *et al.*, 1975) via a transabdominal approach,
thus obviating thoracotomy, gave good clinical results (Hattori *et
al.*, 1980, 1982a,b). These clinical experiences have stimulated us
to design an experiment to test our hypothesis that operative
stress of thoracotomy might enhance the tumor growth in the host
more remarkably than laparotomy.

II. MATERIALS AND METHODS

A. Animals and Tumor

Two-month-old male Donryu rats, weighing 170-200 g, were pur-
chased from Nihon Rat Co., Saitama, Japan. Sato lung cancer (SLC),
kindly provided by Dr. H. Niitani of the National Cancer Center
Hospital (Tokyo, Japan) was maintained by serial subcutaneous transplantation of solid graft biweekly in the backs of Donryu rats. To
obtain the tumor cell suspension, tumor tissue was minced, treated
with 0.25% trypsin at 37° C for 60 min, centrifuged three times at
200 g for 5 min at 4° C and resuspended in Hank's balanced solution.

Size of inoculum was 2.5×10^6, 2.5×10^5, 2.5×10^4, 2.5×10^3, or 10^3 cells for intraperitoneal (ip) inoculation, and 10^5, 10^4, or 10^3 cells for intravenous (iv) inoculation.

B. Operative Procedure

Details were already described in the previous article (Hattori et al., 1977a,b). Rats were anesthetized by intraperitoneal administration of 12.4 mg/kg pentobarbital sodium on Day 2 after inoculation. They were divided into four groups: laparotomy, thoracotomy, laparothoracotomy, and control (no operation). Laparotomy was made by midline incision 7–8 cm in length under spontaneous respiration. Right thoracotomy was made by oblique incision 3 cm in length in the fifth intercostal space. The incised wounds were kept open for 1 hr. Respiration was controlled artificially with the rodent respirator (Harvard Type 680, Harvard, Millis, Cambridge, Massachusetts) by intratracheal intubation in the thoracotomized rats. The tidal volume was adjusted to 2 ml and the respiration rate to 60 per minute.

C. Evaluation of Enhancing Effect on Tumor Growth

The survival period of the rats after inoculation, and the number and percentage area of metastatic nodules on the lungs were examined. The survival period of the test groups was expressed as the percentage in relation to that of the control. Rats surviving over 50 days were calculated as 50-day survivors in the determination of mean survival period. For the determination of the number and percentage area of metastatic nodules on the lungs, rats were sacrificed between 15 and 30 days after inoculation according to the size of inoculum as indicated in Tables I–X. The number of metastatic nodules on the surface of the lungs was calculated macroscopically. The lungs were sectioned in the frontal segment through the pulmonary hilus, stained with hematoxylin-eosin, and subjected to the calculation of segmental area of metastatic nodules. Percentage area was expressed as the percentage of the metastases in relation to the whole area of the section. The values of the preceding three determinations in the test groups were expressed as T:C, the percentage of test values in relation to the control values.

D. Assay for Natural Killer Activity

Spleen cells from rats that had undergone surgery were prepared and used as effector cells. Cytolytic activity of NK cells was evaluated on ^{51}Cr-labeled K562 myeloid cell line targets in 18-hr assay as described previously (Toge and Hattori, 1979).

In brief, target cells (2×10^5) were suspended in 1.0 ml of RPMI-1640 medium (GIBCO, Grand Island, New York) and minced with 200 μCi of ^{51}Cr sodium chromate for 40 min at 37° C. Labeled target cells were washed four times and resuspended in RPMI-1640 medium containing 20% fetal calf serum. Aliquots (0.1 ml) of the cell suspensions were dispensed into the wells of microplates (Towa Co. Ltd., Tokyo, Japan). Effector spleen cells (2×10^6 or 8×10^5) were added to each well to a final volume of 0.3 ml of complete medium, giving effector:target cell ratios of 40:1. Cultures in triplicate were incubated for 18 hr at 37° C. After incubation, the plates were centrifuged, then 0.2 ml of cell-free supernatant fluid in each well was withdrawn and its radioactivity was counted in a γ spectrometer. The cytotoxicity was calculated as follows:

$$\text{cytotoxicity (\%)} = \frac{E - S}{T - S} \times 100$$

where E is ^{51}Cr release from labeled target cells in the presence of effector cells, T is maximum release, and S is spontaneous release.

E.   Assay for Lung Macrophage Cytostatic Activity

Lung macrophages were isolated as described by Olivotto and Bomford (1974). The cytostatic activity of lung macrophages against K562 target cells was measured as described previously (Toge et al., 1979). Effector:target cell ratios of 40:1 were used, and all tests were set up in triplicate.

F.   Assay for Spleen Cell Blastogenesis

Spleen cells were prepared and measured as described previously (Hattori et al., 1976). The results were expressed as stimulation index (SI), which was calculated from the following formula:

$$SI = \frac{\text{cpm of spleen cells with PHA}}{\text{cpm of spleen cells without PHA}}$$

All the assays for NK activity, lung macrophage cytostatic activity, and spleen cell blastogenesis were repeated three times, and comparison of the difference between normal (no operation) and treated rats was carried out by means of Student's t-test.

TABLE I

Effect of Use of Respirator in Laparotomy on Survival Time
and Number of Metastatic Nodules on the Lungs on Donryu Rats
Inoculated with SLC[a]

Experimental group	Survival time in days (mean ± SD)[b]		No. of nodules[c] (mean ± SD)
	2.5×10^3 Cells (ip)	10^3 Cells (iv)	
Laparotomy with respirator	38.4 ± 10.4 (4)	47.2 ± 3.6 (6)	5.5 ± 6.8
Laparotomy without respirator	39.3 ± 11.5 (4)	46.8 ± 4.6 (6)	4.1 ± 4.0

[a]Figures in parentheses show the number of rats surviving over 50 days. Each experimental group consisted of 10 rats. There was no significant difference between the two groups, either in survival time or in the number of metastatic nodules.
[b]Rats surviving over 50 days were calculated as 50-day survivors in the determination of mean survival time.
[c]Rats were sacrificed on Day 20 after intravenous inoculation of 10^3 cells.

III.   RESULTS

A.   Effect of Respirator on Tumor Growth

   To clarify the effect of artificial respiration using intratracheal intubation and a rodent respirator on the tumor growth,
laparotomy was performed under artificial respiration in one group
and under spontaneous respiration in the other on Day 2 after inoculation. As shown in Table I, the survival period after intraperitoneal or intravenous inoculation and the number of metastatic
nodules on the lungs after intravenous inoculation indicated no
difference between the two groups.

B.   Survival Period

   The results are shown in Tables II and III. In both experiments of intraperitoneal and intravenous inoculation, the survival
period was significantly reduced by the stress of thoracotomy and
laparothoracotomy compared with the control, but no significant
difference was observed between these two test groups. Neither
was any significant difference seen between the laparotomy and the
control. The differences were more pronounced in the case of a
smaller size of inoculum.

C.   Number of Metastatic Nodules

   The result is shown in Table III. In the group receiving
10^5-cell inoculation, laparothoracotomy enhanced the increase of
the number of the metastatic nodules on the lungs with significant
difference from the control. In the group receiving a 10^4-cell
inoculation, increase in the number of metastatic nodules was
indicated in the thoracotomy and laparothoracotomy groups with
significant difference from the control.

D.   Percentage Area of Metastatic Nodules

   As shown in Table III, the results obtained were quite similar
to those in the number of metastatic nodules. Laparothoracotomy
enhanced the increase of percentage area of metastatic nodules with
significant difference from the control in both the 10^5-cell and
10^4-cell inoculation groups. It was also indicated with the percentage area was directly proportional to the number of metastatic
nodules with a high coefficient of correlation.

TABLE II

Survival Time of Donryu Rats Inoculated with SLC Intraperitoneally in Relation to Operation Stress[a]

Size of inoculum	Mean survival time in days (± SD)[b]			
	Control	Laparotomy	Thoracotomy	Laparothoracotomy
10^3	50.0 ± 0	49.3 ± 2.2 (98.6)	44.1 ± 7.9 (88.2)[c]	42.1 ± 8.7 (84.0)[d]
2.5×10^3	41.8 ± 9.7	40.1 ± 10.8 (95.9)	35.0 ± 12.0 (83.7)[c]	30.9 ± 8.3 (73.9)[c]
2.5×10^4	38.2 ± 10.4	36.2 ± 11.9 (94.8)	27.8 ± 8.6 (72.8)[c]	24.0 ± 3.4 (62.8)[d]
2.5×10^5	31.8 ± 12.7	28.2 ± 14.9 (88.7)	21.3 ± 7.3 (67.0)	19.4 ± 6.1 (61.0)[c]
2.5×10^6	21.5 ± 10.6	19.4 ± 6.0 (90.2)	17.0 ± 4.9 (79.1)	17.0 ± 3.7 (79.1)
50-day survivors in total	23/50	18/50	9/50[c]	5/50[d]

[a]Figures in parentheses are percentages calculated from the ratio of the mean survival days of the test groups to that of the control. Each experimental group consisted of 10 rats.
[b]Rats surviving over 50 days were calculated as 50-day survivors in the determination of mean survival time.
[c]Significant difference from the control: $p < .05$.
[d]Significant difference from the control: $p < .01$.

TABLE III

Survival Time, Number and Percentage Area of Metastatic Nodules
on the Lungs of Donryu Rats Inoculated with SLC Intravenously in Relation to Operative Stress[a]

Size of inoculum	Control	Laparotomy	Thoracotomy	Laparothoracotomy
		Survival time in days (mean ± SD)[b]		
10^3	47.1 ± 6.1	45.7 ± 6.6 (97.2)	37.3 ± 12.6 (79.4)[c]	35.9 ± 11.8 (76.4)[c]
10^4	35.1 ± 13.1	29.6 ± 9.8 (84.3)	24.0 ± 9.6 (68.4)[c]	21.4 ± 3.7 (61.0)[c]
10^5	26.2 ± 12.7	22.1 ± 9.9 (84.4)	18.8 ± 4.2 (71.8)	17.6 ± 1.4 (67.2)[c]
50-day survivors in total	6/20	2/20	1/20	0/20

Number of metastatic nodules (mean ± SD)[d]

10^3	2.6 ± 3.7	2.8 ± 4.1 (107.7)	10.4 ± 16.8 (400.0)	37.4 ± 69.0 (1438.5)
10^4	22.5 ± 25.8	32.8 ± 21.2 (145.8)	57.8 ± 45.6 (256.9)[c]	59.9 ± 30.9 (266.2)[e]
10^5	149.2 ±141.9	130.3 ± 71.7 (87.3)	204.9 ± 84.4 (137.3)	291.8 ±132.9 (195.6)[c]

Percentage area of metastatic nodules (mean ± SD)[d]

10^3	3.4 ± 3.9	4.7 ± 6.4 (137.2)	9.0 ± 6.7 (262.5)	20.6 ± 28.2 (605.6)[c]
10^4	10.7 ± 11.8	17.3 ± 7.7 (161.7)	32.0 ± 17.6 (299.0)[c]	37.2 ± 10.6 (347.7)[c]
10^5	20.4 ± 17.0	23.1 ± 11.9 (113.2)	41.9 ± 14.5 (205.2)[c]	54.9 ± 9.7 (269.1)[c]

[a] Figures in parentheses are percentages calculated from the ratio of the values of the test groups to those of the control. Each experimental group consisted of 10 rats.

[b] Rats surviving over 50 days were calculated as 50-day survivors in the determination of mean survival time.

[c] Significant difference from the control: $p < .05$.

[d] Rats were sacrificed on Day 20 in the 10^4-cell group and on Day 15 in the 10^3-cell group.

[e] Significant difference from the control: $p < .01$.

E.   Duration of Operation

   In this experiment, laparotomy was performed for 5 hr and
thoracotomy for 1 hr.   In the laparothoracotomy group a 5-hr laparotomy and a 1-hr thoracotomy were combined.   As indicated in
Table IV, survival time and the number of metastatic nodules on
the lungs were almost the same in the 5-hr laparotomy and the 1-hr
thoracotomy groups.   In the laparothoracotomy group, a significant
decrease of survival time and increase of metastatic nodules were
observed compared with the control.

F.   Bleeding Associated with Operation

   As shown in Table V, decrease of survival time and increase
of the number of metastatic nodules were observed in the laparothoracotomy plus bleeding group, but the difference from the control was not significant.

G.   Timing of Operation

   Operations were performed on Days -7, -4, -2, -1, 0, +2, and
+4 from the inoculation.   The results are summarized in Table VI.
Significant reduction of survival time was seen in the laparothoracotomy group when the operation was performed on Days -2, -1,
0, or +2.   In the thoracotomy group, a significant reduction of
survival time was seen when the operation was performed on Days
-1, 0, or +2.

H.   Administration of Immunopotentiators

   OK-432 (50 KE* × 4, ip), PS-K (250 mg/kg × 10, ip), lentinan
(0.5 mg/kg × 5, iv), and C. parvum (20 mg/kg × 2, iv) were administered on the various days indicated in Table VII.   Generally,
reduction of survival time and increase of metastatic nodules on
the lungs after laparothoracotomy were restored by administration
of immunopotentiators.   Significant restoration was observed in
survival time, when OK-432 was given from Days -5 to -2, and also
in the number of metastatic nodules, when lentinan was administered from Days -5 to -1.

---

   *KE represents Klinische Einheit.   One KE is equivalent to
approximately 0.1 mg lyophilized preparation of heat-killed
Streptococcus hemolyticus.

TABLE IV

Survival Time and Number of Metastatic Nodules on the Lungs of Donryu Rats Inoculated with SLC in Relation to Operative Stress and Its Duration[a]

Route and size of inoculum	Control	Laparotomy (5 hr)	Thoracotomy (1 hr)	Laparo-thoracotomy (5 hr + 1 hr)
		Survival time in days (mean ± SD)[b]		
2.5×10^4 ip	40.3 ± 10.5	35.8 ± 13.6 (88.8)	34.5 ± 12.8 (85.6)	26.6 ± 7.5 (66.0)[c]
10^4 iv	43.2 ± 8.5	39.9 ± 10.9 (92.3)	39.6 ± 10.9 (91.6)	31.2 ± 9.6 (72.2)[c]
50-day survivors in total	12/23	7/17	8/20	0/19
		Number of metastatic nodules (mean ± SD)[d]		
10^4 iv	1.9 ± 2.0	4.1 ± 3.5 (215.7)	3.6 ± 3.8 (189.4)	8.1 ± 4.8 (426.3)[e]

[a] Rats were divided into three groups and subjected to a 5-hr laparotomy, a 1-hr thoracotomy, or both on Day 2 after inoculation of tumor cells. Figures in parentheses are percentages calculated from ratio of the values of the test groups to those of the control.
[b] Rats surviving over 50 days were calculated as 50-day survivors in the determination of mean survival time.
[c] Significant difference from the control: $p < .05$.
[d] Rats were sacrificed on Day 20 after inoculation. Each group consisted of 10 rats.
[e] Significant difference from the control: $p < .01$.

TABLE V

Survival Time and Number of Metastatic Nodules on the Lungs of Donryu Rats Inoculated with SLC in Relation to Operative Stress and Bleeding[a]

Route and size of inoculum	Control	Bleeding only	Laparotomy + bleeding	Thoracotomy + bleeding	Laparo-thoracotomy + bleeding
			Survival time in days (mean ± SD)[b]		
2.5×10^4 ip	48.1 ± 7.1	48.0 ± 7.2 (99.7)	45.0 ± 8.4 (93.5)	41.7 ± 11.2 (86.6)	38.1 ± 13.1 (79.2)
10^4 iv	45.7 ± 6.6	43.5 ± 7.2 (95.1)	42.5 ± 10.0 (92.9)	39.0 ± 11.4 (85.3)	35.0 ± 12.1 (76.5)[c]
50-day survivors in total	16/22	13/20	14/20	9/20	8/19
			Number of metastatic nodules (mean ± SD)[d]		
10^4 iv	1.8 ± 3.1	2.3 ± 2.2 (127.7)	2.8 ± 2.1 (155.6)	5.5 ± 5.6 (305.5)	8.1 ± 7.5 (450)[c]

[a] Rats were subjected to a 1-hr operation on Day 2 after inoculation, and 4 ml of blood were withdrawn from the femoral artery during the operation. Figures in parentheses are percentages calculated from the ratio of the values of the test groups to those of the control.
[b] Rats surviving over 50 days were calculated as 50-day survivors in the determination of mean survival time.
[c] Significant difference from the control: $p < .05$.
[d] Rats were sacrificed on Day 20 after inoculation. Each group consisted of 10 rats.

TABLE VI

Survival Time of Donryu Rats Inoculated with SLC Intravenously in Relation
to Operative Stress and Its Timing[a]

Day of operation	Control	Survival time in days (mean ± SD)[b]		
		Laparotomy	Thoracotomy	Laparothoracotomy
-7	50.0 ± 0	50.0 ± 0 (100.0)	44.7 ± 11.3 (89.4)	42.0 ± 13.8 (84.0)
-4	50.0 ± 0	50.0 ± 0 (100.0)	42.3 ± 16.7 (84.6)	42.1 ± 16.7 (84.2)
-2	48.4 ± 5.5	43.1 ± 11.2 (89.0)	38.6 ± 15.3 (79.7)	37.6 ± 16.6 (77.6)[c]
-1	48.0 ± 6.3	41.3 ± 12.7 (86.0)	32.9 ± 14.0 (68.5)[c]	26.8 ± 14.2 (55.8)[d]
0	45.1 ± 8.9	44.1 ± 8.4 (97.7)	37.8 ± 13.0 (83.8)	33.7 ± 14.2 (74.7)[d]
+2	47.0 ± 6.1	45.7 ± 6.6 (97.2)	37.3 ± 12.6 (79.3)[c]	35.9 ± 11.8 (76.3)[c]
+4	49.7 ± 0.7	49.5 ± 1.1 (99.5)	48.3 ± 2.5 (97.1)	44.9 ± 5.8 (90.3)

[a]Rats were inoculated with 10^4 cells intravenously on Day 0 and the operation was performed for 1 hr. Figures in parentheses are percentages calculated from ratio of the survival time of the test groups to that of the control.

[b]Rats surviving over 50 days were calculated as 50-day survivors in the determination of mean survival time.

[c]Significant difference from the control: $p < .05$.

[d]Significant difference from the control: $p < .01$.

TABLE VII

Survival Time and Number of Metastatic Nodules on the Lungs of Donryu Rats
Inoculated with SLC Intravenously in Relation to Laparothoracotomy and Administration of Potentiators[a]

Experimental group[b]	Immunopotentiators		Survival time[c]			Number of metastatic nodules[e]	
	Doses	Administered on days	Days (mean ± SD)	T:C[d] (%)	Survivors at 50 days	(mean ± SD)	T:C (%)
I.							
LT	-	-	36.5 ± 11.5	83.3[f]	3/10	6.6 ± 6.6	471.4
LT + OK-432	50 KE × 4	-5,-4,-3,-2	46.1 ± 8.2	105.3	8/10	5.7 ± 7.5	407.1
LT + OK-432	50 KE × 4	-1, 0,+1,+2	38.2 ± 11.2	87.2	4/10	6.2 ± 6.0	442.8
LT + OK-432	50 KE × 4	+3,+4,+5,+6	39.0 ± 12.2	89.0	5/10	3.8 ± 7.0	271.4
Control	-	-	43.8 ± 11.5	-	9/12	1.4 ± 2.3	-
II.							
LT	-	-	29.7 ± 11.6	68.0	2/10	10.1 ± 6.5	531.6
LT + PS-K	250 mg/kg × 10	-10 to -1	42.0 ± 12.4	96.0	6/10	5.1 ± 3.6	268.4
LT + PS-K	250 mg/kg × 10	-3 to +6	40.1 ± 13.0	91.8	6/10	5.4 ± 4.9	284.2
LT + PS-K	250 mg/kg × 10	+3 to +6	35.4 ± 13.2	81.0	4/10	7.6 ± 7.2	400.0
Control	-	-	43.7 ± 9.7	-	8/10	1.9 ± 3.1	-

III.

LT	—	—	31.3 ± 12.6	72.5	2/10	9.7 ± 6.9	646.7[f]
LT + lentinan	0.5 mg/kg × 5	-5 to -1	25.6 ± 9.4	59.3	1/10	3.4 ± 3.7	226.7
LT + lentinan	0.5 mg/kg × 5	-1 to +3	33.7 ± 14.3	78.0	4/10	5.1 ± 5.6	340.0
LT + lentinan	0.5 mg/kg × 5	+2 to +6	35.0 ± 13.2	81.0	4/10	6.7 ± 7.7	446.7
Control	—	—	43.2 ± 12.5	-	9/12	1.5 ± 1.9	-

IV.

LT	—	—	33.6 ± 14.4	75.2	4/10	7.0 ± 4.8	318.2
LT + C. parvum	20 mg/kg × 2	-4, -3	42.0 ± 10.5	94.0	6/10	3.6 ± 3.2	163.3
LT + C. parvum	20 mg/kg × 2	0, +1	26.4 ± 9.1	59.1	1/10	3.8 ± 3.3	172.7
LT + C. parvum	20 mg/kg × 2	+3, +4	41.7 ± 10.7	93.4	5/10	3.7 ± 3.9	168.2
Control	—	—	44.7 ± 9.9	-	9/10	2.2 ± 2.9	-

[a] Rats were subjected to a 1-hr laparothoracotomy on Day 2 after inoculation of 10^4 SLC cells. OK-432 and PS-K were administered intraperitoneally and lentinan and C. parvum intravenously.

[b] LT, laparothoracotomy.

[c] Rats surviving over 50 days were calculated as 50-day survivors in the determination of mean survival time.

[d] T:C, ratio of the values of test groups to those of the control.

[e] Rats were sacrificed on Day 20.

[f] Significant difference from LT group: $p < .05$.

I.   Natural Killer Activities of Spleen Cells

Natural killer (NK) activities of spleen cells were measured
on Days 1, 3, 7, and 14 after surgical stress. As shown in Table
VIII, NK activities were significantly depressed on Day 1 in all
the test groups compared with the control. They were already
close to or higher than those of normal control rats on day 7 in
both the thoracotomy and laparotomy groups, while they remained
still depressed in the laparothoracotomy group. However, on Day
14, the effects of surgical stress on NK activities have clearly
disappeared.

J.   Proliferative Response to PHA of Spleen Cells

The effects of proliferative response to PHA of spleen cells
was also examined on Days 1, 3, 7, and 14. The results were quite
similar to those obtained with NK activities, but the restoration
on Day 14 was not so clear as it was with NK activities in the
laparothoracotomy group, as shown in Table IX.

K.   Cytostatic Activities of Lung Macrophages

As shown in Table X, the activities were not significantly
depressed on Day 1 in the laparotomy group, while they were significantly depressed on Days 1 and 3 in the thoracotomy and laparothoracotomy groups. In the laparothoracotomy group the restoration
on Day 14 was not so clear as in the laparotomy and thoracotomy
groups.

IV. DISCUSSION

As described in the introduction, we have suspected that the
surgical stress of thoracotomy or laparothoracotomy might depress
general resistance of the patient. However, the direct evidence
that thoracotomy or laparothoracotomy enhances the tumor growth
has not yet been obtained. Surgeons aim at low mortality from
surgery even in the treatment of cancer, and their concern does
not seem to be directed to enhancing the effect of operative
stress itself on the tumor growth.
Many experimental factors have been known to increase the number of metastases in vivo. They are massage (Jonescu, 1931; Knox,
1922; Marsh, 1927), local X-irradiation (Kaplan and Murphy, 1949;
Krebs, 1929), total-body irradiation (Krebs, 1929), elevated environmental temperature (Lucke and Schlumberger, 1949), pregnancy
(Greene, 1950), and surgical stress. Although there has been
speculation as to the possibility that surgical trauma results in

TABLE VIII

Effect of Operative Stress on NK Activity of Spleen Cells in Rats[a]

Days after operation	Control	Laparotomy	Thoracotomy	Laparothoracotomy
		NK activities (%) (mean ± SE)[b]		
Prior to operation	46.8 ± 6.5	—	—	—
1	—	27.3 ± 9.4[c] (58.3)	28.2 ± 1.8 (60.3)[c]	29.4 ± 2.2[c] (62.8)
3	—	41.3 ± 6.9 (88.2)	41.4 ± 6.1 (88.5)	38.8 ± 6.8[c] (81.2)
7	—	44.1 ± 3.9 (94.2)	61.9 ± 6.5 (132.3)	40.3 ± 8.6 (86.6)
14	—	53.1 ± 2.1 (113.5)	49.4 ± 4.0 (105.6)	44.6 ± 4.2 (95.3)

[a]Rats were divided into three test groups, and each group consisted of three rats. Figures in parentheses are percentages calculated from ratio of the NK activities of the test groups to those of the control.

[b]Effector:target cell ratio, 40:1.

[c]Significant difference from the control: $p < .05$.

TABLE IX

Effect of Operative Stress on Proliferative Response
to PHA of Spleen Cells in Rats[a]

Days after operation	Proliferative response to PHA (SI) (mean ± SE)			
	Control	Laparotomy	Thoracotomy	Laparothoracotomy
Prior to operation	12.1 ± 1.9	—	—	—
1	—	4.9 ± 1.2[b] (40.9)	3.9 ± 1.3[b] (32.2)	5.9 ± 1.9[b] (48.8)
3	—	11.6 ± 0.4 (95.9)	8.5 ± 2.8[b] (70.2)	7.8 ± 1.7[b] (64.5)
7	—	11.5 ± 0.3 (95.0)	10.4 ± 4.9 (86.8)	7.7 ± 5.1[b] (63.6)
14	—	13.0 ± 2.9 (107.0)	11.3 ± 5.5 (93.4)	10.4 ± 4.7 (85.9)

[a] Rats were divided into three test groups and each group consisted of three rats. Figures in parentheses are percentages calculated from ratio of SI of the test groups to that of the control.
[b] Significant difference from control: $p < .05$.

70

TABLE X

Effect of Operative Stress on Cytostatic Activities
of Lung Macrophages in Rats[a]

Days after operation	Cytostatic activities (%) of lung macrophages (mean ± SE)[b]			
	Control	Laparotomy	Thoracotomy	Laparothoracotomy
Prior to operation	61.9 ± 3.6	—	—	—
1	—	50.2 ± 6.5 (81.1)	29.9 ± 5.2[c] (48.3)	35.2 ± 6.8[c] (69.9)
3	—	54.3 ± 5.6 (87.7)	40.3 ± 5.3[c] (65.1)	37.5 ± 3.3[c] (60.6)
7	—	57.2 ± 6.5 (92.4)	53.7 ± 5.7 (86.8)	44.3 ± 9.8[c] (71.6)
14	—	57.0 ± 3.9 (92.1)	58.1 ± 9.9 (93.9)	49.7 ± 3.0 (80.3)

[a]Rats were divided into three test groups and each group consisted of three rats. Figures in parentheses are percentages calculated from ratio of the cytostatic activities of lung macrophages of the test groups to those of the control.
[b]Effector:target cell ratio, 40:1.
[c]Significant difference from the control: $p < .05$.

a more rapid growth of tumor, little factual evidence is available.
Schatten (1958) and Lewis and Cole (1958) reported increased incidence of pulmonary metastases following total removal of the primary tumor or amputation of the limb with tumor. Buinauskas *et
al.* (1958) reported an increase in the "take" of Walker-256 cells
by the stress of celiotomy performed just before subcutaneous
inoculation of the cells into rats. Fisher and Fisher (1959) investigated the influence of surgical stress on the incidence of
hepatic metastases after cell inoculation into the portal vein.
Increased incidence was observed when inoculation was immediately
followed by partial hepatectomy. Partial hepatectomy had a lesser
effect when performed 24 hr after inoculation, and no greater incidence of metastases was found in the operated group than in the
control, when hepatectomy was performed 48 hr later. They emphasized a transient time after inoculation as an important factor
for the stress of hepatectomy influencing the rapid growth of
tumor cells. Thus, a few reports on the enhancing effect of abdominal surgery on tumor growth could be seen, but none has been
on the enhancing effect of thoracotomy, probably because of the
difficulty in performing thoracotomy safely in small animals.

    In this study, the reduction of survival time and increased
incidence in the number and percentage area of metastatic nodules
of the lungs were clearly shown by the stress of thoracotomy and
laparothoracotomy after intraperitoneal and intravenous inoculation
of tumor cells. In contrast, laparotomy alone was indicated to
give no significant enhancing effect on the tumor growth. Between
the number and the percentage area of the metastatic nodules on the
lungs, a high statistical correlation was indicated, and in the
later experiments the percentage of the segmental area of the
metastatic nodules was not performed, because it consumed much
time and expense.

    From the experiments on duration of operation, thoracotomy
seems to enhance the tumor growth about five times more effectively than laparotomy. This is of deep import from a clinical standpoint. In operative treatment for esophagocardial cancer, our new
bypass procedure (Hattori *et al.*, 1975) generally requires much
more time than the usual abdominothoracic approach, especially
when the bypass is done with a colonic segment. This was one of
the major points of objection raised by many other surgeons. That
the permissible duration for laparotomy is several times greater
than that for thoracotomy seems to provide persuasive theoretical
support for our new procedure.

    The experimental results concerning the timing of an operation
suggest that the enhancing effects of thoracotomy or laparothoracotomy on tumor growth reach a maximum on the first postoperative
day and then decrease, becoming slight on the fourth postoperative
day. However, operative stress seems to be most effective in
stimulating tumor cells when they are still in the bloodstream 1
or 2 days after inoculation, as already pointed out by Fisher and
Fisher (1959). If tumor cells establish a microfocus in the target organ, the operative stress does not appear to stimulate its

growth significantly. At this time it is still difficult to translate the experimental results into clinical terms, but the data presented here seem to be suggestive in relation to the surgical treatment of a cancer that necessitates thoracotomy.

The mechanism of enhancing effects on tumor growth of operative stress is still not clear. As previously reported (Hattori et al., 1978), the increase in the number of metastatic nodules after thoracotomy or laparothoracotomy was quite similar in all five lobes of both lungs in rats. This suggests that the mechanism of tumor growth enhancement by operative stress mainly depends on general factors of the host rather than on local factors such as pathophysiological changes in the chest. As a general factor associated with operative stress, immunological unresponsiveness following surgery has been well documented, and this functional failure has been demonstrated in many facets of the host response including skin tests (Cooper et al., 1974), leukocyte migration inhibition (Cochran et al., 1972), ADCC (Vose and Moudgil, 1976), and lymphocyte blastogenesis (Toge et al., 1976). Munster (1976) suggested the possibility of activation of the suppressor cell system by major burns or extensive surgical operations. In this article, the stress of thoracotomy and laparothoracotomy indicated a depression of host's immunological reactivities and a delay of their restoration with NK activities of spleen cells, proliferative response to PHA of spleen cells, and cytostatic activities of lung macrophages. Furthermore, administration of several immunopotentiators generally resulted in a recovery from the reduction in survival time and from the increase of metastatic nodules on the lungs after surgical stress. From these results, it seems reasonable to conclude that immunological unresponsiveness is one of the most important factors that enhance tumor growth after operative stress such as thoracotomy or laparothoracotomy.

As another important factor, the possibility of excessive secretions of adrenal steroid hormones cannot be neglected. We are investigating the production of rats without adrenal glands and planning to make comparative studies between tumor-bearing rats with and without adrenal glands associated with operative stress and tumor growth.

V. SUMMARY

To indicate the influence of operative stress on tumor growth, thoracotomy and/or laparotomy were performed prior to or after intraperitoneal or intravenous inoculation of Sato lung cancer cells into Donryu rats. Survival time in the thoracotomy or laparothoracotomy group was significantly reduced compared with that of the control. The results obtained in the number and percentage area of metastatic nodules on the lungs were quite similar to those obtained in the survival period. Correlation between the number and the percentage area of metastatic nodules was highly significant. Enhancing effects on tumor growth were several times more effective in thoracotomy or laparothoracotomy than in laparotomy. As for the operation timing, operative stress of thoracotomy or laparothoracotomy enhanced tumor growth significantly, when the operation was performed on Days -2, -1, 0, or +2. The operative stress of thoracotomy or laparothoracotomy indicated a depression of host's immunological reactivities and a delay of their restoration with NK activities of spleen cells, proliferative response to PHA of spleen cells, and cytostatic activities of lung macrophages. Administration of several immunopotentiators generally resulted in a recovery from the reduction in survival time and from the increase of metastatic nodules on the lungs. From these results, it seems reasonable to conclude that immunological unresponsiveness is one of the major factors enhancing tumor growth in relation to operative stress.

REFERENCES

Buinauska, P., McDonald, G. O., and Cole, W. H. (1958). *Ann. Surg.* 148, 642-648.
Cochran, A. J., Spilg, W. G. S., Mackie, R. M., and Thomas, C. E. (1972). *Br. Med. J. 4*, 67-70.
Cooper, A. J., Irvine, J. M., and Turnbull, A. R. (1974). *Immunology 27*, 393-400.
Fisher, E. R., and Fisher, B. (1959). *Cancer (Philadelphia) 12*, 926-932.
Greene, H. S. N. (1950). *Yale J. Biol. Med. 22*, 611-620.
Hattori, T., Hamai, Y., and Ishii, T. (1975). *Jpn. J. Surg. 5*, 211-221.
Hattori, T., Niimoto, M., Yamagata, S., and Toge, T. (1976). *Gann 67*, 105-110.
Hattori, T., Hamai, Y., Harada, T., Ikeda, H., and Ikeda, T. (1977a) *Jpn. J. Surg. 7*, 258-262.
Hattori, T., Hamai, Y., Harada, T., Ikeda, H., and Ikeda, T. (1977b) *Jpn. J. Surg. 7*, 263-268.
Hattori, T., Hamai, Y., Ikeda, H., Harada, T., and Ikeda, T. (1978). *Gann 69*, 401-406.
Hattori, T., Hamai, Y., Takiyama, W., Hirai, T., and Ikeda, T. (1980). *Gann 71*, 280-284.
Hattori, T., Hamai, Y., Ikeda, T., Takiyama, W., Hirai, T., and Miyoshi, Y. (1982a). *Gann 73*, 132-135.
Hattori, T., Hamai, Y., Ikeda, T., Takiyama, W., Hirai, T., and Miyoshi, Y. (1982b). *Jpn. J. Surg. 12*, 143-147.
Jonescu, P. (1931). *Z. Krebsforsch. 33*, 264-280.
Kaplan, H. S., and Murphy, E. D. (1949). *J. Natl. Cancer Inst. (US) 9*, 407-413
Knox, L. C. (1922). *Ann. Surg. 75*, 129-142.

Krebs, C. (1929). *Acta Radiol. 8 (Suppl.),* 1-133.
Lewis, M. R., and Cole, W. H. (1958). *Arch. Surg. (Chicago) 77,* 621-629.
Lucke, B., and Schlumberger, H. (1949). *J. Exp. Med. 89,* 269-278.
Marsh, M. C. (1927). *Cancer Res. 11,* 101-107.
Munster, A. M. (1976). *Lancet I,* 1329.
Olivotto, M., and Bomford, R. (1974). *Int. J. Cancer 13,* 478-488.
Schatten, W. E. (1958). *Cancer (Philadelphia) 11,* 455-468.
Toge, T., and Hattori, T. (1979a). *Hiroshima J. Med. Sci. 23,* 95-101.
Toge, T., Ikeda, H., Senou, N., Niimoto, M., and Hattori, T. (1976). *Jpn. J. Surg. 6,* 157-163.
Toge, T., Yamada, Y., Ikeda, H., Niimoto, M., and Hattori, T. (1979b). *Gann 70,* 699-703.
Vose, B. M., and Moudgil, G. C. (1976). *Immunology 30,* 123-128.

DISCUSSION

LIOTTA: What is the role of anesthesia and lung atelectasis in the enhancement of lung metastasis following thoracotomy?

HATTORI: (1) Controls received anesthesia and respiratory support. (2) Atelectasis does not play a role, because thoracotomy was done on one side but the effect on metastases was seen in both right and left lungs.

GOLUB: Comment: Dr. Jack Smith and I studied this phenomenon in both cancer patients and cardiac surgery patients. We saw transient (24-48 hr) depression of T cell function. Similar to your findings, this was dependent on type of operation, with thoracotomy being the most suppressive. This phenomenon, which has been developed in a remarkably complete model by Dr. Hattori, deserves serious study and consideration in therapeutic trials.

HOSHINO: Comment: One of my colleagues, Dr. Uchida in Wien, discovered NK-suppressive macrophages or monocytes in blood of surgically operated patients with breast cancer. Because your data on macrophage and NK activity showed depression after the operation, NK-suppressive macrophages might be important as the cause of your data.

KNODO: Generally speaking, blood coagulation is activated after the operation, and as a result fibrinolysis occurs. The more important thing is that complement level decreases after the operation, and the correlation between coagulation and complement should be taken into account for the defense mechanism.

COCHRAN: In a previous study, we (Cochran *et al.*, 1972) found
that postoperative immune suppression lasted longer than
the period of elevation of circulating steroids. Did you
examine the thymus glands of your thoracotomy patients
relative to the changes in the laparotomy group? Does
thoracotomy damage the blood supply to the thymus in humans or animals?

HATTORI: On examination of thymus, the answer is no. In regard to
corticosteroids, examinations are now going on. We made
"rats without adrenal glands," that is, rats were bilat-
erally adrenalectomized and replaced with appropriate
doses of hydrocortisone. Then, experiments on operative
stress and tumor growth were performed, comparing rats
with and without adrenal glands. Interim results suggest
that enhancing effects of thoracotomy on tumor growth were
not observed in rats without adrenal glands.

KONDO: Have you measured corticosteroid levels in serum or excreted into urine during the experiment?

HATTORI: No.

TORISU: Have you measured some kind of skin tests before and
after operation of each group, because skin tests are
easy to measure immunopotencies of the rat?

HATTORI: Yes, we have tried delayed hypersensitivity tests against
SRBC using radioisotopic ear assay method, but the results
were not very clear to indicate the differences between
laparotomy and thoracotomy groups.

WEISS: What happens to blood coagulation after thoracotomy and/or
laparotomy? Does this affect metastasis?

HATTORI: Changes of blood coagulation and fibrinolysis after operation are very complicated, and activated and depressed
phases appear in confusion according to the time after the
operation. But usually these changes are not that big
and we have experienced no troubles with blood coagulation
or lysis after major abdominal surgery. Theoretically, the
hyperlysis phase may enhance the metastases.

PART IIA

Regulations of Metastatic Tumor Cells

Chairpersons

George Poste
Kokichi Kikuchi

CHAPTER 5

TUMOR CELL HETEROGENEITY
AND THE PATHOGENESIS OF CANCER METASTASIS

George Poste

Smith Kline and French Laboratories
Philadelphia, Pennsylvania

and

Department of Pathology and Laboratory Medicine
University of Pennsylvania Medical School
Philadelphia, Pennsylvania

BASIC MECHANISMS AND CLINICAL TREATMENT
OF TUMOR METASTASIS

I. INTRODUCTION

   Despite its overwhelming clinical importance, it is only within the last few years that the problem of cancer metastasis has
attracted the level of intense research interest accorded other
topics in cancer research such as viral and chemical carcinogenesis
and tumor immunology. This stems in part from the technical problems involved in studying this complex phenomenon. However, advances in our understanding of the pathogenesis of metastasis and the
emergence of new experimental methods for studying malignant cells
in vivo and *in vitro* have led to a renaissance of interest in this
important disease. Of crucial importance has been the discovery
that tumor cells within a malignant tumor cell do not have identical metastatic properties but differ markedly in their metastatic
capabilities (see reviews in Poste and Fidler, 1980; Poste, 1982a).
This finding has supplanted the long-held view that if a tumor was
malignant, then any tumor cell from within the tumor was capable of
generating a metastasis. The demonstration that malignant tumors
contain phenotypically heterogeneous subpopulations of tumor cells
with differing metastatic properties, including cells that lack
metastatic ability, has major implications for both experimental
attempts to identify properties unique to metastatic cells and
also for the clinical treatment of metastases (see reviews in Nicolson and Poste, 1982; Poste, 1982a; Poste and Greig, 1982).
   This article presents a brief survey of advances in our knowledge of the extent of cellular heterogeneity within malignant tumors and how such cellular diversity might arise and be regulated
at different stages in the growth of a tumor.

II. THE CELLULAR DIVERSITY OF MALIGNANT TUMORS

   The cellular heterogeneity of neoplasms has been known since
the last century, when histologic studies first identified morphologic differences among cells within the same tumor. Since then
the use of increasingly sophisticated methods has revealed significant heterogeneity in the expression of myriad phenotypic properties by tumor cells in both primary and metastatic lesions in the
same host. These include differences in karyotype, antigenicity,
immunogenicity, biochemical properties, growth behavior, susceptibility to destruction by chemotherapeutic drugs, radiation, and

hyperthermia, and ability to escape recognition and destruction by humoral and/or cell-mediated immune reactions mounted by the host (see reviews in Heppner, 1979; Hart and Fidler, 1981; Fidler and Hart, 1982; Fidler and White, 1982; Fidler and Poste, 1982; Nicolson and Poste, 1982).

A. Animal Tumors

Definitive evidence for the coexistence of clonal cell sub-populations with different metastatic properties within the same tumor was obtained in 1977 by Fidler and Kripke. They showed that clones isolated from the same B16 murine melanoma differed markedly in their ability to form metastases when reinjected into syngeneic C57BL/6 mice. The relevance of these observations to malignant tumors in general was viewed initially with considerable caution, because the B16 melanoma had been maintained since 1954 under diverse *in vitro* and *in vivo* cultivation conditions and its cellular heterogeneity might thus have represented an artifact of its "antiquity." This has proved not to be the case. Comparable extensive clonal heterogeneity has been demonstrated recently by Fidler *et al.* (1981) in another mouse melanoma (K1735) of much more recent origin. In this study, clones were isolated immediately after the tumor was first detected on the skin of a C3H mouse that had been exposed over a 2-year period to UV irradiation and skin painting with croton oil.

Metastatic heterogeneity is not a peculiarity of clonal sub-populations in either melanomas or murine tumors. Similar metastatic heterogeneity has now been described in clones isolated from solid tumors of diverse histologic origin from the mouse, rat, hamster, and chicken (see reviews in Poste and Fidler, 1980; Fidler and Hart, 1982; Poste, 1982a). Additional evidence of metastatic heterogeneity among tumor cells from the same tumor is also provided by experiments showing that cells isolated from individual metastases in the same host have different metastatic properties (Mantovani *et al.*, 1981; Poste *et al.*, 1982a,b; Talmadge and Fidler, 1982).

B. Human Tumors

Clonal heterogeneity is not limited to experimental animal tumors. Studies in my own laboratory have revealed similar metastatic heterogeneity in clones isolated from biopsy specimens of human malignant melanoma, colon carcinoma, breast carcinoma, and in cell lines established from human melanoma and squamous cell carcinoma specimens (G. Poste, N. Hanna, and I. J. Fidler, unpublished). Such studies were previously not possible because of the lack of experimental systems for assaying the *in vivo* behavior of human tumor cells. Transplantation into congenitally athymic nude mice has been used widely to assay the tumorigenic potential

of human cells. However, a consistent finding has been that in
the majority of reported examples the implanted human xenografts
grew but failed to metastasize, including tumor grafts taken directly from metastatic lesions. Similar results have also been
obtained with metastatic animal tumors implanted into nude mice.
However, Hanna (1980, 1982) has shown that the failure of tumors
to metastasize in nude mice is an age-dependent phenomenon. Tumors that are nonmetastatic in nude mice older than 10 weeks of
age will metastasize at a high frequency if inoculated into 3-
week-old animals (see review in Hanna, 1982).

C.   The Concept of the "Metastatic Phenotype"

     Metastases need not be caused by cells with the highest metas-
tatic potential. The basic tenet of the concept of metastatic
heterogeneity is that metastases are caused by cells endowed with
the "metastatic phenotype" and that tumor cells that lack this
phenotype are unable to generate metastases.
     Examination of the literature suggests that this simple con-
cept has apparently caused confusion in some quarters. For example, Mantovani and colleagues (Mantovani et al., 1981) have argued that if metastases are caused by special subpopulations of
metastatic cells, then cells recovered from metastases should
produce more metastases than the parental population, since the
latter would comprise both metastatic and nonmetastatic cells.
On finding that individual metastases from several rodent tumors
expressed a broad spectrum of metastatic behavior, with some producing fewer metastases than the parent line, some more and some
less, Mantovani et al. interpreted this as indicating that metastases do not arise from specific metastatic subpopulations.[1]
This argument completely misinterprets the concept of metastatic
heterogeneity. The data of Mantovani et al. do not refute this
concept. To the contrary, they provide additional experimental
evidence to support the view that malignant tumors are heterogeneous and contain subpopulations of cells with differing metastatic capacities. The results described by Mantivani et al. merely demonstrate that cell subpopulations with both high and low
metastatic properties coexist in tumors and each give rise to
metastases. This confirms the results first reported by Fidler
and Kripke in 1977 and subsequently by many others (see reviews
in Fidler and Hart, 1982; Poste, 1982a).
     In setting out to test the premise that cells from metastases
should produce more metastases than the parental cell population
from which they arose, Mantovani et al. have distorted the hypothesis of metastatic heterogeneity proposed by Fidler and Kripke,
which is eminently straightforward. It states that malignant
neoplasms are heterogeneous and contain metastatic and nonmetas-

---

[1]The same argument was made by L. Weiss at the present meeting.

tatic subpopulations of tumor cells, and that only the former can
give rise to metastases. This hypothesis argues that to produce
a metastasis, tumor cells must be endowed with properties that
suit them to complete all of the potentially destructive steps in
the metastatic process, and that tumor cells that lack these properties will not form metastases. Fidler's hypothesis does *not*
propose that metastases will always arise from subpopulations
with the *greatest* metastatic potential.

D. Influence of Parent Cell Population on Metastatic
    Potential of Tumor Cells

    The question whether tumor cells recovered from individual
metastases will produce more, fewer, or a similar number of metastases than the parent tumor cell population from which they were
derived will depend on the cellular composition of the parent cell
population. For example, if parent tumor cell populations are
used in which all cells, or a very large fraction of the cells,
have high metastatic capacities, then the probability of recover-
ing cells that produce more metastases than the parent population
will be lower than if the parent population contained relatively
few subpopulations with high metastatic abilities. The history
of the parent cell population and the selection pressures to which
it has been exposed will thus determine the frequency with which
cells having greater metastatic abilities than the parent population can be isolated from metastases.
    Experimental evidence illustrating this point has been obtained
in two studies (Poste *et al.*, 1982a; Talmadge and Fidler, 1982).
In experiments from my own laboratory, clonal analysis of a series
of uncloned B16 melanoma cell lines revealed that in a line with a
low metastatic capacity (B16-F1) only 30% of the clones tested
produced more metastases than the parent cell line. However, in
three cell lines that had been selected from the B16-F1 line
(B16-F10, B16-F1-BV8, and B16-F1-BL6) for high metastatic properties, 60-70% of the clones tested produced more metastases than
the original B16-F1 line. In a related series of experiments,
Talmadge and Fidler (1982) showed that cells recovered from lung
metastases arising from sc implants of the weakly metastatic
B16-F1 cell line produced 25-35 times more metastases than the
uncloned parent F1 cell line. In contrast, the metastatic proportion of clones isolated from metastases produced by sc implants
of the highly metastatic B16-F10 and B16-F1-BL6 cell lines did not
differ significantly from the parent cell lines. These data thus
demonstrate that when a weakly metastatic cell line is used as
starting material (e.g., B16-F1), the process of metastasis se-
lects for subpopulations that have well-developed metastatic abilities, even though they represent only a minor fraction of the
total parent cell population. However, the highly metastatic
B16-F10 and B16-F1-BL6 cell lines already contain a large fraction
of highly metastatic cells, and it is therefore difficult, if not

impossible, to select for cells that exhibit greater metastatic
abilities. Consequently, in starting with cell lines that are
already highly metastatic it is not entirely surprising that cells
with even greater metastatic proficiency cannot be easily detected.

E. Tumor Cell "Fitness" to Overcome Selection Barriers

     Metastatic competence can be viewed as the ability of a tumor
cell to complete each of the potentially destructive steps in the
metastatic process. Very few of the cells that are released from
the primary tumor (typically less than 1%) survive to form metastases (see review in Poste and Fidler, 1980). Each step in the
metastatic process represents a potent selection barrier. To
successfully metastasize a tumor cell must possess the appropriate
combination of properties (the metastatic phenotype) to overcome
all of these barriers. To pass each barrier, tumor cells presumably possess specific properties that are lacking in nonmetastatic
cells. Assuming, however, that only a threshold level of "phenotypic fitness" is needed to cross any particular barrier, expression of the necessary properties may vary in different cells,
ranging from extreme or exaggerated fitness to mere sufficiency.
The level of fitness exhibited by any particular tumor cell at
different steps in the metastatic process may also vary.
     Furthermore, at any time the competence of a tumor cell to
complete the various steps in metastasis could be modulated by
changes in cellular properties or tumor-host interactions. For
example, alterations in tumor cell nutrition and/or metabolism
created by proliferative and/or degenerative events taking place
in a solid tumor can modulate a variety of cell properties (see
Weiss, 1980). Phenotypic modulation of this kind could conceivably create a situation in which metastatic subpopulations undergo
transient phenotypic alterations that restrict or enhance their
metastatic competence. Weiss (1980) coined the term "transient
(metastatic) compartments" to describe such events. Metastatic
subpopulations might thus enter and exit such "compartments" many
times depending on the microenvironmental conditions that exist
within a particular focus of tumor cells. The use of the term
compartment does not refer to a single anatomic location within a
tumor but refers instead to space-time zones within a tumor (primary or metastatic tumor) that may differ in their impact on specific metastatic subpopulations.
     Conversely, changes in the nature or the intensity of the se-
lection pressure(s) acting at one or more steps in the metastatic
process could modify metastatic competence in the absence of any
change in cellular properties. For example, therapy introduces
an entirely new selection pressure, and fluctuations in the various
humoral and cell-mediated host defense reactions will presumably
reduce or increase the height of certain selection barriers in
the metastatic sequence.

F. Random and Nonrandom Aspects of the Metastatic
    Process

In emphasizing that metastasis appears to be a nonrandom process in which only certain subpopulations of tumor cells complete
all of the steps in the metastatic process, it is important to
stress that random (chance) events will continue to play a role.
Subpopulations of tumor cells endowed with metastatic properties
will be at constant risk throughout the metastatic process of
perishing because of random events. For example, it is easy to
envisage a situation in which a metastatic cell in transit in the
circulation could easily be killed as a result of a random col-
lision with a blood cell or the vessel wall, yet in a different
situation in time and space it might survive to complete the
metastatic process and generate a metastatic tumor.
    The purpose of using the term "nonrandom" to describe the
metastatic process is prompted by the need to make a clear dis-
tinction from the traditional interpretation of metastasis as a
"random" process in which all the cells in a malignant tumor were
believed to be endowed with metastatic potential, and thus any
cell at random could form a metastasis at a distant tissue site.

G. Subpopulation Diversity in Heterogeneous Tumors

The exact number of phenotypically distinct subpopulations
present in different types of malignant tumors is not known. The
number is probably very high. It is probably also dynamic, with
the number and nature of the subpopulations changing during progressive growth of the tumor as different selection pressures act
on the constituent subpopulations.
    Tumor cell subpopulations that express metastatic capacity and
subpopulations that are tumorigenic but noninvasive may merely
represent the two extremes of a broad spectrum of subpopulation
diversity in heterogeneous tumors. The presence of tumor cell subpopulations that are invasive but are nonmetastatic has already
been demonstrated (Poste et al., 1980). The possibility must
therefore be considered that additional subpopulations exist that
can complete many, but not all, steps in the metastatic process.
For example, subpopulations may exist that can invade and enter
the blood but are not "fit" to survive their journey in the circulation. Other invasive subpopulations might survive transit in
the circulation but do not possess the properties needed for
efficient arrest in the microcirculation. Consequently, a minimum
number of subpopulations can probably be defined in terms of competence to complete each successive stage in the metastatic process
(see Poste, 1982a). However, this is a minimum value. Coexisting
with such subpopulations would be an unknown number of metastatic
subpopulations of increasing aggressiveness that produce increasing
levels of metastatic disease. At the other extreme, the tumori-

genic but noninvasive phenotype may also represent a graded spectrum of phenotypic progression toward the eventual acquisition of
invasive potential.

In addition to the coexistence of cell subpopulations with
different metastatic capabilities within the same tumor, these,
in turn, can be subdivided further on the basis of their diversity
for other phenotypic characteristics (e.g., antigens, karyotypic
changes, enzyme alterations). Of particular importance from a
clinical standpoint is that individual tumor cell subpopulations
with different metastatic properties also differ significantly in
their susceptibility to killing by host defense mechanisms and the
various therapeutic modalities currently employed in cancer therapy (see reviews in Fidler and Poste, 1982; Fidler and White, 1982).

Malignant tumors in advanced progression may thus represent an
extraordinary mosaic of diverse cellular subpopulations that display almost limitless patterns of phenotypic variation.

The major challenge now facing cancer research is how best to
approach the formidable experimental problem of analyzing tumor
cell subpopulations of defined metastatic potential to identify
the panel of phenotypic changes that confer metastatic competence.
As discussed in detail elsewhere (Nicolson and Poste, 1982; Poste,
1982a), the technical demands of this task are considerable. Characterization of the metastatic phenotype requires that a distinc-
tion be made between cellular changes that are obligatory for
metastatic behavior and cellular alterations that are not obligatory for metastatic behavior but that may confer significant
adaptive advantage. These would include changes that would facilitate cell survival in the face of adverse environmental factors
(e.g., limited nutrients, pH extremes, anoxia) and changes that
might predispose tumor cells to the development of changes in obligatory metastatic properties (e.g., genetic alterations, defect-
ive DNA polymerase activity, altered DNA methylation or DNA re-
pair).

These issues, and other aspects of the experimental analysis
of the metastatic phenotype, are discussed in detail in Poste
(1982a).

III. EVOLUTION OF TUMOR CELL HETEROGENEITY
     IN MALIGNANT TUMORS AND REGULATION
     OF METASTATIC TUMOR CELL SUBPOPULATIONS

Cellular diversity could arise in tumors by two nonexclusive
mechanisms. For tumors of multicellular origin, diversity would
be present from the outset. However, even in these tumors, and
certainly for tumors of unicellular origin (this is believed to be
the mode of origin of most human tumors), the available evidence
suggests that additional diversity is generated by the emergence
of cell variants during progressive tumor growth.

A. Generation of Cell Variants

Nowell (1976), elaborating on the concept advanced earlier by
Foulds (1956), proposed that generation of cell variants is an inevitable and fundamental feature of progressive tumor growth. He
proposes that tumor progression occurs via a series of multiple
yet independent changes in many different cellular properties, resulting in rapid generation of clonal subpopulations with widely
differing phenotypes. This diversity is amplified by the fact
that tumor progression toward autonomy from host control may pro-
ceed simultaneously along many pathways and need not follow a set
"program" of inevitable phenotypic progression.
    At any time during progression, the number of subpopulations
present in a tumor, and the extent of their phenotypic diversity,
will reflect the selection pressures encountered during the life-
time of the tumor. Selection pressures can be natural (e.g., assault by host defense mechanisms, limiting nutritional conditions)
or applied (e.g., therapy). Even though the kinetics for the generation of cell variants may vary in tumors of differing histologic
origin, as well as in tumors of common histologic origin in different patients, the probability is high that by the time of initial clinical presentation most tumors will exhibit extensive cellular heterogeneity for a wide range of phenotypes.

B. Genetic Instability

Nowell's concept of tumor progression also proposes that as
successive clonal subpopulations emerge they will display increasing genetic instability. This, coupled with the selection
pressures imposed by host defense and/or therapy, will favor relentless emergence of new subpopulations with enhanced metastatic
capacities.
    The relationship between genetic instability and metastatic
ability has been studied by Cifone and Fidler (1981) using clones
with low and high metastatic potential isolated from three murine
tumors: the UV2237 fibrosarcoma; the SF19 fibrosarcoma; and the
Kl735 melanoma. In all cases the rate of spontaneous cellular
mutation to acquire resistance to ouabain or thioguanine was found
to be significantly higher (five to seven times) in the highly
metastatic clones.

C. Interaction of Different Tumor Cell
    Subpopulations

Given the role of tumor progression as a mechanism for generating cellular diversity within tumors, and the apparent increasing genetic instability of the new variants generated by this process, how is it that the metastatic properties of uncloned, polyclonal tumor cell lines can remain so constant? For example, the

murine B16 melanoma cell lines, B16-F1 (low metastatic ability)
and B16-F10 (high metastatic ability) isolated originally by
Fidler (1973) have maintained their relative metastatic capacities
during 8 years of serial passaging *in vitro* and also after long
periods of *in vivo* transfer (see Poste *et al.*, 1980, 1981). What
has prevented these differences from being obliterated by the generation of new variants with different metastatic properties? One
reason may be that tumor cells within a polyclonal population do
not behave as autonomous units but are affected by the presence of
other tumor cells. Support for this concept has been obtained in
studies from my own laboratory that show that different subpopulations of B16 melanoma cells isolated from the B16-F1 and B16-F10
cell lines can affect each other's behavior and influence the stability of the metastatic phenotype in individual subpopulations
(Poste et al., 1981).

Studies on individual clones isolated from the heterogeneous,
polyclonal B16-F1 and B16-F10 lines revealed that their metastatic
phenotypes were highly unstable during serial passage *in vitro* and
in vivo, and variant subclones with diverse metastatic phenotypes
emerged quickly (Poste *et al.*, 1981). In contrast, the metastatic
properties of the uncloned parent cell lines were stable when exposed to the same culture conditions. "Destabilization" of the
metastatic phenotype in individual clones did not occur, however,
when replicate populations of the same clones were cocultivated
together. The stability of the metastatic phenotype in individual
clones during this experiment was verified by using clones bearing
stable, drug-resistant markers and by showing that subclones exhibiting resistance to particular drugs had identical metastatic
phenotypes to the original clones with the same drug resistance
phenotype (Poste *et al.*, 1981).

The role of clonal interactions in regulating the stability of
the metastatic phenotype is not unique to melanomas. Similar instability of the metastatic phenotype has been identified in clones
of the mouse UV2237 fibrosarcoma (Cifone and Fidler, 1981), mouse
RAW 117 lymphosarcoma, 13762 mammary adenocarcinoma (Nicolson,
1982), and the rat 1AR6 hepatocarcinoma (Talmadge and Fidler,
1982).

The "stabilizing" effect is not produced by mixing clones from
tumors of different histologic origin. Single clones of B16 melanoma cocultivated with clones from the Lewis lung carcinoma or
UV2237 fibrosarcoma show marked phenotypic instability and rapidly
generate subclones with widely differing metastatic properties
(Poste *et al.*, 1981). Similarly, non-neoplastic cells from syngeneic C57BL/6 mice cannot "quench" the metastatic instability of
B16 melanoma clones grown in isolation (Poste, 1982a).

However, clones isolated from tumors of similar histologic
origin arising in different hosts can interact to stabilize their
metastatic properties, although the responsiveness of individual
clones in these heterologous interactions are more variable than
between clones isolated from the same tumor. For example, single
clones from the B16 melanoma that exhibit unstable metastatic

phenotypes when cultivated as single clones exhibit stable metastatic phenotypes when cocultivated with a series of clones from
the mouse K1735 melanoma (and vice versa), even though these tumors arose in different mouse strains (B16 in C57BL6/N mice and
K1735 in C3H/HeN mice). However, clones have been identified that
are unresponsive to regulation by clones from the heterologous tumor. These clones do, however, show stable metastatic phenotypes
when cocultivated with clones from their homologous tumor (G.
Poste, unpublished).

The proportion of clonal subpopulations that display unstable
metastatic phenotypes when deprived of interactions with other
clonal subpopulations may vary, however, in different tumors. As
shown in Table I, virtually all of the B16 melanoma clones examined to date exhibit unstable metastatic properties when grown as
single clones but not when cocultivated with other B16 clones. In
contrast, several clones isolated from the UV2237 fibrosarcoma cell
line exhibit stable metastatic phenotypes when grown in isolation
and thus do not appear to require clonal interactions to maintain
a stable metastatic phenotype.

As described later, maintenance of polyclonal tumor cell populations *in vitro* or *in vivo* can alter the fraction of "unstable"
clones in the overall population. More important, however, it has
been shown that the instability of metastatic properties in clones
deprived of polyclonal interactions is not limited to "antique"
cell lines that have been serially passaged *in vitro* or *in vivo*
for considerable periods. The same phenomenon has been identified
in clones isolated from newly induced tumors and subjected to a
minimum period of cultivation before assay of their metastatic
properties. As shown in Table I, clones isolated from several
UV-induced fibrosarcomas and methylcholanthrene-induced tumors
that were excised within 3 months of their initial detection each
contained a small fraction of clones with unstable metastatic properties. The fraction of unstable clones in these populations increased during further passage in culture and serial transplantation in syngeneic mice (Table I). Of more interest, however, is
the finding that the proportion of unstable clones is significantly
higher in cell populations harvested from tumors that had been allowed to reach an advanced stage of progression before excision
(Table I). This indicates that unstable clones evolve *in situ* and
that the proportion of such clones increases with tumor progression. As in the case of clones isolated from "early" tumors, serial passage of cells from "advanced" tumors increases the fraction of unstable clones in the population. The term "unstable
clone(s)" as used here refers to the expression of unstable metastatic properties in clones maintained in the absence of other
clones and does not mean that similar instability will occur when
the clone was growing within the heterogeneous, polyclonal tumor
mass *in situ* or when mixed with other clones during serial transfer
in vitro or *in vivo*. A few examples have been identified, however,
of clones isolated from "advanced" tumors that display unstable

TABLE I

Incidence of Unstable Metastatic Phenotypes in Tumor Cell Clones
Isolated from Tumors of Different Ages and from Tumor Cell Lines

Sample	Number of passages[a]		Number of unstable clones/total clones tested[b]
	In vitro	In vivo	
B16 melanoma	>40	–	104/114
K1735 melanoma	>40	–	32/36
UV2237 fibrosarcoma	>40	–	21/39
UV2237-HPM fibrosarcoma[c]	>40	8	16/18
UV6487-3/12 fibrosarcoma[d]	3	–	2/14
UV6487-HPC fibrosarcoma[e]	>20	–	11/20
UV6487-HPM fibrosarcoma[c]	5	8	18/19
UV5175-6/12 fibrosarcoma[d]	4	–	16/23
UV5175-HPC fibrosarcoma[e]	>20	–	18/20
MC 118-3/12 fibrosarcoma[d]	3	–	3/14
MC 118-HPC fibrosarcoma[e]	>20	–	10/17
MC 224-5/12 fibrosarcoma[d]	4	–	15/18
MC 224-HPC fibrosarcoma[e]	>20	–	10/16

^{a}The indicated cell populations were serially passaged *in vitro* or *in vivo* for the number of transfers shown. The subcultivation intervals for the melanoma and fibrosarcoma lines were 5 and 7 days, respectively. For serial passage *in vivo*, single-cell suspensions (1×10^6 cells) were injected sc into the flanks of syngeneic mice and nodules excised on reaching a size of 2 cm or greater.

^{b}Clones were classified as exhibiting an unstable metastatic phenotype if they yielded subclones with significantly different metastatic properties within 10 serial subcultivations after cloning. Clones were isolated at the end of the indicated period of serial passaging *in vitro* and/or *in vivo*.

^{c}HPM, high passage in the mouse. The suffix HPM represents the tumor cell population isolated from the indicated tumor after serial passage in syngeneic mice after a minimum of eight transfers.

^{d}The designations 3/12, 5/12, and 6/12 refer to the number of months between initial macroscopic detection of the indicated tumor and its subsequent excision for preparation of cell cultures.

^{e}The suffix HPC represents the same tumor cell population shown on the preceding line after passage *in vitro* for a minimum of 20 subcultivations.

metastatic properties and generate variants with altered metastatic properties even when maintained in a polyclonal population
(G. Poste, unpublished).

Collectively, the experiments described in the preceding para-
graphs suggest that the stability of the metastatic phenotype in
clonal tumor cell subpopulations and the rate at which they give
rise to new cell variants with altered metastatic properties is
influenced by interactions between the different subpopulations.
In polyclonal populations that contain multiple clonal subpopulations of cells, the rate of formation of metastatic variants is
significantly lower than when the constituent subpopulations exist
in isolation and fail to interact with other subpopulations.

Further evidence to support the role of subpopulation diversity
in regulating the stability of the metastatic phenotype has come
from studies in which B16 melanoma clonal subpopulations bearing
specific drug resistance markers were cocultivated with a series of
wild-type B16 melanoma clones and treated with different drugs to
restrict subpopulation diversity by killing wild-type clones and
clones carrying the inappropriate resistance marker. Following
drug-induced elimination of the majority of clones, the surviving
one or two clones generated variants with altered metastatic properties at a very high frequency (10^{-3}-10^{-4} per cell per generation) (Poste et al., 1981). With time, the formation of new cell
variants recreated substantial subpopulation diversity, and the
rate of variant formation returned to a low level ($>1 \times 10^{-6}$ per
cell per generation) and remained at this low level until another
selection pressure was imposed to restrict subpopulation diversity
and the cycle began again.

The mechanism(s) by which clonal subpopulations interact to
regulate each other's behavior is not known. As discussed at this
meeting by Gloria Heppner (Chapter 1, this volume), a complex combination of soluble factors released by the cells, cell-to-cell
contact, and factors contributed by host cells appears to be involved, with different subpopulations exhibiting different responses
to regulation by each mechanism.

The precise extent of subpopulation diversity needed to "stabilize" the metastatic phenotype is not known. In vitro experiments using B16 clones indicate that the exact number varies from
clone to clone (G. Poste, unpublished). In addition, it may well
vary in different tumors and also at different stages in progression of the same tumor. The time at which sufficient subpopulation heterogeneity is created within a polyclonal population to
limit the rate of formation of new metastatic variants has been
referred to as T_{pt} (pt = plateau). In previous publications from
this laboratory (Poste, 1982a; Poste and Greig, 1982), the term
T_{eq} (eq = equilibrium) had been used for this time point. The
term equilibrium is misleading, however, since it implies that an
equilibrium state is reached in which the rate of formation of new
cell variants is matched by the demise of a similar number of subpopulations. No experimental evidence is available to suggest that
this is occurring. Rather, on achieving a given level of subpop-

ulation heterogeneity it appears that the rate of formation of new variants slows dramatically to establish a plateau (T_{pt}) relative to the preceding phase of rapid formation of new variants.

The phenomenon of rapid destabilization of the metastatic phenotype may also be occurring in vivo (Poste et al., 1982b). Isolation of multiple clones from individual lung metastases produced by the B16 melanoma has revealed that in "early" metastases excised after 6-25 days, clones isolated from the same metastasis typically show indistinguishable metastatic properties (i.e., intralesional clonal homogeneity). This situation was found in approximately 80% of the early metastases tested, although the metastatic phenotypes of clones isolated from different metastases in the same animal do differ significantly (i.e., interlesional clonal heterogeneity). In contrast, in "late" metastases excised after 40-45 days, intralesional clonal homogeneity was found in only 20-30% of metastases; the majority of the remaining metastases yielded two or more clonal subpopulations with differing metastatic properties (i.e., intralesional heterogeneity). These data suggest that B16 melanoma metastases are populated initially by cells with a uniform metastatic phenotype. This is in agreement with data showing that the majority of experimental metastases result from the arrest and proliferation of a single tumor cell (Poste et al., 1982a). This in vivo situation is therefore analogous to the in vitro experiments described earlier in which individual B16 clones grown in isolation from other clones quickly generated variant subclones with altered metastatic properties (Poste et al., 1981).

Although these observations are the first to document an interaction between tumor cell subpopulations affecting metastatic behavior, work by Heppner and colleagues has shown that cellular subpopulations isolated from the same mammary tumor exert growth-regulatory restraints on each other (Miller et al., 1980). The interaction pattern is complex, however, with different patterns of uni- and bidirectional response occurring between different subpopulations. The same subpopulations also exhibit equally complex interactions affecting immunogenicity and sensitivity to cytotoxic drugs (Miller et al., 1980). Similarly, nontumorigenic clones of B16 melanoma have been reported to suppress the tumorigenicity of other B16 clones when mixed together before implantation into mice (Newcomb et al., 1978). The mechanism(s) underlying these fascinating events is not known. The numerous reports showing that the presence of the primary tumor can restrict the growth of metastases in certain tumors might also represent an analogous phenomenon (see review in Sugarbaker, 1979).

Irrespective of the mechanism involved, identification of these interactions between different subpopulations from the same tumor suggests that a full understanding of the role of tumor cell heterogeneity in determining the behavior of tumors and in predicting their response to therapy cannot be achieved by simple analysis of the individual component subpopulations but will require more sophisticated analyses of subpopulation interactions.

Such interactions among different subpopulations also argue against anarchic progression of tumors (Fidler and Hart, 1982). The apparent role of subpopulation diversity in regulating the rate at which new variant subpopulations of cells appear may provide a mechanism whereby tumors can sustain extensive cellular diversity in the face of fluctuations in the variability of different subpopulations caused by destructive selection pressures acting on the tumor. Such a mechanism would have two important advantages.

On the one hand, the ability to generate rapidly new subpopulations of tumor cells with novel phenotypes under conditions where subpopulation diversity is restricted would ensure that the tumor will not be at risk of becoming dominated by a small number of subpopulations or even a single subpopulation. This has the advantage for the tumor that it reduces the likelihood that a destructive assault mounted against the tumor by host defense mechanisms or by the oncologist would be successful in eliminating all of the subpopulations present. On the other hand, the apparent stimulation of subpopulation diversification caused by events that reduce subpopulation diversity would provide a potentially potent mechanism for the relentless generation of new variants when the tumor is exposed to an assault that destroys a significant fraction of the subpopulations present. This concept will be discussed later in the context of the possible effect of therapeutic assaults on the dynamics of tumor cell subpopulations.

In addition to ensuring the rapid recovery of cellular diversity in tumors exposed to potent destructive selection pressures, the same mechanism could also serve to prevent "domination" of the tumor by a single subpopulation of tumor cells. For example, if a subpopulation were to emerge during tumor growth whose "fitness" enabled it to proliferate at the expense of other subpopulations, the tumor would eventually become clonally homogeneous and thus be at risk to destruction by any assault(s) that was effective against the particular subpopulation. However, in gaining dominance, a "superfit" subpopulation would restrict subpopulation diversity and might thus immediately stimulate the generation of new variants. Dominance of an individual subpopulation(s) would thus be expected to be temporary, and the tumor would quickly become heterogeneous again. If this is so, then tumors may have a "self-correcting" mechanism to counter the risk of dominance of the population by tumor cells of limited phenotypic diversity.

Stimulation of the rate of formation of tumor cell variants by restriction of subpopulation diversity may also provide an explanation for the rapid evolution of cellular diversity within individual metastases mentioned earlier (Poste et al., 1982b). Diversification of the cellular phenotypes present in a metastasis formed by the arrest and proliferation of a single tumor cell could occur by two mechanisms. The first would be if the cell involved was intrinsically unstable and had been generating new variants at a high frequency even while in the primary tumor. The alternative possibility is that transport of a single tumor cell from a heterogeneous polyclonal primary tumor to a distant organ where it now exists in isolation from other clonal subpopulations could destabilize phenotypic regulation. In the primary tumor, interactions between the heterogeneous constituent subpopulations act to impose relative phenotypic stability and restrict the rate of formation of new variants. However, as a single cell in a newly established metastasis, these interactions would be absent. This would thus stimulate the rate of formation of new tumor cell variants, quickly covering the initially clonally homogeneous metastasis to a clonally heterogeneous lesion. The composition of the tumor cell embolus from which a metastasis arises might therefore be important in determining its subsequent cellular composition (see Poste, 1982a).

Neither the nature nor the intensity of the selection pressures operating in any two hosts bearing tumors of similar histologic origin will be identical. Consequently, the panel of tumor cell subpopulations present in any two experimental animal hosts inoculated with the same tumor, or two cancer patients with ostensibly the same type of tumor, will inevitably be different.

Tumors of the same histologic type tend to follow a relatively predictable and reproducible pattern of clinical progression in most hosts. Indeed, much of the clinical practice of oncology is based on these precepts. Knowledge of the different, yet relatively constant, behavioral patterns exhibited by human malignancies of defined histologic type is used in the diagnosis, clinical staging, and prognosis of disease. This constancy suggests that the selection pressures operating against tumors of similar histologic origin at equivalent body sites in different hosts are of a relatively similar nature and intensity. If so, this would mean that the tumor cell subpopulations present in such tumors should not be overwhelmingly different in different patients at comparable stages in disease progression. As emphasized, subtle qualitative and quantitative differences in the selection pressures in different hosts will produce inevitable phenotypic variation in the tumor cell subpopulations present in any two hosts. However, notwithstanding differences that could arise at any time because of random generation of variant tumor cells with extremely different phenotypes, similarities appear to outweigh dissimilarities with regard to the nature of the selective environment that will drive the evolution of tumor cell diversity in different patients. However, differences in the therapies administered to different patients may profoundly alter this situation.

D.   Influence of Timing in Emergence
     of Metastatic Subpopulations

In addition to our lack of knowledge of the range of selection pressures that can shape the cellular composition of a malignant tumor, we remain also completely ignorant about the fundamental question of when metastatic variants first make their appearance in a tumor. Are they present from the very early life of a tumor?

Are variant subpopulations with metastatic potential present in
certain tumors from the very outset of neoplastic conversion?
Once metastatic subpopulations are present do they have adaptive
advantage over nonmetastatic subpopulations, so that their contribution to the overall population will increase with progressive
growth of the tumor? Answers to these questions are lacking, and
they represent obvious topics for future research.

Differences in the time at which metastatic subpopulations
first emerge in primary tumors, and/or differences in the timing
with which they fully express their metastatic potential, may explain the relatively consistent differences in metastatic behavior
observed in human malignancies arising in different tissues. For
example, certain tumors carry a high risk of metastatic disease
developing very early in the growth of the primary lesion. In
small cell carcinoma of the ling, undifferentiated carcinoma of
the thyroid, and pancreatic carcinoma, widespread dissemination
has often occurred by the time of initial diagnosis (see review in
Sugarbaker, 1979). Similarly, multiorgan involvement is a characteristic feature of the so-called liquid cancers--the leukemias
and the lymphomas. In the most common solid epithelial tumors in
the United States (breast, lung, and colon), a statistical relationship has been defined between the risk of metastasis and increasing size of the primary tumor (see Sugarbaker, 1979). These
tumors are classified as having a "moderate" metastatic potential.
In contrast, at the least aggressive end of the metastatic spectrum, tumors such as basal cell carcinoma, lip carcinoma, desmoids,
and chondrosarcoma can attain huge sizes without metastasizing (see
Sugarbaker, 1979). Although of some general predictive value, this
classification is not absolute. Within any population of patients
with histologically similar tumors, individual cancers can be found
whose behavior falls at either end of the metastatic spectrum.

The factors responsible for these relatively consistent patterns of metastatic behavior are not known. In malignant neoplasms
that carry a high risk of early metastasis, metastatic subpopulations must presumably be present from very early in the life of the
primary tumor. In tumors of moderate metastatic potential, the increasing risk of metastasis accompanying progressive enlargement of
the primary tumor may reflect emergence of a larger number of increasingly aggressive metastatic subpopulations. In addition, the
dose of tumor cells released from many tumors is known to increase
with progressive enlargement (see Sugarbaker, 1979).

IV. CONCLUSIONS

Research done in many laboratories over the last few years has
provided important new insights into the cell biology of cancer
metastasis. Beginning with observations made in the late 1970s,
a large body of experimental evidence has been assembled showing

that malignant tumors contain multiple subpopulations of cells
with widely differing metastatic abilities, including subpopulations that lack this ability. These studies have shown that metastases are caused by specific subpopulations of tumor cells and
that not all cells in a tumor have this capacity. The demonstration of heterogeneity in the metastatic competence of different
cellular subpopulations coexisting in the same tumor has now focused attention on how such cellular diversity is generated, how
it is regulated, and how improved therapies could be devised to
circumvent the equally heterogeneous responses of different cellular subpopulations to the range of therapeutic modalities currently used in cancer treatment. Although research on these important questions is only just beginning, evidence is emerging
that suggests that the rate of formation of new subpopulations of
cells with novel phenotypes is influenced by interactions occurring between the constituent cell subpopulations that coexist
within tumors. These findings suggest that a tumor is more than
the sum of its parts and that experimental analysis of tumors
must address the question of how such interactions influence both
the properties displayed by individual subpopulations and the
behavior exhibited by the entire tumor.

These issues introduce a new level of technical complexity to
the task of identifying the cellular properties that are responsible for metastatic behavior (see reviews in Nicolson and Poste,
1982; Poste, 1982a). Detailed understanding of the factors involved in the evolution and control of cellular diversity within
malignant tumors is also crucial for the design of more effective
protocols for the treatment of metastatic disease. Successful
therapy of multiple metastases populated by tumor cells with differing responses to antineoplastic agents will require treatment
regimens that are able to circumvent such cellular heterogeneity.
In addition, the demonstration that the extent of subpopulation
heterogeneity within a neoplastic lesion can influence the rate
at which new subpopulations of cells with novel properties are
formed raises the disturbing question whether restriction of cellular diversity via therapeutic elimination of susceptible cellular subpopulations might stimulate the rate of formation of new
variant tumor cells from any surviving subpopulations (see reviews
in Fidler and Poste, 1982; Poste, 1982a; Poste and Greig, 1982).

ACKNOWLEDGMENT

The personal research cited in this article was supported by
USPHS Grants CA13393, 18260, and 30192 from the National Cancer
Institute.

REFERENCES

Cifone, M., and Fidler, I. J. (1981). *Proc. Natl. Acad. Sci. USA*
78, 6949-6952.
Fidler, I. J. (1973). *Nature (London) New Biol. 242*, 148-149.
Fidler, I. J., and Hart, I. R. (1982). *Science (Washington, D.C.)*
217, 998-1003.
Fidler, I. J., and Kripke, M. L. (1977). *Science (Washington,*
D.C.) 197, 893-895.
Fidler, I. J., and Poste, G. (1982). *In* "Tumor Cell Heterogeneity"
(A. H. Owens, D. S. Coffey, and S. B. Baylin, eds.), pp. 127-145.
Academic Press, New York.
Fidler, I. J., and White, R. J. (1982). "Design of Models for
Testing Cancer Therapeutic Agents." Van Nostrand, New York.
Fidler, I. J., Gruys, E., Cifone, M. A., Barnes, Z., and Bucana,
C. (1981). *J. Natl. Cancer Inst. (US) 67*, 947-956.
Foulds, L. (1956). *J. Natl. Cancer Inst. (US) 17*, 713-756.
Hanna, N. (1980). *Int. J. Cancer 26*, 675-680.
Hanna, N. (1982). *In* "Cancer Metastasis Reviews")I. J. Fidler,
ed.), Vol. 1, pp. 45-64. Nijhoff, Amsterdam.
Hart, I. R., and Fidler, I. J. (1981). *Biochim. Biophys. Acta*
651, 37-50.
Heppner, G. H. (1979). *In* "Commentaries on Research in Breast
Cancer" (R. D. Bulbrook and D. J. Taylor, eds.), pp. 177-191.
Liss, New York.
Mantovani, A., Giavazzi, R., Alessandri, G., Spreafico, F., and
Garattini, S. (1981). *Eur. J. Cancer 17*, 71-76.
Miller, B. E., Miller, F. R., Leith, J., and Heppner, G. H. (1980).
Cancer Res. 40, 3977-3981.
Newcomb, E. W., Silverstein, S. C., and Silagi, S. (1978). *J.*
Cell. Physiol. 95, 169-177.
Nicolson, G. L. (1982). *Biochim. Biophys. Acta,* in press.
Nicolson, G. L., and Poste, G. (1982). *Curr. Probl. Cancer 8*,
4-83.
Nowell, P. C. (1976). *Science (Washington, D.C.) 194*, 23-28.
Poste, G. (1982a). *In* "Cancer Metastasis Reviews" (I. J. Fidler,
ed.), Voo. 1, pp. 141-200. Nijhoff, Amsterdam.
Poste, G. (1982b). *In* "Tumor Invasion and Metastasis" (I. R. Hart
and L. Liotta, eds.), pp. 148-177. Nijhoff, Amsterdam.
Poste, G., and Fidler, I. J. (1980). *Nature (London) 283*, 139-146.
Poste, G., and Greig, R. (1982). *Invasion Metastasis 2*, 137-176.
Poste, G., Doll, J., Hart, I. R., and Fidler, I. J. (1980). *Cancer*
Res. 40, 1636-1644.
Poste, G., Doll, J., and Fidler, I. J. (1981). *Proc. Natl. Acad.*
Sci. USA 78, 6226-6230.
Poste, G., Doll, J., Brown, A. E., Tzeng, J., and Zeidman, I.
(1982a). *Cancer Res. 42*, 2770-2778.
Poste, G., Tzeng, J., Doll, J., Greig, R., Rieman, D., and Zeidman,
I. (1982b). *Proc. Natl. Acad. Sci. USA 79*, 6574-6578.
Sugarbaker, E. V. (1979). *Curr. Probl. Cancer 3*, 3-59.

Talmadge, J. E., and Fidler, I. J. (1982). *J. Natl. Cancer Inst. (US) 69*, 975-980.
Weiss, L. (1980). *In* "Pathology Annual" (H. Ioachim, ed.), Vol. 10, pp. 51-81. Raven, New York.

DISCUSSION

LIOTTA: Do you have evidence for soluble factors that mediate clonal interactions?

POSTE: Yes, we do in experiments employing cocultivation of media from cultured clones. These factors appear to be very labile.

KOBAYASHI: I wonder if you know any kind of antimutagenic substances (mutagen suppressors) that subsequently inhibit the rapid progression and subsequent heterogeneity of metastatic tumor?

POSTE: This is an interesting proposal. However, no research has been done to date that I am aware of.

GOLUB: What types of variants follow these rules? Are growth rate and other characteristics similar to drug resistance?

POSTE: We have studied instability of only one "metastatic" phenotype. It is clear from our experiment that the instability of the metastatic phenotype seen in our clones is not a generalized phenotypic stability, since the drug-resistance phenotypes of these clones remain stable under conditions where the metastatic phenotype is unstable.

HEPPNER: In regard to mechanisms of clonal interactions that limit diversification, you seem to imply that they occur locally within a tumor mass, rather than at a distance, say between a primary and its metastasis. Do you have any direct evidence for this?

POSTE: No, I did *not intend* to imply this. As you stated this morning, I think that both humoral and cell contact mechanisms may be operating. The primary tumor undoubtedly influences the growth of lung metastases in the B16 system used here. Removal of the primary tumor enhances the growth of metastases. However, the rate of emergence of intralesional clonal heterogeneity in lung

metastases is compensative, irrespective of whether
the primary tumor is amputated or allowed to remain in
place.

WEISS: How universal is the emergence of "metastatic pheno-
            types"? My colleagues and I found no difference in the
            metastatic capacities in mice of punch biopsies taken
            from heterogeneous B16 wild-type tumors of different
            ages. Could your observations be related to the anti-
            genicity/immunogenicity of the UV-induced tumors?

POSTE: The existence of clonal subpopulations with differen-
            tial metastatic properties has now been demonstrated in
            a variety of animal tumors of differing histologic ori-
            gin. Recently, the same phenomenon has been demonstra-
            ted in human melanoma and colon. My comments on the
            emergence of metastatic phenotypes in new UV-induced
            tumors referred to the "stability" of the metastatic
            phenotype rather than the emergence of specific sub-
            populations. Also, it is impossible to compare trans-
            planted B16 tumors of different ages with the situation
            of newly induced UV donors, since the former represent
            "antique" cell lines in which cell clones tend to (over
            100) show unstable metastatic phenotypes. In contrast,
            as shown in "early" UV-induced tumors, only very few
            clones exhibit unstable metastatic phenotypes.

CHAPTER 6

MOLECULAR MECHANISM OF ADHESIVENESS
AND DISSOCIATION OF CANCER CELLS

Hideo Hayashi
Yasuji Ishimaru
Ryuichi Hattori
Shinya Kurano

Department of Pathology
Kumamoto University Medical School
Kumamoto, Japan

I. INTRODUCTION

    Intercellular adhesion is of fundamental importance in the
physiology of multicellular organisms, but our knowledge of the
molecular mechanisms of this phenomenon is still limited. However,
evidence indicating that this phenomenon may be mediated by specific binding between cell surface-associated molecules in a re-
ceptor-ligand type of interaction has been accumulated. The first
successful demonstration of a specific adhesive substance was in
marine sponges (Humphreys, 1963). The substance was released from
sponge cells, which were dissociated mechanically in Ca^{2+}- and
Mg^{2+}-free seawater and then purified (Cauldwell et al., 1973; Henkart et al., 1973); it was a proteoglycan with a molecular weight
of 2×10^{6}. The tissue-specific adhesive component was separated
from conditioned medium of embryonic chick neural retina cells and
then purified (Lilien and Moscona, 1967; Lilien, 1968); it was a
glycoprotein with a molecular weight of approximately 50,000
(Hausman and Moscona, 1975). Cell-aggregating protein with tissue-specific effects has also been obtained from embryonic mouse
cerebrum, optic tectum, and spinal cord (Garber and Moscona, 1972;
Hausman et al., 1976), and embryonic chick liver (Kuroda, 1968).
    As is well known, histopathology of malignant tumor cells (of
epithelial cell origin) indicates that cells termed "differentiated
type" exhibit a tendency for cell-to-cell adhesion in varying degrees, while the cells termed "undifferentiated type" show a tendency to proliferate as single cells, indicating loss of cellular
recognition. Electron-microscopically, the adhesion of differentiated tumor cells is characterized by development of junctional
complexes to different extents and with different distributions.
Accordingly, it is of special importance to confirm whether any
adhesive substance(s) associated with cellular adhesion exists in
the differentiated tumor cells but not in the undifferentiated tumor cells. In other words, the presence of such adhesive sub-
stance(s) may be concerned in the problem of tumor cell differentiation.
    Rat ascites hepatoma cell lines, established by Yoshida and
associates, exhibited subpopulations of cells with different growth
capabilities, adhesive capacities, and antigenicities. Among the
strains, island-forming strains (called the differentiated type)
such as AH136B cells can be favorably utilized for separation of
the putative adhesive factor. We (Tasaki and Hayashi, 1969, 1971;
Kudo et al., 1974, 1976a,b; Kudo and Hayashi, 1976) have successful
ly separated a previously undescribed adhesive substance from the
tumor cells and purified it, as described later. In contrast, the
cells of rat ascites hepatoma AH109A strain (called the undifferentiated type) are present as single cells in vivo and lack the ability to synthesize the adhesive substance. The purpose of the present article is to define the scope of the biological significance
and biochemical properties of this adhesive substance.

II. ADHESIVENESS OF CANCER CELLS

AH136B cell islands were composed of approximately 30-40 cells; the cell island was usually round or oval, and individual cells showed close contact. The close contact in the apical portion of the cell islands was characterized by tight junctions, while that in the inner portion consisted of simple apposition, interdigitation of plasma membranes, intermediate junctions, and desmosomes. The mean number of tight junctions, desmosomes, and intermediate junctions in the cell islands, when counted for 150 nuclei in cross sections, was 100, 24, and 28, respectively (Ishihara et al., 1977).

A. Biochemical Characterization
    of Adhesive Factor Separated

On the basis of the observations just mentioned, separation of the adhesive factor, which is involved in the aggregation and adhesiveness of the hepatoma cells, was performed as reviewed by Hayashi and Ishimaru (1981). The active substance was released from AH136B cells, which were suspended in Hanks' balanced salt solution (free of Ca^{2+} and Mg^{2+}), gently pipetted, and then allowed to stand for 3 hr in the cold. The substance in the cell-free supernatant fluids was partially purified by chromatography with a DEAE-Sephadex and Bio-gel A-5m (Kudo et al., 1974) (Table I). This substance was noncytotoxic and clearly effective for aggregation of the rat ascites hepatoma cells mentioned earlier, but not liver cells and red blood cells from normal rats. Cell aggregation at a similar grading was induced by dissociated AG136b cells (5 × 10^5 cells/ml) or AH109A cells (1.5 × 10^6 cells/ml); aggregation became visible after 10 min of incubation with the substance at $37^{\circ}C$ (but not at $4^{\circ}C$).

The adhesive preparation noted previously was found to contain a considerable quantity of serum proteins (Kudo et al., 1976a). For removing the serum proteins, the adhesive preparation was eluted through an immunoadsorbent column coupled with anti-rat serum antibody (Table I) (Kudo et al., 1976a). As a result, the preparation was revealed to be a mixture of two types of adhesive factors with different antigenic determinants: One, which is clearly more potent for induction of cell aggregation, is not absorbed by the antibody, and the other, which is apparently less active, is absorbed by the antibody; these are called the unabsorbed factor and the absorbed factor, respectively.

In this connection, it was of interest that the serum from AH136B tumor-bearing rats became much more potent for induction of cell aggregation according to the duration after intraperitoneal inoculation of the cells. The increase in potency was found to be due to an increased quantity of the unabsorbed factor in the serum, indicating the release by the cells of the unabsorbed factor into the body fluids. However, the quantity of the absorbed factor in

TABLE I

Procedures of Separation and Purification
of Adhesive Factors

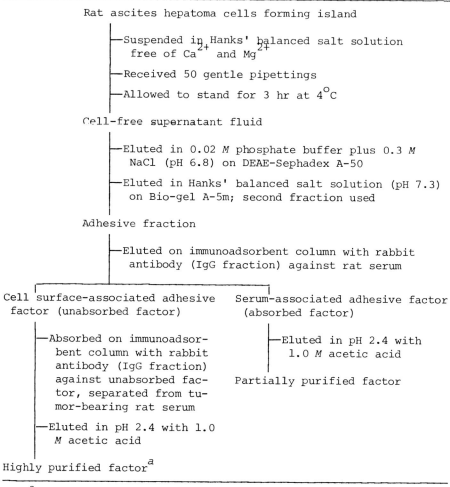

Rat ascites hepatoma cells forming island

—Suspended in Hanks' balanced salt solution free of Ca^{2+} and Mg^{2+}

—Received 50 gentle pipettings

—Allowed to stand for 3 hr at $4^{\circ}C$

Cell-free supernatant fluid

—Eluted in 0.02 M phosphate buffer plus 0.3 M NaCl (pH 6.8) on DEAE-Sephadex A-50

—Eluted in Hanks' balanced salt solution (pH 7.3) on Bio-gel A-5m; second fraction used

Adhesive fraction

—Eluted on immunoadsorbent column with rabbit antibody (IgG fraction) against rat serum

Cell surface-associated adhesive factor (unabsorbed factor)

—Absorbed on immunoadsorbent column with rabbit antibody (IgG fraction) against unabsorbed factor, separated from tumor-bearing rat serum

—Eluted in pH 2.4 with 1.0 M acetic acid

Highly purified factor[a]

Serum-associated adhesive factor (absorbed factor)

—Eluted in pH 2.4 with 1.0 M acetic acid

Partially purified factor

[a]Approximately 220 μg of the factor can be obtained from cell-free supernatant fluid (containing 40.0 mg protein from 1.5×10^{9} AH136B cells).

the serum remained unchanged, independent of the duration after inoculation of tumor cells. Serum from healthy rats contained the absorbed factor (similarly less active) but not the unabsorbed factor, indicating that the absorbed factor was not tumor cell specific in nature. As mentioned later, since the localization of the unab-

sorbed factor on the cell surfaces was confirmed by the immunofluorescence technique, this unabsorbed factor was termed the *cell
surface-associated adhesive factor,* while the absorbed factor was
termed the *serum-associated adhesive factor.*

The unabsorbed factor gave two distinct precipitin lines when
tested by agar immunodiffusion with rabbit antibody against the
factor, while the adhesive factor, which was separated from tumor-
bearing rat serum following the same procedures noted earlier, gave
only one distinct precipitin line, which obviously corresponds to
one of the two precipitin lines demonstrated. Accordingly, the
adhesive factor (from tumor cells) was applied to an immunoadsorbent column coupled with rabbit antibody against the adhesive factor (from tumor-bearing rat serum). The substance was absorbed
on the column and then eluted without loss of its activity in an
acid condition (Table I) (Kudo and Hayashi, 1976). The adhesive
factor recovered from the column produced only one distinct precipitin line, which is obviously common to the two adhesive factors (from tumor cells and tumor-bearing rat serum) when assayed
by agar immunodiffusion with the rabbit antibody (Kudo *et al.,*
1976b). Polyacrylamide gel electrophoresis in the presence of SDS
revealed that this factor shows a single band with a molecular
weight of 70,000 (Hayashi and Ishimaru, 1981). This substance was
a heat-stable and acid-stable glycoprotein (quantitative analysis
of the sugars in the molecule is in progress). Thus, approximately
220 µg of the purified factor could be obtained from the cell-free
supernatant fluids (containing 40.0 mg protein) prepared from
1.5×10^9 AH136B cells. Its minimum effective dose for induction
of aggregation of AH109A cells (1.5×10^6/ml) at 30 min incubation
was approximately 10.0 µg (Kudo *et al.,* 1976b). This factor aggregated hepatoma cells but not erythrocytes (untreated or trypsin-
treated, glutaraldehyde-fixed) from rats, rabbits, or guinea pigs.

It seemed reasonable that the aggregating effects of the cell
surface- and serum-associated adhesive factors may be concerned
with the protein portions in their molecules, not with the carbohydrate portions, because these factors were similarly sensitive
to trypsin but resistant to periodate (Hanaoka *et al.,* 1978). The
retina cell-adhesive substance was also sensitive to trypsin but
resistant to periodate (McClay and Moscona, 1974; Hausman and Moscona, 1975). Accordingly, it was supposed that the aggregating
effects of these adhesive factors may be initiated by interaction
of the protein portions in their molecules with some components at
the surface of the tumor cells. Furthermore, it was found that
D-mannose and α-methyl-*D*-mannoside specifically inhibited hepatoma
cell aggregation by the cell surface factor: these sugars (100 m*M*)
resulted in a complete inhibition of cell aggregation (Hanaoka *et
al.,* 1978). In contrast, the potency of the serum factor was inhibited specifically by *N*-acetyl-*D*-glucosamine; this sugar (100 m*M*)
resulted in a complete inhibition of cell aggregation. Thus, it
seemed reasonable to suppose that adhesion of rat ascites hepatoma
cells due to the cell surface factor may be a consequence of the
interaction of the protein structure in the molecule with certain

carbohydrate molecules such as D-mannose at the cell surface,
whereas that due to the serum factor may operate by interaction of
the protein portion in the molecule with certain carbohydrate molecules such as N-acetyl-D-glucosamine at the cell surface.

B. Biological Characterization
    of Adhesive Factor Separated

    It was of special interest that the hepatoma cells aggregated
in 30-min or 2-hr incubation with the cell surface factor, could
easily be dissociated by pipetting, whereas those incubated for
12 or 24 hr with the factor mostly could not be dissociated by
pipetting, indicating a distinct difference in the development of
binding structures in the aggregated cells. Such a difference in
the binding manner was more conveniently analyzed by the use of
aggregated AH109A cells, which required no previous dissociation
before aggregation.
    The most common sort of aggregated cell contact observed at
the 2-hr stage was simple apposition of plasma membranes. Apposed
plasma membranes were separated by a space of 20 to 30 nm showing
no electron density, resembling those observed in the island-forming tumor cells (Ishimaru et al., 1975, 1976). The cell contact
became closer and more distinct at the 12-hr stage; a distinct increase in intermediate junctions was noticed. The junctions consisted of two outer leaflets disposed in a parallel fashion and
separated by an intercellular space of 10 to 15 nm exhibiting low
electron density, resembling those observed on the island-forming
tumor cells. In the cytoplasm subjacent to the inner leaflets,
moderate electron density was revealed (Ishimaru et al., 1975,
1976). The desmosome-like and tight junction-like structures were
found in the limited surface regions of close cell contact. The
desmosome-like structure consisted of two outer leaflets running in
a parallel fashion and separated by an intercellular space of approximately 20 nm containing a central disk of electron-dense materials. In the cytoplasm subjacent to each inner leaflet, electron-
dense laminar plaques running parallel to the inner leaflets were
observed. A few tonofilaments were frequently found in the cytoplasm, but they were unrelated to the laminar plaques. Such
structures seemed to correspond to that of desmosomes in the process of development. Tight junctions, corresponding to the focal
tight junctions described by Staehelin (1974), were revealed less
frequently at this stage; they were characterized by a narrow gap
of less than 4 nm in distance that was formed by close approxima-
tion and punctate fusion of the outer leaflets.
    At the 24-hr stage of incubation, cell contact became closer
and more characteristic. The cell surface regions showing close
contact clearly increased: The cell contact was characterized by
an increase in desmosomes and tight junctions. Well-defined desmosomes observed at this stage were characterized by one distinct
laminar plaque accompanied by prominent tonofilaments (Ishimaru

et al., 1975, 1976). Tight junctions showed a tendency to develop
in the apical portion of the cell aggregates. The development by
this adhesive factor of tight junctions, desmosomes, and intermediate junctions was strongly inhibited in the presence of actinomycin D during 24 hr of cultivation (Ishimaru *et al.*, 1976). The
failure to develop junctional complexes was associated with inhibition of RNA synthesis by actinomycin D, exclusively resulting in
failure to synthesize the proteins required for the development of
junctional complexes.

In contrast, the cell contact observed at 24 hr incubation
with the serum factor with a similar aggregating activity consisted of only simple apposition. The intercellular spaces of the
aggregated cells were larger, and the areas of cellular apposition were smaller; the aggregated cells were easily dissociated by
pipetting. These experiments indicated a distinct functional difference between the cell surface and serum factors in the induction of junctional complexes. Thus, it was clear that the cell
surface factor is undoubtedly involved in the development of junctional complexes.

As mentioned earlier, the cell surface factor induced not only
aggregation of hepatoma cells but also adhesiveness of the cells.
In order to act on the cells, this factor must bind to their surfaces, presumably through specific surface receptors. The factor
was labeled with ^{125}I. The labeled product was homogeneous and
its biological activity remained unchanged after purification by
affinity chromatography; its binding to the cells (AH109A cells)
was specifically inhibited by *D*-mannose. The binding to the cells
exhibited a simple saturation pattern, reaching its peak at a concentration of 50 µg/ml. By plotting the binding data according to
the Steck and Wallach (1965) equations, the total numbers of binding sites per cell were calculated to be 6×10^5, and the affinity
constant (K_a) was 1.1×10^6 (Hayashi and Ishimaru, 1981; Kurano,
1981b). The binding of this factor to the cells was also demonstrated by the indirect immunofluorescence technique using rabbit
antibody against the factor; this bound factor was found localized on the cell surface.

C. Biological Characterization
    of Adhesive Factor Synthesized

As mentioned earlier, the cell surface factor functioned as a
trigger factor to develop junctional complexes in tumor cells,
provided it was exogenously applied to the cells. In order to
form cell islands characterized by junctional complexes without
any addition of this component, AH136B cells must synthesize this
adhesive component. It seemed possible that if the tumor cells
could be maintained under physiological conditions but prevented
from aggregating at a reasonably low cell density, the cells might
continue to synthesize this component. The dissociated cells were
suspended at a density of 2×10^4 cells/ml for cultivation. The

regeneration of this component was examined using ^{125}I-labeled
rabbit antibody (IgG fraction) against the adhesive factor. The
synthesis (as shown in the form of increased radioactivity specifically bound to the cells) began to rise rapidly; it increased
eightfold in 12 hr of cultivation, reaching its peak, that is, a
10-fold increase, in 24 hr of cultivation (Hayashi and Ishimaru,
1981; Kurano, 1981a). The regeneration of the factor was strongly
inhibited by addition of actinomycin D or puromycin, indicating
that the regeneration required protein synthesis.

In contrast, this type of adhesive component was not detectable
in AH109A cells during 24 hr of cultivation, although there remained some questions that this component might exist in an inac-
cessible state (hidden within the surface membrane layer or sit-
uated at the submembrane layer), or in a smaller quantity not
demonstrable by this technique. However, biochemical evidence
that this component could not be separated from the tumor cells
by the same procedures as noted earlier (Table I) strongly suggested that this component may not be synthesized by the cell;
from the cells only the serum factor was separated (Ishimaru et
al., 1979).

Localization of the regenerated adhesive component was examined by the indirect immunofluorescence test using the immune IgG
described earlier and FITC-labeled goat anti-rabbit IgG. The surface localization of this component was reasonable; the intensity
and distribution of the immunofluorescence increased in parallel
to the duration of cultivation (Hayashi and Ishimaru, 1981;
Kurano, 1981a). The cells at 2 hr culture exhibited faint patch-
like fluorescence at the limited small area of the cell surface;
those at 6 hr culture showed bright fluorescence at the larger
(but limited) area of the cell surface; those at 12 hr culture
showed conspicuous fluorescence, which was diffusely distributed
on the whole cell surface; and those at 24 hr culture showed a
similar but more conspicuous fluorescence. Such an increase in
immunofluorescence seemed to correspond to the radioimmunologically
detected increase in the synthesis of this component mentioned
previously. Thus, the tumor cells could recover from the disso-
ciative effect by at least 24 hr; such recovery did not occur in
the presence of puromycin or actinomycin D. No immunofluorescence
was revealed in AH109A cells.

AH136B cells, which had completed the regeneration of the adhesive factor at 24 hr cultivation, adhered to each other, finally
resulting in the development of junctional complexes, provided
they were cultured at a reasonably high cell density (2×10^6
cells/ml) capable of inducing cell contact (Hayashi and Ishimaru,
1981; Koga, 1981). In contrast, the cells, which had failed to
regenerate this adhesive factor in the presence of actinomycin D
or puromycin, did not adhere to each other. The process of cell
adhesiveness observed was divided into three stages:

1. The cells aggregated in the form of a linear or branched
   chain within 3 hr of incubation; such cell aggregation

was specifically suppressed by the antibody (Fab fraction) against the adhesive factor.

2. The cell aggregates became grape cluster-like in shape as a result of fusion at 6 hr of incubation, and the contact of aggregated cells consisted of simple apposition of plasma membranes.

3. The cell aggregates became oval in shape at 12 to 24 hr of incubation, closely resembling the shape of AH136B cell islands (floating in the ascitic fluids), and the contact of aggregated cells was characterized by the development of junctional complexes.

Tight junctions were found only in the apical portion of the cell aggregates, while intermediate junctions and desmosomes were found in the inner portion; such development of junctional complexes were more frequent at 24 hr of incubation. In contrast, AH109A cells failed to adhere under the same condition of incubation, because of their lack of potency in synthesizing the adhesive factor.

Further study confirmed the existence of an adhesive component cross-reactive with the aforementioned factor in extracts of embryonic rat liver by single radial immunodiffusion test using the same rabbit antibody as noted previously; this component became detectable in extracts prepared at 15 days gestation, and its quantity became maximal in those prepared at 19 days gestation, but became undetectable in those prepared at about 10 days after birth (T. Kako and H. Hayashi, unpublished). The synthesis of this component by the embryonic cells was examined using the same ^{125}I-labeled rabbit antibody as mentioned earlier. The synthesis began to rise rapidly, reaching its peak at 24 hr of cultivation; the cells could recover from trypsinization at least for 24 hr, resembling the recovery of AH136B cells (T. Kako and H. Hayashi, unpublished). Its regeneration required protein synthesis because of its strong inhibition by puromycin or actinomycin D. This component was also found located on the cell surface.

D. Immunological Characterization
   of Adhesive Factor Separated

As is well known, plant lectins serve as a most attractive tool in biological research. The main characteristics of lectins are their ability to bind sugars and to agglutinate cells. In all their activities, lectins exhibit varying degrees of specificity. The target sites for lectins such as PHA and Con A are fully exposed on the cell surface, while the sites for soybean agglutinin (SBA) and peanut agglutinin (PNA) are masked by sialic acid residues and require treatment with neuraminidase before activation of lymphocytes. Lectins are also of great interest to immunologists, mainly because of their ability to interact with lymphocytes and to induce blast cell formation. The morphological changes and biochemical events occurring in lectin-stimulated lymphocytes *in vitro* have been said to resemble many of the antigen-induced immune reactions that take place *in vivo*. Moreover, lectin-activated lymphocytes are capable of synthesizing lymphokines with different biological functions, which may mediate cell-mediated immune reactions. Lectins thus belong to the large group of polygonal activators of polyclonal ligands.

It is important to point out that the cell surface adhesive factor (from tumor cells) also exhibits the power to bind certain sugar structures, to agglutinate tumor cells, and to activate lymphocytes (as noted later); such activities of this adhesive factor clearly represented the main characteristics of lectins as outlined earlier. Its potency was compared with that of lectins, including PHA, Con A, SBA, pokeweed mitogen (PWM), and lipopolysaccharide (LPS), in the form of increased DNA and protein synthesis, blast transformation, and mitosis (Kuratsu *et al.*, 1978). In such experiments, rat lymphocytes (from thymus, lymph node, and spleen) were utilized because the adhesive factor tested was separated from rat hepatoma cells. Synthesis of DNA was increased even by a small quantity (0.1 µg/culture) of the adhesive factor, but no suppression of DNA synthesis was revealed even when greater quantities (10-30 µg/culture) of the adhesive factor were applied. In contrast, the mitogenic effect of PHA and Con A was stronger than that of the adhesive factor, but their responses sharply decreased at doses over 10 µg/culture. The kinetics of DNA synthesis induced by the adhesive factor appeared to differ from that by PHA and Con A; the response to the adhesive factor became maximal at 6 days after stimulation, whereas that to PHA or Con A became maximal at 3 days after stimulation. This adhesive factor stimulates T lymphocytes, because no stimulation was revealed with antithymocyte serum (ATS)-resistant spleen cells.

It has been shown that the stimulating effect of SBA (Novogrodsky and Katchalski, 1973) and PNA (Novogrodsky *et al.*, 1975) on murine and human lymphocytes was similarly weak, but their effect increased when the cells had been treated with neuraminidase to expose hidden target sites for them. A hepatic binding protein also exhibited a weak mitogenic activity on human T lymphocytes, but its effect was enhanced by previous treatment with neuraminidase (Novogrodsky and Ashwell, 1977). In contrast, the effect of the adhesive factor on rat lymphocytes was not influenced by treatment with the enzyme, suggesting the existence of the receptor sites at the cell surface, which differed from those for the hepatic binding protein, SBA, or PNA. Like PHA, the adhesive factor stimulated protein synthesis in an early stage (6-12 hr) of lymphocyte activation, and it induced blast transformation and mitosis like Con A. The mechanism by which plant lectins exert their stimulating effect is completely obscure, but it is generally accepted that the initial step or first signal is binding of the lectin through its sugar-binding site(s).

As is well known, soon after activation by lectins (PHA and Con A) or specific antigens, lymphocytes release a variety of biologically active products, called *lymphokines*. The better known

of the lymphokines are migration-inhibitory factor (MIF), macrophage-chemotactic factor, macrophage-aggregating factor (MAF),
lymphotoxin, and interferon. When stimulated by a small quantity
of the cell surface-adhesive factor, rat lymphoid cells, or T
lymphocytes, cultured in serum-free RPMI-1640, clearly released a
macrophage-chemotactic factor (Hifumi and Hayashi, 1983). This
chemotactic factor released was stable for heat or acid, and its
molecular weight was approximately 12,500 when estimated by gel
filtration. Since the release of this chemotactic factor from
lymphocytes was strongly suppressed in the presence of puromycin,
the synthesis of this chemotactic factor by activated lymphocytes
was suggested.

It was of interest that this chemotactic lymphokine closely
resembles previously described macrophage-chemotactic lymphokines, which are, respectively, released from guinea pig lymphocytes stimulated by PHA (Snyderman et al., 1972; Altman et al.,
1973; Honda et al., 1982), purified protein derivative of tuberculin (PPD) (Snyderman et al., 1972; Altman et al., 1973; Hayashi
et al., 1979; Honda et al., 1982), and bovine γ-globulin (Postlethwait and Snyderman, 1975; Hayashi et al., 1979). The macrophage-
chemotactic lymphokines mentioned earlier were all stable for heat
or acid, and their molecular weights were approximately 12,500.

Histopathological comparison of the proliferation of AH136B
cells (forming cell islands in vivo) and AH109A cells (present as
single cells in vivo) subcutaneously transplanted was of special
importance. When examined at 5 days after transplantation, the
developed AH136B tumor was small in size, but the skin site was
characterized by marked mononuclear cell reaction; the developed
AH109A tumor was much larger in size, but the mononuclear cell
reaction in the skin site was apparently less marked (Hayashi and
Ishimaru, 1981). The mononuclear cell reaction included macrophages (characterized by many lysosomal acid phosphatase granules
stained histochemically) and lymphocytes (characterized by a few
acid phosphatase granules). The finding suggested a possible involvement of macrophage-chemotactic lymphokine as one of the biochemical mechanisms underlying the macrophage reaction in the skin
site, because AH136B cells could release the adhesive factor capable of activating T lymphocytes and of producing macrophage-chemotactic lymphokine. In contrast, AH109A cells were unable to synthesize the adhesive factor.

Although the mechanism underlying the lymphocyte reaction noted earlier was not clear, production of lymphocyte-chemotactic
lymphokine(s) in the skin site was expected as one of the conditions concerned. Our study has suggested the release of lymphocyte-chemotactic lymphokine by rat T lymphocytes stimulated by the
cell surface adhesive factor in a small quantity (S. Harita, Y.
Shimokawa, and H. Hayashi, unpublished). It has been found that
guinea pig lymphocytes stimulated by PPD clearly released two
types of chemotactic factors responding to lymphocytes of rat and
guinea pig; one was labile for heat but stable for acid, and the
other was labile for both heat and acid. Both factors chemotac-

tically affect T lymphocytes. Both these lymphocyte-chemotactic
lymphokines were isolated from the skin site of cell-mediated immune response induced by PPD and then highly purified by column
chromatography (Shimokawa *et al.*, 1979, 1981). Similar lymphocyte-
chemotactic lymphokines were also produced by guinea pig lymphocytes stimulated by Con A (Harita *et al.*, 1983). Accordingly, it
would be important to verify which type of factor may be similar
to the chemotactic lymphokine produced by the adhesive factor stimulation.

It has been generally known that lymphocytes and macrophages
play an important role in the clinical and pathological state defined as cellular immunity; they are crucial in host defense and
they presumably function in the process of tumor surveillance.
Many lymphocyte functions, as mentioned earlier, may be affected
by biologically active molecules released as a consequence of
lymphocyte activation. Lymphocyte reaction in tumor tissues has
been described as an immune response to tumor cells (Blacker *et
al.*, 1953; Underwood, 1974) or a favorable prognostic indicator
(Black *et al.*, 1953). T lymphocytes, among the infiltrated
lymphocytes, have been considered to be necessary as the source
of effector cells in immune response against tumor cells (Plata
et al., 1973; Epstein *et al.*, 1976). In various types of tumor
tissues, T lymphocytes have been found to accumulate intensively
toward the tumor cells, while B lymphocytes infiltrate apart from
the tumor cells. Moreover, the response of T lymphocytes is more
intense than that of B lymphocytes (Kikuchi *et al.*, 1976). In
this report, it is of primary importance that the survival of animals inoculated with AH136B cells is much longer than that of the
animals inoculated with AH109A cells.

III. DISSOCIATION OF CANCER CELLS

In the foregoing section, a possible mechanism underlying tumor cell adhesiveness was discussed from the viewpoint of biological function of the cell surface-associated adhesive factor. As
mentioned earlier, AH136B cell islands are generally composed of
approximately 30-40 cells in number, while AH7974 cell islands are
composed of approximately 5-10 cells in number. First, there occurs the question why these tumor cells may develop characteristic
islands consisting of nearly constant numbers of the cells, respectively. It seems possible that the regulation in the number of
the cells forming the respective islands must be required for favorable function of the individual cells or for favorable social
behavior of the cells. However, it has been known that dissociation of tumor cells is primarily responsible for the initial stages of invasion or metastasis. In fact, histopathological examination of tissue surrounding a tumor frequently reveals single
tumor cells, or small clumps of tumor cells, with no obvious con-

nection to the parent tumor. Moreover, it has been suggested that
tumor cells, if still alive after dissociation, show an increased
locomotion that accounts for their invasive capacity or for their
reactivity to chemotactic stimulation.

A. Effect of Calcium Depletion

     For measurements of the forces required to dissociate compar-
able normal and malignant cells, Coman (1944) has suggested that
the malignant cells show less mutual adhesiveness than normal cells.
Using more reproducible techniques involving standardized conditions of agitation or aspiration, McCutheon *et al.* (1948) and
Tjernberg and Zajicek (1965) have confirmed Coman's original observations. The demonstration by Carruthers and Suntzeff (1944)
of a decrease in the calcium content of normal epithelium after an
initial application of 3-methylcholanthrene, followed by a further
decrease when tumors developed, has led Coman (1944) to emphasize
that the lower calcium content of tumor is responsible for the
decreased mutual adhesiveness of tumor cells. Calcium ions are
known to be involved in establishment and maintenance of adhesion
between the cells of many tissues by forming direct or indirect
linkages between adjacent cells, by reducing electrostatic repul-
sion, or by influencing the function of cytoplasmic contractile
elements involved in cell motility and detachment.
     Subsequent work has complicated Coman's original hypothesis.
For instance, Hickie and Kalant (1967) have demonstrated that the
calcium content of Morris hepatoma in rats is twice as high as
that of normal liver, although this may have been a consequence of
high extracellular binding of calcium in regions of necrosis. The
calcium content of the whole tissue is not, however, necessarily
relevant to cell adhesion; tumor cells may possess a decreased
concentration of calcium-binding groups at their surface, which are
not detectable in measurements of the total calcium content in a
tissue (Coman, 1961). Measurement of the calcium-binding capacity
of cell surfaces has not revealed any significant differences between comparable normal and cancer cells (Bangham and Pethica,
1960; Patinkin *et al.*, 1970). The measurements provide only an
average for the whole cell surface; some calcium-binding sites may
be involved in cell-to-cell adhesions, while others are not. Thus,
although there is a conviction that calcium associated with the cell
surface and cytoplasmic structures plays an important role in the
adhesive properties of cells, it is of interest to clarify the relationship between calcium ions and the reduced adhesiveness of
tumor cells for each other.
     In this respect, electron-microscopic observations by Sedar
and Forte (1964) are of value. They have demonstrated that simple
apposition, intermediate junctions, and desmosomes in the oxyntic
cells of frog gastric glands are respectively dissociated under
calcium-depleted conditions by EDTA, but tight junctions remain
intact. Similar events have also been observed in the structures

in the cardiac muscle cells of rat embryos (Muir, 1967) and in the simple columnar epithelial cells of rat (Cassidy and Tidball, 1967). Accordingly, it would be of interest to investigate whether any electron-microscopic changes in the binding structures of tumor cells may occur under calcium-depleted conditions. AH136B and AH7974 cells (forming islands *in vivo*) were also convenient for the experiments. Treatment with EDTA (2 m*M*) of these tumor cells induces a distinct separation of apposed membranes of the adherent cells in the inner portion of the cell islands, but tight junctions in the apical portion remain unchanged (Ishihara *et al.*, 1977). Such separation of apposed membranes occurs at the regions of simple apposition, intermediate junctions, and desmosomes, as shown by a decreased number of these structures; the mean number of tight junctions, desmosomes, and intermediate junctions in the AH136B cell islands was approximately 100, 0, and 0 in that order, respectively, per 150 nuclei in cross section, while that of those structures in the AH7974 cell islands was approximately 100, 9, and 6. Such separation was clearly temperature dependent; it was induced at 37°C but not at 4°C.

The electron-microscopic changes in desmosomes occur in the following steps: (1) the central disk of electron-dense materials becomes obscure, (2) the central disk disappears, intercellular space dilates to more than 30 nm, and endoplasmic laminal plaque becomes obscure, and (3) widely dilated intercellular space develops with active formation of microvilli, and endoplasmic laminar plaque disappears. However, endoplasmic tonofilaments remain almost intact. The electron-microscopic changes in intermediate junctions are characterized by dilation of intercellular space to more than 45 nm and by decrease in the electron-dense materials in the cytoplasm subjacent to the inner leaflets. However, the altered structures in the inner portion of the cell islands can be reconstructed after 1.5 hr of readministration of calcium ions, as shown by an increased number of the structures; the mean number of tight junctions, desmosomes, and intermediate junctions in the AH136B cell islands was approximately 100, 12, amd 19 in that order, while that of these structures in the AH7974 cell islands was 100, 55, and 40. Thus, it seems reasonable that a decrease in calcium ions on the tumor cell surfaces may cause a reduced adhesiveness of tumor cells, as shown in the form of partial separation of tumor cells held together by simple apposition, intermediate junctions, and desmosomes. Therefore, the separation of the apical portion of the cell islands composed of tight junctions needs other conditions, as will be described.

In a systematic investigation of the effects of proteolytic enzymes (trypsin), chelators (EDTA), and detergents (sodium desoxycholate, DOC) on desmosomes originating in a variety of tissues, Borysenko and Revel (1973) have divided desmosomes into broad categories: One group, sensitive to trypsin or DOC but insensitive to EDTA, is functionally stable in maintaining cell-to-cell contacts for long periods, as seen in stratified squamous and many glandular epithelia; the other group, sensitive to EDTA but insensitive to trypsin or DOC, is physiologically labile or plastic, and allows intercellular passage of substances, as seen in simple columnar epithelia. The fact that the extracellular components of desmosomes from simple columnar epithelia are sensitive to EDTA (Borysenko and Revel, 1973) seems to be comparable to the initial disappearance by EDTA of the central disk of electron-dense materials in the AH136B and AH7974 cells. Thus, it is assumed that desmosomes observed in those tumor cells may belong to the group sensitive to EDTA. However, Polak-Charcon *et al.*, (1978) have shown that desmosomes in human adenocarcinoma cell line are sensitive to trypsin and broken up by the enzyme.

B. Effect of Intrinsic Protease Activation

It is known that many different enzymes can induce cell dissociation *in vitro,* and in the laboratory, proteolytic enzymes are used routinely for this purpose. Lysosomal hydrolases released from embryonic cells *in vitro* digest intercellular matrix and promote cell detachment from glass substrates. Sylvén (1968, 1973) has also demonstrated the facilitation of such cell detachment by lysosomal cathepsin B and other enzymes. Hypervitaminosis A, which is known to activate lysosomes, has been shown to promote cell separation from glass surfaces *in vitro* (Weiss, 1962), and to induce cell dissociation and metastasis in mice carrying spontaneous tumors (Weiss and Holyoke, 1969). However, the most direct method of analyzing the role of the putative proteases in the cell dissociation is to use highly specific inhibitors to the enzymes because well-characterized proteases may give reasonable explanations for their biological functions required.

As is well known, the tumor cell invasion is often associated with areas of tissue lysis and stromal disruption, suggesting that extensive hydrolytic activity occurs at the invading edge of a growing tumor. Since the hydrolytic activity appears to take place extracellularly, the enzymes must be released by the tumor cells themselves, by damaged or activated adjacent normal cells, or even by sequestered cells such as lymphocytes or macrophages. The substrates may include globular proteins, membrane-bound proteins, fibrous proteins, and collagen-like proteins. In addition, the pH and ionic composition in the microenvironment of the invasive zone can vary depending on the cell or tissue type, the extent of damage and lysis to surrounding tissue, and the secretory properties of the tumor cell. From these suppositions, it is presumed that the increase in tumor-induced proteolytic activity at the invasive zone may be a result of the action of a relatively large number of highly specific proteases and peptidases (Quigley, 1979). The purification and characterization of the putative proteases concerned with the dissociation or invasion of tumor cells are strongly required.

As one of the conditions concerned with tumor cell dissociation (particularly separation of the apical portion in the tumor
cell islands), activation of a certain neutral protease in the
tumor cells has been proposed (Katsuya et al., 1978). Our protease, which is optimally active in neutral pH range when assayed
for casein or hemoglobin, is separated from the AH136B cells just
mentioned and partially purified by column chromatography with
DEAE-Sephadex, DEAE-cellulose, and hydroxyapatite, in that order
(Koono et al., 1974a). Treatment with the enzyme of the cell
islands at 37°C for 30 min provokes in vitro electron-microscopic
changes in the apical portion of the cell islands, which are characterized by disappearance of punctate fusion in tight junctions
(occurring from the outer side of the structures to the inner
side) and by distinct dilation of the intercellular spaces; such
changes can be induced by a low activity of the enzyme. After a
further 30-min treatment with the enzyme, a well-defined structure
of tight junctions is scarcely found. In the cytoplasm adjacent
to the inner leaflets of altered tight junctions, electron-dense
materials are scarcely found. At this stage of the enzyme treatment, little or no morphological alteration in intermediate junctions and desmosomes is revealed. Morphological change by the
protease in tight junctions is clearly temperature dependent,
being provoked at 37° C but not at 4°C. The activity of the enzyme applied was almost negligible when assayed at 4°C. The action
of this protease for inducing tight-junctional change seems to be
specific, because alkaline protease, acid protease, and another
neutral protease isolated from the same tumor cells did not cause
tight-junctional alteration.

Although the enzyme has not yet been well defined, it appears
to resemble chymotrypsin because of its strong inactivation by di-
isopropyl fluorophosphate (DFP), phenylmethyl sulfonyl fluoride
(PMSF), or chymostatin. From the viewpoint of observations that
this enzyme may be lysosomal in origin, the work by Staehelin
(1973) is of interest. Investigating the fine structures of
freeze-cleaved tight junctions from epithelia of rat small intestine, he has postulated that the fragments of tight junctions can
be internalized and broken down in lysosome-like vesicles. Many
of the proteases that have been observed to be increased on malignant transformation in vitro appear to be lysosomal enzymes. Extracellular release of lysosomal enzymes seems to take place
through fusion of the lysosome with the plasma membrane (Dingle
and Fell, 1969). If such enzymes were to gain access to the cell
surface, they would be capable of chemically altering the structure of cell surface glycoproteins and proteins that may serve as
cell recognition and cell-regulatory molecules. Since lysosomes
release their contents at or near the cell surface, it has been
proposed that lysosomal induced changes in the cell periphery do
occur and are a regulatory factor in cell recognition or cell
growth.

A subsequent important problem is how the lysosomal chymotrypsin-like enzyme can be activated within the tumor cells, resulting

in the morphological change in tight junctions as described earlier. The enzyme has been demonstrated to be activated in and released from the tumor cells by a certain peptide (Koono *et al.*, 1974b), which was extracted from AH136B tumor-transplanted skin, 3-methylcholanthrane-induced rat mammary cancer tissue, and human lymph nodes with metastatic mammary cancer cells, and then partially purified by ultrafiltration followed by gel filtration. Our peptide is heat stable and dialyzable; it is characterized by a prompt release of the enzyme and by noncytotoxicity for the cells. Treatment with this peptide of AH136B cell islands at 37°C (but not at 4°C) for 60 min clearly provokes electron-microscopic alterations in the apical portion of the cell islands, fundamentally resembling those observed after treatment with the chymotrypsin-like enzyme separated from the cells. Interestingly, disappearance of punctate fusion in tight junctions occurs from the inner side of the structure to the outer side, differing from the effect of the enzyme exogenously applied (Katsuya *et al.*, 1978; Ishimaru *et al.*, 1979). Thus, it seems evident that activation of this intrinsic enzyme induces tight-junctional disruption, but its activation does not cause a complete dissociation of the tumor cells, because intermediate junctions and desmosomes remain intact. Depletion of calcium ions on the cell surfaces induces intermediate junctional and desmosomal disruptions, but it does not cause a complete dissociation of the cells, because tight junctions remain unchanged. Accordingly, a complete dissociation of the cells may require combined conditions, that is, calcium depletion and protease activation. Tumor cells, which were dissociated under the combined conditions, are mostly still alive and show smooth surfaces accompanied by a small number of cytoplasmic projections.

Activation of the intrinsic enzyme, as mentioned earlier, appears to be controlled by the peptide present in the tumor site, which is a mixture of host and tumor cells. Essentially, the proposed system is an example of host-tumor interaction; the activated protease causes the disruption of tight junctions, while its own activation is controlled by the peptide, possibly produced as a result of interactions between host and tumor cells. Such an *in vitro* mechanism underlying the complete dissociation of tumor cells seems to be applicable to the process of *in vivo* dissociation of AH136B and AH7974 cells subcutaneously proliferated. Although these tumor cells form cell masses, respectively, the principal development of AH136B cell masses tends to be composed of the adhered cells (characterized by development of tripartite junctional complexes) less than about 40 in number, and that of AH7974 cell masses composed of the adhered cells less than about 10 in number. Suggesting a possible regulation in number of the cells forming the respective masses, there is observed the dissociation of tumor cells from the masses exhibiting various stages of electron-microscopic changes, which fundamentally resemble those seen *in vitro*. The dissociated cells exhibit smooth surfaces accompanied by cytoplasmic projections in varying number.

IV.   CONCLUDING REMARKS

As mentioned previously, it seems reasonable that the cell
surface-associated adhesive factor (but not the serum-associated
factor) from tumor cells may play a key role in tumor cell adhesiveness. The factor can be synthesized by well-differentiated
tumor cells (characterized by development of junctional complexes)
but not by undifferentiated tumor cells (present as single cells).
This finding also suggests that this adhesive factor may represent
an expression of tumor cell differentiation. The main question
regarding the factor that remains open concerns its adhesive *se-
lectivity,* because the present research was limited to the hepatoma cells of rats. Its demonstration in embryonic rat liver cells
suggests that this adhesive factor might be one of the carcinoembryonic proteins; the factor is also associated with the embryonic cell adhesiveness (characterized by development of junctional
complexes). The adhesive factor, when it is further characterized,
may provide an important model system in the study of the phenomenon associated with gene expression. Such investigation is
likely to further the general understanding of the expression of
fetal proteins in cancer. In relation to these observations, it
is of value of study whether or not the cell surface-associated
adhesive factors, corresponding to the origin of malignant or embryonic cells, can be separated from the respective cells.
     It is also important to clarify whether any adhesive substance
associated with adhesiveness in adult rat liver cells can be separated from the cells, because the cell-to-cell contact is also
characterized by development of junctional complexes as described
earlier. The substance, if present, may share different antigenicity with the adhesive factor from malignant and embryonic rat
liver cells, because the adhesive factor referred to cannot be revealed immunologically in the adult cells; a different gene expression for this adhesive protein is expected.
     This adhesive factor possesses a mitogenic activity, as shown
by increase in DNA and protein synthesis or blast transformation
and mitosis of T lymphocytes. T lymphocytes activated by this
factor can release chemotactic lymphokines capable of attracting
macrophages or lymphocytes. Release by this factor of other
lymphokines with different biological functions, which may concern
a local tumor immunity, is also expected.
     The dissociation of tumor cells can be induced under the com-
bined conditions of depletion of calcium ions on the cell surface
and activation of lysosomal chymotrypsin-like enzyme. Such a type
of tumor cell dissociation can be observed *in vivo*. Dissociated
tumor cells are assumed to locomote directionally under the influence of chemotactic stimuli into the surrounding normal stroma
at the initial stages of invasion. Our chemotactic factors, which
can also induce an extravasation of tumor cells, may be produced
extracellularly by chymotrypsin-like enzyme released from tumor
cells; and precursors of the chemotactic factors can be found in

normal serum and tissue. Further information on this enzyme is required to determine the mechanism underlying the invasion by tumor cells or metastasis.

ACKNOWLEDGMENTS

The authors are very grateful to Drs. R. Kurano and M. Hifumi for their invaluable discussion. Our investigations referred to in this article were performed in a thankful collaboration with the past and present staffs in this laboratory, and fruitfully supported by grants from the Japanese Ministry of Education, Science and Culture, the Biological Institute of Shionogi Pharmaceutical Company, Osaka, and the Society for Metabolism Research, Tokyo. Our thanks are also due to Miss Yoshimi Hoshiko for typing this manuscript.

REFERENCES

Altman, L. C., Snyderman, R., Oppenheim, J. J., and Mergenhagen, S. E. (1973). *J. Immunol.* 110, 801-810.
Bangham, A. D., and Pethica, B. A. (1960). *Proc. R. Soc. Edinburgh Sect. A 28,* 43-50.
Black, M. M., Kerpe, S., and Speer, F. D. (1953). *Am. J. Pathol. 24,* 505-521.
Borysenko, J. Z., and Revel, J. P. (1973). *Am. J. Anat. 137,* 403-421.
Carruthers, C., and Suntzeff, V. (1944). *Science (Washington, D.C.) 99,* 245-247.
Cassidy, M. M., and Tidball, C. S. (1967). *J. Cell Biol. 32,* 685-698.
Cauldwell, C. B., Henkart, P., and Humphreys, T. (1973). *Biochemistry 12,* 3051-3055.
Coman, D. R. (1944). *Cancer Res. 4,* 625-629.
Coman, D. R. (1961). *Cancer Res. 21,* 1436-1438.
Dingle, J. T., and Fell, H. B. (1969). "Lysosomes in Biology and Pathology," Vols. 1 and 2. North-Holland, Amsterdam.
Epstein, R. S., Lopez, D. M., Oritz-Muniz, G., and Siegel, M. M. (1976). *Int. J. Cancer 18,* 458-461.
Garber, B. B., and Moscona, A. A. (1972). *Dev. Biol. 27,* 235-243.
Hanaoka, Y., Kudo, K., Ishimaru, Y., and Hayashi, H. (1978). *Br. J. Cancer 37,* 536-544.
Harita, S., Shimokawa, Y., and Hayashi, H. (1983). *Int. Arch. Allergy Appl. Immunol. 70,* 118-123.
Hausman, R. E., and Moscona, A. A. (1975). *Proc. Natl. Acad. Sci. USA 72,* 916-920.
Hausman, R. E., Knapp, L. W., and Moscona, A. A. (1976). *J. Exp. Zool. 198,* 417-422.

Hayashi, H., and Ishimaru, Y. (1981). *Int. Rev. Cytol. 70,* 139-215.

Hayashi, H., Honda, M., and Shimokawa, Y. (1979). *In* "Immunology '79" (Y. Yamamura and T. Tada, eds.), pp. 141-151. Nakayama, Tokyo (in Japanese).

Henkart, P., Humphreys, S., and Humphreys, T. (1973). *Biochemistry 12,* 3045-3050.

Hickie, R. A., and Kalant, H. (1967). *Cancer Res. 27,* 1053-1057.

Hifumi, M., and Hayashi, H. (1983). *Immunology 49,* 245-253.

Honda, M., Miura, K., Kuratsu, J., and Hayashi, H. (1982). *Cell. Immunol. 67,* 213-228.

Humphreys, T. (1963). *Dev. Biol. 8,* 27-47.

Ishihara, H., Ishimaru, Y., and Hayashi, H. (1977). *Br. J. Cancer 35,* 643-656.

Ishimaru, Y., Ishihara, H., and Hayashi, H. (1975). *Br. J. Cancer 31,* 207-217.

Ishimaru, Y., Kudo, K., Ishihara, H., and Hayashi, H. (1976). *Br. J. Cancer 34,* 426-436.

Ishimaru, Y., Kudo, K., Koga, Y., and Hayashi, H. (1979). *J. Cancer Res. Clin. Oncol. 93,* 123-136.

Katsuya, H., Ishimaru, Y., Koono, M., and Hayashi, H. (1978). *Virchows Arch. B 27,* 159-172.

Kikuchi, K., Ishii, Y., Ueno, H., and Koshiba, H. (1976). *Ann. N.Y. Acad. Sci. 276,* 188-206.

Koga, Y. (1981). *Kumamoto Med. J. 34,* 79-90.

Koono, M., Ushijima, K., and Hayashi, H. (1974a). *Int. J. Cancer 13,* 105-115.

Koono, M., Katsuya, H., and Hayashi, H. (1974b). *Int. J. Cancer 13,* 334-342.

Kudo, K., and Hayashi, H. (1976). *In* "Lectins" (T. Osawa and R. Mori, eds.), pp. 155-172. Kodansha, Tokyo (in Japanese).

Kudo, K., Tasaki, I., Hanaoka, Y., and Hayashi, H. (1974). *Br. J. Cancer 30,* 549-559.

Kudo, K., Hanaoka, Y., and Hayashi, H. (1976a). *Br. J. Cancer 33,* 79-80.

Kudo, K., Hanaoka, Y., and Hayashi, H. (1976b). *Br. J. Cancer 33,* 88-89.

Kurano, R. (1981a). *Kumamoto Med. J. 34,* 164-173.

Kurano, R. (1981b). *Kumamoto Med. J. 34,* 174-183.

Kuratsu, J., Yoshinaga, M., and Hayashi, H. (1978). *Br. J. Cancer 38,* 224-232.

Kuroda, Y. (1968). *Exp. Cell Res. 49,* 626-637.

Lilien, J. E. (1968). *Dev. Biol. 17,* 657-678.

Lilien. J. E., and Moscona, A. A. (1967). *Science (Washington, D.C.) 157,* 70-72.

McClay, D. R., and Moscona, A. A. (1974). *Exp. Cell Res. 87,* 438-443.

McCutheon, M., Coman, D. R., and Fontaine, B. M. (1948). *Cancer (Philadelphia) 1,* 460-467.

Muir, A. R. (1967). *J. Anat. 101,* 239-261.

Novogrodsky, A., and Ashwell, G. (1977). *Proc. Natl. Acad. Sci. USA 74*, 676-678.
Novogrodsky, A., and Katchalski, E. (1973). *Proc. Natl. Acad. Sci. USA 70*, 2515-2518.
Novogrodsky, A., Lotan, R., David, A., and Sharon, N. (1975). *J. Immunol. 115*, 1243-1248.
Patinkin, D., Zaritsky, A., and Doljanski, F. (1970). *Cancer Res. 30*, 498-503.
Plata, F., Gomard, E., Leclerc, J. C., and Levy, J. P. (1973). *J. Immunol. 111*, 667-671.
Polak-Charcon, S., Shoham, J., and Ben-Shaul, Y. (1978). *Exp. Cell Res. 116*, 1-13.
Postlethwait, A. E., and Snyderman, R. (1975). *J. Immunol. 114*, 274-278.
Quigley, J. P. (1979). *In* "Surfaces of Normal and Malignant Cells" (R. O. Hynes, ed.), pp. 247-285. Wiley, New York.
Sedar, A. W., and Forte, J. G. (1964). *J. Cell Biol. 22*, 173-188.
Shimokawa, Y., Harita, S., and Hayashi, H. (1979). *Proc. Jpn. Soc. Immunol. 9*, 337-338.
Shimokawa, Y., Harita, S., and Hayashi, H. (1981). *Proc. Jpn. Soc. Immunol. 11*, 661-662.
Snyderman, R., Altman, L. C., Hausman, M. S., and Mergenhagen, S. E. (1972). *J. Immunol. 108*, 857-860.
Staehelin, L. A. (1973). *J. Cell Sci. 13*, 763-786.
Staehelin, L. A. (1974). *Int. Rev. Cytol. 39*, 191-283.
Steck, T. L., and Wallach, D. F. H. (1965). *Biochim. Biophys. Acta 97*, 510-522.
Sylvén, B. (1968). *Eur. J. Cancer 4*, 559-562.
Sylvén, B. (1973). *In* "Chemotherapy of Cancer Dissemination and Metastasis" (S. Garattini and G. Franchi, eds.), pp. 129-138. Raven, New York.
Tasaki, I., and Hayashi, H. (1969). *Proc. Jpn. Cancer Assoc. 28*, 154.
Tasaki, I., and Hayashi, H. (1971). *Trans. Soc. Pathol. Jpn. 60*, 124-125.
Tjernberg, B., and Zajicek, J. (1965). *Acta Cytol. 9*, 197-202.
Underwood, J. C. E. (1974). *Br. J. Cancer 30*, 538-548.
Weiss, L. (1962). *J. Theor. Biol. 2*, 236-250.
Weiss, L., and Holyoke, E. D. (1969). *J. Natl. Cancer Inst. (US) 43*, 1045-1053.

DISCUSSION

KONDO: Have you ever treated animals bearing AH109 by your chymotrypsin-like enzyme?

HAYASHI: No, I have never attempted *in vivo* experiments as you suggest.

LIOTTA: Is the chymotrypsin-like enzyme cell surface bound?

HAYASHI: The enzyme is lysosomal in origin and was released into
          the culture media when AH136B or AH109A cells were stim-
          ulated by the peptide. The peptide may be a product of
          interactions between host and tumor cells.

OKADA: You have demonstrated that the adhesive glycoprotein ag-
          gregates only tumor cells but not normal cells. On the
          other hand, normal lymphocytes were shown to be stimula-
          ted by the glycoprotein. Why can normal lymphocytes be
          stimulated without being aggregated?

HAYASHI: Our glycoprotein binds the surface of AH109A cells. Num-
          bers of receptor sites are estimated about 600,000 per
          cell. I imagine the presence of similar (but not iden-
          tical) receptor structure on the lymphocyte surface.
          Binding of the glycoprotein to the cell surface receptor
          is primarily required for AH109A cell aggregation or
          lymphocyte activation, but those phenomena may be advanced
          by different biochemical processes.

WEISS: Agents promoting cell dissociation can act directly on
          cell surfaces, or alternatively, can act through lyso-
          some labilization. These effects can be discriminated
          from each other by using lysosome stabilizers such as
          hydrocortisone. Does your peptide promote cell dissocia-
          tion in the presence of hydrocortisone?

HAYASHI: Our chymotrypsin-like enzyme is lysosomal in origin and
          induces chemical structural changes of cell surface
          proteins associated with the tight-junction structure
          when passed through the cell surface, I think. Dingle
          et al. have described that enzymes, when they were re-
          leased from lysosome after or near the cell surface,
          cause chemical structural changes of cell surface glyco-
          proteins and proteins. I wish to examine the effect of
          hydrocortisone in an experimental system. Thank you for
          your comment.

CHAPTER 7

SYSTEMIC AND LOCAL REGULATION
OF HUMAN NATURAL KILLER CYTOTOXICITY

*Sidney H. Golub, Peter M. Moy, J. Dixon Gray,
Linda M. Karavodin*

Division of Oncology
Department of Surgery
University of California at Los Angeles
School of Medicine
Los Angeles, California

*Norihiko Kawate
Masayuki Niitsuma*

Department of Surgery
Tokyo Medical College
Tokyo, Japan

Martyn W. Burk

Division of Surgical Oncology
John Wayne Clinic
Jonsson Comprehensive Cancer Center
University of California at Los Angeles
School of Medicine
Los Angeles, California

BASIC MECHANISMS AND CLINICAL TREATMENT
OF TUMOR METASTASIS   123

I. INTRODUCTION

     Considerable interest is being focused on natural killer (NK)
cells. Natural killer cells have been implicated in natural resistance to tumors, but the actual contribution of NK cells to host
resistance against established and growing tumors is not clear.
Natural killer activity is apparently depressed in patients with
large tumor burdens (Pross and Baines, 1976; Takasugi *et al.*,
1977), and it may well be much more than coincidental that two of
the most extensively studied and interesting modes of immunotherapy for cancers, Bacillus Calmette-Guérin (BCG) and interferon
(IFN), are both associated with augmentation of NK activity. Thus,
the observations that NK is apparently depressed in patients with
progressively growing tumors and can be augmented by agents known
to have both antitumor effects and immune modulating effects infer
a role for NK cells in resistance to further spread and proliferation of tumor cells. However, direct proof that NK cells can contribute to restriction of clinically apparent tumors is difficult
to obtain.
     Our studies have focused on possible regulatory mechanisms in
NK cytotoxicity. A number of systems have been reported that indicate cellular or humoral mechanisms for regulation of NK cytotoxicity. For example, interferon has been shown to increase NK
activity of mouse cells (Djeu *et al.*, 1978a), and this increase is
apparently dependent on the presence of macrophages (Djeu *et al.*,
1978b). Similarly, intraperitoneal administration of BCG in mice
results in elevated NK activity of peritoneal exudate cells (Wolfe
et al., 1977), and this augmentation of NK activity is apparently
dependent on a macrophage, as administration of silica to mice
prevents BCG augmentation of NK (Tracey, 1979). There is limited
evidence for the involvement of accessory cells in the development
of human NK cytotoxicity, although one *in vitro* model has suggested
a T cell control of the development of NK-like cytotoxicity in
culture (Ortaldo *et al.*, 1979). Conversely, there is some evidence
that cells are able to assert suppressive effects on NK cells.
Spleen cells from *Corynebacterium parvum*-treated or newborn mice
can suppress NK function (Savary and Lotzova, 1978), as can prostaglandin-secreting macrophages (Droller *et al.*, 1978). Thus, a
number of model systems have pointed to both positive and negative
regulation by non-NK cells of NK cytotoxicity.
     We studied the significance of NK activity in the human cancer
patient from three approaches. The questions we have addressed
are: (1) What are the cellular regulatory events involved in aug-

mentation or suppression of NK activity in patients being treated with IFN or BCG? Is NK function regulated by interactions with other cell types? (2) What factors regulate NK function at the site of human tumors? Can such factors be manipulated by induction of an inflammatory response at the tumor site with BCG? (3) What are the regulatory events and what lineage of cells is involved in generating NK or NK-like cytotoxicity *in vitro*? We feel that these three approaches may provide us with a broad view of the biological significance of NK activity in the patient with malignant disease.

This report will attempt to provide an overview of the first two of these three lines of investigation. We are greatly indebted to our colleagues within the Division of Surgical Oncology, UCLA School of Medicine, for their contributions to these studies. In particular, we extend our thanks to Drs. E. Carmack Holmes and Alistair Cochran for their help and encouragement in our studies of local immune responses, and to Dr. Donald Morton for his support and advice concerning the BCG and IFN studies.

II. SYSTEMIC REGULATION OF NK

A. Effects of Interferon

Considerable interest has been focused on the use of IFN as an antineoplastic agent in humans (Strander, 1977; Merigan et al., 1978; Gutterman et al., 1980). Thus far, IFN has not been used extensively for patients with metastatic malignant melanoma. We are participating in a multiinstitutional trial sponsored by the American Cancer Society to investigate the possible therapeutic benefit of human leukocyte IFN (IFN-α) for the treatment of malignant melanoma. Systemic administration of IFN to cancer patients results in a marked increase in NK activity shortly after first administration (Einhorn et al., 1978; Huddlestone et al., 1979). We investigated the effect of daily doses of IFN given over a 42-day period. The purpose of these studies was to determine how long and at what level elevated NK activity could be maintained.

Natural killer activity in these patients is of interest for several reasons. First, NK cells are cytotoxic to tumor cells, and may contribute to the host defenses against the neoplastic disease. Whether the therapeutic benefits of IFN are due to elevated NK activity or to some other mechanism, such as direct antineoplastic effects, is difficult to determine. However, NK activity is an easy and convenient means to measure the biological activity of IFN. Thus, measurement of NK activity in a systematic fashion following administration of IFN may prove useful in the adjustment of dosage and time schedules for the use of this agent.

Sixteen patients with metastatic malignant melanoma were entered into the study. Patients had metastases to subcutaneous tissues and/or lungs. The patients received daily doses of 1×10^6, 3×10^6, or 9×10^6 units IFN for 42 consecutive days. The IFN was human leukocyte IFN (IFN-α) provided by the American Cancer Society as part of a multiinstitutional trial. The patients were randomly assigned to dosage, and the IFN was administered by an injection. Toxicity and therapeutic benefit is the subject of a separate report (Krown et al., 1981) and will only be briefly summarized. Of the 35 evaluable patients treated at UCLA, Memorial Sloan-Kettering, and Yale Cancer Centers, six had evidence of tumor regression. One patient with skin disease had objective partial tumor regression; two patients with lung metastases showed minor tumor regression in 20 of 23 cutaneous lesions while simultaneously developing two new cutaneous nodules. Two other patients with cutaneous disease displayed intense inflammatory reactions around melanoma nodules; this phenomenon was associated with partial regression of two of eight nodules in one patient. Seven patients were stable and 22 progressed. Toxicity was generally dose related and most frequently manifested as reversible leukopenia, thrombocytopenia, and increased liver enzyme levels. Fever and chills early in the course of treatment, plus weakness, malaise, and anorexia, were also common.

While these results are not dramatic, they do indicate that IFN has some activity against melanoma. Further study is clearly required to determine if more effective doses and schedules can be found.

Peripheral blood lymphocytes (PBL) were obtained daily for 2 days before initiation of IFN treatment, daily for 3 days after initiation of treatment, and weekly thereafter. Natural killer cytotoxicity of PBL was measured against K562 myeloid leukemia cells. For all cytotoxicity assays a microcytotoxicity ^{51}Cr-release assay was used as described previously (Seeley and Golub, 1978). Effector:target cell (E:T) ratios were 100:1, 50:1, 25:1, and 12.5:1 with all targets. Results are expressed as percentage cytotoxicity. Spontaneous release was determined in the wells containing targets without added lymphocytes; total release was calculated from wells containing targets and 5% Nonidet P40 detergent. All tests were performed in RPMI-1640 medium, supplemented with antibiotics and 10% pooled human AB serum. One lot of serum was used, and this lot had been screened and showed no activity in antibody-dependent cellular cytotoxicity (ADCC) and no augmentation or diminution of NK cytotoxicity when compared to other serum supplements. To assure ourselves that the cytotoxicity assay was working properly each day, we thawed a sample of cryopreserved PBL from a single batch from one donor and tested it during each experiment. These data were used simply as a quality control on the cytotoxicity test and as a means of searching for systematic variations, such as those due to day of the week, in the assay system. No systematic variations were found in analysis of day-to-day or week-to-week differences in control samples. Thus, the assay was sufficiently reproducible to allow for comparisons over time from a single group of patients.

TABLE I

Changes in NK Cytotoxicity during IFN Treatment

Days of IFN treatment	Average change in mean cytotoxicity to K562[a] (%)	Number of patients with increased cytotoxicity/number tested[a]
1	-7.0	6/15
2	+3.8	8/14
3	+7.7	9/15
7	+15.3	13/16
14	+6.6	10/15
21	+3.9	9/16
28	+3.5	9/15
35	+1.0	7/14

[a] Compared to average of two pretreatment samples.

1. Natural Killer Cytotoxicity

Results from these 16 patients are summarized in Table I. The general pattern is quite apparent. Natural killer activity tends to decline at 24 hr after the first administration of IFN. Subsequently, NK activity rises, with peak activity found at 7 days of continuous daily treatment. After the first week of treatment, NK activity again declines toward pretreatment baseline levels, although it tends to remain slightly elevated. Results in this table are expressed as mean cytotoxicity, which is the average of four different effector:target ratios in the assay. Similar results were obtained in all four ratios; therefore, we have simply summarized the data with the mean of the four ratios.

Two points are particularly interesting in the pattern illustrated in Table I. First of all, there is an apparent decline in NK activity at the first day of treatment. This decline has also been noted in healthy volunteers treated with similar doses of human leukocyte IFN (Kariniemi et al., 1980). The reasons for this decline are not immediately apparent, although several possibilities deserve examination. There may be a redistribution of NK cells in the immediate post-treatment period, so that they are not available in the peripheral blood. Alternatively, NK activity may be depressed by the fever that usually accompanies the first treatment with IFN. Regardless, the NK activity promptly recovers, and peak activity was seen at Day 7 of treatment. This was a very consistent finding, with 13 of the 16 patients having NK activity elevated at Day 7. In fact, this is the only time period with a statistically significant increase in NK activity.

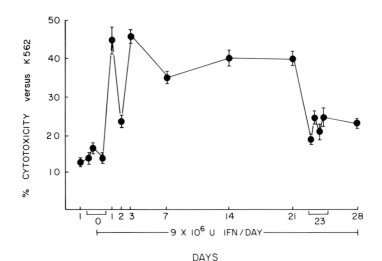

DAYS

Fig. 1. Sequential tests of NK cytotoxicity versus K562 in
the ^{51}Cr-release assay for patient 16. Vertical bars indicate SE
for cytotoxicity tested at effector:target ratio of 100:1. Samples
were tested 1 day prior to the initial treatment, immediately before and 2 and 12 hr following the first treatment; on Days 1, 2,
3, 7, 14, 21, and 28 at 24 hr after treatment; and on Day 23 immediately before and 3, 6, and 8 hr following treatment.

An example of changes in NK cytotoxicity during IFN treatment
is shown in Fig. 1. This demonstrates the NK activity detected in
patient 16 through the course of IFN treatment, and several important features are illustrated in this example. Although NK cytotoxicity was elevated longer in this patient than in most others
we studied, the NK activity did return to baseline levels after 3
weeks of treatment despite continued high-dose IFN treatment.
Furthermore, this lack of response cannot be explained as a change
in kinetics of IFN activation to more rapid activation, as samples
drawn on Day 23 at times before the usual 24-hr post-treatment sample also showed low NK activity.

Our results are slightly in contrast to other laboratories that
have studied NK activity in patients who received IFN (Huddlestone
et al., 1974; Einhorn et al., 1978). Other investigators have
usually seen peak NK activity after 12 to 48 hr following intramuscular injection of IFN, whereas our results suggested a much
later peak in activity. We would tend to attribute this difference to the fact that we were studying melanoma patients whereas
other groups were studying a variety of cancer patients, including
a large proportion with lymphoproliferative malignancies. These
patients are likely to have impaired immune functions. In contrast, we have shown previously that patients with malignant melanoma, even patients with widespread metastases, have only a modest
impairment of cellular immune functions (Golub et al., 1977).

It is possible that these patients would show different kinetics of response to IFN. In fact, reports of NK changes in healthy individuals show responses more similar to those we saw in melanoma patients than have been reported in other disease states.

Increased NK activity was not confined to activity against the K562 target cell. We also saw concurrent increased cytotoxicity against other NK-sensitive targets and moderately sensitive targets along with concurrent increases in ADCC. However, NK-resistant targets, most importantly including melanoma cells, remained unaffected throughout the course of treatment.

We have examined the dose of IFN used. All three doses that were employed in this trial were effective in elevating NK activity, and all three showed peak activity at 7 days of treatment. However, the lowest dose used (1×10^6 units/day) was actually slightly more effective at maintaining elevated levels of NK activity past Day 7 of treatment, whereas the higher dose levels (3×10^6 or 9×10^6 units/day) were more likely to have a decline in activity after the seventh day of treatment. These differences in pattern of activity according to dose are based on rather small patient groups (five to six patients per dose level), but they at least suggest that 1×10^6 units are sufficient to elevate NK activity and that higher doses are unlikely to be more effective for augmenting this form of cellular cytotoxicity. This does not imply that higher doses are less likely to be effective therapeutically, but simply indicates that as far as the NK system is concerned, lower doses appear to be sufficient. Additional information on the effects of IFN on NK activity in melanoma patients can be found in Golub et al. (1982a).

2. Regulation of NK Cytotoxicity

Since our results showed both positive and negative effects of IFN on NK activity, we had good reasons to search for complex regulatory events. To examine NK regulation in this situation, we asked two specific questions: (1) What events in the maturation of NK cells are involved in the increase in NK activity seen during the first week of treatment? (2) Why does NK activity decline after the first week of treatment despite continued IFN administration? With regard to the first question, there is good evidence that NK cytotoxicity requires a sequence of events. The first event is the binding of target cells to the potential killer cells, followed by the actual cytolysis process. However, only about one-half of the binding cells ordinarily will kill the targets. In vitro studies by Targan and colleagues (Targan and Dorey, 1980) have shown that treatment of lymphocytes with IFN in vitro results in an increase in the proportion of those binding cells that can actually kill. However, IFN in vitro does not generally affect the proportion of cells that can actually bind the target. This as well as other evidence suggests that IFN primarily affects the most mature NK cells and not the less mature precursors of NK cells.

TABLE II

Single-Cell Analysis of Nylon Fiber Column (NFC)-Passed PBL
from IFN-Treated Melanoma Patients[a]

Patient	Day 0		Day 2		Day 7		Day 35	
	B	NK	B	NK	B	NK	B	NK
12	15	0	22	4	25	10	17	4
13	13	3.6	14	5.6	19	7.6	12	1.6
14	14	2.5	16	2.2	24	5.7	11	1.0
6	11	n.t.[b]	9	n.t.	16	n.t.	9	n.t.

[a]B, Target-binding lymphocytes (%); NK, lytic lymphocytes
(% binders × % binders that kill).
[b]n.t., Not tested.

When we monitored for changes in binding and killing of NK-
sensitive targets using the single-cell assay developed by Grimm
and Bonavida (1979), we found that both the number of target-binding cells and the number of target-killing cells increased during
the first week of IFN treatment. The increase in binding was confined to NK-sensitive targets, as there was no increased number of
binders to NK-resistant target cells. Throughout the course of
treatment the NK cells that actually mediated target-cell killing
retained the usual characteristics of NK cells (nonadherence to
nylon fiber columns and adherence to antigen-antibody complexes).
Several examples of such results are shown in Table II. Thus, our
data suggested that the *in vivo* treatment with IFN resulted in a
different type of change than *in vitro* treatment of lymphocytes
with IFN. In addition to the well-documented increase in cytotoxicity by mature NK cells, our data suggest that additional cells
are recruited from precursors of NK cells into the NK differentiation pathway. Presumably, such precursors come from the bone marrow, or perhaps from the spleen, and are obviously not readily
available when one tests for *in vitro* responses of peripheral blood
lymphocytes to IFN.
    The single-cell results suggest that IFN affects the recruit-
ment of NK cells from precursors, but we had to use indirect means
to confirm this. To determine if there is any increase in the number or activity of NK inactive precursors of NK cells during IFN
treatment, we attempted to generate NK activity *in vitro*. Cryopreserved PBL from various points during treatment were depleted
of NK activity by passage over EAγ monolayers. The nonadherent
cells were then stimulated in microwell plates with allogeneic
lymphoblastoid cell line cells. After 6 days of culture, sets of
microwell plates were assayed for proliferation, and other sets
were assayed for cytotoxic activity against K562 targets. The

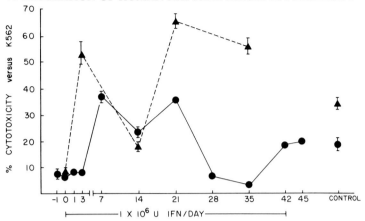

DAYS POST INITIAL TREATMENT

Fig. 2. Natural killer (NK) and cell-mediated lymphocytotoxicity (CML) responses of PBL from patient 4. Peripheral blood lymphocytes were tested for NK cytotoxicity (●——●) versus K562 at various times during treatment with 1×10^6 units IFN/day. Also, PBL were cryopreserved, depleted of NK activity by passage over a EAγ monolayer, and stimulated for 6 days with allogeneic lymphoblasts. Cells were tested in CML assay versus K562 (▲---▲). Vertical bars, SE. Control is the NK and CML responses of a simultaneously tested healthy donor.

results of a representative experiment of this type are given in Fig. 2. The ability to generate NK activity *in vitro* shows a similar time course as the original NK activity detected in the peripheral blood. No differences in proliferative activity were observed at any point during treatment, although differences were detected in cytotoxicity. Nonstimulated control PBL showed no cytotoxicity. In four such series of experiments with the use of PBL from four IFN-treated patients, increased anti-K562 cytotoxicity could be generated from PBL drawn at the time of peak NK activity or at times just preceding peak NK activity. These data supported, although did not directly prove, the concept that IFN treatment is associated with an increase in NK precursors.

We do not think that our results conflict with those of *in vitro* studies, but describe an additional biological activity in the IFN-NK system. In agreement with our hypothesis that IFN systemic administration promotes the differentiation of NK precursors into mature NK cells is our finding that lymphocytes drawn from IFN-treated patients (and depleted *in vitro* of mature NK cells) have an augmented ability to generate new cytotoxic cells. These data are at least consistent with the concept that IFN affects both precursors of NK cells and mature NK cells.

We also examined the events involved in the decline in NK activity after the first week of treatment. One can visualize several possible explanations for this decline, including (a) the

depletion of precursors from the pool of available cells, presumably located in the bone marrow, (b) redistribution of NK cells
from the circulation to other sites, or (c) activation of suppressor cells able to suppress NK activity. Thus far, we have been
unable to find any evidence for the development of suppressor cell
activity that is associated with the period of declining NK cytotoxicity. Lymphocytes obtained late in IFN treatment, when NK activity had declined, failed to inhibit NK activity of either normal lymphocytes or pretreatment lymphocytes from the same patient.
Since macrophages have often been shown to suppress various cellular functions, including NK cytotoxicity, we performed experiments to determine if adherent cells could be suppressing the NK
activity. Removal of adherent cells caused a slight increase in
NK activity, but this increase was no greater in the period of
low NK activity than in other time points during IFN treatment.
Furthermore, inhibitors of prostaglandin synthesis, such as indomethacin, failed to restore responsiveness. Thus, it is unlikely
that a prostaglandin-secreting macrophage is responsible for the
low NK cytotoxicity late in IFN treatment. This does not mean that
there are no suppressor cells for NK activity, but simply that activation of suppressor cells is not a likely explanation for the
low NK activity after the first week of IFN treatment.

When lymphocytes from IFN-treated patients were tested for
their response to IFN in vitro, a marked difference was found between lymphocytes drawn before or early in treatment and those
drawn late in treatment. One standard dose of IFN (60-min treatment with 100 units) resulted in a consistent increase in cytotoxicity for pretreatment lymphocytes, averaging 8.2% increase in the
chromium release assay. A similar level of increase was found
with samples drawn during the first week of treatment (7.6%). However, samples drawn from the period of peak cytotoxicity through
the rest of treatment had a very poor response to leukocyte IFN
in vitro (1.4%). This response promptly returned to normal after
in vivo treatment was terminated (13.7%). These results, along
with our other results (Golub et al., 1982b), indicate that cellular resistance to IFN activation is probably a key event in the
IFN-induced decline in NK activity.

One other possibility that should be considered is that IFN
induces changes in the types of lymphocytes in the circulation.
We were unable to find any significant differences in total lymphocyte counts, or proportions of cells with E receptors, complement
receptors, or FcY receptors (Golub, 1982a). However, our most recent data do indicate that the proportion of cells bearing the
"HNK-1" antigen detected by the monoclonal antibody developed by
Abo and Balch (1981) may reflect the changes in cytotoxicity. Drs.
Abo and Balch generously provided antibody to us, and our preliminary results are presented in Table III. We assessed the portion
of HNK-1 positive (HNK-1+) cells among nylon nonadherent PBL at
selected time points during IFN treatment. The trend is toward
increased numbers of HNK-1 positive cells at peak NK cytotoxicity

TABLE III

Percentage of HNK-1[+] Cells in NFC-Passed PBL
of IFN-Treated Melanoma Patients

Patient	Day 0 (%)	Day 2 or 3 (%)	Day 7 (%)	Day 21 or 35 (%)
6	16%	18%	23%	15%
12	22	8	14	26
13	12	15	17	14
14	6	3	9	6
16	16	23	21	n.t.[a]

[a] n.t., Not tested.

(Day 7), although this was not the case in all samples tested.
Further studies are in progress to determine if the phenotype of
the circulating NK cell changes during IFN treatment.

B. Effects of BCG

It has been shown that BCG augments NK cytotoxicity in mice
(Wolfe et al., 1977), in healthy humans (Thatcher and Crowther,
1978), and in melanoma patients (Thatcher et al., 1979). In our
preliminary results, we have also observed an augmentation of NK
activity against K562 target cells in melanoma patients treated
with intravenous BCG or intralesional BCG (Golub, 1981).
Our results with the ^{51}Cr-release assay indicated that BCG
augmented PBL-mediated cytotoxicity against K562 target cells.
This could be a result of more cytotoxic cells or greater cytotoxicity per NK cell. To address this question, we utilized the single-cell cytotoxicity analysis. We examined a group of 14 stage
II and III melanoma patients treated with intralymphatic immunotherapy (ILI) consisting of intradermal BCG and intralymphatic administration of either an irradiated tumor-cell vaccine or vaccine
plus BCG. Further details of the immunization procedure are given
in Ahn et al. (1982). As can be seem in Table IV, these treatments
resulted in an increased number of K562-binding cells, and this
increase persisted throughout the treatment. However, the proportion of cells lytic for K562 among the binders did not increase.
This indicates that more NK cells are recruited rather than more
lytic activity per cell, and is similar to our IFN results. It is
interesting to note that the number of cells able to bind to the
M14 melanoma target also increased during treatment. This target
is resistant to NK cells, and BCG or IFN treatment alone does not
increase cytotoxicity against this target (Golub, 1981). However,

TABLE IV

Single-Cell Analysis of Melanoma Immunotherapy Patients

	PBL obtained prior to treatment no.				
	1	2	3	4	5 to 8
K562 binders (%)	8.3 ± 0.6	10.3 ± 0.8	13.0 ± 1.1	11.9 ± 0.9	12.6 ± 0.9
K562 binders that kill (%)	22.3 ± 3.0	21.7 ± 2.3	21.5 ± 2.8	20.4 ± 2.1	19.8 ± 1.7
NK (%)	1.9 ± 0.3	2.2 ± 0.2	2.6 ± 0.3	2.4 ± 0.3	2.5 ± 0.3
M14 binders (%)	6.5 ± 0.9	11.3 ± 1.3	11.0 ± 1.3	12.5 ± 2.0	11.1 ± 1.6
Number of samples tested	14	13	13	10	12

the M14 line was included in the vaccine used to treat the patients, and the increased number of cytotoxic cells probably represents allospecific T cells rather than NK cells.

The design of this experimental immunotherapy protocol precluded assessment of the relative roles of the BCG and vaccine in altering NK activity, since all patients received both agents. However, the route of administration of the BCG seemed to affect only slightly the increase in activity against K562. Of the 14 ILI patients we studied, 7 received intralymphatic BCG plus intradermal BCG, while 7 received only intradermal BCG. The intralymphatic group showed an increase from $8.9 \pm 0.9\%$ binders (pretreatment) to $14.4 \pm 1.6\%$ (after two treatments), while the intradermal BCG group showed an increase from $7.7 \pm 0.6\%$ to $10.8 \pm 1.0\%$ in the same time period. Thus, either the ILI or the BCG or both were capable of augmenting PBL NK activity. These results again indicate that PBL NK activity can be modulated, although proving that this results in clinical effects is difficult. These results also suggest that alloimmunization may augment NK cytotoxicity and provide an *in vivo* counterpart to our observation that mixed lymphocyte culture (MLC) generates NK activity (Seeley and Golub, 1978).

III. LOCAL AND REGIONAL REGULATION OF NK

A. Tumor-Infiltrating Lymphocytes (TIL)

1. *Natural Killer Activity*

One of the general assumptions among those studying NK cells is that these cells are important in the host defense against tumors. However, little evidence is available to indicate that NK cells actively restrict tumor growth of established tumors or can lead to tumor regression. One approach to this question has been to study the cells at the actual tumor site. Such studies have generally shown that the human lymphoid cells infiltrating tumor sites have little NK activity (Vose *et al.*, 1977; Totterman *et al.*, 1978; Moore and Vose, 1981). Our purpose was to determine if NK cells are even present at tumor sites as well as the influence of the tumor microenvironment on NK function. To do this, we studied both tumor-infiltrating lymphocytes (TIL) from human pulmonary tumors and TIL from human tumors that had received an intralesional injection of BCG. As BCG can augment NK activity in humans (Thatcher and Crowther, 1978), and since this agent can provoke intense granulomatous reactions at injected tumor sites, we felt that this would be a useful way to study the regulation of NK activity in the presence of a tumor mass.

We have previously reported (Niitsuma *et al.*, 1981) that TIL from human pulmonary tumors have decreased proportions of T cells and decreased activity in assays of T cell function including alloantigen-induced proliferation and generation of cytolytic T cells.

However, we did find considerable proportions of cells with Fcγ
receptors among these TIL (average of 18.8% EAγ rosette-forming
cells), and therefore it is possible that NK activity would be
present among TIL. However, ^{51}Cr-release assays against K562 targets showed low activity among TIL from pulmonary tumors. The TIL
were obtained by mechanical disaggregation, Ficoll-Hypaque density
gradient centrifugation, and further fractionated by filtration
through nylon monofilament mesh to remove tumor cells. We have
shown that removal of residual tumor cells did not result in improvement of NK activity (Niitsuma et al., 1981), indicating that
the low NK activity is not due to cold-target competition by residual tumor cells. However, TIL obtained from tumors injected 2
weeks prior to surgery with intralesional BCG did exhibit higher
levels of NK activity than TIL from uninjected tumors (20.5 ± 7.7%
for 5 BCG-injected tumors compared to 7.7 ± 1.9% at 50:1 for TIL
from 20 uninjected tumors). Similarly, hilar lymph node lymphocytes (LNL) and peripheral blood lymphocytes (PBL) from the same
BCG-injected patients showed modestly higher NK activity. It is
interesting to note that in three cases we were able to obtain
BCG-injected TIL and uninjected TIL from the same patients. These
patients had multiple pulmonary metastases, only one of which was
BCG injected. In these cases, the NK activity of uninjected TIL
remained low (5.7%), while the NK activity of TIL from the adjacent
BCG-injected tumors was high (24.8%). These preliminary results
suggest that the induction of augmented NK activity at one tumor
site, even in combination with augmented systemic NK activity among
PBL and LNL, does not necessarily ensure the delivery of active NK
cells at other tumor deposits. In this sense, our results are
compatible with the suggestion of Hanna and Fidler (1980) that NK
activity is most effective against circulating tumor cells and of
less relevance in defenses against established tumor deposits.

We then asked whether there were target-binding and killing
cells among the TIL. For this assessment we utilized the single-
cell assay of Grimm and Bonavida (1979). Results of this analysis
are shown in Table V. Thus far, we have seen equivalent numbers
of target-binding cells among TIL as we see among PBL from the
same patients. The proportion of those binding cells actually
mediating cytolysis in a 3-hr assay is also similar among TIL as
compared to PBL. Thus, the low activity in ^{51}Cr-release assays
is probably not due to a lack of NK cells among the TIL but instead appears to be due to a functional impairment of these cells.
Since the proportion of K562-killing cells among the binders is
comparable to PBL, the functional impairment is most likely in the
kinetics of lysis or in the recycling ability of the NK cells among
the TIL. In line with this hypothesis are the results of Moore and
Vose (1981) and our unpublished observations that TIL cannot be ac-

TABLE V

Single-Cell Analysis of TIL and PBL NK Activity
(21 Patients)

	PBL	TIL
K562-Binding cells (%)	11.8 ± 1.0	11.9 ± 1.1
Binders that kill (%)	11.6 ± 2.2	15.0 ± 3.4
NK (%)[a]	1.3 ± 0.2	1.5 ± 0.3

[a]Product of % binders × % binders that kill.

tivated to further NK activity with interferon. Interferon, which
has been shown to accelerate the kinetics of NK-induced lysis (Silva et al., 1980), would presumably promote recycling and might have
little effect on cells unable to mediate repeated lytic events.

2. *Suppressor Cell Activity in TIL*

One possible mechanism for the suppressed activity in NK assays of TIL would be the presence of suppressor cells of NK function. We have examined this possibility by the addition of TIL
to autologous PBL and have not found the mixtures to show significantly diminished cytotoxic activity relative to the PBL. Although TIL have been reported to contain suppressor cells for proliferative responses (Vose and Moore, 1979), our results (Table
VI) show very little suppressive influence of the TIL on NK activity. Furthermore, removal of adherent cells on nylon fiber columns also failed to restore NK activity (Niitsuma et al., 1981),
indicating that an adherent suppressor of NK activity appears to
be unlikely in this situation. Furthermore, incubation in the
presence of indomethacin for 18 hr failed to restore NK activity
of TIL. Of course, it is possible that suppressor cells for the
development of NK cells from their precursors exist or that the
conditions we chose to test for suppressor cells are not able to
detect their presence. However, it is also possible that suppressor functions, like proliferative and cytotoxic functions, are not
fully expressed by TIL. The microenvironment of the tumor may not
be conducive to any differentiated cell functions, including suppression. Presumably, the environment in carcinomatous effusions
allows the development of suppressor cells for NK activity (Mantovani et al., 1980), although even those suppressor cells require
24 hr to exert their activity.

TABLE VI

Lack of Suppression of NK by TIL[a]

Lung tumor patient no.	TIL 50:1	TIL 25:1	PBL 50:1	PBL + TIL	50:1 50:1	50:1 25:1
1	5	n.t.[c]	56		49	n.t.
2	2	0	30		24	27
3	0	0	9		10	11
4	2	n.t.	43		n.t.	44
5	1	n.t.	31		25	n.t.
6[b]	8	0	43		39	n.t.

Column header group: Lysis of K562 (%) at E:T ratio of

[a] In ^{51}Cr-release microassay.
[b] BCG-injected tumor.
[c] n.t., Not tested.

B. NK Activity in Regional Lymph Nodes

Human lymph node lymphocytes (LNL) are generally regarded as low in NK activity (Moore and Vose, 1981). However, the primary source of LNL has been axillary or inguinal nodes. In our studies of pulmonary tumors we have examined hilar nodes. The hilar nodes of these patients exhibited significant NK activity in ^{51}Cr-release assays (Table VII) with average activity approaching that of PBL from these patients (average ^{51}Cr release by PBL, 27.3%).

TABLE VII

NK Activity of Lymph Node Cells

	Hilar nodes (7)	Axillary nodes[a]
^{51}Cr Release (50:1)	15.4 ± 4.8	5.3 ± 0.7 (36)
K562 Binders (%)	11.8 ± 3.1	11.3 ± 0.7 (34)
Binders that kill (%)	19.6 ± 3.9	7.4 ± 0.4 (19)
NK (%)	2.2 ± 0.7	1.0 ± 0.4 (19)

[a] From five patients. Number of nodes individually tested given in parentheses.

In contrast to these hilar nodes are the axillary nodes from melanoma patients (Table VII). The axillary LNL are quite low in the ^{51}Cr-release assay, with many nodes exhibiting no detectable activity. It should be pointed out that none of these nodes contained tumor and none were from BCG-treated patients. Even so, this comparison is of limited validity, for we cannot determine if the difference is due to anatomical location, tumor type, or other parameters.

Despite these limitations, our single-cell analyses of LNL have provided an interesting hint at a different mechanism for regulation of NK expression. The predominant difference between the hilar and axillary LNL in NK activity appears to be in the higher proportion of hilar K562-binding cells that can kill these targets. Hilar and axillary LNL had equivalent proportions of K562-binding cells, but more than twice as many of the hilar binders were lytic as compared to the axillary binders (Table VII). This suggests that NK activity of LNL may be a function of degree of maturation of NK cells from nonlytic but target binding "pre-NK" cells. Our preliminary results indicate that NK or NK-like activity can be developed from noncytolytic LNL by culture in the presence of T cell growth factor (J. D. Gray and S. H. Golub, unpublished). Thus, NK activity of LNL can be modulated.

IV. CONCLUSIONS

Our studies indicate several types of *in vivo* regulation of NK cytotoxicity. Systemic activation of NK by IFN or BCG was associated with an increase in the number of cytotoxic cells. Other evidence, such as the quantitation of MLC-generated NK activity, is in agreement with the single-cell data, and together they indicate that a major mode of "up-regulation" is the development of more cytotoxic cells from noncytotoxic precursors. Whether other cells or factors modulate this process, or if it is a direct response of precursor cells to the stimulus, has yet to be determined.

"Down-regulation" of NK appears to be a complex process. We have identified three different manifestations of decreased NK activity. After a week or more of systemic IFN treatment, NK activity returned from high levels to pretreatment levels. This decline was associated with less target-binding cells and the development of cellular resistance to IFN activation. The second instance is the low NK activity of axillary LNL, which is associated with normal binding activity but poor lytic function. The third situation is TIL that have levels of target binding and killing that are comparable to PBL but display poor activity in ^{51}Cr-release tests. This could be a result of impaired kinetics of lysis or impaired recycling. It is interesting to note that none of these three situations was clearly associated with suppressor cell functions. A better understanding of how these various forms of down-regulation are mediated may provide us with better opportunities to utilize NK cells as antitumor effectors.

ACKNOWLEDGMENTS

These studies were supported by NIH Grants CA-12582 and CA-29938. The authors thank Mr. Dean Hara and Ms. Veronica Routt for technical help and Ms. Lisa DeTournay for assistance in preparation of the manuscript.

REFERENCES

Abo, T., and Balch, C. M. (1981). *J. Immunol. 127,* 1024-1029.
Ahn, S. S., Irie, R. F., Weisenburger, T. H., Jones, P. C., Juillard, G., Roe, D. J., and Morton, D. L. (1982). *Surgery (St. Louis) 92,* 362-367.
Djeu, J. Y., Heinbaugh, J. A., Holden, H. T., and Herberman, R. B. (1978a). *J. Immunol. 122,* 175-181.
Djeu, J. Y., Heinbaugh, J. A., Holden, H. T., and Herberman, R. B. (1978b). *J. Immunol. 122,* 182-188.
Droller, M. J., Schneider, M. V., and Perlmann, P. (1978). *Cell. Immunol. 39,* 165-177.
Einhorn, S., Blomgren, H., and Strander, H. (1978). *Acta Med. Scand. 204,* 477-483.
Golub, S. H. (1981). In "Fundamental Mechanisms in Human Cancer Immunology" (J. P. Saunders, J. C. Daniels, B. Serrou, C. Rosenfeld, and C. B. Denney, eds.), pp. 477-479. Elsevier-North Holland, New York.
Golub, S. H., Rangel, D. M., and Morton, D. L. (1977). *Int. J. Cancer 20,* 873-880.
Golub, S. H., Dorey, F., Hara, D., Morton, D. L., and Burk, M. (1982a). *J. Natl. Cancer Inst. (US) 68,* 703-710.
Golub, S. H., D'Amore, P., and Rainey, M. (1982b). *J. Natl. Cancer Inst. (US) 68,* 711-717.
Grimm, E., and Bonavida, B. (1979). *J. Immunol. 123,* 2861-2869.
Gutterman, J. U., Blumenschein, G. R., Alexanian, R., Yap, H. Y., Buzdar, A. U., Cabanillas, R., Hortobagyi, G. N., Gersh, E. M., Rasmussen, S. L., Harmon, N., Kramer, M., and Pestka, S. (1980). *Ann. Intern. Med. 93,* 399-406.
Hanna, N., and Fidler, I. J. (1980). *J. Natl. Cancer Inst. (US) 65,* 801-809.
Huddlestone, J. R., Merigan, T. O., Jr., and Oldstone, M. B. (1979) *Nature (London) 282,* 417-420.
Kariniemi, A. L., Timonen, T., and Kousa, M. (1980). *Scand. J. Immunol. 12,* 371-374.

Krown, S. E., Burk, M., Kirkwood, J. M., Kerr, D., Nordlund, J. J., Morton, D. L., and Oettgen, H. F. (1981). *Proc. Am. Assoc. Cancer Res.* 22, 158.

Mantovani, A., Allavena, P., Sessa, C., Bolis, G., and Mangioni, C. (1980). *Int. J. Cancer 25*, 573-582.

Merigan, T. C., Sikora, K., Breeden, J. H., Levy, R., and Rosenberg, S. A. (1978). *N. Engl. J. Med. 299*, 1449-1453.

Moore, M., and Vose, B. M. (1981). *Int. J. Cancer 27*, 265-272.

Niitsuma, M., Golub, S. H., Edelstein, R., and Holmes, E. C. (1981). *J. Natl. Cancer Inst. (US) 67*, 997-1003.

Ortaldo, J. R., MacDermott, R. P., Bonnard, G. D., Kind, P. D., and Herberman, R. B. (1979). *Cell. Immunol. 48*, 356-368.

Pross, H. F., and Baines, M. G. (1976). *Int. J. Cancer 18*, 593-604.

Savary, C. A., and Lotzova, E. (1978). *J. Immunol. 120*, 239-243.

Seeley, J. K., and Golub, S. H. (1978). *J. Immunol. 120*, 1415-1422.

Silva, A., Bonavida, B., and Targan, S. (1980). *J. Immunol. 125*, 479-484.

Strander, H. (1977). *Blut 35*, 279-299.

Takasugi, M., Ramseyer, A., and Takasugi, J. (1977). *Cancer Res. 37*, 413-418.

Targan, S., and Dorey, F. (1980). *J. Immunol. 124*, 2157-2161.

Thatcher, N., and Crowther, D. (1978). *Cancer Immunol. Immunother. 5*, 105-107.

Thatcher, N., Swindell, R., and Crowther, D. (1979). *Clin. Exp. Immunol. 36*, 227-233.

Totterman, T. H., Hayry, P., Saksela, P., Timonen, T., and Eklund, B. (1978). *Eur. J. Immunol. 8*, 872-875.

Tracey, D. E. (1979). *J. Immunol. 123*, 840-845.

Vose, B. M., and Moore, M. (1979). *Int. J. Cancer 24*, 579-585.

Vose, B. M., Vanky, R., Argov, S., and Klein, E. (1977). *Eur. J. Immunol. 7*, 753-757.

Wolfe, S. A., Tracey, D. E., and Henney, C. S. (1977). *J. Immunol. 119*, 1152-1158.

DISCUSSION

WEISS: You showed "NK activity" against K562 targets, but the same "NK cells" had no activity against M14 targets. How can one tell which estimate of activity is relevant to the patient's own tumor?

GOLUB: Unfortunately, we can't. Probably both are, as there may be considerable heterogeneity of both NK cells and target cells. That is, some but not all NK cells may react to M14 cells, although this is not usually associated with lysis, but they can be made to kill M14 by long incubation (18 hr) plus IFN activation *in vitro*.

Similarly, this meeting has emphasized the heterogeneity of the tumor cells. In any case, I do not have a direct answer to your question, but this is an important problem that needs to be addressed.

KONDO: High NK activity in hilar lymph nodes seems to be due to exposure of the lungs to viruses. Is it possible to think that the effect of IFN on NK cells is due to inhibition of naturally infected viruses that reduced immune reaction of the host?

GOLUB: I think that the NK-IFN system is clearly related to the infection history of the host, particularly with respect to viruses. I do not know if viral infections and immune suppression are modulated by NK cells.

HOSHINO: (1) How did you measure the target-binding cells? We discovered one NK cell binds to a target and then moves to the other target. Therefore, target binding itself probably has no relation to activity of cytotoxicity. (2) Did you count LGL? (3) Our study showed IFN does not accelerate autologous killing, but OK632 produce a capacity of autologous killing.

GOLUB: (1) With an agarose assay that prevents recycling. We use both the single-cell assay and the ^{51}Cr assay to allow us to assay both binding and killing as well as recycling. (2) Not yet, these studies are in progress. (3) This is an interesting result. I do not doubt that there are other means of regulating NK cytotoxicity besides IFN. Your result agrees with our thinking that NK cells are quite heterogeneous.

ISHIKAWA: Do you have some evidence whether NK cells, activated either by IFN or by BCG, can kill the autologous tumor cells?

GOLUB: We have some very preliminary evidence that BCG-activated NK cells may kill autologous tumors, but our experience is very small. We have no data on IFN-activated NK cells. This is an important problem and we are trying to study it.

CHAPTER 8

SIGNIFICANCE OF LOCAL T CELL RESPONSE
TO HUMAN CANCER[1]

Kokichi Kikuchi
Kiyoshi Kasai
Hiroyoshi Hiratsuka
Tomoaki Usui
Hirofumi Kamiya
Izuru Shimokawara

Department of Pathology
Sapporo Medical College
Sapporo, Japan

[1]Supported by Grant-in-Aid by the Ministry of Education, Science, and Culture, and the Ministry of Welfare of Japan.

BASIC MECHANISMS AND CLINICAL TREATMENT
OF TUMOR METASTASIS

I. INTRODUCTION

    Our previous experiments with the autochthonous tumor system
of the rat showed clearly that the intensity of the lymphocyte infiltration in the tumor tissue correlated well with the tumor-
specific immune resistance and *in vitro* cytotoxic tests (Kikuchi
et al., 1972, 1974). It was further shown by electron microscopy
and immunofluorescence studies that the majority of infiltrating
lymphocytes were T cells, which often located themselves intimately
to the target autologous tumor cells and finally rejected the tumor cells (Kikuchi *et al.*, 1976).
    On the basis of the results, we extended our experiments to
the investigation of human cancer. Lymphocyte subpopulations and
subsets infiltrating in cancer tissues of the stomach, breast,
uterine cervix, and oral cavity were identified with immunoperoxidase technique using anti-human lymphocyte monoclonal antibodies.
Intensity of infiltration of T and B cells and their subsets in
the marginal part of the tumor invasion was semiquantified, and
the relationship between the grade of lymphocyte infiltration,
especially of T cells, in cancer tissue and clinical and immunologic parameters were studied.

II. PATIENTS AND METHODS
     USED IN THIS STUDY

    Forty-six patients with breast cancer, 68 patients with gas-
tric cancer, 15 patients with uterine cancer, and 38 patients with
oral cancer were studied. Biopsy specimens and surgical specimens
of the cancer tissues were examined. Clinical stages and histologic types were determined according to the Japanese Research Society for each cancer.
    Monoclonal antibodies used mainly in this study are listed in
Table I. Their mouse homologues and distribution and known function of cells recognized by these monoclonal antibodies are also
shown. HTL, HLy-1, HLy-2,3, DR, HLB-1, and HLB-2 were monoclonal
antibodies produced in our laboratory. The specificity was well
investigated. HTL shows the same specificity as OKT-6, HLy-1 the
same as Leu-1 (OKT-1), and HLy-2,3 as Leu-2a,b (OKT-5,8). DR
recognizes the framework of human Ia antigens. HLB-1 is pan-B
specific and does not recognize plasma cells, lymphocytes of T
cell lineage, or lymphoid stem cells. HLB-2 is reactive only to
mature B cells.
    Frozen sections were fixed in periodate-lysine-paraformalde-
hyde (PLP) fixative (McLean and Nakane, 1974) for 15 min at 4°C.
After washing with PBS for 30 min, the sections were reacted with
monoclonal antibodies for 1 hr at room temperature. The sections
were then washed three times with PBS for 30 min and reincubated
with rabbit anti-mouse Ig serum for 1 hr at room temperature.

TABLE I

Monoclonal Antibodies Used for Immunohistology

| Human | | Mouse | Chemical | Distribution |
Sapporo	Leu	homolog	nature	and function[a]
HTL		TL	gp48K + β 2m	Thymic cortex
HLy-1	1	Lyt-1	gp65-72K	Thy (cortex < medulla), pan-T
HLy-2,3	2a,b	Lyt-2,3	gp30K	Tc/s, Thy 80%, T 20%,
	3a,b		gp62-55K	Ti/h, Thy 80%, T 60%,
	4		gp19-20K	MLC, pan-T
DR		Ia	gp33K + 28K	B, Mφ, stem, activated T,
HLB-1			n.d.	pan-B,
HLB-2			n.d.	peripheral B

[a]Tc/s, cytotoxic/suppressor T cells; Ti/h, inducer/helper T cells; Mφ, macrophages.

After washing with PBS for 30 min, the sections were stained by a biotin-avidin-horseradish method using biotinized goat anti-rabbit Ig antibody and avidin-peroxidase conjugate (Warnke and Levy, 1980). The enzyme reaction was developed with 0.05% 3,3',5,5'-diaminobenzidine tetrahydrochloride and 0.01% hydrogen peroxide in 0.05 M Tris-HCl buffer (pH 7.6).

Grading of lymphocyte infiltration in cancer tissue was made according to the following standards: none (-), slight (+), moderate (++), and marked (+++), considering the predominant picture and neglecting cellular reactions to necrosis or infection. Usually, two trained pathologists were engaged independently in evaluating and classifying the histology.

III. DISTRIBUTION OF THE ANTIGENS DEFINED
      WITH MONOCLONAL ANTIBODIES IN THE HEMATOPOIETIC
      CELL LINES AND NORMAL LYMPHOID TISSUES

The reactivity of the monoclonal antibodies used in this study to hematopoietic cell lines is shown in Table II. HLy-1 is reactive to all T cell lines, and HTL is reactive to the immature T cell lines, such as RPMI-8402, CCRF-CEM, and MOLT-4F. HLB-1 antigen distributes all cell lines of B cell lineage, whereas HLB-2 antigen is expressed only in the mature B cell lines.

TABLE II

Reactivity of Monoclonal Antibodies
to Hematopoietic Cell Lines

Cell lines	DR	cALL	SmIg	HLB 1	HLB 2	HTL	HLy-1	Leu 1	Leu 2	Leu 3
Non-T, non-B ALL										
KM-3, Reh	+	+	-	-	-	-	-	-	-	-
Pre-B										
NALM-18	+	+	+[a]	+	-	-	-	-	-	-
NALM-6	+	+	+[a]	+	-	-	-	-	-	-
Burkitt's and B-ALL										
Raji	+	+	+	+	-	-	-	-	-	-
Daudi	+	+	+	+	-	-	-	-	-	-
SU-DHL-4	+	+	+	+	-	-	-	-	-	-
BALM-1	+	-	+	+	-	-	-	-	-	-
BALM-3	+	-	+	+	-	-	-	-	-	-
EBV-transformed B										
RPMI-8075	+	-	+	+	+	-	-	-	-	-
RPMI-6410	+	-	+	+	+	-	-	-	-	-
Myeloma										
ARH 77	+	-	+	+	+	-	-	-	-	-
RPMI-8226	+	-	+	-	-	-	-	-	-	-
U226	+	-	+	-	-	-	-	-	-	-
Oda	+	-	+	-	-	-	-	-	-	-
T-Leukemia										
RPMI-8402	-	+	-	-	-	+	+	+	+	+
CCRF-CEM	-	+	-	-	-	+	+	+	-	+
MOLT-4F	-	-	-	-	-	+	+	+	+	+
Peer	-	-	-	-	-	-	+	+	-	+
MT-1	+	-	-	-	-	-	+	+	-	-
SKW-3	-	-	-	-	-	-	+	+	+	+

[a] CyIg.

    Immunohistological examination of the thymus revealed that HTL antigen was expressed only on the cortical cells. HLy-1 was expressed on both cortical and medullary thymocytes; however, the expression on the medullary cells was more intensive. HLy-1-positive cells were distributed in the paracortical area of the lymph node (Fig. 1) and in the periarterial sheath of the spleen. HLB-1 antigen was expressed mainly on the cells comprising lymphoid follicles of the lymph node (Fig. 2) and the spleen, and HLB-2 antigen was expressed more intensively on the cells in the mantle zone

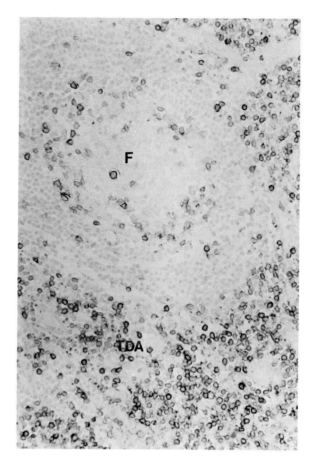

Fig. 1. Immunoperoxidase staining of lymph node sections with HLy-1 (Leu-1). Whereas lymphocytes in the paracortical area (TDA) were stained with HLy-1, most of the follicular cells were not stained except a few cells in the area between germinal center and mantle zone. The sections were counterstained lightly with methyl green. F, follicular cells.

of the lymphoid follicle and on the peripheral B cells. Monoclonal DR antibody was also sometimes useful as a B cell marker. On the section of the normal lymph node, DR-positive cells and HLy-1 (Leu-1)-positive cells were reciprocally located in the lymphoid follicle and the paracortical area. T cell subsets could be identified with HLy-1 (Leu-1), HLy-2,3 (Leu-2), Leu-3, and Leu-4 on the tissue sections. In the lymph node, HLy-2,3, which is considered to be expressed on killer/suppressor T cells, was expressed on about 20% of paracortical cells. Leu-3, which is considered to be expressed on inducer/helper T cells, was expressed on about 70% of paracortical cells.

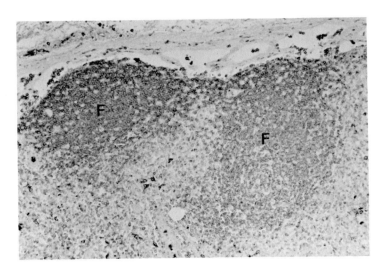

Fig. 2. Immunoperoxidase staining of lymph node sections with HLB-1. Follicular (F) cells were stained, but majority of the paracortical cells were not stained.

IV. T AND B CELLS IN CANCER TISSUES

Normal or benign lesions of the uterine cervix sometimes showed an abundant lymphocyte reaction. Most of them were proved to be HLB-1 and 2 and DR positive, that is, B cells. *In situ* cancer of the cervix is sometimes accompanied by subepidermal lymphoid cell infiltration. Most of these cells were not B cells but HLy-1- and 2,3-positive T cells. Early invasive cancer of the cervix was also accompanied with lymphoid infiltration, which was proved to be T cell response by immunoperoxidase study with monoclonal antibodies. In the advanced cancer of the uterine cervix, T cell infiltration was dominant compared with B cell infiltration. HLy-2,3-positive cells tended to decrease in advanced cancer of the cervix.

About the same results were obtained in breast cancer (Shimokawara *et al.*, 1982). Lymphocytes infiltrating in the normal breast or in the benign lesions were mostly B cells with surface IgA without exception. However, in breast cancer tissues, T cells were dominant in most cases (Fig. 3). In a few cases, T cells infiltrated to the same degree as B cells. There was no case of B cell-dominant infiltration in the breast cancer tissue examined. Macrophage infiltration was usually slight. Lymphocytes in a case of the medullary carcinoma with lymphoid infiltration were mostly HLy-1$^+$2,3$^+$HTL$^+$ T cells.

The same was true in the cancer of the stomach. B cells were the major lymphocyte in the lamina propria mucosa of normal stomach, chronic gastritis, or gastric ulcer; however, T cells became dominant in gastric cancer tissue, even in the early mucosal cancer

148

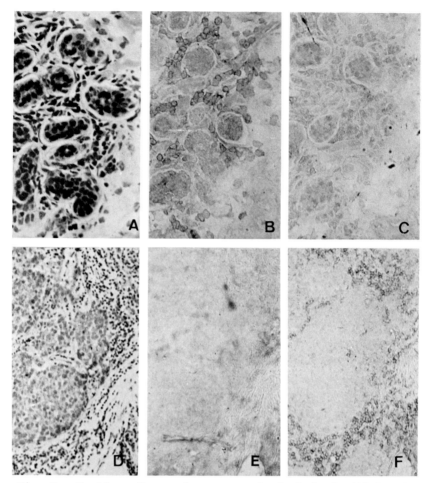

Fig. 3. Section of normal mammary gland stained with hematoxylin-eosin (H-E) (A), by immunoperoxidase technique with anti-B serum (B), and anti-T serum (C). Lymphoid cells around mammary tubule proved to be T cells. Section of cancer of the breast (medullary carcinoma with lymphoid infiltration) was stained with H-E (D), by immunoperoxidase technique with anti-B serum (E), and with anti-T serum (F). Numerous lymphocytes in cancer tissue proved to be T cells.

(Kikuchi *et al.*, 1979) (Fig. 4). Phenotype of these T cells was either Leu-2 (HLy-2,3) or Leu-3. We counted T and B cells in the randomly chosen microscopic fields, and T:B ratio was calculated. Figure 5 indicates a summary of T:B ratio in gastric cancer tissue and in other (benign) gastric lesions. Most of normal mucosa or chronic gastritis revealed T:B ratio of less than 1, that is, B cells were dominant over T cells. The T:B ratio in peptic ulcer was also less than 1. T:B ratios of the advanced cancer cases

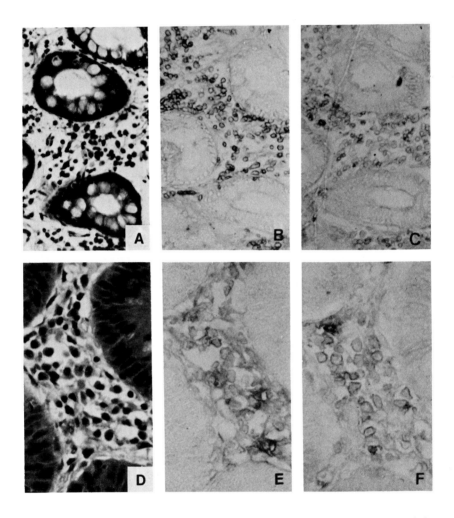

Fig. 4. Sections of chronic gastritis stained with H-E (A),
by immunoperoxidase technique with HLB-1 (B) and HLy-1 (C). B
cells are scattered predominantly over T cells. Sections of gastric atypia stained with H-E (D), by immunoperoxidase technique
with HLB-1 (E) and HLy-1 (F). In the atypical mucosa, both T and
B cells were found. Section of early mucosal gastric cancer
stained with H-E (G), by immunoperoxidase technique with HLB-1 (H)
and HLy-1 (I). T cell infiltration was dominant already. Sections
of advanced gastric cancer stained with H-E (J), by immunoperoxidase technique with HLB-1 (K) and HLy-1 (L). In the cancer tissue
T cells infiltrated but B cells were hardly seen.

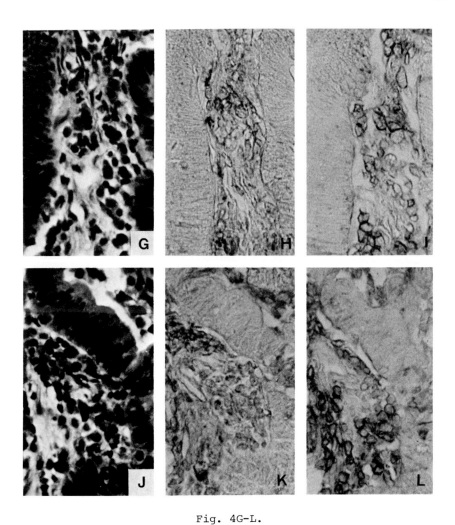

Fig. 4G–L.

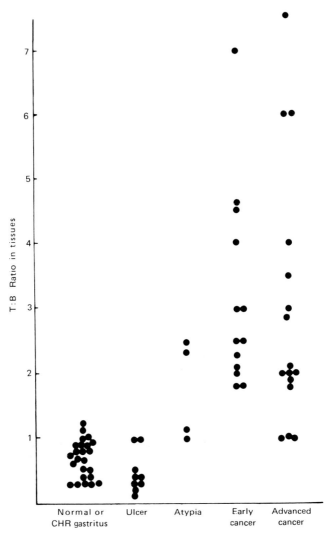

Fig. 5.   T:B cell ratios in lymphocytes infiltrating in cancer
tissues and benign lesions of the stomach.

Fig. 6.   Histopathology of squamous cell carcinoma of the
tongue infiltrated with many lymphocytes (A).   Immunoperoxidase
staining with HLB-1 (B) and HLy-1 (C) showed that the infiltrating
lymphocytes were T cells.   Invasive cancer of the tongue (D) was
surrounded by numerous lymphocytes that were Leu-1 (HLy-1) positive (E) by immunoperoxidase technique.   In this particular case,
majority of T cells had Leu-2 (HLy-2,3)-positive phenotype (F).
Leu-3-positive T cell was minor population (G).

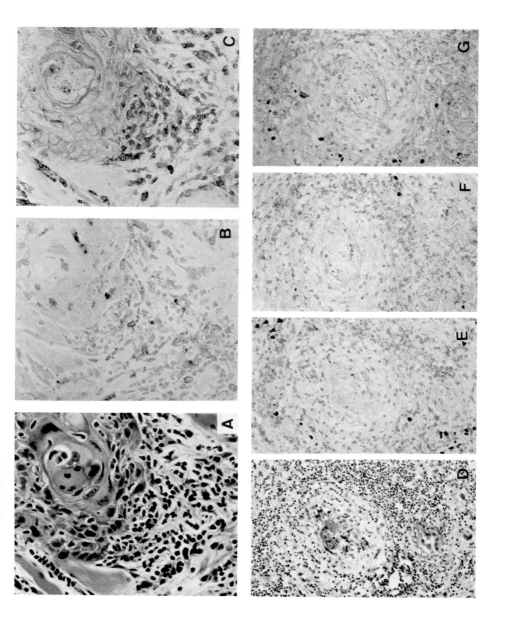

were variable, but they were more than 1--namely, T cell dominant--
in all cases. Even in the early cancers, T:B ratios were significantly high.

In the oral cancer, especially cancer of the tongue had relatively intensive macrophage and plasma cell response; however, the
similar tendency of T and B cell frequency was observed (Fig. 6)
as other cancers examined.

The pattern of T and B cell accumulation was different. T
cells tended to infiltrate around cancer cells and around blood
vessels, whereas B cells tended to accumulate at some distance
from cancer nests.

V.   FUNCTIONAL ROLE OF INFILTRATING T CELLS

Intensity of T cell infiltration in gastric cancer tissue was
correlated with mixed lymphocyte tumor cell interaction (MLTI) of
the identical patient (7). The ratios of Leu-2-positive cells
(suppressor/killer T cells) to Leu-3 cells (inducer/helper T cells)
in cancer tissues were variable from case to case. There was a
tendency for Leu-2-positive cells to be predominant over Leu-3-
positive cells in cancers of the uterine cervix and the stomach,
when lymphocyte response was high, especially in early stages.
However, the reverse was observed in cancers of the breast. No
significant correlation has been found between infiltrating T
cell subsets and clinical course. HTL$^+$ T cells were never found
in cancer tissues examined. It was difficult to delineate the
functional role of infiltrating T cells, since no suitable monoclonal antibodies have been developed to distinguish killer, suppressor, and helper T cells.

Lymphocytes were isolated from gastric cancer tissue and normal tissues, and *in vitro* functions were examined (Sakai and Koizumi, 1982). Cytotoxicity of the isolated lymphocytes from gastric cancer tissue against allogeneic cancer cell line, KATO-III,
was significantly high compared with those from noncancerous gastric mucosa. No K cell activity was found in the isolated lymphocytes.

VI.   CARCINOGENIC PROCESS AND T CELL RESPONSE

It is worthwhile to note that even the very early stage
of cancer, such as cancer *in situ* of the uterine cervix and early
mucosal cancer of the stomach, was infiltrated with T cells, in
contrast to B cell dominancy in the normal or benign lesions.
This phenomenon could be interpreted as a morphologic manifestation of immunologic surveillance of transformed cells. Interestingly, in some leukoplakia, lesion of the tongue was accompanied
with T cell infiltration (Fig. 7).

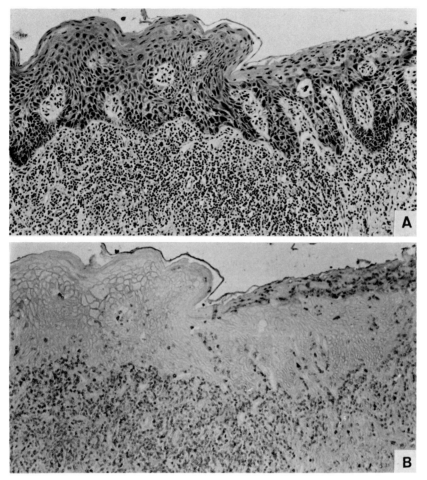

Fig. 7. Leukoplakia-like lesion near the cancer of the tongue was infiltrated with numerous lymphocytes (A), which were proved to be T cells by immunoperoxidase staining with HLy-1 (B).

Experimental gastric carcinoma induced by the oral administration of MNNG (N-methyl-N-nitroso-N'-nitrosoguanidine) in the rat showed the same host response to cancer cells as in human cancers. Immunoperoxidase studies with anti-rat T cell monoclonal antibodies of the early mucosal adenocarcinoma of the stomach revealed the similar T cell infiltration among cancer cells. Time course studies of lymphoid cell responsiveness against experimentally induced carcinoma are being carried out using various anti-rat lymphocyte monoclonal antibodies in order to clarify the dynamic aspects of host response to cancer cells during carcinogenesis and to determine the relevance of immune response in carcinogenesis.

TABLE III

Relationship between T Cell Infiltration
and Clinical Stage

| Stage | Grade of T cell infiltration in cancer | | | | | |
| | Breast | | | Tongue | | |
	-,+	++	+++	-,+	++	+++
I	4	3	2	1	2	1
II	3	1	1	1	3	3
III	10	1	0	2	2	3
IV	4	0	0	6	2	0
Total	21	5	3	10	9	6

VII. CLINICAL SIGNIFICANCE OF T CELL
      INFILTRATION IN CANCER TISSUE

The relationship between the intensity of T cell infiltration
in breast and oral cancer and clinical stages is shown in Table
III. There was a significant reverse correlation between clinical
stages and the grade of T cell infiltration in both cancers. T
cell infiltration was scanty in the advanced clinical stages.
This correlation was significant to $p < .05$ by Mann-Whitney's U
test.

Table IV shows the relationship between T cell infiltration
and lymph node metastasis. Breast and oral cancer patients with
lymph node metastasis tended to have a slight infiltration of T
cells. This correlation was also significant to $p < .025$ by Mann-
Whitney's U test.

T categories of TNM (Tumor Node Metastasis) classification of
the oral cancer and the grade of T cell infiltration were compared.
There was a significant ($p < .005$) correlation between them
(Table V).

More interestingly, sensitivity of the cancer of the tongue
to bleomycin, a chemotherapeutic agent, was parallel to the grade
of T cell infiltration in the primary cancer. In this project,
the size of the primary cancer was measured and cancer tissue was
biopsied. Immunoperoxidase study with antilymphocyte monoclonal
antibodies on lymphoid cells was done on the biopsy specimen, and
the grade of T cell infiltration was determined. The patient was
then given bleomycin, a total of 90 mg for 9 weeks. The tumor
size was measured after chemotherapy was finished, and operation

TABLE IV

Relationship between T Cell Infiltration
in Primary Cancer and Metastasis

Grade of T cell infiltration	Metastasis of cancer			
	Breast		Tongue	
	−	+	−	+
None, slight	3	15	4	6
Moderate	4	2	7	2
Marked	2	1	6	0

TABLE V

T Categories of TNM Classification
and Grade of T Cell Infiltration in Oral Cancer

Grade of T cell infiltration	T categories			
	T1	T2	T3	T4
None	0	0	0	2
Slight	1	1	2	4
Moderate	2	4	1	2
Marked	1	6	0	0

was carried out. Regression rate of the tumor by the treatment
was calculated and compared with the grade of T cell infiltration
in the primary cancer tissue. The relationship between the grade
of T cell infiltration and the regression rate, in which there
was a significant correlation, is shown in Fig. 8. Therefore, one
might predict the sensitivity of cancer to some anticancerous
agent, and this might mean the relevance of host responsiveness
in cancer treatment, which is manifested directly in the place of
cancer proliferation.

Although the follow-up study of the patients is still under-
way, the facts just outlined suggest the clinical significance of
T cell responsiveness in cancer tissue.

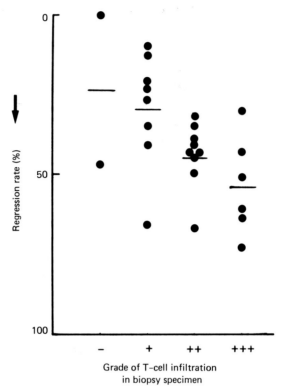

Fig. 8. Relationship between regression rates of the cancer of the tongue by bleomycin treatment and the grade of T cell infiltration in the primary cancer. There was a significant correlation between them.

VIII. CONCLUSIONS

The intimate correlation between lymphocyte infiltration in human cancer tissue and the clinical prognosis of the patients has been noticed for many years (Moore and Foote, 1949; Berg, 1971; Black and Leis, 1971), however, the significance of the phenomenon has not been completely elucidated. Progress in immunology has made it possible to analyze the histology more in detail. Advanced techniques of immunohistochemistry with a variety of monoclonal antibodies have permitted the identification of the origin of lymphocytes and their functional subsets.

It was evident that in normal or benign lesions, B cells were predominant over T cells, whereas in cancer tissues, T cells were predominant over B cells in all cases examined. There was some clinical significance of T cell response in cancer tissue. In short, the earlier the clinical stages of the patients, the greater the T cell response in cancer tissue was. The greater the T cell response in cancer tissue, the less frequent metastasis the patients had. Killer activity of isolated lymphoid cells from gastric cancer tissue to an allogeneic gastric cancer cell line was significantly high.

The functional role of infiltrating T cells is a problem that should be elucidated by using newly developed monoclonal antibodies or by isolating and propagating lymphocytes using TCGF (T Cell Growth Factor) or other agents. However, all the results obtained in this study and in the previous animal experiments support the hypothesis that T cells react to autochthonous cancer cells and that T cells infiltrating into cancer tissue are reacting directly to target cancer cells.

REFERENCES

Berg, J. W. (1971). *Cancer (Philadelphia)* 28, 1453-1456.
Black, M. M., and Leis, H. P. (1971). *Cancer (Philadelphia)* 28, 263-273.
Kikuchi, K., Kikuchi, Y., Phillips, M. E., and Southam, C. M. (1972). *Cancer Res.* 32, 516-521.
Kikuchi, K., Ishii, Y., Ueno, H., Kanaya, T., and Kikuchi, Y. (1974). *Gann Monogr. Cancer Res.* 16, 99-116.
Kikuchi, K., Ishii, Y., Ueno, H., and Koshiba, H. (1976). *Ann. N.Y. Acad. Sci.* 276, 188-206.
Kikuchi, K., Shimokawara, I., Takami, T., Yamanaka, N., and Ishii, Y. (1979). *In* "Immunobiology and Immunotherapy of Cancer" (W. Terry and Y. Yamamura, eds.), pp. 263-275. Elsevier-North Holland, New York.
McLean, I. W., and Nakane, P. K. (1974). *J. Histochem. Cytochem.* 22, 1077-1085.
Moore, O. S., Jr., and Foote, F. W., Jr. (1949). *Cancer (Philadelphia)* 2, 635-642.
Sakai, Y., and Koizumi, K. (1982). *Gastroenterology* 82, 1374-1380.
Shimokawara, I., Imamura, M., Yamanaka, N., Ishii, Y., and Kikuchi, K. (1982). *Cancer (Philadelphia)* 49, 1456-1464.
Warnke, R., and Levy, R. (1980). *J. Histochem. Cytochem.* 28, 771-776.

DISCUSSION

ISHIKAWA: Would you explain the meaning of the correlation between sensitivity to BLM and accumulation of T cells?

KIKUCHI: Any cancer therapy, including chemotherapy, should require immunological responsiveness to cancer cells in the background, I think. T cell response is a direct manifestation of host reactivity to cancer. Therefore, it is natural we found the correlation between the intensity of T cell response and regression rate of tumor. We observed the significance of T cell response in radiation therapy.

KONDO: It was my great surprise that even in the early gastric cancer tissue there was a high T:B ratio. Have you experienced the time course of T:B ratio in the same patient who did not receive chemotherapy?

KIKUCHI: No, we have not experienced any case of serial biopsy of gastric cancer, which was investigated immunohistologically. The first biopsy of early mucosal cancer revealed T cell infiltration without exception. We have an animal model of induction of gastric cancer in the rat. In this experiment, we are examining an infiltration lymphocyte subset using various newly produced monoclonal anti-rat T subset antibodies during carcinogenesis. The results will answer your question.

COCHRAN: We have similar studies in progress and would confirm your elegant findings. Marc Nestor, in my laboratory, finds T cell predominance in breast cancer, lung cancer, and melanoma. There is usually a T helper predominance, but we have observed a reversal to cytotoxic/suppressor cell predominance in Kaposi's sarcoma in immunosuppressed patients. Have you considered immune competence in your patients?

KIKUCHI: We have no data concerning the relationship between immunocompetence of the patients and T cell subsets infiltrating in cancer. Our results showed the ratio of Tc/s to Ti/h infiltrating was variable from case to case. There was a tendency that Tc/s (Leu-2$^+$T) was predominant over Ti/h when the infiltrating cells were abundant, especially at early stages; however, the reverse tendency was observed in breast cancer and oral cancer.

GOLUB: This is a very important approach, but showing the presence of a T subpopulation does not define the functional abilities of these cells. Have you examined T helper functions of lymphocytes purified from T helper-predominant tumors?

KIKUCHI: At this moment, we cannot show the functional abilities of infiltrating T cell subsets immunohistologically, because we have no monoclonal antibodies that distinguish suppressor T cells and helper T cells. *In vitro* tests of isolated lymphoid cells from gastric cancer tissue showed a significant cytotoxicity against allogeneic

gastric cancer cell line; however, the tests were un-
satisfactory to elucidate completely the functional role
of infiltrating cells.

HEPPNER: Comment: In our series of mouse mammary tumors, T cells
also predominate over B cells. With tumors produced by
the mammary tumor subpopulations described earlier, the
T killer-suppressor phenotype generally is greater than
the T helper phenotype. However, in one tumor the T
helper predominates, and this is by far our slowest
growing tumor. Among the tumors in which the T killer-
suppressor phenotypes predominate, there are both high-
and low-metastasizing tumor subpopulations. We have
used isokinetic gradient separation as a means to isolate the tumor-infiltrating T cells.

CHAPTER 9

NATURAL AND INDUCED RESISTANCE TO METASTASIS
FROM MOUSE MAMMARY CARCINOMAS

Jan Vaage

Department of Experimental Pathology
Roswell Park Memorial Institute
Buffalo, New York

I. INTRODUCTION

    Evidence from mouse mammary tumor studies suggests that host
defense reactions against immunogenic tumors may affect the incidence of metastatic spread (Vaage, 1973, 1974; Vaage and Agarwal,
1977). But nonimmunogenic and weakly immunogenic tumors probably
represent the majority of mouse mammary carcinomas (Hewitt and
Blake, 1975; Van de Velde *et al.*, 1977; Vaage, 1978a), and this
class was once considered outside of control by the host. However, natural protective factors are also known that may prevent
metastasis independently of specific antitumor immunity (Apffel,
1976; Vaage, 1978b; Bishop and Donald, 1979). There are, therefore, most likely several different biologic factors and mechanisms that prevent circulating, viable cancer cells from developing
into metastases. But one cannot yet generalize whether natural
resistance factors or induced resistance factors are the most important, or whether any resistance factors are as important in
preventing metastases as is the basic unacceptability of cells in
heterotopic locations. This review will not attempt to present a
comprehensive analysis of cell-mediated and humoral immunity to
mouse mammary tumors, because this topic has been exhaustively
treated in the reviews by Blair (1981) and Stutman (1982). Instead
it will focus primarily on information from *in vivo* investigations
of the role of host resistance in the control of mammary tumor
cells at successive stages of metastasis, starting with the release of cells from the primary tumor, through vascular dissemination, to resistance to secondary growth.

II. RESISTANCE TO METASTASIS
     AT THE PRIMARY TUMOR

    While the majority of primary mouse mammary tumors grow pro-
gressively, defensive processes may be activated that have the
potential to limit the spreading of tumor cells and the formation
of metastases. The infrequency of metastases in mouse mammary
tumor hosts, except when the animal is approaching death with overwhelming primary tumor burden, suggests the existence of an effective, but mainly unidentified defense mechanism. Since the original observations by DaFano (1912) and Murphy (1926), the accumulation of mononuclear cells in the stroma of a primary tumor has been
considered a host defense reaction (reviews by Underwood, 1974;
Evans, 1976). An inverse correlation between metastatic potential
and monocytic infiltration has been described in a rat tumor system
(Eccles and Alexander, 1974; Alexander, 1976). In the T1699 mammary carcinoma system of DBA/2 mice, the local accumulation of
lymphocytes, macrophages, and eosinophils was dependent on the status of immune reactivity against this immunogenic tumor (Parthenais

and Haskill, 1979). Treatment of tumor recipients with antilymphocyte IgG suppressed infiltration by all of these cell types, and
in thymectomized Tl699 hosts, the local reaction resembled immediate hypersensitivity, neutrophils being the major component. It
appeared that antibody-dependent, macrophage-mediated cytotoxicity
most effectively restricted Tl699 carcinoma size and invasion into
surrounding normal tissues. Inhibition of primary tumor growth
and invasion were related to metastatic frequency, because only
4% of normal mice developed pulmonary metastases, while 79% of
immunologically crippled mice developed pulmonary, lymphatic, and
hepatic metastases (Parthenais and Haskill, 1979). Lymphocytes
and other reactive cells such as macrophages may, however, accumulate at any site of inflammation. Their presence does not therefore necessarily demonstrate specific host recognition of and reaction to tumor antigens.

The fibrous tissue formation often associated with mammary carcinomas suggests that collagen formation is a defense mechanism
that, when successful, contains a primary tumor in a capsule. The
fibrous encapsulation can inhibit the release of potentially metastatic tumor cells and can, by collagen fiber shrinkage (Benjamin
et al., 1977), lead to a tumor's dormancy or destruction by con-
striction and occlusion of its vascular supply (Vaage and Ghandbhir, 1978; Vaage, 1979a). The mammary carcinoma MC2 may be rejected by about 20% of syngeneic, unimmunized, untreated female
implant recipients after a period of subcutaneous (sc) growth to
as much as 8 mm diameter. This tumor is therefore a convenient
model to study the local expression of a primary immune rejection
reaction, and the histologic characteristics of the local tumor-
host confrontation that results in 20% rejection. Typically,
small- and medium-sized lymphoid cells migrate from venules near
the sc tumor implant and are easily recognizable as perivascular
cuffing. Peritumor accumulation of lymphocytes occurs within 48
to 72 hours after implantation. These lymphoid cells show no
tendency to enter into the tumor implant but spread out along and
close to the surface of the implanted tumor tissue. The arrival
of lymphoid cells at the tumor implant is closely associated in
time and location with the formation of a fibrous capsule around
the tumor. An intact, continuous fibrous capsule is a typical
histologic feature of any MC2 implant that is examined during regression or prolonged constant size (dormancy?). Because no open
blood vessels can be found in serial sections of "dormant" or regressing tumors, it is suggested that vascular occlusion, caused
by a tightening fibrous capsule, could be an effective mechanism
of tumor destruction.

The growth of MC2 in syngeneic nu/nu athymic C3H/He mice, and
the histology of the local host reaction, present a different picture. Small lymphoid cells do not accumulate at MC2 implants, and
a fibrous capsule does not develop. Subcutaneous MC2 implants
spread very rapidly in nude mice, and after a few days of growth
they cannot be successfully excised because of extensive invasion
into surrounding tissues. Pulmonary metastases are commonly found

in nude C3H/He mice carrying sc MC2 implants, a significant dis-
tinction from normal C3H/He mice, in which metastases from primary
mammary carcinomas are very rarely found, except when a primary
tumor is very large and the host is close to death (Ashburn, 1937;
Wexler et al., 1965; Anderson et al., 1974; Pitelka et al., 1980).
By simple and alluring logic it may be suggested, then, that in
normal C3H/He mice, the release of cells from a primary MC2 implant
is obstructed when the process of fibrous capsular containment of
the primary tumor is complete. The process of tumor containment
involves peritumor lymphoid cell accumulation and collagen fiber
deposition in a relationship that is not yet understood, but the
importance of the relationship is indicated by its absence in
athymic nu/nu hosts.

The immunogenic MC2 and T1699 tumor systems are examples of
vigorous reactions against tumor-associated immunogens. These two
tumor models may represent the high side of a scale of effectiveness of resistance to primary tumor growth, invasion, and metastatic spread.

III. RESISTANCE TO TUMOR CELL DISSEMINATION

A. Vascular Dissemination

The vascular stage of tumor dissemination is probably critical
to the metastatic progress and may for that reason be the most
amenable to experimentation. Systemic analyses of the kinetics
and quantitation of cancer cells shed spontaneously from solid tumors into the circulation are limited (Liotta et al., 1974; Butler
and Gullino, 1975; Gullino, 1978) and, unfortunately, do not include mouse mammary adenocarcinomas. The numbers of circulating
cancer cells shed from a rat mammary carcinoma reached 10^6 cells/g
of tumor tissue per day, yet no overt metastases were reported
(Butler and Gullino, 1975). However, the fate of tumor cells introduced into the circulation by intravenous injection has become
a useful model of the postintravasation phases of metastases, namely, vascular distribution and subsequent growth in target organs.
Using intravenous (iv) inoculation, it was shown many years ago
(Iwasaki, 1915; Warren and Gates, 1936) that few of the cancer
cells introduced directly into the circulation survived to produce
"metastases." By the use of radiolabeled cancer cells it has been
shown that the low incidence of experimental "metastases" is largely due to the intravascular death of over 90% of the original cancer cell inoculum within 24 hr of iv injection (Fidler, 1970; Vaage
1978b; Bishop and Donald, 1979; Glaves, 1980). It has also become
apparent that, although many cancer cells may undergo seemingly
spontaneous lysis within the circulation (Bishop and Donald, 1979)
a number of immunologic (Proctor et al., 1979) and nonspecific
factors (Vaage, 1978b) may determine the fate of cancer cells duri

vascular dissemination. Studies that monitored radiolabeled T1699 mammary tumor cells injected into the tail veins of normal or tumor-bearing mice showed that arrested cells were subsequently cleared at a faster rate from the lungs of tumor-bearing mice (Proctor *et al.*, 1979). The authors concluded that specific antitumor humoral factors mediated cancer cell death within the circulation.

Based on *in vitro* observations, resistance to disseminating tumor cells could also be mediated by the cytotoxic action of peripheral blood lymphocytes (Blair, 1981; Stutman, 1982) or granulocytes (Fisher and Saffer, 1978). Although the hemodynamics of blood flow makes collisions between *sensitized* lymphocytes and circulating cancer cells unlikely, some cancer cells may be eliminated if lymphocytes become impacted against cancer cell emboli arrested in the microvasculature of the lungs or other organs.

Nonspecifically induced cell-mediated and humoral factors may also make a major contribution to host resistance against disseminating mammary carcinoma cells. For instance, pretreatment of normal mice with the microbial adjuvants glucan, *Corynebacterium parvum*, and bacillus Calmette Guérin (BCG) was associated with an accelerated pulmonary clearance of radiolabeled T1699 mammary during the 8 hr following intravenous injection (Proctor *et al.*, 1978). The mechanism of these accelerated clearance processes was not related to specific immune responses, since the recipients were nonimmunized, normal mice. The results of a similar series of studies with a mouse melanoma showed that appropriately timed injections of bacterial endotoxin or zymosan either increased or decreased the clearance of radiolabeled cells from the lungs (Glaves, 1980). These modulations in clearance processes were associated with concomitant stimulation or suppression, respectively, of host reticuloendothelial system (RES) activity, which was expressed systemically as changes in carbon clearance efficiency. It was also shown that changes in clearance of tumor cells from the lungs were correlated with a decreased or increased incidence of tumor nodules in RES-modified hosts, and it is possible that the microbial adjuvants glucan, *C. parvum*, and BCG had produced similar effects in the T1699 mammary tumor system described previously (Proctor *et al.*, 1978).

Potential metastasis enhancement by tumor-specific serum components considered to be free antigen (Vaage and Agarwal, 1976) or blocking factor (Wexler *et al.*, 1976) has been described in mouse mammary tumor systems. Circulating excess tumor antigen or antigen-antibody complex will cause declining resistance to tumor growth by neutralizing humoral and cellular resistance factors (Vaage and Agarwal, 1976). Conversely, passively transferred immune serum promotes immune recovery by neutralizing excess free antigen (Vaage, 1974). The presence of excess free tumor antigen in a tumor host may well be the most significant negative factor in immune resistance to tumor growth, because it may impair resistance at a critical time, such as the time of implantation of disseminated tumor cells. Thus, a condition may develop where,

analogous to presulfonamide lobar pneumonia, the parasitic or neoplastic mass has grown large enough to shed excessive amounts of
antigenic material into the circulation, resulting in systemic
neutralization of immune cellular and humoral resistance factors,
with a corresponding loss of effective resistance to tumor/microbe
dissemination.

While it is true that the emphasis in tumor immunology is on
cell-associated factors and phenomena, the apparent subsidence of
theories describing antibodies as promoters of tumor growth, and
the demonstration of the protective effect of humoral factors
against metastatic dissemination of cancer (Kassel et al., 1972;
Proctor et al., 1973; Vaage, 1973, 1976, 1978b; Vaage and Agarwal,
1977; Rein and Gibbins, 1979) makes a more intensive study of
humoral factors in cancer particularly pertinent.

B. The Lymph Node Barrier

Different opinions have surrounded the so-called barrier
function of regional lymph nodes draining primary tumors, especially mammary tumors (Fisher and Fisher, 1967; Perez and Stewart,
1980; Glaves, 1980), and there has often been the tacit assumption
that lymph nodes can prevent or delay the transit of cancer cells
by mounting antitumor defense reactions (Mitchell, 1980). A natural corollary of this hypothesis would be that nonantigenic cancer cells would traverse the regional lymph nodes unimpeded. Indeed, Hewitt and Blake (1975) concluded that nonantigenic WHT
mammary carcinoma cells continually streamed through the regional
nodes without accumulating in them or establishing metastatic
growth. Similarly, excision of regional lymph nodes before inoculation of the nonantigenic 2661 adenocarcinoma had no effect on
the incidence of metastases, compared with the incidence of metastases in intact tumor bearers (Van de Velde et al., 1977). These
examples indicate that there was little tumor-specific and also
little nonspecific resistance to cancer cell passage through the
regional nodes. Positive evidence of lymph node resistance to
antigenic mammary tumors comes from in vitro studies only, one
example being the earlier proliferative response of lymphocytes
from proximal compared to distal nodes, when incubated with tumor
cells (Goldfarb and Hardy, 1975). Whether this reactivity modified
the course of metastasis was not determined. Morphologic, inflammatory changes in draining lymph nodes have also been considered
as indicators of host resistance to cancer cells (Fisher et al.,
1977). In other studies, however, both immunogenic and nonimmunogenic tumors elicited lymphoid hyperplasia (Van de Velde et al.,
1978; Vaage, 1979b), as did sc implants of pieces of autochthonous
liver or syngeneic liver and kidney (Vaage, 1979b).

Mammary cancer cells can no longer be assumed to disseminate
preferentially via the lymphatics, except possibly in very early
stages of the disease, because complex patterns of metastasis cannot be explained by single-route dissemination. There are also

extensive lymphaticovenous connections that cancer cells have been
seen to traverse within minutes of iv injection (Fisher and Fisher,
1966). It appears, therefore, that although some cancer cells no
doubt succumb to host resistance within the lymphatic system, lymph
nodes can perhaps best be regarded as meters of mammary tumor
metastasis rather than as regulators of secondary disease (Fisher
and Fisher, 1966; Weiss, 1980).

C. The Early Development of Systemic Immunity

     The concept of concomitant immunity is described as the ability
of a host with a progressively growing immunogenic primary tumor to
become, by virtue of the primary tumor, able to resist experimental
secondary implants of the same tumor and conceivably, therefore,
also to resist spontaneous metastases derived from the primary tumor. Conversely, the secondary growth of cancer cells disseminated
from nonantigenic tumors should be unimpaired, and it has been
found (Tarin and Price, 1979) that tumor cells inoculated into the
tail veins of mice bearing nonimmunogenic spontaneous primary mammary carcinomas, grew in the lungs with the same frequency as tumor cells injected into the circulation of nontumor bearers.
     The dissemination of potentially metastatic cancer cells may
begin early in the growth of a primary tumor, possibly before an
immunogenic primary tumor has had the time and/or has acquired
sufficient mass to stimulate an effective systemic immune status
in the host. It is therefore important to know how early, under
favorable circumstances, a host with a primary mammary tumor does
develop systemic immune protection against metastasis.
     In a series of experiments that will be described in this
section (Vaage and Pepin, 1983) the relationship between the development of systemic resistance against metastasis and the local
reaction against a primary tumor implant was investigated. In
the first experiment, the schema and results of which are summarized in Fig. 1, the development of systemic resistance against
artificial metastases was determined in the following manner: At
the same time (Day 0), seven experimental groups plus one group
of control mice were injected via the left ventricle with 2×10^4
viable cells of the C3H/He mammary carcinoma MC2. The experimental groups had been implanted from 1 to 8 days (see Fig. 1) before
Day 0 with a 3-mm piece of viable MC2 sc in the right flank, about
1 cm anterior to the inguinal lymph node. The sc implants were
excised without disturbing the inguinal lymph node after 21 days.
When some of the mice showed loss of vitality, 35 days after the
intracardiac implantation, all of the mice were killed by CO_2
asphyxiation and their visceral organs examined for tumor growth.
The results in Fig. 1 show that systemic immunity was clearly expressed against MC2 cells injected into the left ventricle on the
sixth day (and later) after the sc implantation of MC2.
     In parallel with the investigation of the development of con-
comitant systemic immunity, implants of the mammary carcinoma MC2

JAN VAAGE

Metastases found in

	Unsensitized Mice 27/30	1 Day Sensitized Mice 16/20	2 Day Sensitized Mice 18/20	4 Day Sensitized Mice 16/20	5 Day Sensitized Mice 11/20	6 Day Sensitized Mice 7/20	7 Day Sensitized Mice 5/20	8 Day Sensitized Mice 5/20
Number of Metastases	155	95	103	99	81	29	14	18

SCHEMA

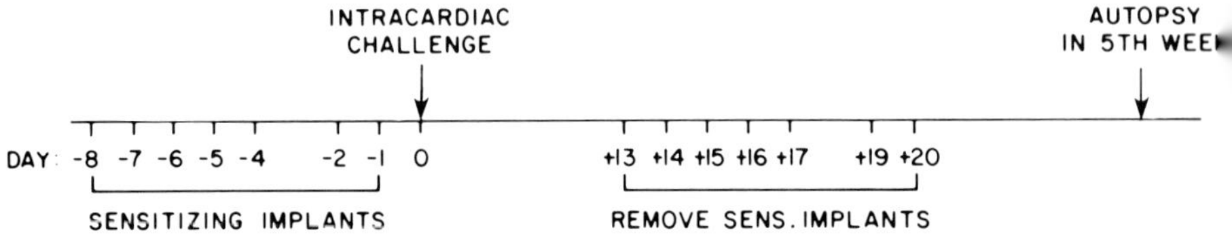

Fig. 1.   Development of systemic resistance against the growth of MC cells injected intra-arterially.   A summary of the number of mice per group with visceral tumor growth, and a summary of the total number of metastases per group.   The mice had been immunized by a sc tumor implant 1-8 days before the intracardiac injection of 2×10^4 tumor cells.   (From Vaage and Pepin, 1983.)

were removed at daily intervals for histologic examination.   The stromal reaction typically contained two lymphoid components: One was a small lymphocyte that arrived at the implant in substantial numbers within 2 to 3 days.   They would infiltrate the stroma surrounding the implant and accumulate at its periphery but showed no tendency to infiltrate the body of the tumor.   A second, larger lymphoid cell would appear at the tumor implant 1 or 2 days later than the small lymphocytes.   This lymphoid cell was associated with numerous plasma cells; some were scattered throughout the stromal reaction, but most were seen in small accumulations by venules near the tumor.   This second lymphoid cell type was also never seen to infiltrate the body of the tumor.

Because the accumulation of lymphoid cells at the MC2 primary implant was a constant feature of often substantial proportions, the implant and its surrounding stroma were surgically removed to observe the effects of interference with the local antitumor reaction.   To determine whether the surgical removal of the primary tumor implant together with its immediately surrounding lymphocytic reaction would have an effect on the resistance against disseminated tumor cells, a number of experiments were done that will be described in brief outline: Figure 2 shows the summarized results and schema of an experiment where mice were cured of immunizing sc tumor implants 6 days after implantation (early surgery) or 19 days after implantation (late surgery).   Two groups of mice were given 450 rad of whole-body irradiation 2 days before the immunizing sc tumor implants, and were then subjected to early or late

Metastases found in

	Group 1 irrad. and early surgery 20/20	Group 2 irrad. and late surgery 19/20	Group 3 early surgery 6/15	Group 4 late surgery 2/15	Group 5 irradiated controls 10/10	Group 6 untreated controls 11/15
Number of Metastases	152	142	30	5	78	70

SCHEMA

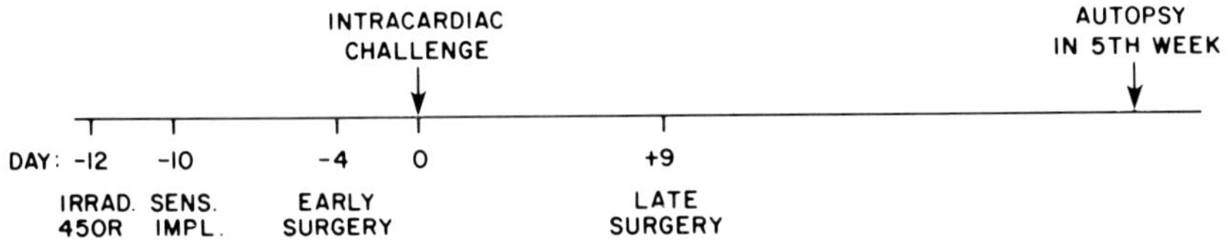

Fig. 2. Effect of primary tumor removal on the disseminated growth of MC. A summary of the number of mice per group with visceral tumor growth, and a summary of the total number of metastases per group. Early surgery, sc implants removed after 6 days; late surgery, sc implants removed after 19 days. All mice were injected with 2×10^4 tumor cells into the left ventricle 10 days after the sc implantation. (From Vaage and Pepin, 1983.)

surgery. In two control groups, the mice received irradiation only or no treatment. All groups of mice were challenged via the left ventricle 10 days after the immunizing sc implant. The results in Fig. 2 show that there was a significant increase in the number of metastases found in unirradiated mice when the immunizing sc tumor implant had been removed after 6 days of growth, 4 days before the intracardiac injection of tumor cells (group 3 vs. group 4, $p < .05$). This effect was greatly reduced if the immune response to the primary sc tumor implant had been prevented by whole-body irradiation (group 1 vs. group 2). Histologic examinations of sc MC2 implants removed at daily intervals from normal and from irradiated hosts had shown that the irradiation had caused a marked reduction in the lymphocytic elements of the stromal reaction, and had enhanced the growth of the implants.

The reduced resistance to artificial metastases that was observed after early removal of a primary, immunizing tumor could conceivably have been the result of (a) removal of the source of tumor antigen or (b) removal of the cells of the local host reaction against the tumor. To compare the importance of (a) the tumor itself as antigen source and (b) the peritumor accumulation of immunocytes in the early development of systemic resistance, the following two experiments were done. In the first, the mice had a sc immunizing tumor excised after 6 or after 19 days of growth, and were challenged via the left ventricle 10 days after the im-

Metastases found in

	Group 1 early surgery 9/20	Group 2 late surgery 3/20	Group 3 early surgery tumor cells 11/20	Group 4 late surgery tumor cells 2/20	Group 5 untreated controls 18/20
Number of Metastases	51	7	56	8	97

SCHEMA

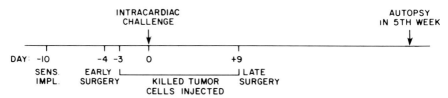

Fig. 3.   Effect of primary tumor removal and killed tumor cell injections on the disseminated growth of MC. See legend for Fig. 2. The mice in groups 3 and 4 received 13 daily ip injections of 2×10^5 killed tumor cells from Day 7 to Day 19 after the sc tumor implant. (From Vaage and Pepin, 1983.)

munizing tumor was implanted sc. The mice with early (6 days) excision of the sc tumor then received, from the seventh to nineteenth day after the sc implant, daily ip injections of 0.1 ml saline containing 2×10^5 freshly prepared, washed, radiation-inactivated (4250 rad) MC2 cells. Each daily inoculation of tumor cells was equivalent to 1% of the average mass of a 14-day sc tumor implant. The ip route of injections was used to provide systemic access for soluble components of tumor cells, without the toxicity of iv injections (Vaage, 1978b) or the re-establishment of lymphoid accumulations at sc injection sites. The control mice received only the intracardiac injection of tumor cells. The results presented in Fig. 3 show that the ip injection of antigen in the form of radiation-killed tumor cells did not support the development of systemic resistance, nor did it adversely affect the development of systemic resistance in mice that carried their sc tumors for 19 days.

In the second experiment, early and late excision of the sc tumor and intracardiac challenge followed the schedule of the first experiment. This experiment studied the effect of transfers of plasma from MC2 hosts to mice with early (6 days) excision of tumors. The mice received 13 daily ip injections of 0.5 ml of plasma taken from mice carrying 6- to 19-day-old sc implants of MC2. The control plasma was collected from mice carrying 6- to 19-day-old sc implants of an antigenically unrelated C3H/He mammary carcinoma. The normal control mice received only the intracardiac injection of

Metastases found in

	Group 1 early surgery 7/10	Group 2 late surgery 3/10	Group 3 early surgery MC2 host plasma 7/10	Group 4 early surgery control plasma 9/10	Group 5 untreated controls 8/10
Number of Metastases	51	9	17	59	68

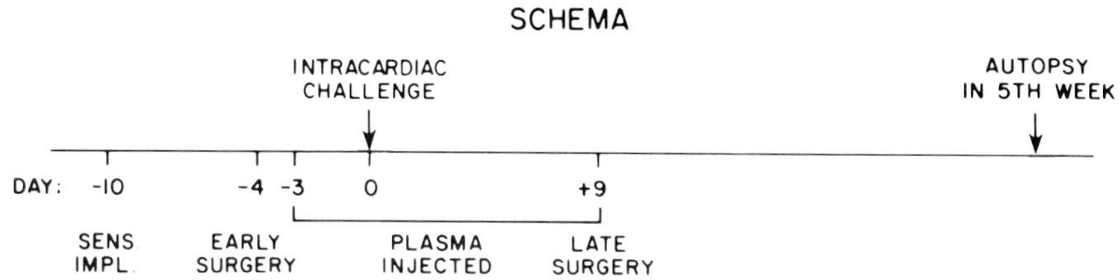

SCHEMA

Fig. 4.   Effect of primary tumor removal and plasma therapy on the disseminated growth of MC.   See legend for Fig. 2.   The mice in group 3 received 13 daily injections of 0.5 ml of MC2 host plasma, whereas the mice in group 4 received equal injections of plasma from mice carrying tumor 21-6.   (From Vaage and Pepin, 1983.)

tumor cells.   The results presented in Fig. 4 show that the effect of early excision of the immunizing tumor was partially corrected by the injection of MC2 host plasma, but not by control plasma.

According to the results of these experiments, it appears possible that tumor-specific resistance factors could be produced by the cells of the lymphocytic infiltrate surrounding an immunogenic tumor, and that this lymphocytic organoid may have an important function in the early development of systemic concomitant immune resistance against metastases.   Morphometric quantitation of plasma cells by the immunoperoxidase staining technique produced a low estimate of 10,000 IgG-producing cells in the stromal reaction surrounding a 5-mm, 4-week-old MC2 implant.   Using data from the studies of Van Furth (1966) showing that a single plasma cell may produce $1-2 \times 10^3$ IgG molecules/sec, I arrived at the conclusion that antibodies directed against MC2 immunogens may, in this case at least, have been produced by the peritumor plasma cells in the remarkable quantity of 2×10^7 antibody molecules/sec!   These morphologic parameters of host resistance are also particularly relevant to the earlier discussion of the nature of host resistance to primary tumor growth (Section II).   It is tempting to speculate that antibodies found associated with tumors (Ran et al., 1980) may have been secreted by antibody-producing cells associated with the tumor rather than absorbed by the tumor from antibodies in the circulation.

D. Antimetastatic Factors in Normal Plasma

The following study was motivated by a frequent observation
during iv injection of tumor cells into normal and immunized mice,
that the mice would frequently die in acute dyspnea within less
than a minute of the injection (Vaage, 1978b). Because the carefully washed cells were free of clumps, and no signs of embolism
were found at autopsy, the possibility had to be considered that
the rapid deaths were the results of intravascular cell destruction and therefore toxic in nature. The purpose of the study was
to investigate whether blood may contain factors that can cause
lysis of neoplastic cells that enter the circulation.

Many of the mice survived the immediate toxic effect of iv
inoculation of tumor cells and subsequently developed tumors in
the lungs. It was therefore obvious that if intravascular cell
lysis was indeed the cause of the toxicity, only a portion of the
cells could have been lysed. Accordingly, it seemed that iv inoc-

TABLE I

Susceptibility of Tumor Cells to Damage
by Normal Blood Factors[a,b]

Tumor cell type	Treatment	Unstained cells (%) by incubation time (min)		
		15	30	60
MCa1	PBS	19	19	19
	WB	4	4	3
	NS	3	1.5	1
	NP	4	1	0.25
MC2	PBS	20	20	20
	WB	16	15	14
	NS	15	12.5	9
	NP	10	6	1.5
MC2 ascites	PBS	95	95	95
	WB	92	89	85
	NS	90	84	84
	NP	82	77	77.5

[a] From Vaage (1978b).
[b] Cytotoxic effect (trypan blue staining) on tumor cells treated
with whole normal blood (WB), normal serum (NS), normal heparinized
plasma (NP), and PBS as control. The data for each tumor are the
results of five separate, repeated tests.

ula of cancer cells would be most toxic if all the cells were rup-
tured just before the suspension was injected. This was found to
be the case. For each of several different C3H/He mammary carcinomas tested, the lethal effect of iv inoculation of otherwise
similar cell suspensions was much greater if the cells had first
been disrupted by sonication. The cause of death was presumed to
be respiratory failure because of the observed dyspnea and because
death could sometimes be prevented if an animal in distress was
given O_2 resuscitation.

Aliquots of the cell suspensions that were used for iv injections were also at the same time treated with whole blood or cell-
free fractions of blood and tested for membrane damage by trypan
blue exclusion. Freshly prepared suspensions of 10^6 cells/ml were
incubated at room temperature for 15 min to 1 hr in PBS or in 1
ml PBS containing 0.2 ml of the following: (1) fresh whole C3H
blood (diluted 1:5 with PBS in the syringe at the time of bleeding
by cardiac puncture, (2) fresh normal serum from clotted whole C3H
blood, or (3) fresh heparinized C3H plasma. The results in Table
I show that MC1 and MC2 were susceptible to damage *in vitro* but
that the ascites form of MC2, which had low toxicity when injected
iv as whole cells, was less affected by the treatment *in vitro* than
cells from the solid MC2. With the greater resistance to damage by
plasma factors, the ascites form of MC2 had also acquired a greater
ability to form pulmonary tumors after iv injection. Tests using
the standard ^{99}Tc-release assay (Vaage and Agarwal, 1978) and cells
from MC1, found that the cytolytic activity in normal blood was
not in the isolated IgG fraction.

The rapid death of normal mice injected iv with tumor cell
preparations is only a laboratory phenomenon, probably in the same
class as the Jarisch-Herxheimer effect,[1] and is caused by the release of a large quantity of toxic cytoplasmic material from the
large number of cells deliberately introduced into the circulation.
Natural release of disseminating malignant cells would be gradual
and unlikely to provide lethal levels of free toxic material. The
significant deduction from the observation is, however, that normal, protective molecular factors in the blood can recognize and
interact effectively with intruding neoplastic cells. The observations support work by others who have described antitumor activity in normal plasma (Bessis, 1949; Kochen et al., 1975; Apffel,
1976; Kassel et al., 1977; Lichtiger, 1977; Bishop and Donald,
1979).

The lower lytic activity in diluted whole blood (which formed
fibrin during the test) and in serum, compared with heparinized

---

[1]Increase in syphilitic symptoms after administration of anti-
syphilitic drugs. Also related to the fatal release of bacterial
endotoxin following single, rather than fractionated, curative
doses in antibiotic treatment of *Pasteurella pestis* infection.

plasma (Table I), suggests that the factors that were active against cells of solid tumors were related to, or identical with, the normal plasma factors that Kassel et al. (1977) found to be active against leukemia in several species of animals. The active factors bind to fibrin and are believed to include some of the components of complement. The traditional view of cell lysis by complement considers it necessary that specific antibody binds to cell surface receptors before the components of complement can implement the events of membrane damage. If components of complement are low in a tumor host, however, tumor cells with attached antibodies may remain intact. The transfer of tumor cells to the blood or plasma of normal mice may then provide the necessary factors for the lysis of sensitized cells.

Alternative mechanisms for complement activation probably exist. According to Müller-Eberhard (1968), free fragments of combined C5, 6, 7 can bind to cells in the absence of antibody, and once bound, can in turn bind the terminal components of C8 and C9. If fibrin is deposited on the surface of tumor cells arrested in vascular channels (Wood et al., 1961), it can bind C5, 6, 7, the complex of which can in turn bind the lytic elements C8 and C9 (Müller-Eberhard, 1968). This could well be an example of one of nature's ways of performing complement-mediated cytolysis before or without specific antibody. It would then follow that the deposition of fibrin on a potentially metastatic cancer cell may not always be the event that, by popular theory, promotes the development of metastases, and a patient may not always benefit from anticoagulant therapy.

IV.   RESISTANCE TO SECONDARY TUMOR GROWTH

A.   Metastasis-Forming Potential of Tumor Cells

The majority of the cancer cells disseminated from a primary tumor apparently fail to survive their vascular passage, and the survival of the remainder after extravasation is also not ensured. At least one factor that may determine the success or failure of metastases is the intrinsic capacity of cancer cells originating in one organ to grow in distant, heterotopic sites. Some measure of the overall potential of mouse mammary tumors to grow in other organs can be inferred from surveys of the frequency of pulmonary growth that has followed the iv injection of the mechanically dissociated cells of primary tumors. The frequency of pulmonary growth has been reported as 93% (26 of 28) among DBA/2 and CBA mammary tumors (Tarin and Price, 1979), and as 68% (34 of 50) among C3H/He mammary tumors (Vaage, 1978a). A second survey using CBA mice compared the organ colonization potential of 23 primary mammary tumors following intravenous, intraperitoneal, subcutaneous, and hepatic

portal vein injections.   Nine tumors grew in all four sites, but
the combination of sites colonized by the remaining 14 tumors varied considerably (Tarin and Price, 1981).

By repeatedly testing the growth characteristics of mammary
tumors maintained by serial sc passage, it has been observed that
the ability to form secondary colonies is a characteristic that
may be acquired by a tumor during the course of progressive growth
(Vaage, 1980).   By comparing the changing sc growth rates, the sc
transplantation immunogenicity, and pulmonary (iv) transplantability during six to nine transplant generations, the relationships
between these characteristics were determined for 10 tumors.   The
ability to grow in the lungs, which appeared in most tumors only
after repeated sc passages, coincided mainly with increased growth
rate and not with loss of immunogenicity and/or gain of endogenous
growth-stimulating factors.   When 3 of the 10 tumors were retested
in serial passages started again from pieces of the primary tumors
stored in liquid N_2, the identical changes recurred in the same,
or in nearly the same, transplant generations.   This was interpreted to indicate that certain variable neoplastic characteristics
such as growth rate, which may influence metastasizing potential,
may be inherent and will appear during progressive growth, not hap-
hazardly but according to a genetically predetermined schedule
(Vaage, 1980).

In an earlier investigation (Vaage, 1978a), which did not
primarily study changes in tumor characteristics but which tested
the frequency and strength of immunogenicity among 100 C3H/He
mammary tumors, the pulmonary transplantability (by iv injection)
of 50 of the tumors was also tested.   The observation was then
made that the ability to grow in the lungs occurred more frequently
among the moderately immunogenic tumors than among the strongly
immunogenic or the nonimmunogenic tumors.   By re-examining the
data for the 50 tumors that were tested for pulmonary growth, it
was found that the average sc growth rate at the time of the pulmonary tests was 3.5 mm/month for the 34 tumors that grew in the
lungs and 2.5 mm/month for 16 tumors that did not grow in the
lungs ($p < .05$).   Accordingly, while a case can be made for immuno-
regulation and even immunostimulation (Fidler, 1974) of metastasis,
it seems that a rapid growth rate is more critical in determining
metastasizing potential among mouse mammary tumors.

B.   The Time Factor in Resistance
     to Metastasis

Under natural conditions, an immunogenic, spontaneous primary
tumor will, by definition, at some stage of its progression, initiate a systemic immune response in the host.   The effectiveness
of the response against metastases is in most instances of greater
importance to survival than the effectiveness of the response
against the primary.   It may be imagined that it is the balance of
opposing forces involving tumor growth potential (depending on

many tumor characteristics) and the destructive potency of host
resistance factors that determines the outcome of the tumor-host
confrontation. It can be shown that the factor of time, when it
allows a metastatic microfocus to establish itself, soon tips the
balance in favor of progressive growth.

An experiment was designed to determine the time, relative to
challenge, at which transfer of immune cells would provide protection against intravenously implanted tumor cells. The test animals were irradiated to preclude a primary immune response that
could easily obscure the moderate protection provided by passive
immunization. The mice were challenged with iv or sc injections
of tumor cells and subsequently treated with ip injections of
lymph node cells as indicated in Table II. The mice that were
given injections of lymph node cells each received the equivalent
of one-half the quantity of cells obtained from two axillary, two
brachial, and two inguinal lymph nodes, approximately 5×10^6
lymph node cells per injection. The incidence and size of tumors
at the sc injection sites were recorded at weekly intervals. Following injection of tumor cells into the tail vein, tumor growth
was found almost exclusively in the lungs. The amount of tumor
growth found in the lungs was rated on a scale of 0 to 3, according to the number and size of nodules found.

The results presented in Table II show that tumor growth in
the lungs and also sc was not significantly inhibited unless the
passive transfer of immune lymph node cells was started within 3
days of tumor cell injection (groups 1 to 4 vs. groups 5 to 8).
Also, passive immunization gave greater protection the earlier it
was started (groups 1-4). Transfers of normal lymph node cells
from the day before challenge (group 9) had no apparent protective
effect.

The reduced vulnerability of the tumor implants 3 days after
implantation may be one example of the general concept in tumor
growth called "sneaking through" by Klein (1966), which was based
on the original observation by Old et al. (1962). The results
also indicate that there is a sharp, rather than a gradual, change
when conditions in a host change to favor tumor growth.

At least two different but compatible explanations may be offered for this apparent change from immunosensitivity to relative
immunoresistance of "metastatic" growth. Those injected tumor
cells with clone-forming potential may, on the third day after implantation, have achieved sufficient mass to render the clone ref-
ractory to immune rejection. Alternatively, or additionally, progressive tumor growth beyond an aggregation of at most 10^6 cells
or about 1 mm^3 is not considered possible without vascularization
(Tannock, 1970; Folkman, 1974). Accordingly, it seems quite likely that vascularization is the event that gives micrometastases
greater resistance to rejection by host defenses. The observed
time of this event, about the third day after implantation, is
within the 1- to 4-day range observed by Algire (1954) in his studies of vascularization of implanted pieces of a mouse mammary
carcinoma.

TABLE II

Effect of Time of Lymphocyte Transfer on Passive Immunity
to the Pulmonary Growth of Injected Mammary Carcinoma Cells[a]

Group	Immune status	Treatment[b]	iv Challenge[c] (Day 0) No. of mice with tumors/no. treated	%	Average tumor growth	sc Challenge[c] (Day 0) No. of tumors/no. treated	%	Average tumor size (mm)
1	Irradiated	Immune LNC Day −1,+1,+3	5/15	35	0.67	17/30	57	2.0
2	Irradiated	Immune LNC Day 0,+2,+4	7/15	47	0.91	20/30	67	2.3
3	Irradiated	Immune LNC Day +1,+3,+5	8/15	53	0.94	21/30	70	2.3
4	Irradiated	Immune LNC Day +2,+4,+6	16/30	53	0.98	39/60	65	2.2
5	Irradiated	Immune LNC Day +3,+5,+7	23/30	77	1.85	50/60	83	3.4
6	Irradiated	Immune LNC Day +4,+6,+8	29/30	97	2.70	60/60	100	4.4
7	Irradiated	Immune LNC Day +5,+7,+9	15/15	100	2.55	30/30	100	4.5
8	Irradiated	Immune LNC Day +7,+9,+11	15/15	100	2.65	29/30	97	4.1
9	Irradiated	Normal LNC Day −1,+1,+3	10/10	100	2.25	20/20	100	4.0
10	Irradiated	n.t.	30/30	100	2.70	57/60	95	4.6
11	Unsensitized	n.t.	27/30	90	1.22	60/60	100	3.6
12	Sensitized	n.t.	2/30	7	0.11	24/60	40	1.6

[a] From Vaage (1977).
[b] For description of treatment procedures, see text. LNC, lymph node cells; n.t., no treatment.
[c] All the mice were challenged with sc injections of 10^5 tumor cells at the left shoulder and hip, and with injections of 3.3×10^4 tumor cells into the tail vein.

C. Systemic Immunity against Metastasis

As has been reported (Vaage and Agarwal, 1976), the immune resistance against mouse mammary carcinoma cells injected into the circulation appears to be significantly more effective than the immune resistance facing tumor cells that have been deposited sc. It was observed that the number of tumor cells that would just give 100% growth sc in normal mice, would give tumor growth in about 50% of immunized mice. However, if a number of cells of the same tumor, sufficient to give 100% growth in the lungs after iv injection into normal mice, were injected iv into immunized mice, tumor growth would occur in less than 10% of the animals. In other words,

TABLE III

Effect of a Growing Mammary Carcinoma
on the Resistance of the Host to iv and sc Mammary
Carcinoma Challenge[a,b]

		Challenge			
Group	Mammary carcinoma removed on day (tumor size in mm)	Challenge route	No. of mice with tumor	Average tumor growth[c]	Rejection response (%)
1	13 (3.5)	iv	14/15	1.80	21
2	13 (3.5)	sc	26/30	9.80	11
3	16 (4.0)	iv	5/15	0.47	80
4	16 (4.0)	sc	17/30	6.13	45
5	22 (6.0)	iv	3/15	0.20	91
6	22 (6.0)	sc	13/30	4.93	55
7	28 (9.0)	iv	2/20	0.10	96
8	28 (9.0)	sc	19/40	5.55	50
9	37 (15.0)	iv	5/20	0.30	87
10	37 (15.0)	sc	31/40	8.73	21
11	41 (18.0)	iv	11/15	1.20	48
12	41 (18.0)	sc	23/30	9.00	19
13	Unsensitized	iv	35/35	2.29	0
14	Unsensitized	sc	64/70	11.06	9

[a] From Vaage and Agarwal (1976).
[b] Live sensitizing tumors were implanted sc in the right flank. After various periods of growth, the implants were excised on the third day after challenge.
[c] The average sc growth values are expressed in millimeters. The average tumor growth in the lungs is expressed in values from 0 to 3 (see text).

immune resistance appeared to be 40% more effective against tumor
cells in the blood and/or in the lungs, than against tumor cells
that had been deposited sc.

In order to make a direct comparison of the relative effectiveness of subcutaneous and pulmonary resistance to tumor growth, mice
were sensitized with sc implants of living pieces of mammary carcinoma tissue, which were excised after various predetermined periods of growth. The level of resistance in the various groups
was tested by iv or sc challenge implants of living tumor cells in
suspension. The challenge implants were always made 3 days before the immunizing tumors were removed. Each group received
1×10^5 cells injected sc at the left shoulder and at the left hip,
or received 3.3×10^4 cells injected iv.

The results in Table III show that resistance to challenge
was detectable after a sensitization period of 10 days (immunizing
tumor removed Day 13) and was fully developed in 13 days (tumor
removed Day 16). Fully immunized animals challenged iv were able
to reduce by 96% the amount of tumor growth found in the lungs of
unimmunized control animals compared to maximum reduction of 55%
in immunized mice challenged sc. The results also show that the
antitumor resistance in the lungs remained effective longer than
did the sc resistance, before declining with the increasing tumor
load.

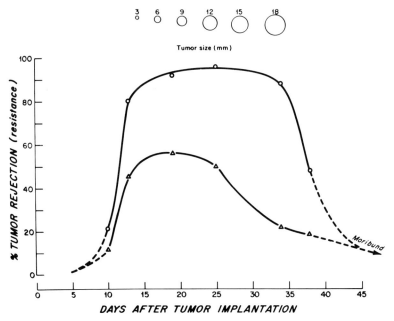

Fig. 5. Development and decline of immune resistance in the
lungs (O, iv) and sc (Δ) under the influence of a progressively
growing mammary carcinoma. Curves constructed from the values in
Fig. 2. (From Vaage and Agarwal, 1976.)

TABLE IV

Effect of Active Immunization on the Growth of Mammary
Carcinoma Cells Injected Intra-arterially

| Location of tumor | Incidence[a] | | Reduction (%) |
	Normal	Immunized	
Adrenals	21	0	100
Ovaries	22	1	93
Lungs	14	0	100
Kidneys	9	0	100
Liver	1	0	100
Spleen	0	0	–
Mesentery	16	0	100
Mediastinum	12	0	100
Myocardium	17	4	65
Diaphragm	10	4	40
Chest wall	17	3	74
Retroperitoneal	16	2	81

[a]Number of mice with tumors. Total normal mice with tumors,
27 of 30; total immunized with tumors, 7 of 20.

By tracing the two curves of Fig. 5 (constructed from the values in Table III) on pieces of paper covering an area of the graph
from Day 5 to 45, and from 0 to 100%, and then cutting out and
weighing the areas under the curves, an idea of the relative effectiveness of sc and pulmonary immune resistance to challenge was
derived for the period from primary tumor onset to terminal disease. The average of several such estimates gave the value for sc
immune resistance as 30% and the value for pulmonary resistance as
65% of the theoretical total resistance.

The observation that induced systemic resistance is more effective against cancer cells injected iv than against cancer cells
implanted sc has no ready explanation. It may be that different
and more effective resistance mechanisms operate in the blood than
under the skin, or it could simply be that resistance factors are
more readily and more abundantly available in the blood than in
subcutaneous connective tissue spaces. Resistance against cancer
cells injected iv is also not as readily inactivated by a large
primary tumor mass as is resistance against cancer cells implanted
sc (Vaage and Agarwal, 1976).

A similar comparison was also made (J. Vaage, unpublished) between normal and immunized mice that had been injected with mammary
carcinoma cells into the left ventricle, in order to ensure vascular distribution of tumor cells to all organs and tissues. The
results of this test, presented in Table IV, show that the tumor

had a high frequency of growth in the adrenals and ovaries compared to much larger organs such as the lungs, kidneys, and the liver. This may be related to the initial dose of tumor cells delivered to the adrenals and ovaries which have a higher rate of blood flow per gram of tissue than the larger visceral organs. This has been interpreted by Weiss et al. (1980) as the basis for the high frequency of metastases in these organs. The observed immune resistance to tumor growth was not expressed equally in all organs. There was a greater reduction in the number of tumors found in visceral organs than in the mesentery and mediastinum of immunized mice.

In the T1699 mouse mammary carcinoma system, host defense plays a definitive role in resisting the progressive outgrowth of spontaneous metastases. The tumor is highly antigenic; antibody-dependent, cell-mediated reactions restrict the growth and also the invasiveness of the primary neoplasm, and systemic immunity may reduce the intravascular survival of T1699 cells. Despite the host resistance, some T1699 cells do survive and form lung colonies in most animals. However, the growth is transient and micrometastases almost invariably regress. The contribution of host defense to this regression is shown by the fact that the pulmonary metastases grow progressively in 80 to 100% of mice immunologically crippled by thymectomy and irradiation (Parthenais and Haskill, 1979). Why even transient growth of pulmonary metastases occurs in the face of demonstrable immune reactions is an interesting question. It is possible that a critical mass of antigenic cells must be present to attract sufficient inflammatory cells and humoral factors to implement rejection.

The demonstration of covert or dormant cancer cells in various organs is often taken to imply host restraint of metastatic growth (Alexander, 1976; Wheelock, 1981), and covert cancer cells were detected by bioassays in the thymus, spleen, and liver of mice bearing sc transplants of a carcinogen-induced mammary carcinoma (Haran-Ghera et al., 1981). However, growth inhibition by inadequate vascular supply should also be considered in this context (Folkman, 1974; Vaage and Ghandbhir, 1978).

D. Immunotherapy and Metastasis

The demonstrated existence of host defense mechanisms against cancer has prompted numerous attempts to increase the level of reactivity against primary tumors and metastases by means of both specific and nonspecific immunotherapy. I am aware of only a few studies that have attempted to use immunotherapeutic procedures to control the growth of metastases from mouse mammary tumors. The variable results reported could be related to the lack of uniformity in agents, doses, routes, and timing used in treatment regimens. While avoiding generalizations regarding the relative efficacy of any particular treatment, the following report is an example of success in immunotherapeutic control of metastasis.

The injections of nonspecific adjuvants directly into the primary
mammary carcinomas of C3HBA mice induced extensive necrosis of the
primary tumor and also reduced the incidence of spontaneous hepatic and pulmonary metastases (Heggers et al., 1979). The authors
attributed this inhibition to increased infiltration by mononuclear
cells. A similar phenomenon may have been observed when intratumor injections of C. parvum increased the survival of C3H mice
bearing sc transplants of a spontaneous mammary tumor and concomitantly inhibited a second inoculation of cancer cells at another
sc site (Fisher et al., 1979). In three other mammary tumor systems, very little objective response to immunotherapy was detected
(Purnell et al., 1975; Hewitt and Blake, 1978; Vaage, 1979c).

The unspectacular result of attempted immunostimulation against
cancer is not so surprising considering that there are no examples
from clinical medicine in general of successful use of immunostimulation during active, diagnosable disease. Vaccination may be
effective prophylactically but never after symptoms appear. Rabies
vaccination, for example, must be started directly after suspected
infection, well ahead of symptoms. Tetanus vaccine may be used as
a therapeutic booster in already immunized individuals, but before
symptoms appear. The only medical situation where immunostimulation
is still attempted during disease is in cancer. The remarkable
and unexplained cases of tumor regression after intralesion injection of BCG is a separate phenomenon not thought to involve immune mechanisms, because the local reaction is not associated with
demonstrable systemic resistance (Sparks and Breeding, 1974;
Piessens et al., 1977).

CONCLUDING REMARKS

When considering the mouse mammary carcinoma system as a model
for metastasis, two points may need emphasis.

1. The best available evidence suggests that humoral factors
are particularly and maybe uniquely effective in resisting the
dissemination of cancer cells. The mechanisms of control of metastasis are probably in fundamental ways different from the clearly
demonstrated cellular nature of host reactions against established
neoplastic growth. Analogous duality of defense mechanisms may be
found in the inflammatory and cellular-granulomatous reaction at
points of infection, and the antibody- and complement-dependent
control of bacteremia. This consideration leads to the speculation
that prognostic forecasts based on histopathologic evaluations of
biopsy specimens of primary tumors may have little value, because
the resistance factors that may most resist dissemination, are not
displayed in such histologic preparations.

2. The effectiveness of metastatic control mechanisms may be
inferred from the general observation that mouse mammary carcinomas
very rarely metastasize, except when the primary tumor burden has

become very large and the host is approaching death. The important point to consider here is not that mouse strains with a high primary mammary tumor incidence and infrequent metastases are poor models for metastasis research, but that they are good models to study the nature of host resistance to metastasis, and to study the tumor-related factors that abrogate resistance. The balance of tumor growth potential *versus* host resistance involves more than excess antigen *versus* immune resistance factors, because metastases are infrequent and nonimmunogenic mouse mammary tumors common.

REFERENCES

Alexander, P. (1976). *In* "Fundamental Aspects of Metastasis." (L. Weiss, ed.), pp. 227-239. North-Holland, Amsterdam.

Algire, G. H. (1954). *J. Natl. Cancer Inst. (US) 15*, 483-488.

Anderson, J. J., Fugman, R. A., Stolfi, R. L., and Martin, D. S. (1974). *Cancer Res. 34*, 1916-1920.

Apffel, C. A. (1976). *Cancer Res. 36*, 1527-1537.

Ashburn, L. L. (1937). *U.S. Public Health Rep. 52*, 915-929.

Benjamin, S. P., Mercer, R. D., and Hawk, W. A. (1977). *Cancer (Philadelphia) 40*, 2342-2352.

Bessis, L. (1949). *Blood 4*, 324-328.

Bishop, C. J., and Donald, K. J. (1979). *Br. J. Exp. Pathol. 60*, 29-37.

Blair, P. (1981). *In* "Mechanisms of Immunity to Virus-Induced Tumors" (J. W. Blasecki, ed.), pp. 181-257. Dekker, New York.

Butler, T. P., and Gullino, P. M. (1975). *Cancer Res. 35*, 512-516.

DaFano, C. (1912). *Int. Cancer Res. Found. Sci. Rep. 5*, 2296-2309.

Eccles, S., and Alexander, P. (1974). *Nature (London) 250*, 667-669.

Evans, R. (1976). *In* "The Macrophage in Neoplasia" (M. A. Fink, ed.), pp. 27-42. Academic Press, New York.

Fidler, I. J. (1970). *J. Natl. Cancer Inst. (US) 45*, 773-782.

Fidler, I. J. (1974). *Cancer Res. 34*, 491-498.

Fisher, B., and Fisher, E. R. (1966). *Science (Washington, D.C.) 152*, 1397-1398.

Fisher, B., and Fisher, E. R. (1967). *Cancer (Philadelphia) 20*, 1907-1913.

Fisher, B., and Saffer, E. A. (1978). *J. Natl. Cancer Inst. (US) 60*, 687-691.

Fisher, B., Gebhardt, M., and Saffer, E. (1979). *Cancer (Philadelphia) 43*, 451-458.

Fisher, E. R., Fisher, B., and Saffer, E. (1977). *Arch. Pathol. Lab. Med. 101*, 152-155.

Folkman, J. (1974). *Adv. Cancer Res. 19*, 331-358.

Glaves, D. (1980). *Int. J. Cancer 26*, 115-122.

Goldfarb, P. M., and Hardy, M. A. (1975). *Cancer (Philadelphia) 35*, 778-783.

Gullino, P. M. (1978). *J. Natl. Cancer Inst. (US) 61,* 639-643.

Haran-Ghera, N., Krauthgamer, R., and Peled, A. (1981). *J. Immunol. 126,* 1241-1244.

Heggers, J. P., Robson, M. C., Yetter, J. F., Kreig, R. E., and Jennings, P. B. (1979). *J. Surg. Oncol. 11,* 161-169.

Hewitt, H. B., and Blake, E. R. (1975). *Br. J. Cancer 31,* 25-35.

Hewitt, H. B., and Blake, E. R. (1978). *Br. J. Cancer 38,* 219-223.

Iwasaki, T. (1915). *J. Pathol. Bacteriol. 20,* 85-105.

Kassel, R. L., Old, L. J., Carswell, E. A., Fiore, N. C., and Hardy, W. D. (1972). *J. Exp. Med. 138,* 925-938.

Kassel, R. L., Old, L. J., Day, N. K., and Hardy, W. D. (1977). *Proc. Soc. Exp. Biol. Med. 155,* 230-233.

Klein, G. (1966). *Annu. Rev. Microbiol. 20,* 233-252.

Kochen, J., Radel, E., and Nathenson, G. (1975). *Pediatr. Res. 9,* 389-395.

Lichtiger, B. (1977). *Cancer (Philadelphia) 27,* 194-199.

Liotta, L. A., Kleineman, J., and Saidel, G. M. (1974). *Cancer Res. 34,* 997-1004.

Mitchell, M. S. (1980). *In* "Lymphatic System Metastasis" (L. Weiss, H. A. Gilbert, and S. C. Ballon, eds.), pp. 74-79. Hall, Boston.

Müller-Eberhard, H. J. (1968). *In* "Textbook in Immunopathology" (P. A. Miescher and H. J. Müller-Eberhard, eds.), pp. 33-47. Grune & Stratton, New York.

Murphy, J. B. (1926). *Monogr. Rockefeller Inst. Med. Res. 21,* 168-189.

Old, L. J., Boyse, E. A., Clarke, D. A., and Carswell, E. (1962). *Ann. N.Y. Acad. Sci. 101,* 80-106.

Parthenais, E., and Haskill, S. (1979). *J. Immunol. 123,* 1334-1338.

Perez, C. A., and Stewart, C. C. (1980). *In* "Lymphatic System Metastasis" (L. Weiss, H. A. Gilbert, and S. C. Ballon, eds.), pp. 170-195. Hall, Boston.

Piessens, W. F., Campbell, M., and Churchill, W. H. (1977). *J. Natl. Cancer Inst. (US) 59,* 207-211.

Pitelka, D. R., Hamamoto, S. T., and Taggart, B. N. (1980). *Cancer Res. 40,* 1588-1599.

Proctor, J. W., Rudenstam, C. M., and Alexander, P. (1973). *Nature (London) 242,* 29-30.

Proctor, J. W., Stiteler, R. D., Yamamura, Y., Mansell, P. W. A., and Winters, R. (1978). *Cancer Treat. Rep. 62,* 1873-1880.

Proctor, J. W., Mastromatteo, W. P., Antos, M., and Hedderson, E. D. (1979). *Oncology 36,* 49-54.

Purnell, D. M., Kreider, J. W., and Bartlett, G. L. (1975). *J. Natl. Cancer Inst. (US) 55,* 123-128.

Ran, M., Yaakubowicz, M., Amitai, O., and Witz, J. P. (1980). *Contemp. Top. Immunobiol. 10,* 191-208.

Rein, G. H., and Gibbins, J. R. (1979). *Cancer Res. 39,* 4724-4731.

Sparks, F. C., and Breeding, J. H. (1974). *Cancer Res. 34,* 3262-3269.

Stutman, O. (1982). *Springer Semin. Immunopathol. 4,* 333-372.

Tannock, I. F. (1970). *Cancer Res. 30,* 2470-2476.

Tarin, D., and Price, J. E. (1979). *Br. J. Cancer 39*, 740-754.
Tarin, D., and Price, J. E. (1981). *Cancer Res. 41*, 3604-3609.
Underwood, J. C. E. (1974). *Br. J. Cancer 30*, 538-548.
Vaage, J. (1973). *Cancer Res. 33*, 1957-1965.
Vaage, J. (1974). *Cancer Res. 34*, 2979-2983.
Vaage, J. (1976). *Isr. J. Med. Sci. 12*, 334-343.
Vaage, J. (1977). *Cancer Res. 37*, 1064-1067.
Vaage, J. (1978a). *Cancer Res. 38*, 331-338.
Vaage, J. (1978b). *Cancer Immunol. Immunother. 4*, 257-261.
Vaage, J. (1979a). *Proc. Am. Assoc. Cancer Res, 20*, 1.
Vaage, J. (1979b). *Cancer Immunol. Immunother. 6*, 185-189.
Vaage, J. (1979c). *Cancer Immunol. Immunother. 7*, 185-189.
Vaage, J. (1980). *Cancer Res. 40*, 3495-3501.
Vaage, J., and Agarwal, S. (1976). *Cancer Res. 36*, 1831-1836.
Vaage, J., and Agarwal, S. (1977). *Cancer Res. 37*, 3556-3560.
Vaage, J., and Agarwal, S. (1978). *Methods Cancer Res. 14*, 1-27.
Vaage, J., and Ghandbhir, L. (1978). *Cancer Immunol. Immunother. 4*, 263-268.
Vaage, J., and Pepin, K. G. (1983). *J. Natl. Cancer Inst. (US) 71*, 147-155.
Van de Velde, C. J. H., Van Putten, L. M., and Zwaveling, A. (1977). *Eur. J. Cancer 13*, 555-565.
Van de Velde, C. J. H., Meyer, C. J. L. M., Cornelisse, C. J., Van de Velde, E. A., Van Putten, L. M., and Zwaveling, A. (1978). *Cancer Res. 38*, 661-667.
Van Furth, R. (1966). *Immunology 11*, 13-18.
Warren, S., and Gates, P. (1936). *Am. J. Cancer 27*, 485-492.
Weiss, L. (1980). *In* "Lymphatic System Metastasis" (L. Weiss, H. A. Gilbert, and S. C. Ballon, eds.), pp. 1-40. Hall, Boston.
Weiss, L., Haydock, K., Pickren, J. W., and Lane, W. W. (1980). *Am. J. Pathol. 101*, 101-114.
Wexler, H., Minton, J. P., and Ketcham, A. S. (1965). *Cancer (Philadelphia) 18*, 985-994.
Wexler, H., Sindelar, W. F., and Ketcham, A. S. (1976). *Cancer (Philadelphia) 37*, 1701-1706.
Wheelock, E. F. (1981). *Adv. Cancer Res. 34*, 107-140.
Wood, S. R., Holyoke, E. D., and Yardley, J. H. (1961). *Proc. Can. Cancer Res. Conf. 4*, 167-223.

DISCUSSION

KOBAYASHI: (1) Are the tumors used in your experiment transplanted tumor or autochthonous tumor? There may be some difference between the two groups. (2) Are there any differences between big and small sizes of tumors even in the same group of early surgery, for example, in terms of pulmonary metastasis? What is the definition of early or late? Is it "time" or the "size" of the tumor?

VAAGE: The answer to your first question is that the tumor used
            in these experiments is a syngeneic C3H/He tumor used in
            early transplant generations. Tissue from the original
            primary tumor is kept in liquid N$_2$ to avoid using a tu-
            mor of too ancient an origin. Comparisons between host
            reactions to primary autochthonous tumors *in situ* and
            transplanted to sc and intramammary sites in the ori-
            ginal and syngeneic hosts are being done, but are pro-
            gressing slowly because of the time needed to accumulate
            spontaneous tumor hosts among the breeding mice. In
            response to your second question, the restricted size
            range of tumors removed early in their sc growth, avoids
            the effect of small versus large tumor burden on the
            host's immune status. The difference between "early"
            and "late" surgery groups is related to time only, and
            at the stage of tumor development studied, was not af-
            fected by tumor burden.

KONDO: By the immunohistochemical method you showed that plasma
            cells surrounding the tumor synthesized IgG. Why were
            the tumor cells not stained by IgG if IgG was specific
            to the tumor cell? Another question is, what did you
            say regarding the plasma containing platelets?

VAAGE: The answer to your first question is that the tumor
            cells inside the cellular fibrous capsule were not
            reached by the antibodies produced by the plasma cells
            in the capsule. The capsule, which slowly destroys a
            tumor, probably by interrupting its blood supply, also
            prevents some systemic host resistance factors from
            reaching the tumor. The rapid destruction of additional
            tumor implants placed sc into the same host, is an ex-
            ample of two distinct defense mechanisms functioning
            simultaneously--one locally, the other systemically--in
            the same animal. In answer to your second question, the
            heparizined blood (2 units/ml) was centrifuged twice to
            remove all cells and platelets from the plasma.

COCHRAN: Plasma cell infiltration in primary malignant melanoma
            in humans has been studied by Little in Queensland, and
            he found plasma cells only in ulcerated tumors, implying
            that they are reactive to infection rather than tumor-
            associated antigens. Would you care to comment on this?

VAAGE: Plasma cell accumulation has, of course, been observed
            in a variety of nonneoplastic and neoplastic lesions.
            In my tumor system, ulcerated tumors were not studied
            histologically, because a significant portion of the
            stromal reaction would be missing. The capacity of the
            plasma cells of the stromal reaction surrounding the
            tumor to produce antitumor antibodies is indicated by

the reduced resistance to metastasis in the mice subjected to "early" surgery and the partial restoration
of resistance by transfusions of plasma from tumor
hosts.

OKADA: Is there specificity to tumor cells in the effect of
immune plasma in the prevention of metastasis in your
in vivo experiment? In immune plasma, lymphokines such
as γ-IFN are possibly present, and they might also have
had some effect in your experiment.

VAAGE: Lymphokines and other factors are certainly involved in
the display of *in vivo* immune resistance. The specificity of the protective effect of transfused tumor-host
plasma was controlled, as you saw in the last slide, by
the group of mice transfused with plasma from hosts of
an antigenically unrelated C3H/He mammary carcinoma.

PART IIB

Chairpersons

Takeshi Yoshida
Hideo Hayashi

CHAPTER 10

THE CELL SURFACE MARKERS
OF TUMORICIDAL MACROPHAGES

Tohru Tokunaga
Kiyoko S. Akagawa
Tadayoshi Taniyama

Department of Tuberculosis
National Institute of Health
Tokyo, Japan

BASIC MECHANISMS AND CLINICAL TREATMENT
OF TUMOR METASTASIS

I. INTRODUCTION

A. Role of Tumoricidal Macrophages
    in Cancer Immunotherapy

        The most convincing therapeutic effects of immune potentiating
agents on human cancer have been reported mostly in "local" or "adjuvant contact" immunotherapy, where an immunotherapeutic agent is
introduced into the tumor site. For instance, intralesional injection with bacillus Calmette-Guérin (BCG) caused regression of
animal autochthonous tumors (Tokunaga et al., 1974; Bast and Bast,
1976; Kleinschuster et al., 1977) and human cutaneous cancers
(Morton et al., 1970; Mastrangelo et al., 1976). For controlling
the growth of microscopic metastases, intralesional injection with
BCG prior to surgery was shown to be effective in a guinea pig
model (Zbar et al., 1976), and injection of a BCG-tumor cell mixture was effective in rat models (Baldwin et al., 1976).
        We proposed that the process of tumor regression and metastasis
inhibition caused by intralesional injection of BCG can be conceptually divided into three sequential steps, where three different
effector cells work against tumor cells, respectively (Tokunaga
et al., 1978). The first step is an immediate-type inflammation
elicited by BCG, where macrophages activated directly by BCG are
the major effector cells against tumor cells. The second step is
a delayed-type hypersensitivity (DTH) reaction induced by BCG,
where the effector cells are also macrophages, but they are activated by lymphokines (LK) released from BCG-sensitized T cells
(Mackaness, 1969; Zbar et al., 1976; Tokunaga et al., 1978). Both
steps take place in response to BCG, but not to tumor cells; tumor
cells are destroyed as bystanders being involved in these inflammatory reactions. The third step is a tumor-specific immune reaction, in which the effector cells are tumor-specific killer T cells
and/or DTH T cells. In the latter, the direct effector cells for
destroying tumor cells are macrophages activated by LK released
from the DTH T cells.
        In all of the steps, tumoricidal macrophages play a very im-
portant role. The strongest cytocidal activity is seen in the
second step; those macrophages activated by LK released from BCG-
sensitized T cells have a very strong destructive action on tumor
cells in a nonspecific manner. In vitro cytotoxicity of those
macrophages is usually seen at a much lower cell ratio of effector
to target (E:T) than that of killer T cells.
        Macrophages play another important role in the second and
third steps. They process and present BCG antigen to T cells in
the second step, and tumor antigen, if it exists, to T cells in
the third step. At the place of the DTH reaction to BCG, antigens
and adjuvant-active substances from BCG, T cells and their products,
and macrophages and their products are all accumulated, and the
place possesses a strong adjuvant activity for a weakly antigenic
substance existing at the same place. A model experiment sup-

TABLE I

Induction of DTH to BSA Given Intradermally
Together with PPD in BCG-Sensitized Guinea Pigs[a]

Intradermal injection	DTH skin reaction at the injection site[b] (mm)	DTH skin reaction to BSA after 2 weeks[b] (mm)
BSA 100 µg alone	0	0 (0/8)[c]
BSA 100 µg + PPD 2 µg	23.5 ± 0.8	9.3 ± 7.9 (4/6)
BSA 100 µg + PPD 0.2 µg	20.1 ± 1.1	17.9 ± 4.6 (6/6)

[a]BCG-sensitized guinea pigs were injected intradermally with bovine serum albumin (BSA) with or without PPD. Skin reactions at the injection sites were measured after 24 hr. Two weeks later, the animals were skin-tested with 5 µg of BSA.
[b]Skin reactions were expressed as the mean (mm) ± SD.
[c]Number of animals with positive skin reaction (larger than 10 mm)/number of animals tested.

porting this idea is shown in Table I (Kataoka and Tokunaga, 1979). We can easily imagine that the DTH reaction elicited at the site of the tumor offers the most suitable condition for inducing tumor-specific cellular immunity, if the tumor cells possess their own antigen.

In addition, it should be pointed out that macrophages may play a key role in deviating the immune response in either a positive or negative direction. For instance, we found that macrophages from a mouse strain that gives a low response to BCG presented BCG antigen dominantly to suppressor T cells but not to DTH T cells (Nakamura and Tokunaga, 1980); I-J molecules on their macrophage surface seemed to be a key (Nakamura et al., 1982).

Systemic immunotherapy with various agents including BCG has failed to produce complete regression of palpable neoplasms, with a few significant exceptions. Systemic passive transfer of activated macrophages is also much less effective than intralesional injection with the same macrophages, according to the reports by many investigators, including our own experience with mouse tumors. One possible explanation for this is that, since macrophages cannot recognize tumor cell surface specifically, in contrast to specific T cells, they cannot accumulate at the tumor site unless DTH T cells dispatch a lymphokine signal to them. To overcome this weak point of macrophages as the effector cells against tumors, many approaches are under study, such as using liposomes containing macrophage activators (Fidler, 1980; Fidler et al.,

1981) or monoclonal antibodies conjugated with macrophage activators (K. Tokunaga, T. Kataoka, and K. Nemoto, unpublished).

B. Differentiation Markers of Macrophage
    Activation

     Macrophages are well known to possess diverse functions. Be-
sides their phagocytic capacities, they show a series of effector
functions, such as bactericidal or tumoricidal activity (Blanden
et al., 1966; Evans and Alexander, 1970; Hibbs *et al.*, 1972; Keller, 1973). They have also received attention as secretory cells
(Morahan, 1980) and immunoregulatory cells (Nelson, 1976). For
example, they induce differentiation and clonal expansion of T
cells, release colony-forming factors, and act themselves as suppressor cells. At present, whether such a functional heterogeneity
can be ascribed to different subsets of macrophages, like lymphocyte subsets, or to different stages of maturation is not thorough-
ly understood. However, reports from several laboratories have
provided evidence that macrophage activation for tumor cytotoxicity
requires the completion of a series of reactions (Hibbs *et al.*,
1977; Meltzer, 1981). This reaction sequence can be conceptually
divided into several phases, and activation of cytotoxic macrophages is the final result of a cascade of short-lived intermedi-
ary reactions. It is conceivable that each stage of macrophage
activation is dependent on the activation signal and the responsive precursor cells, both of which are different in nature from
stage to stage (Meltzer, 1981). We reported that both Ia-positive
and Ia-negative mouse peritoneal macrophages could be activated for
tumor cytotoxicity equally well by incubation with LK (Tanaka *et
al.*, 1981). However, since little is known about cell surface markers distinguishable for each step of the sequential activation of
macrophages for tumor cytotoxicity, it is necessary to have such
markers for accomplishment of these lines of study.
     Among macrophages from various organs of various animal species,
mouse peritoneal macrophages have been studied relatively extensively, and several cell surface markers that may be useful for
distinguishing resident and inflammatory peritoneal macrophages
have been reported (Edelson, 1981). For instance, 5'-nucleotidase
is strongly positive in resident peritoneal macrophages and mouse
alveolar macrophages, but its activity is reduced in cells from
mice infected with BCG and challenged with the antigen (Edelson,
1981). The enzyme activity is lacking in thioglycollate (TGC)-in-
duced macrophages (Edelson, 1981). Leucine aminopeptidase activity
is much higher in TGC-elicited macrophages and is also elevated in
macrophages from animals injected with *Corynebacterium parvum* or
pyran copolymer. Alkaline phosphatase (APD) activity of TGC-elicited macrophages is about threefold higher than that of resident
cells (Edelson, 1981). Besides such biochemical approaches with
the plasma membrane, serological studies have been performed. Monoclonal antibodies, such as Mac-1, 2, 3, and 4 (Springer *et al.*,

1979; Ho and Springer, 1981), 2.6 (Mellman *et al.*, 1980), F4/80 (Austyn and Gordon, 1981), and 54.2 (LeBlanc *et al.*, 1980), defined mouse macrophage cell surface markers. However, none of these monoclonal antibodies have been able to discriminate activated macrophages from elicited or resident macrophages. Such a selective antibody was reported only as a heterologous rabbit antiserum against the P388D$_1$ mouse macrophage cell line that, after extensive absorption with the proper cells, detected a cell surface antigen associated with macrophages induced by *C. parvum* or pyran.

We therefore intended to search for biochemical and serological markers characteristic for tumoricidal macrophages. The results are reviewed in the following sections.

II. A NEW BIOCHEMICAL MARKER OF TUMORICIDAL
     MACROPHAGES IN MICE

A.   Glycosphingolipids as Differentiation Markers
     of a Macrophage Lineage Cell Line, M1

One approach to searching for cell surface markers of macrophage differentiation is to determine the chemical basis for the differences between normal and activated cells. For such an approach, macrophage lineage cell lines have merit as the cell source, because, for instance, possible contamination with other types of cells can be excluded.

We chose the M1 cell line established by Y. Ichikawa from a myeloid leukemia of an SL strain mouse (Ichikawa, 1969), because the M1 cells have been shown to differentiate into macrophage-like cells possessing such characteristics as Fc and C3 receptors, phagocytosis, motility, adhesiveness, and macrophage-like morphology, when they are incubated with various agents including lipopolysaccharides (LPS) (Hozumi *et al.*, 1979). We found that a culture supernatant of mouse spleen cells stimulated with concanavalin A-agarose (lymphokines, LK) was one of the agents (Akagawa *et al.*, 1981b). When the original M1 cells were incubated with 10% LK at 37°C for 2 days, the cells became activated and showed cytotoxicity for EL4 leukemic cells *in vitro*, when tested by an 18-hr ^{51}Cr-release assay at an E:T ratio of 30:1. The M1 cells incubated with LPS 10 µg/ml for 2 days also showed a significant level of cytotoxicity. We compared glycosphingolipids extracted from matured-type M1 cells preincubated with either LK or LPS with those from control M1 cells preincubated with medium alone (Akagawa *et al.*, 1981b). These extracts were subjected to tritiation, and [^{3}H]glycosphingolipids from 10^6 cells were applied on a high-performance silica gel thin-layer plate (Merck, Darmstadt), which was developed with chloroform-methanol-water (60:30:5, by volume). Autoradiofluorography of the glycosphingolipids showed almost the same band patterns, except for three bands. The cells preincubated with

either LK or LPS showed two dense bands corresponding to monohex-
osylceramide and gangliotriaosyl ceramide, and also a weak but significantly visible band corresponding to gangliotetraosyl ceramide
(asialo GM_1), whereas these bands were not seen or were seen only
faintly in the control M_1 cells. Among these three glycolipids,
we studied asialo GM_1 first; the other two are currently under in-
vesitgation.

Antiserum to asialo GM_1 (anti-asialo GM_1) prepared by means of
ammonium sulfate precipitation of the whole serum from a rabbit
given repeated injections of purified asialo GM_1 was provided by
M. Kasai (Kasai *et al.*, 1980). This antiserum reacted with asialo
GM_1 but not with the related glycolipids. The $F(ab')_2$ fraction of
anti-asialo GM_1 was purified by passage through a protein A-Sepha-
rose 4B column.

We tried to stain Ml cells preincubated with medium alone, LK,
or LPS with the $F(ab')_2$ fraction and assayed them by immunofluorescence microscopy. The results indicate that 47.3 or 13.2% of
the Ml cells preincubated with LK or LPS were stained with the
antiserum, respectively, while none of the control Ml cells were
stained (Akagawa *et al.*, 1981b).

Saito *et al.* (1980) observed that the sialylated glycosphingo-
lipid of asialo GM_1 was induced in Ml cells by preincubation with
LPS. These results and ours strongly suggest that the pathway of
asialo GM_1 synthesis is essentially present on Ml cells and that
asialo GM_1 synthesis-related glycosyl transferase is primarily induced during the activation.

B.   Asialo GM_1 as a Marker of Mouse Peritoneal
     Tumoricidal Macrophages

The findings just described led us to test whether mouse peritoneal macrophages generally become able to express asialo GM_1 on
the cell surface during activation.

Adherent fractions of resident peritoneal cells (PC) obtained
by washing out normal mouse peritoneal cavities, and peritoneal
exudate cells (PEC) obtained from mice receiving an ip injection
of proteose peptone 4 days earlier, or viable BCG or heat-killed
C. parvum 6 days earlier were tested for immunofluorescence staining with anti-asialo GM_1 and for killing with antiserum plus complement (Akagawa and Tokunaga, 1982). These adherent cells were
also tested for their cytotoxicity for EL4 leukemic cells *in vitro*.
Cytotoxicity was assayed by ^{51}Cr release from labeled target cells
during 18 hr of incubation, and the test results were expressed as
percentage tumor cell lysis by the formula:

$$\frac{\text{experimental release - spontaneous release}}{\text{maximal release - spontaneous release}} \times 100 \ (\%)$$

The results are shown in Table II. Peritoneal macrophages induced
by either BCG or *C. parvum* were stained with anti-asialo GM_1, killed

TABLE II

Percentage of Anti-Asialo GM_1-Reactive Cells
in Peritoneal Macrophages Induced with Various Agents,
and Cytotoxicity of the Macrophages for EL4 Tumor Cells

Macrophage-eliciting agent	Anti-asialo GM_1-reactive cells (%)		Cytotoxicity for EL4 (% ± SD)
	Staining	Killing	
None	1.8	1.8	-1.6 ± 1.8
Proteose peptone	8.6	4.8	-2.1 ± 0.6
BCG	37.4	23.0	28.2 ± 1.8
Heat-killed *C. parvum*	47.6	34.2	42.5 ± 2.3

by the antiserum plus complement, and showed strong cytotoxicity
for EL4, while resident and peptone-induced macrophages showed no
or very weak reactions.

Proteose peptone-induced macrophages were incubated with 10%
LK, 10 µg/ml LPS, or medium alone for 20 hr at 37°C. These cells
were stained with anti-asialo GM_1 and also tested for their cytotoxicity for EL4 cells *in vitro*. As shown in Table III, both the
percentages of cells stained with anti-asialo GM_1 and of target
cell lysis were markedly increased by incubation with LK or LPS.

TABLE III

Percentage of Anti-Asialo GM_1-Reactive Cells
and Cytotoxic Activity of Peritoneal Macrophages
Activated with LK or LPS

In vitro treatment	Cells stained with anti-asialo GM_1 (%)	Cytotoxicity for EL4 (% ± SD)
None	9.3	0.6 ± 3.5
LK	37.3	19.0 ± 6.1
LPS	30.6	23.3 ± 5.6

When peptone-induced macrophages were incubated with LK or LPS
for 20 hr at 37°C, and then treated with anti-asialo GM$_1$ plus complement for 40 min at 37°C, the cytotoxic activity of the remaining
macrophages was markedly reduced. In contrast, pretreatment of
peptone-induced peritoneal macrophages with anti-asialo GM$_1$ plus
complement did not affect the ability of the macrophages to be
activated by LK. The results suggest that mouse peritoneal cytotoxic macrophages activated either *in vivo* or *in vitro* selectively
express asialo GM$_1$ (Akagawa and Tokunaga, 1982).

It is known that asialo GM$_1$ is also a cell surface marker glycolipid of mouse natural killer (NK) cells (Kasai *et al.*, 1980),
and that PEC induced by BCG or *C. parvum* contain not a small number
of NK cells (Wolfe *et al.*, 1976; Ojo and Haller, 1978). In order
to certify that the asialo GM$_1$-positive cytotoxic cells induced by
BCG or *C. parvum* are macrophages as well as NK cells, we used two
different assay systems (Akagawa and Tokunaga, 1982). One is the
assay of ^{51}Cr released from labeled YAC cells during 4 hr of incubation, by which only NK activity is measurable. The other is
the assay of ^{51}Cr released from labeled EL4 cells during 18 hr of
incubation, by which only cytotoxic macrophage activity is detectable. As the effector cells for these assays, both whole PEC and
adherent macrophages induced by BCG 6 days earlier, in addition to
normal spleen cells, were used. The cells were incubated with normal rabbit serum plus complement (C), anti-asialo GM$_1$ plus complement, or medium alone for 30 min at 37°C, washed, and then tested
for their cytotoxicity. The results are shown in Table IV.

TABLE IV

Effects of *in Vitro* Treatment of BCG-Induced PEC
and Normal Spleen Cells with Anti-Asialo GM$_1$ Plus Complement (C)
on Their Cytotoxic Activity

Effector cells	Treatment	Cytotoxicity (% ± SD)	
		YAC	EL4
BCG-Induced whole PEC	None	23.7 ± 8.7	21.7 ± 1.9
	Normal serum + C	29.0 ± 5.1	22.1 ± 1.5
	Anti-asialo GM$_1$ + C	2.9 ± 3.6	5.3 ± 4.9
BCG-Induced macrophages	None	0.2 ± 0.7	16.6 ± 0.6
	Normal serum + C	-0.1 ± 0.5	18.0 ± 1.0
	Anti-asialo GM$_1$ + C	-1.0 ± 0.8	4.3 ± 1.6
Normal spleen cells	None	11.7 ± 1.9	-0.4 ± 1.6
	Normal serum + C	7.4 ± 0	-3.6 ± 6.5
	Anti-asialo GM$_1$ + C	-2.8 ± 0.6	-4.5 ± 9.0

Natural killer activity was detected in normal spleen cells
and BCG-induced whole PEC, but not in the adherent fraction of
BCG-induced PEC. Cytotoxic macrophage activity was detected in
whole cells and the adherent fraction of BCG-induced PEC, but not
in normal spleen cells. After treatment with anti-asialo GM_1 plus
complement, both NK and macrophage tumoricidal activities were
diminished.

Although the data are not shown, an intraperitoneal injection
of a very small amount of anti-asialo GM_1 into mice given BCG or
C. parvum 6 days earlier markedly reduced the cytotoxic activity
of both NK cells and macrophages (Akagawa and Tokunaga, 1982).

C. Significance of Asialo GM_1 as a Differentiation
    Marker of Macrophages

The distribution of anti-asialo GM_1-reactive macrophages was
investigated by means of staining with the F(ab')$_2$ fragment of the
antiserum. Only less than about 10% of the macrophages derived
from different tissues were stainable, except for lung macrophages
(Akagawa *et al.*, 1981a). Almost 100% of the lung macrophages from
various inbred mouse strains were stained with anti-asialo GM_1.
They were also killed by the antiserum plus complement. These
facts forced us to think about the possibility that lung macrophages express asialo GM_1 because they were already activated by
continuous stimulation with infecting microorganisms. However,
this was not true, because our subsequent experiments showed that
all of the lung macrophages from specific pathogen-free mice, germ-
free mice, mice 1 day after birth, and fetal mice at 18 days gestation were stained with anti-asialo GM_1. In contrast, lung macrophages from rat, guinea pig, monkey, and human were not stained
(Akagawa *et al.*, 1981).

An alternative possibility that we considered was that the
mouse lung macrophage surface molecule that is reactive with anti-
asialo GM_1 is not asialo GM_1 itself, but a kind of glycoprotein
possessing the same sugar residue as Galβ(1→3)GalNacβ of asialo
GM_1, because Momoi *et al.* (1982) found that this antiserum reacted with glycophorin pretreated with neuraminidase. However, this
possibility was also excluded. Our observation by autoradiofluorography of [^{3}H]glycosphingolipids extracted from mouse lung macrophages clearly indicated the existence of a large amount of asialo
GM_1 (T. Momoi, K. Akagawa, and T. Tokunaga, unpublished).

Subsequently, we found that mouse lung macrophages were not
cytotoxic for EL4 cells *in vitro*, even after incubation with either
10% LK or 10 µg/ml LPS for 20 hr, while peritoneal resident or peptone-induced macrophages could be activated for cytotoxicity with
either of them. Interestingly, incubation of lung macrophages
together with both 10% LK and a small amount of LPS rendered them
strongly cytotoxic (K. S. Akagawa, K. Sano, and T. Tokunaga, unpublished). The presence of anti-asialo GM_1 without complement

during the cytotoxicity test period did not block the cytotoxic
activity of BCG-induced macrophages. These facts suggest that
asialo GM_1 is not a critical molecule for cytotoxicity.

There are reports showing that some fractions of murine immature T cells (Habu et al., 1980), mature T cells, suppressor T
cells (Stein et al., 1978), and bone marrow cells (Kasai et al.,
1980) are reactive with anti-asialo GM_1. When these facts are
considered together, the significance of asialo GM_1 as a differentiation marker of macrophages is somewhat limited. We can say
that asialo GM_1 is a useful differentiation marker for mouse tumoricidal macrophages, except for lung macrophages.

III. NEW SEROLOGICAL MARKERS FOR TUMORICIDAL
      MACROPHAGES

To unravel the complexity of activation or differentiation of
macrophages for tumor cytotoxicity, we attempted to obtain hybridomas that secrete monoclonal antibodies specific for mouse macrophages in different stages of activation for tumor cytotoxicity
(Taniyama and Watanabe, 1982; Taniyama and Tokunaga, 1983).

Peritoneal macrophages of C3H/HeN or CBA/N mice induced by
TGC or pyran were injected ip into LOU/CN rats, and the immune
spleen cells were fused with P3U1 myeloma cells (Köhler and Milstein, 1975; Gefter et al., 1977). Screening for a hybridoma
secreting a monoclonal antibody was carried out by a ^{125}I-labeled
protein A or rabbit anti-rat IgG-binding assay or complement-dependent cytotoxicity with appropriate target cells. Target cells
for macrophage-mediated cytotoxicity test were ^{51}Cr-labeled L1210
cells.

Three monoclonal antibodies thus prepared, designated MM9,
WE15, and AcM.1, were cloned at least twice. The immunoglobulin
classes of these antibodies were IgM, IgG_{2b}, and IgG_{2c}, respectively. Table V summarizes the reactivity of the monoclonal antibodies, determined by immunofluorescence microscopy. Three patterns of reactivity were noted. WE15 antibody reacted with resident, TGC-induced, and pyran- or C. parvum-activated PEC, in
parallel with the macrophage content. MM9 antibody reacted with
only resident and TGC-induced PEC. AcM.1 antibody reacted with
only pyran- or C. parvum-activated PEC. However, none of the
three monoclonal antibodies reacted with spleen cells or thymocytes. These results were confirmed by complement-mediated cell
lysis by those antibodies and by binding assay with ^{125}I-labeled
rabbit anti-rat IgG.

Pyran- or C. parvum-activated macrophages abolished most cytotoxicity for tumor cells after treatment with AcM.1 and WE15 monoclonal antibodies plus complement, but not with MM9 monoclonal
antibodies plus complement. However, none of these three monoclonal antibodies blocked the cytotoxicity of the macrophages when

TABLE V

Reactivity of MM9, WE15, and AcM.1 Monoclonal Antibodies
with Mouse PEC Induced by Various Agents
and with Spleen and Thymus Cells

Cells	Cells stained (%)		
	MM9	WE15	AcM.1
Resident PEC	53	64	5
TGC-induced PEC	60	78	5
Pyran-induced PEC	7	70	73
C. parvum-induced PEC	8	67	62
Spleen cells	7	10	5
Thymocytes	5	5	5

they were present during the cytotoxicity assay period. Figure 1
shows fluorescence-activated cell analysis of PEC induced by TGC,
proteose peptone, or pyran, stained with AcM.1 monoclonal antibodies. It is clearly seen that the antibodies reacted with only
pyran-induced macrophages. The results of fluorescence-activated
cell analysis with MM9 and WE15 monoclonal antibodies also agreed
with the results just described.
    Taking these findings together, we conclude that WE15 antigen
is consistently expressed on macrophages during activation, MM9
antigen is present on resident and TGC-induced macrophages but not
on tumoricidal macrophages, and AcM.1 antigen exists on only pyran-
or C. parvum-activated macrophages (Taniyama and Tokunaga, 1983).
A heterologous antiserum prepared by injecting rabbit with the
P388D$_1$ mouse macrophage cell line has been reported to react only
with macrophages induced by pyran or C. parvum but not with resident macrophages or macrophages induced by TGC (Kaplan and Mohanakumar, 1977). The AcM.1 antigen is the first unique marker of tumoricidal macrophages recognized by monoclonal antibody. Relationship between AcM.1 and AMϕCSA antigen of Kaplan and Mohanakumar
(1977) and Kaplan et al. (1978) has not been clarified yet.

IV. CONCLUDING REMARKS

    Table VI summarizes all of our results presented here and some
of the results of other investigators. As Edelson (1981) stated,
identification of the activated state may require the demonstration of coordinate changes in a whole panel of markers, rather

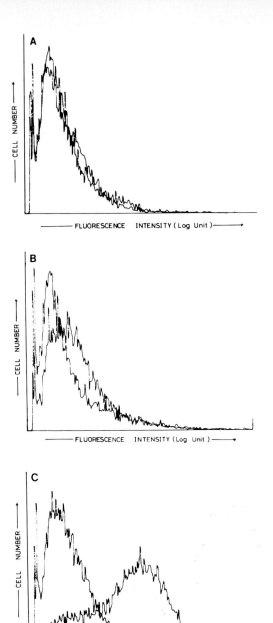

Fig. 1. Fluorescence-activated cell analysis of mouse peritoneal exudate cells stained with AcM.1 monoclonal antibody. The cells induced by (A) TGC, (B) proteose peptone, or (C) pyran were stained with biotinylated monoclonal antibody and FITC-avidin, and then cytofluorometry was performed with the EPICS V cell sorter (Coulter Electronics Inc., Hialeah, Florida). (From Taniyama and Watanabe, 1982; Taniyama and Tokunaga, 1983.)

TABLE VI

Cell Surface Markers of Macrophages

Markers	Peritoneal macrophages			Lung macrophages	References
	Resident	TGC-induced	C. parvum-induced		
Biochemical[a]					
5'-nucleotidase	++	−	±	++ [b]	Edelson (1981)
LAP	+	++	++	n.t.	Edelson (1981)
APD I	+	++	±	n.t.	Edelson (1981)
Asialo GM_1	−	−	++	++	Akagawa and Tokunaga (1982)
					Akagawa et al. (1981a)
Serological					
MM9	+	+	−	−	Taniyama and Tokunaga (1983)
WE15	+	+	+	−	Taniyama and Tokunaga (1983)
AcM.1	−	−	+	−	Taniyama and Watanabe (1982)
Tumor cytotoxicity	−	−	++	−	Taniyama and Tokunaga (1983)

[a]LAP, Leucine aminopeptidase; APD I, alkaline phosphatase I.
[b]n.t., Not tested.

than an isolated change in one particular characteristic. Undoubtedly, further efforts to obtain new biochemical and serological markers of activation or differentiation of macrophages including human macrophages promise much better understanding of the dynamic role of macrophages in host defense against tumors, and may finally allow the control of tumor metastasis.

REFERENCES

Akagawa, K. S., and Tokunaga, T. (1982). *Microbiol. Immunol. 26,* 831–842.
Akagawa, K. S., Maruyama, Y., Takano, M., Kasai, M., and Tokunaga, T. (1981a). *Microbiol. Immunol. 25,* 1215–1220.
Akagawa, K. S., Momoi, T., Nagai, Y., and Tokunaga, T. (1981b). *FEBS Lett. 130,* 80–84.
Austyn, J. M., and Gordon, S. (1981). *Eur. J. Immunol. 11,* 805–815.
Baldwin, R. W., Hopper, D. G., and Pimm, M. V. (1976). *Ann. N.Y. Acad. Sci. 277,* 124–134.
Bast, R. C., Jr., and Bast, B. S. (1976). *Ann. N.Y. Acad. Sci. 277,* 60–92.
Blanden, R. V., Mackaness, G. B., and Collins, S. M. (1966). *J. Exp. Med. 124,* 585–600.
Edelson, P. J. (1981). *In* "Lymphokines" (E. Pick, ed.), Vol. 3, pp. 57–83. Academic Press, New York.
Evans, R., and Alexander, P. (1970). *Nature (London) New Biol. 288,* 620–622.
Fidler, I. J. (1980). *Science (Washington, D.C.) 208,* 1469–1471.
Fidler, I. J., Sone, S., Fogler, W. E., and Barnes, Z. L. (1981). *Proc. Natl. Acad. Sci. USA 78,* 1680–1684.
Gefter, M. C., Margulies, D. H., and Sharff, M. D. (1977). *Somatic Cell Genet. 3,* 231.
Habu, S., Kasai, M., Nagai, Y., Tamaoki, N., Tada, T., Herzenberg, L. A., and Okumura, K. (1981). *J. Immunol. 125,* 2284–2288.
Hibbs, J. B., Jr., Lambert, L. H., Jr., and Remington, J. S. (1972) *Nature (London) New Biol. 235,* 48–50.
Hibbs, J. B., Jr., Taintor, R. R., Chapman, H. A., Jr., and Weinberg, J. B. (1977). *Science (Washington, D.C.) 197,* 279–282.
Ho, M. K., and Springer, T. A. (1981). *In* "Monoclonal Antibodies and T-Cell Hybridomas. Perspectives and Technical Advances" (G. Hammerling, U. Hammerling, and J. Kearney, eds.), pp. 53–61. Elsevier, Amsterdam.
Hozumi, M., Homma, Y., Tomida, M., Okabe, J., Kasukabe, T., Sugiyama, K., Hayashi, K., Takenaga, K., and Yamamoto, Y. (1979). *Acta Haematol. 42,* 941–952.
Ichikawa, Y. (1969). *J. Cell. Physiol. 74,* 223–234.
Kaplan, A. M., and Mohanakumar, T. (1977). *J. Exp. Med. 146,* 1461–1466.

Kaplan, A. M., Bear, H. D., Kirk, L., Cummins, C., and Mohanakumar, T. (1978). *J. Immunol. 120,* 2080-2085.
Kasai, M., Iwamori, M., Nagai, Y., Okumura, K., and Tada, T. (1980). *Eur. J. Immunol. 10,* 175-180.
Kataoka, T., and Tokunaga, T. (1979). *Kekkaku 54,* 413-417.
Keller, R. (1973). *J. Exp. Med. 138,* 625-644.
Kleinschuster, S. J., Rapp, H. J., Lueker, D. C., and Kainer, R. A. (1977). *J. Natl. Cancer Inst. (US) 58,* 1807-1814.
Köhler, G., and Milstein, C. (1975). *Nature (London) 256,* 495-497.
LeBlanc, P. A., Katz, H. R., and Russell, S. W. (1980). *Infect. Immun. 29,* 520-525.
Mackaness, G. B. (1969). *J. Exp. Med. 129,* 973-992.
Mastrangelo, M. J., Berd, D., and Bellet, R. E. (1976). *Ann. N.Y. Acad. Sci. 277,* 94-122.
Mellman, I. S., Steinman, R. M., Unkeless, J. C., and Cohn, Z. A. (1980). *J. Cell Biol. 86,* 717-722.
Meltzer, M. S. (1981). *In* "Lymphokines" (E. Pick, ed.), Vol.3, pp. 319-343. Academic Press, New York.
Momoi, T., Tokunaga, T., and Nagai, Y. (1982). *FEBS Lett. 141,* 6-10.
Morahan, P. S. (1980). *J. Reticuloendothel. Soc. 27,* 223-239.
Morton, D. L., Eilber, F. R., Malmgren, R. A., and Wood, W. C. (1970). *Surgery (St. Louis) 68,* 158-164.
Nakamura, R. M., and Tokunaga, T. (1980). *Infect. Immun. 28,* 331-335.
Nakamura, R. M., Tanaka, H., and Tokunaga, T. (1982). *Immunol. Lett. 4,* 295-299.
Nelson, D. S. (1976). "Immunobiology of the Macrophage." Academic Press, New York.
Ojo, E., and Haller, O. (1978). *J. Cancer 21,* 444-452.
Saito, M., Nojiri, H., and Yamada, M. (1980). *Biochem. Biophys. Res. Commun. 97,* 452-462.
Springer, T. A., Galfré, G., Secher, D. S., and Milstein, C. (1979). *Eur. J. Immunol. 9,* 301-306.
Stein, K. E., Schwarting, G. A., and Marcus, D. M. (1978). *J. Immunol. 120,* 676-679.
Tanaka, H., Tsuru, S., and Tokunaga, T. (1981). *Immunol. Lett. 2,* 251-255.
Taniyama, T., and Tokunaga, T. (1983). *J. Immunol. 131,* 1032-1037.
Taniyama, T., and Watanabe, T. (1982). *J. Exp. Med. 156,* 1286-1291.
Tokunaga, T., Yamamoto, S., Nakamura, R. M., and Kataoka, T. (1974). *J. Natl. Cancer Inst. (US) 53,* 459-463.
Tokunaga, T., Kataoka, T., Nakamura, R. M., Yamamoto, S., and Akagawa, K. S. (1978). *Gann Monogr. Cancer Res. 21,* 59-72.
Wolfe, S. A., Tracey, D. E., and Henney, C. S. (1976). *Nature (London) 262,* 584-586.
Zbar, B., Ribi, E., Kelly, M., Dranger, D., Evans, C., and Rapp, H. J. (1976). *Cancer Immunol. Immunother. 1,* 127-137.

DISCUSSION

YOSHIDA: Is the same factor (MAF?) in crude lymphokine prepara-
           tions responsible for both induction of asialo GM_1 and
           cytotoxicity? Is the activity in LK preparations res-
           ponsible for asialo GM_1 induction due to LPS activity?

TOKUNAGA: For the first question, we do not know yet whether the
           same factor is responsible for both induction of asialo
           GM_1 and cytotoxicity. We also do not know about the
           significance of asialo GM_1 in the cytotoxicity. At
           least, anti-asialo GM_1 antiserum, without complement,
           does not block the cytotoxicity. For the second ques-
           tion, my answer is no, because, for instance, LPS at
           any dose could not induce cytotoxicity of lung macro-
           phages, but could if the cells were pretreated crude
           lymphokines.

OKADA: Is it not possible that the inhibitory effect of anti-
           GM_1 on cytotoxic activity of macrophages (on EL4) was a
           result of secondary effect of immune complex formed by
           some other GM_1-positive cell and anti-GM_1? $F(ab')_2$ an-
           tibodies still have some biological function such as a
           capacity to activate Cl via the alternative pathway.

TOKUNAGA: I do not think so, because we used the $F(ab')_2$ fraction
           of anti-asialo GM_1 antiserum with complement to elim-
           inate asialo GM_1-positive macrophages. Also, we took
           anti-Thy-1 antibody as a control to exclude a possible
           nonspecific effect of immunoglobulin.

CHAPTER 11

HUMAN AMNION AS A NEW QUANTITATIVE MODEL
FOR TUMOR INVASION *IN VITRO*

Lance A. Liotta
Unnur P. Thorgeirsson
Raymondo G. Russo

Laboratory of Pathology
National Cancer Institute
National Institutes of Health
Bethesda, Maryland

I. INTRODUCTION

    Local invasion and secondary dissemination are the two most
reliable criteria for the definition of a "malignant" tumor. Although the phenomenon of cancer invasion has been recognized for
centuries, we are now only beginning to explore the basic biochemical and genetic mechanisms of this process. Our ability to study
the mechanism of invasion has been hampered by the lack of a simple, quantitative, reproducible *in vitro* assay for measuring invasive capacity. The majority of previous investigators studying
invasion *in vitro* have cocultivated organ fragments with tumor
cells and used histology to score invasion potential (Table I).
These systems are nonquantitative. The few previous quantitative
assays have used chorioallantoic membrane, canine veins, and urinary bladder (Table I). These assays have not been ideal because
the tissue being used is highly complex, containing multiple host
tissue layers and host immune cells. Other investigators have
quantitated the ability of tumor cells to degrade cultured extracellular matrix or isolated matrix components (Table I). These
assays are incomplete because they do not use native matrix and do
not measure the ability of the tumor cell to move through the invaded tissue.
    We have therefore developed a new quantitative invasion assay
that measures the ability of the tumor cell to migrate through the
three basic human tissue barriers separating the tissue compartment from the circulatory compartment. These are (1) parenchymal
cells, (2) native basement membranes (BM), and (3) native interstitial stroma. The BM is a continuous structure composed of
types IV and V collagen, laminin, entactin, and proteoglycan
(Kefalides and Denduchis, 1969; Vracko, 1974; Timpl *et al.*, 1979,
1981; Roll *et al.*, 1980; Garbisa *et al.*, 1981; Carlin *et al.*,
1981; Hascall and Hascall, 1982). The interstitial stroma consists
of a dense meshwork of collagen types I and III, elastin, and proteoglycan and does not contain open spaces large enough for cells
to pass through (Pearce and Laurent, 1977; Bornstein and Sage,
1980).
    Human amnion is the tissue used as the invasion barrier
(Liotta *et al.*, 1980b). This tissue is a translucent membrane
available in large quantities (one amnion can be used for 50 assays) from human placenta. It is composed of an epithelium resting
on a continuous basement membrane overlying an interstitial stroma.
It contains no inflammatory cells, nerves, or blood vessels. For
the assay, tumor cells are placed on one side of the amnion membrane and the number penetrating through to the other side are
collected and counted. The amnion matrix can also be radiolabeled
for degradation studies.

TABLE I

EXAMPLES OF *IN VITRO* INVASION ASSAY SYSTEMS

Assay	Reference
Chick blastoderm	Mareel *et al.* (1975)
Chick chorioallantoic membrane	Easty and Easty (1976); Scher *et al.* (1976); Hart and Fidler (1978)
Chick embryonic mesonephros	Porreau-Schneider *et al.* (1977)
Chick embryonic skin	Noguchi *et al.* (1978)
Chick embryonic heart	Mareel *et al.* (1979)
Chick wing bud	Tickle *et al.* (1978)
Human decidual tissue	Schleich *et al.* (1976)
Mouse lung	Schirrmacher *et al.* (1979)
Rat embryo yolk sac	Maignan (1979)
Canine vein	Poste *et al.* (1980)
Extracted bovine articular cartilage	Pauli *et al.* (1981)
Cultured cell matrix	Jones and DeClark (1980)

II. AMNION INVASION ASSAY

A. Histology of the Human Amnion

The fetal membranes consist of a chorion and an amnion, the latter facing the fetus. The amnion is a transparent uniform membrane, less than 1 mm in thickness. It is composed of a single layer of columnar epithelium, a thick basement membrane, and a collagenous stroma that is easily separable from the chorion. The amnion BM is structurally and immunologically identical to BM elsewhere in the body (Van Herendael *et al.*, 1978; Kefalides *et al.*, 1979; Alitalo *et al.*, 1980; Russo *et al.*, 1981). The underlying avascular stroma contains banded collagen fibers and scattered fibroblasts.

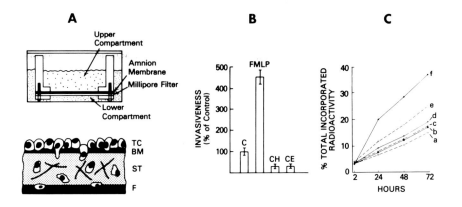

Fig. 1. Summary of studies using the *in vitro* amnion invasion assay. (A) Diagram of the amnion invasion model (cross-sectional representation). The amnion with the attached filter divides the chamber into an upper compartment and a lower compartment where the chemoattractant is added. The tumor cells (TC) are placed in the upper compartment, where they attach to the basement membrane (BM) of the amnion, penetrate by focal proteolytic degradation of the BM and the stroma (ST), and are finally trapped on a Millipore filter (F) that is in close contact with the amnion stroma. (B) Summary of invasion studies with M5076 cells are presented as a bar graph. The chemoattractant FMLP stimulates invasion 450% compared to control (C), but cycloheximide (CH) and bovine cartilage extract (CE) inhibit invasion even in the presence of FMLP. (C) The data from invasion assays using radiolabeled amnion show time course of radioactive counts released by tumor cells presented as percentages of the total counts incorporated into the amnion. Curve a, cultured bovine endothelium; b, human rhabdomyosarcoma (A-675); c, cultured human skin fibroblasts (BUD-8); d, human melanoma (A-375); e, human metastatic melanoma (A-2058); f, human rhabdomyosarcoma (A-204). It can be concluded that tumor cell protein synthesis and extracellular matrix degradation are required for invasion, whereas tumor cell proliferation, serum factors, and living host cells are not required.

B. Preparation of Assay

Term placentas were used within 24 hr of normal delivery. The amnion was aseptically separated from the chorion and the umbilical cord, and rinsed three times in PBS containing antibiotics (penicillin 50 μg/ml; streptomycin 50 μg/ml). Blood and extra mucus was gently wiped off with sterile gauze. For experiments with polymorphonuclear leukocytes (PMN) requiring a living epithelium, the amnion was used immediately. For experiments using the BM surface for tumor cell attachment, the epithelial layer was removed by treatment with 0.2 *M* ammonium hydroxide at room temperature for 30 min. Following the chemical treatment, the epithelial surface was gently wiped with sterile gauze to remove cellular debris. The de-epithelialized amnion was stored refrigerated in Eagle's MEM up to 3 weeks in the presence of the antibiotic mixture (as described earlier).

The invasion chambers were composed of two Lucite rings (Fig. 1). The rings measured 3.2 cm outside diameter and 1.2 cm inner diameter. The upper ring was 1.0 cm in height and the lower 0.2 cm in height. The amnion was layered over the upper rings, and Millipore filters (5 or 8 μm pore size) were placed on the stromal surface. Both were fixed between the two Lucite rings with four screws and placed in a six-well Costar tissue culture plate. The presence of the amnion with the closely attached filter divided the invasion chamber into two compartments, the upper facing the epithelial or BM side of the amnion and the lower compartment facing the Millipore filter. In experiments where a chemoattractant, N-formylmethionyl-leucyl-phenylalanine (FMLP) was used, it was added to the medium (2.5 ml) of the lower compartment of the invasion chamber. The cells were added onto the amnion in the upper compartment in a concentration of 5×10^5 to 1×10^6 cells in 1.5 ml of medium. For PMN and M5076 tumor cell invasion assays (up to 24 hr), no serum was used, but for other tumor cells, 2% Nu serum (Collaborative Research) was used. The invasion assays were carried out at $37^{\circ}C$ (5% CO_2, 95% air) for variable lengths of time depending on cell types. The number of cells that had passed through the entire thickness of the amnion and onto the Millipore filter were counted after routine hematoxylin and eosin (H+E) staining of the amnion with the attached filter. The cells adherent to or within the Millipore filter after clearing in xylene could easily be identified. The whole filter (0.76 cm^2) was scanned (400×), and the total number of cells counted. In each experiment triplicate samples were used. The number of cells attached to the amnion were calculated by using an ocular micrometer (the number of cells within 15 squares were counted).

The second approach to measure tumor cell invasion of the amnion was to use radiolabeled amnion. A fresh amnion (less than 1 hr after delivery) was cleaned as described previously. The amnion was then placed in 80 ml of DMEM medium without glutamine, with penicillin-streptomycin mixture (as described earlier), ascorbic acid (10 mg), β-amino-propionitrile (BAPN) (10 mg), dialyzed fetal bovine serum (20 ml), and 125 μCi of ^{14}C proline (in 2.5 ml). The labeling medium was filtered and incubated with the amnion in a 250-ml tube at $37^{\circ}C$ for 36 hr with gentle shaking. Following the incubation the epithelial layer of the amnion was removed, and the amnion assay was set up as described previously. Tumor matrix degradation was quantitated by measuring the soluble radioactive counts released into the media at different time points. At the end of the experiment the amnion was degraded in 1 mg/ml bacterial collagenase, and the total radioactivity of the membrane was measured. The counts released were recorded as percentages of the total counts incorporated.

III. MIGRATION OF POLYMORPHONUCLEAR LEUKOCYTES
      (PMN) THROUGH THE AMNION

     Inflammatory cells and tumor cells have in common the capacity
to migrate through tissue barriers (Showell *et al.*, 1976; Ryan and
Majno, 1977; Zigmond, 1978). In the amnion invasion assay system,
we first tested spontaneous and chemotactically stimulated penetration of PMN through an untreated fresh amnion (Russo *et al.*,
1981). The PMN were demonstrated by electron microscopy to attach
to the epithelial surface and migrate between the epithelial cells.
As they passed through the BM, the cells formed pseudopodia at the
point of penetration of the BM where a focal dissolution of the
membrane was noted. At the stromal site a local clearing of the
collagen fibers adjacent to the migrating PMN was noted. One of
the most potent chemoattractants for PMN and macrophages is FMLP,
which exerts its activity by binding to specific cell surface receptors. The chemotaxis of PMN through the amnion was concentration
dependent with the optimal concentration of 10^{-8} *M* FMLP, where up to
12-fold increase in number of invading cells was measured. At
a lower concentration (10^{-10} *M*), only a three-fold increase was
detected, but excess concentration (10^{-5} *M*) FMLP caused PMN to
aggregate on the amnion, which led to inhibition of migration
(O'Flaherty and Ward, 1978). Diffusion studies with ^{3}H-labeled
FMLP across the amnion demonstrated that the most rapid migration
was within the first few hours (50% of the equilibrium value was
reached by 4 to 5 hr), and equilibrium across the membrane was
reached by 17 hr. From these measurements a 3-hr assay was chosen
for the PMN invasion. Previous investigators have shown that FMLP
can attract PMN to move through a porous artificial layer. These
amnion studies were the first to demonstrate that FMLP can attract
PMN to move through whole human native tissue barriers.

IV. MIGRATION OF TUMOR CELLS THROUGH
     THE AMNION

     In contrast to PMN, which readily adhered to the living amnion
epithelium, the tumor cells attached poorly to the epithelium but
adhered avidly to the denuded BM (Russo *et al.*, 1981). A number
of normal cells and cultured tumor cell lines have been tested in
the amnion invasion assay (Russo *et al.*, 1982; Thorgeirsson *et
al.*, 1982). Cells that did not invade the amnion within 6 days of
incubation were human fibroblasts, human and bovine endothelial
cells, and rat hepatocytes. Cells that invaded the amnion were
human breast carcinoma (MCF-7 and ZR-75-1), Ewing's sarcoma, human
squamous carcinoma (A431), mouse reticulum cell sarcoma (M5076),
mouse BL6 melanoma (B16 variant), mouse PMT sarcoma, human PMN, and
mouse macrophages. Generally, only a small proportion ($\leq 0.1\%$) of

the attached tumor cells migrated through the entire thickness of
the amnion and entered the Millipore filter. Light microscopy
focusing at different levels of the amnion stroma revealed many
more tumor cells in various stages of invasion. Tumor cells varied
in their rate of invasion, but some, such as M5076 cells, passed
through the entire thickness of the amnion in significant numbers
within 24 hr. Studies with MCF-7 demonstrated a threefold increase
in number of cells from Day 2 to Day 7. Another study of MCF-7
cells showed a fivefold increase in the rate of migration after
the invasive cells were grown up and recycled through the amnion.
Time course studies suggested that most types of tumor cells tra-
versed the amnion as single cells and later grew as colonies on
the filter. Tumor cells on the filter were quantitated as the
total number of single cells or colonies per filter.

The use of radiolabeled amnion indicated that the release of
soluble radioactive counts was associated with tumor cell invasion
of the amnion. Release of degraded amnion basement membrane products into the culture media was dependent on the tumor cell type
and the time of incubation. Many human tumor cell lines degraded
up to 30% of the labeled amnion matrix within 72 hr. Type IV
collagen, which is a major constituent of amnion basement membrane,
is not susceptible to the classic mammalian collagenase, which
degrades collagen I, II, and III. A separate collagenase is required to degrade type IV collagen (Mainardi *et al.*, 1980). A
tumor cell-derived type IV collagenase was purified that produced
specific cleavage products of type IV collagen (Fig. 2) (Liotta
et al., 1979, 1980a). This enzyme is expressed by invasive murine
and human tumors.

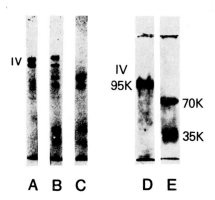

Fig. 2. Cleavage of basement membrane-specific type IV collagen by a metalloprotease isolated from metastatic tumor cells.
(A) "Pro" type IV collagen substrate; (B) substrate + enzyme 5 hr,
35°C; (C) substrate + enzyme 15 hr, 35°C; (D) pepsinized type IV
collagen substrate; (E) substrate + enzyme 18°C, 40 hr.

V. THE EFFECT OF A CHEMOATTRACTANT (FMLP)
    AND NATURAL PROTEASE INHIBITORS ON TUMOR CELL
    INVASION OF THE AMNION

    It has been postulated that tumor cell chemotaxis may be rel-
evant in metastases formation. Several factors have been identified that induce a chemotactic response by tumor cells (Romualdez
and Ward, 1975; Wass *et al.*, 1981). One of these factors, FMLP, is
a potent chemoattractant for PMN and macrophages as mentioned earlier. We studied the effect of FMLP on migration of the murine
reticulum cell sarcoma line M5076 (Hart *et al.*, 1981) through the
amnion. From a series of concentrations tested, a fivefold increase in M5076 cell invasion was measured in response to the optimal concentration of 10^{-7} M FMLP. This stimulation was not associated with an increase in the secretion of type IV collagenase
per cell. It can therefore be concluded that the major effect of
FMLP was to stimulate directed locomotion of the tumor cells
through the amnion.
    Many types of tumor cells produce proteolytic enzymes that may
facilitate invasion (Dresden *et al.*, 1972; Liotta *et al.*, 1977,
1982). Cartilage, which is known to be highly resistant to tumor
invasion *in vivo,* is known to contain various types of protease
inhibitors. We studied the effect of a bovine cartilage extract
on M5076 invasiveness in the amnion assay. When the tumor cells
were placed on the amnion in the presence of the cartilage extract
(100 μg/ml), a significant decrease in invasion was demonstrated.
Because inhibitors to both metalloproteases and serine proteases
are found in the cartilage extract, we had to assess separately
the importance of the two types of inhibitors. A purified metalloprotease inhibitor (TIMP) of a molecular weight of 28,000 (Cawston *et al.*, 1981) was tested in a concentration of 10 μg/ml and
found to inhibit the M5076 cell invasion to the same degree as the
cartilage extract. In contrast to the metalloprotease inhibitor,
a serine protease inhibitor (soybean trypsin inhibitor) had no effect on invasion. Bovine serum albumin, which served as a negative
control, was also ineffective. Cell viability, cell attachment,
or cell growth was not affected by the presence of the FMLP or the
inhibitors. These data (Thorgeirsson *et al.*, 1982) support the
hypothesis that metalloproteases play an important role in tumor
cell invasion.

VI. THE EFFECT OF INHIBITORS TO PROTEIN
     AND DNA SYNTHESIS ON TUMOR CELL INVASION
     OF THE AMNION

    Although cell proliferation is required for expansive tumor
growth, there is no evidence for direct relationship between tumor
growth and invasive behavior (Fidler, 1978). We decided to measure

invasiveness of tumor cells (M5076) treated with inhibitors to protein or DNA synthesis (Thorgeirsson et al., 1984). Treatment of M5076 cells with a low concentration of cycloheximide (10^{-6} M) (Timberlake and Griffin, 1973) selectively blocked protein synthesis and resulted in a fivefold decrease in tumor cell invasiveness. For inhibition of DNA synthesis and cell division, the cells were treated with sodium butyrate (1 mM), which prolongs the G_1 phase of the cell cycle (Fallon and Cox, 1979). Butyrate treatment led to a slight increase in invasion as well as in type IV collagenase production. The second DNA inhibitor, aphidicolin (10 μg/ml), selectively blocks the α-DNA polymerase (Sugino and Nakayama, 1980). It had no effect on the M5076 cell invasion. These data indicate that protein synthesis is required for production of proteolytic enzymes and other factors necessary for invasion, but tumor cells do not need DNA synthesis and cell proliferation to invade host connective tissues.

VII. CONCLUSIONS

The amnion invasion model offers a simple quantitative approach to measure tumor cell invasion in vitro. It is not considered to simulate the complete in vivo situation but to focus on one important step in the invasive process, that is, penetration of tumor cells through a native human BM and connective tissue stroma. The assay can be used to study basic biochemical mechanisms of the invasion process (see legend to Fig. 1). We are currently using the assay to study the genetic basis of tumor cell invasion. The assay also has potential clinical applications.

REFERENCES

Alitalo, E., Kurkinen, M., and Vaheri, A. (1980). Cell 19, 1053-1062.
Bornstein, P., and Sage, H. (1980). Annu. Rev. Biochem. 49, 957-1003.
Carlin, B., Jaffe, R., Bender, B., and Chung, E. E. (1981). J. Biol. Chem. 256, 5209-5214.
Cawston, T. E., Galloway, W. A., Merger, E., Murphy, G., and Reynolds, J. J. (1981). Biochem. J. 195, 159-165.
Dresden, M. H., Heilman, S. A., and Schmidt, J. D. (1972). Cancer Res. 32, 993-996.
Easty, D. M., and Easty, G. C. (1976). In "Organ Culture in Biochemical Research" (M. Balls and M. Monnickendam, eds.), pp. 379-392. Cambridge Univ. Press, Cambridge.
Fallon, R. J., and Cox, R. P. (1979). J. Cell. Physiol. 100, 251-262.

Fidler, I. J. (1978). *Cancer Res. 38,* 2651-2660.
Garbisa, S., Liotta, L. A., Tryggvason, K., and Siegal, G. P. (1981). *FEBS Lett. 127,* 257-262.
Hart, I. R., and Fidler, I. J. (1978). *Cancer Res. 38,* 3218-3224.
Hart, I. R., Talmage, J. E., and Fidler, I. J. (1981). *Cancer Res. 41,* 1281-1287.
Hascall, V. C., and Hascall, G. K. (1982). *In* "Cell Biology of Extracellular Matrix" (E. D. Hay, ed.), pp. 39-63. Plenum, New York.
Jones, P. A., and DeClark, Y. A. (1980). *Cancer Res. 40,* 3222-3227.
Kefalides, N. A., and Denduchis, B. (1969). *Biochemistry 8,* 4613-4621.
Kefalides, N. A., Alper, R., and Clark, C. C. (1979). *Int. Rev. Cytol. 61,* 167-228.
Liotta, L. A., Kleinerman, J., Catanzaro, P., and Rynbrandt, D. (1977). *J. Natl. Cancer Inst. (US) 58,* 1427-1431.
Liotta, L. A., Abe, S., Gehron-Robey, P., and Martin, G. R. (1979). *Proc. Natl. Acad. Sci. USA 76,* 2268-2272.
Liotta, L. A., Tryggvason, K., Garbisa, S., Hart, I., Foltz, C. M., and Shafie, S. (1980a). *Nature (London) 284,* 67-68.
Liotta, L. A., Lee, C. W., and Morakis, D. J. (1980b). *Cancer Lett. 11,* 141.
Liotta, L. A., Garbisa, S., and Tryggvason, K. (1982). *In* "Tumor Invasion and Metastases" (L. A. Liotta and I. R. Hart, eds.), pp. 319-335. Martinus Nijhoff, The Hague, Netherlands.
Maignan, M. F. (1979). *Biol. Cell. 35,* 229-232.
Mainardi, C. L., Dixit, S. N., and Kang, A. G. (1980). *J. Biol. Chem. 255,* 5435-5441.
Mareel, M., DeRidder, L., DeBrabander, M., and Vakaet, L. (1975). *J. Natl. Cancer Inst. (US) 54,* 923-929.
Mareel, M., Kint, J., and Meyvisch, C. (1979). *Virchows Arch. B 30,* 95-111.
Noguchi, P. D., Johnson, J. B., O'Donnel, R., and Petricciani, J. C. (1978). *Science (Washington, D. C.) 199,* 1980-1983.
O'Flaherty, J. T., and Ward, P. A. (1978). *Inflammation 3,* 177-194
Pauli, B. U., Memoli, V. A., and Kuettner, K. E. (1981). *Cancer Res. 41,* 2084-2091.
Pearce, R. H., and Laurent, T. C. (1977). *Biochem. J. 163,* 617-625
Poste, G., Doll, J., Hart, I. R., and Fidler, I. J. (1980). *Cancer Res. 40,* 1636-1644.
Pourreau-Schneider, N., Felix, H., and Haemmerli, G. (1977). *Virchows Arch. B 23,* 257-264.
Roll, R. J., Madri, J. A., Alberta, J., and Furthmayr, H. (1980). *J. Cell Biol. 85,* 597-616.
Romualdez, A. G., and Ward, P. A. (1975). *Proc. Natl. Acad. Sci. USA 172,* 4128-4132.
Russo, R. G., Liotta, L. A., Thorgeirsson, U., Brundage, R., and Schiffman, E. (1981). *J. Cell Biol. 91,* 459-467.

Russo, R. G., Thorgeirsson, U., and Liotta, L. A. (1982). *In* "Tumor Invasion and Metastases" (L. A. Liotta and I. R. Hart, eds.), pp. 173-187. Martinus Nijhoff, The Hague, Netherlands.

Ryan, G. B., and Majno, G. (1977). *Am. J. Pathol. 86,* 185-276.

Scher, C. D., Handenschild, C., and Klagsbrun, M. (1976). *Cell 8,* 373-382.

Schirrmacher, V., Shantz, G., Clauer, K., Komitowski, D., Zimmerman, H. P., and Lohmann-Matthes, M. L. (1979). *Int. J. Cancer 23,* 233-244.

Schleich, A. B., Frick, M., and Mayer, A. (1976). *J. Natl. Cancer Inst. (US) 56,* 221-225.

Showell, H. J., Freer, R. J., Zigmond, S. H., Schiffman, E., Aswanikumar, S., Corcoran, B., and Becker, E. L. (1976). *J. Exp. Med. 143,* 1154-1169.

Sugino, A., and Nakayama, K. (1980). *Proc. Natl. Acad. Sci. USA 77,* 7049-7053.

Thorgeirsson, U. P., Liotta, L. A., Kalebic, T., Margulies, I. M., Thomas, K., Rios-Candelore, M., and Russo, R. G. (1982). *J. Natl. Cancer Inst. (US) 69,* 1049-1054.

Thorgeirsson, U. P., Turpeenniemi-Hujanen, T., Neckers, L. M., Johnson, D. W., and Liotta, L. A. (1984). *Invasion Metastasis 4,* 73-83.

Tickle, A., Crawley, A., and Goodman, M. (1978). *J. Cell Sci. 31,* 293-322.

Timberlake, W. E., and Griffin, D. H. (1973). *Biochem. Biophys. Res. Commun. 54,* 216-221.

Timpl, R., Rhode, H., Gehron Robey, P., Rennard, S. I., Foidart, J. M., and Martin, G. R. (1979). *J. Biol. Chem. 254,* 9933-9937.

Timpl, R., Wiedemann, H., VanDelden, V., Furthmayr, H., and Kuhn, K. (1981). *Eur. J. Biochem. 120,* 203-211.

Van Herendael, B. J., Oberti, C., and Brosens, I. (1978). *Am. J. Obstet. Gynecol. 131,* 872-880.

Vracko, R. (1974). *Am. J. Pathol. 77,* 313-346.

Wass, J. A., Varani, J., Pointek, G. E., Goff, D., and Ward, P. A. (1981). *J. Natl. Cancer Inst. (US) 66,* 927-933.

Zigmond, S. H. (1978). *J. Cell Biol. 77,* 269-287.

DISCUSSION

YOSHIDA: Is the extravasation step in hematogenic metastasis essential? How about the possibility of intravascular proliferation?

LIOTTA: Electron microscopy studies of extravasation demonstrate that the majority of tumor cells exit the blood vessel in single-cell form; nevertheless, some types of tumors may indeed use alternative mechanisms to penetrate basement membranes.

WEISS: (1) Does collagenase IV degrade laminin?   (2) What about
            fibronectin?   Two years ago, the literature was flooded
            with extravagant claims that the key to invasion and
            metastasis was fibronectin.   (3) Would you comment on the
            apparent paradox that crawling cells require attachment
            to a substratum in order to move, but collagenase IV,
            which is required for penetration of the basement membrane,
            also destroys the substratum through which the cells move?

LIOTTA: (1) Collagenase type IV cleaves type IV collagen under
            conditions in which there is little or no cleavage of
            laminin.   (2)   Metastatic tumor cells in our studies do
            not preferentially use fibronectin to attach to type IV
            collagen.   Fibronectin is abundant in the serum, whereas
            laminin is not; therefore, circulating tumor cells would
            be bathed in fibronectin, and it would seem logical that
            laminin in the basement membrane would be a more specific
            factor for mediating attachment.   (3)   Electron micro-
            scopy studies show that the tumor cell is attached at one
            region and extends a cell pseudopodium through the basement
            membrane at a different location.   Basement membrane de-
            gradation is highly localized.

MATHÉ: Don't you think it would be worthwhile to search if vinca
            alkaloids do not work on invasiveness by cutting laminin
            into fragments?

LIOTTA: Yes, this would be a worthwhile study.

POSTE: (1) Have you performed your interesting experiments on
            inhibition of metastasis with the P_1 fragment of laminin
            with nonsyngeneic tumors?   (2) Are there amino acid se-
            quence data available for the P_1 fragment?

LIOTTA: We are now initiating experiments in nude mice with MCF-7
            human breast carcinoma.   We expect human laminin frag-
            ments to behave in identical fashion.   A pharmacologic
            analog to the laminin fragment could be of potential clin-
            ical use.

MORTON: Will tumor cells invade through amnion with epithelium
            intact?

LIOTTA: Yes, the tumor cells move between the epithelial cells.

COHEN: If collagenase is important, then cells that invade but
            don't have collagenase must "hitchhike" along.   Are pos-
            itive and negative invading cells always in close proxi-
            mity in tissue sections, or do they sometimes segregate?

LIOTTA: It is certainly possible that some tumor cells could
         "follow the leader" behind other invading tumor cells.
         Tumor cells immunologically negative for collagenase may
         have arrived by a "hitchhike" means or they may be no
         longer actively invading. They may have "switched off"
         collagenase production.

COHEN: The amnion assay seems ideal to study the role of col-
         lagenase, since you can obtain three populations of cells:
         those that don't stick, those that stick but don't penet-
         rate, and those that penetrate. Have you studied whether
         these have different collagenase content?

LIOTTA: We have not performed those experiments. We might expect
         a different collagenase content.

KONDO: In your experiment with amnion membrane, could you neglect
         the participation of gravity? What will happen if you
         reverse the membrane after attaching tumor cells to the
         membrane?

LIOTTA: Gravity is not important. We can flip the amnion over
         and invasion still takes place.

WEISS: Are the cells selected for invasiveness stable with res-
         pect to this porperty, or are they unstable as shown by
         Poste, Harris *et al.*, and Hill for metastasis?

LIOTTA: We have found that continuous selection pressure is re-
         quired to keep the same level of invasive rate.

CHAPTER 12

EFFECT OF REGIONAL ADMINISTRATION OF NONSPECIFIC
IMMUNOSTIMULATORS ON THE LYMPH NODE METASTASIS

Genshichiro Fujii
Masazumi Eriguchi*
Yoju Miyamoto
Morimasa Sekiguchi

Department of Clinical Oncology
Institute of Medical Science
University of Tokyo
Tokyo, Japan

*Department of Surgery.

BASIC MECHANISMS AND CLINICAL TREATMENT
OF TUMOR METASTASIS

223

I. INTRODUCTION

   Among various methods of administration of nonspecific immunostimulators (NSI) in cancer immunotherapy, "local immunotherapy"
by Zbar *et al.* (1976) and "adjuvant contact therapy" by Baldwin
et al. (1976) have been reported to be most efficacious. They
introduced bacillus Calmette-Guérin (BCG) into the area of tumor.
Clinically, Morton *et al.* (1974) employed intratumoral injection
of BCG in metastatic skin lesions of malignant melanoma and reported remarkable regression of small lesions. McKneally *et al.*
(1976, 1978) reported, first in nonrandomized and second in randomized trials of intrapleural administration of BCG as an adjuvant to surgery in patients with stage I non-small cell lung
cancer, a highly significant improvement in survival after surgery.
Their results, however, have not yet been independently confirmed
(Wright *et al.*, 1979).
   We have been interested in local immunotherapy, particularly
in determining whether nonspecific stimulation of the regional
lymph nodes can be an effective measure to prevent lymph node
metastasis associated with surgical removal of the tumor. The
preventive effect observed in a syngeneic animal tumor model in
mice developed in our department stimulated us to evaluate oral
administration of BCG as a local immunotherapy of gastrointestinal
cancers.

II. MATERIALS AND METHODS

   Animals: Female C3H/HeJms mice 8-10 weeks old were used.
   Tumor: The tumor used was mouse ascites hepatoma, MH134. This
syngeneic tumor, which originated as a carbon tetrachloride-in-
duced liver tumor in a C3H female mouse, had been converted into
the ascites form by Sato *et al.* (1956). The tumor was derived
from the Department of Oncology of this institute in 1971 and has
been maintained in C3H/HeJms mice by serial intraperitoneal passage in our department.
   Allogeneic mouse erythroblastoma: An ascites form of FA/C/2
tumor was used as a nonspecific immunostimulator (NSI). This
tumor was originally induced with Friend's virus in C57BL/6Jms
mouse by T. Odaka of the Department of Genetics of this institute.
   BCG: Lyophilized BCG manufactured by Japan BCG Laboratory,
Tokyo, was suspended in physiological saline and adjusted to an
appropriate concentration. In 80 mg of the lyophilized BCG, there
were approximately 2×10^6 colony-forming units (CFU) of BCG.
   OK-432 (Picibanil, Chugain Pharmaceutical Co. Ltd., Tokyo):
OK-432 is a lyophilized preparation of penicillin G-treated Su
strain *Streptococcus pyogenes* (Sakurai *et al.*, 1972). The unit
used is the klinische Einheit (KE), which corresponds to 0.1 mg
of the dried streptococci.

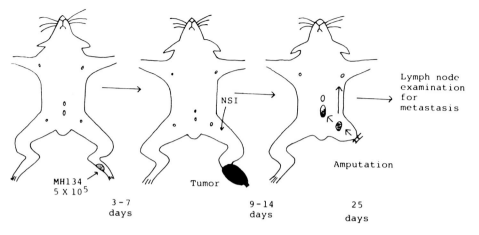

Fig. 1.   Schedule of regional lymph node stimulation by local
intramuscular injection of nonspecific immunostimulators (NSI).

A.   Animal Experiments

1.   *Stimulation of Regional Lymph Nodes
     by Intramuscular Injection of Nonspecific
     Immunostimulators*

The schedule of animal treatment is illustrated in Fig. 1.
Mice were inoculated with 5×10^5 MH134 cells, otherwise indicated
at the left foot pad.   Immunostimulators were injected intramuscularly at the middle of the ipsilateral femur in 3 to 7 days after
tumor inoculation, when the tumor had grown to a footpad thickness
of 5 to 7 mm.   After intervals of several days, approximately 10
days after tumor inoculation, the tumor-bearing limb was ligated at
the middle level of the femur and amputated below the ligation.
Approximately 4 weeks after tumor inoculation, the mice were sacrificed under ether anesthesia and examined both macroscopically
and microscopically for metastatic spread to lymph nodes of various
regions.   Hematoxylin and eosin (H-E)-stained specimens were prepared for microscopic examination.   As immunostimulators, BCG,
allogeneic tumor cells, and OK-432 were used.
     In an additional experiment, survival of mice treated with
removal of tumor and local OK-432 injection was followed for 90
days after surgery.

2.   *Stimulation of Mesenteric Lymph Nodes
     by Oral Administration of BCG*

Schedule of experiment is shown in Fig. 2.   Two weeks before
tumor inoculation at the cecum, 5 mg of BCG were injected intramuscularly in seven C3H/HeJms mice.   Then, 1×10^5 MH134 cells
were inoculated intramurally into the cecum wall by using a sur-

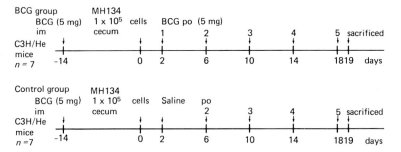

Fig. 2.   Schedule of oral administration of BCG in mice.

gical microscope and a 1/6-gauge needle. On Day 2, 5 mg of BCG
dissolved in 0.5 ml saline were administered into the stomach
through the esophagous by using a stainless-steel tube. Thus,
BCG was given initially 2 days after tumor inoculation, and then
four times with intervals of 4 days. To control mice, 0.5 ml of
physiological saline was administered into the stomach on the same
days. All mice were sacrificed under ether anesthesia.

B.   Clinical Study

     A total of 42 patients with gastrointestinal cancers were given
BCG orally as an adjuvant immunotherapy to surgery from 1978 to
1981. Of the 42 patients, 11 underwent laparotomy for the intestinal obstruction due to tumor recurrence or intestinal adhesion,
and mesenteric lymph nodes were biopsied. The patients were given
orally four capsules containing a total of 80 mg of BCG from 1 to
2 weeks after surgery once a week for 1 month, and then once a
month.

III.   RESULTS

A.   Stimulation of Regional Lymph Nodes
     by Local Administration of Nonspecific
     Immunostimulators

1.   BCG

     On Day 8, 2 mg of BCG were injected and the mice were subjected
to surgical removal of the tumor grown at the footpad. As shown
in Table I, percentage of metastasized nodes in the regional lymph
nodes was 55.6 and 26.1 for the left inguinal and para-aortic
nodes, respectively. These figures were lower than those in controls, that is, 100 and 81.3% for the left inguinal and the para-

TABLE I

Effect of BCG on Lymph Node Metastasis of MH134 Tumor

Experimental Protocol

MH134 cells (1×10^6)   NSI   Amputation of left leg   Sacrifice

Day   0   6 8   28

Group	NSI	Number of mice	Metastasized nodes (%)					
			Left inguinal	Para-aortic	Left axillary	Right axillary	Right inguinal	All nodes
A	BCG (2 mg)	9	55.6 (5/9)	26.1^a (6/23)	33.0 (3/9)	0 (0/9)	0 (0/9)	23.7^a (14/59)
B	Saline	6	100 (6/6)	81.3 (13/16)	66.7 (4/6)	0 (0/6)	0 (0/6)	57.5 (23/40)

[a] $\chi^2 > .005$.

TABLE II

Effect of Allogeneic and Syngeneic Tumor on Lymph Node Metastasis of MH134 Tumor

Experimental Protocol

MH134 cells (5×10^5)	Stimulation	Amputation of left leg	Sacrifice
Day 0	7	11	26

Metastasized nodes (%)

Group	NSI	Number of mice	Left inguinal	Para-aortic	Left axillary	Right axillary	Right inguinal	All nodes
A	FA/C/2 (C57BL/6) 2×10^6	7	0^a (0/7)	10.5^b (2/19)	0 (0/7)	0 (0/7)	0 (0/7)	4.2 (2/47)
B	MH134 (6000 rad) 1×10^7 IFA[c]	6	33.3 (2/6)	20.0 (3/15)	16.7 (1/6)	0 (0/6)	0 (0/6)	15.4 (6/39)
C	Saline	7	42.9 (3/7)	38.1 (8/21)	28.6 (2/7)	0 (0/7)	0 (0/7)	26.5 (13/49)

$^a \chi^2 > .005.$
$^b \chi^2 > .050.$
[c] IFA, Incomplete Freund's adjuvant.

aortic nodes, respectively. The difference in the para-aortic nodes was statistically significant. Metastatic spread in the distal nodes was also lower in BCG group than in controls.

2. *Allogeneic Tumor*

As a strong inducer of cell-mediated immunity, allogeneic tumor, FA/C/2, erythroblastoma of C57BL/6 mouse was employed as NSI. In group A, 2×10^6 FA/C/2 cells were injected on Day 7, and tumor was removed on Day 11. As shown in Table II, percentages of metastasis in the regional lymph nodes in group A were 0 and 10.5 in the left inguinal and para-aortic nodes, respectively. These were significantly lower than those in group C as control. In the distal left axillary nodes, similar results were observed. Instead of allogeneic tumor cells, normal lymph node cells from C57BL/6 mice also exhibited inhibition of metastatic spread of tumor cells into the regional lymph nodes (data not shown).

In group B, 1×10^7 isologous MH134 tumor cells that were irradiated with ^{60}Co in a dose of 6000 rads were used as a stimulator. No significant inhibition of tumor metastasis was observed. This meant that MH134 tumor-specific immunity was not induced strongly enough to inhibit lymph node metastasis.

3. *OK-432*

OK-432 was injected on Days 3 and 7, and the left leg was amputated on Day 13. Group B, injected with 2 KE of OK-432 twice, exhibited significantly lower rates of metastasis than Group C as control in both the regional and distant lymph nodes. Group A, injected with 0.5 KE of OK-432, as compared with control group C, showed a lower percentage metastasis in the regional (para-aortic) and distant (left axillary) lymph nodes, although the differences between groups A and C were not significant. The data are shown in Table III.

4. *Metastatic Spread in the Lymph Node Stimulated with NSI*

In microscopic examination, it was found that metastatic spread was likely to be localized in the cortical sinus area in BCG and OK-432-treated groups. As seen in Fig. 3, in most of the control lymph nodes, tumor cells appeared to spread from cortical sinus directly into the medullary sinus.

In the OK-432-treated group, metastatic spread into the medullary sinus was lower than control in para-aortic nodes and especially extremely low in left axillary nodes. A high density of cells including lymphoid cells and macrophages in the lymph nodes that were induced and activated by NSI stimulation appeared to inhibit the spread of tumor cells in the lymph nodes.

TABLE III

Effect of OK-432 on Lymph Node Metastasis of MH134 Tumor

Experimental Protocol

MH134 cells (5 × 10^5)		OK-432		Amputation of left leg		Sacrifice
Day	0	3	7	13		28

Group	Dose of OK-432	Number of mice	Metastasized nodes (%)					
			Left inguinal	Para-aortic	Left axillary	Right axillary	Right inguinal	All nodes
A	0.5 KE × 2	9	55.6 (5/9)	17.4 (4/23)	11.1 (1/9)	0 (0/9)	0 (0/9)	16.9 (10/59)
B	2 KE × 2	9	11.1^b (1/9)	8.0^b (2/25)	0^b (0/9)	0 (0/9)	0 (0/9)	4.9^a (3/61)
C	Saline	10	50.0 (5/10)	25.9 (7/27)	20.0 (2/10)	0 (0/10)	0 (0/10)	20.9 (14/67)

^{a} $\chi^2 > .010$.
^{b} $\chi^2 > .100$.

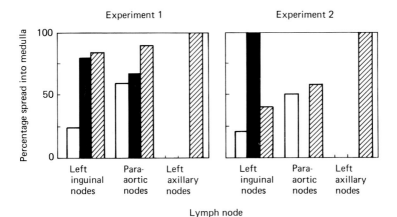

Fig. 3.   Metastatic spread from cortical into medullary sinus. OK-432 dosage (KE): 0.5 (open bar); 2.0 (solid bar); none (hatched bar).

5. *Effect of Preoperative Stimulation*
    of Regional Lymph Nodes with NSI
    on the Survival of Mice

After confirming the preventive effect of OK-432 on the metastatic spread in the lymph nodes, survival was followed without sacrificing the animals for metastasis examination.   Figure 4 shows the results.   Survival at 90 days after amputation of tumor-bearing limb was approximately 60% in the OK-432-treated groups, while only 13% of the control mice remained alive in comparison.   The difference was highly significant statistically.   All the mice that died during the follow-up period had positive lymph node metastasis. These data indicated that preventive effect of local administration of NSI on the lymph node metastasis was also confirmed from the survival of the mice pretreated with the identical NSI.

B. Stimulation of Mesenteric Lymph Nodes
    by Oral Administration of BCG

1. *Effect of Oral Administration of BCG*
    on the Metastasis in the Mesenteric
    Lymph Nodes in Mice

As seen in Fig. 5, metastasis in the cortical sinus was 100% in controls and 50% in the oral BCG group.   In addition, tumor cells spread widely into the medullary sinus in 100% of five control mice.   Contrary to this, only 25% of four mice treated with oral BCG revealed metastatic spread into cortical and then medullary sinuses.   The results indicated that oral BCG stimulated the

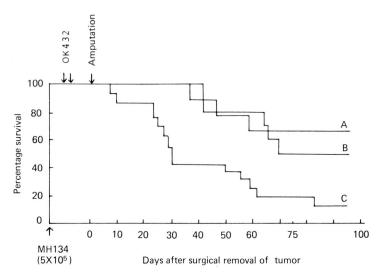

Fig. 4.   Effect of preoperative stimulation of regional lymph nodes with OK-432 on the survival of mice.   Curve A: OK-432 (0.5 KE) on Days 3 and 7 + amputation ($p = .01$).   Curve B: OK-432 (2 KE) on Days 3 and 7 + amputation ($p = .01$).   Curve C: amputation only. p Values by Taguchi's precise accumulation analysis.

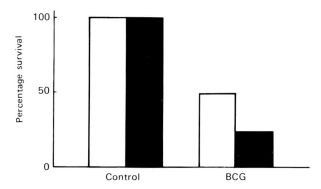

Fig. 5.   Metastasis to the mesenteric lymph nodes.   Cortical sinus (open bar); medullary sinus (solid bar).

TABLE IV

Effect of Oral Administration of BCG and PPD Skin Test
and Cell Response in Mesenteric Lymph Nodes

Patient number	Sex	Age	Organ site of carcinoma	BCG	PPD	Sinus histiocytosis	Follicular hyperplasia
1	M	46	Stomach	7	+ → ++	+[a]	+[a]
2	F	64	Stomach	2	- → ++	-	-
3	F	51	Stomach	2	- → -	-	-
4	M	32	Stomach	12	+ → ++	++	+
5	M	73	Stomach	2	- → +	+	+
6	F	77	Stomach	2		++	+
7	F	79	Stomach	50	- → +	++	+++
8	F	66	Rectum	5	- → +	+	+
9	F	44	Rectum	14	- → ++	++	++
10	F	64	Rectum	5	+ → -	++	+++
11	F	66	Rectum	9	++ → → ++	+	++

[a]Metastasis to lymph node.

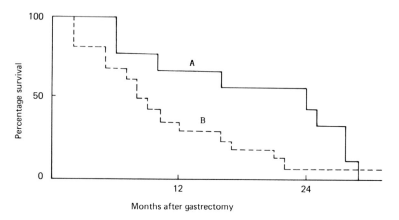

Fig. 6. Survival of patients with stage IV gastric cancer treated with oral BCG (curve A, 9 patients). Control group (curve B, 16 patients).

mesenteric lymph nodes to suppress metastatic spreading in the lymph nodes. By estimating chemiluminescence reaction of intraperitoneal macrophages to zymosan, marked activation of macrophage potentiality by oral BCG was demonstrated in our laboratories (Eriguchi *et al.*, 1982).

2. *Oral Administration of BCG in Patients
    with Gastrointestinal Cancers*

Eleven of 42 patients with gastrointestinal cancers underwent laparotomy in various periods of oral administration of BCG. PPD skin reaction, sinus histiocytosis, and follicular hyperplasia are summarized in Table IV. In most patients except for two (patients 2 and 3), marked improvement of sinus histiocytosis was observed. Prominent (++) sinus histiocytosis was observed in five (patients 4, 6, 7, 9, and 10), or 45%. This rate of prominent histiocytosis (45%) was higher than 23% of the same patients at the time of primary surgery. Patients receiving oral BCG treatment for longer periods appear to show stronger histiocytosis.

3. *Effect of Oral Administration of BCG
    on the Survival of Patients with Stage IV
    Gastric Cancer: Nonrandomized Study*

All of nine patients with stage IV gastric cancer given both oral BCG and anticancer chemotherapy died within 29 months after surgery. The survival curve of the 9 patients was compared with that of 16 patients with stage IV gastric cancer concurrently given only chemotherapy. The 2-year survival rate was 44.4% in oral BCG group. This is higher than 6.3% of the control group (Fig. 6). The difference is significant, although the stratification was not randomized.

IV. DISCUSSION

For the immunotherapy of cancer, tumor bulk should preferably be of a minimal size. It is the case in macroscopically curable surgical operation of cancers. Among various methods of administration of BCG as a nonspecific immunostimulator (NSI), intratumoral administration has been reported to be most efficacious in animal experiments (Zbar et al., 1976; Baldwin et al., 1976) and in clinical trials (Morton et al., 1974). In such cases, the NSI should be administered close to the tumor in the drainage area of the regional lymph nodes. In the surgical treatment of cancer, such adjuvant therapies should be focused first on the micrometastasis that might be caused by surgical manipulation of cancer, and second on the late local recurrence.

In this study, NSI such as BCG, OK-432, and allogeneic cells were administered proximately to the footpad tumor. The NSI used in this study stimulated the regional lymph nodes to inhibit tumor metastasis into the lymph nodes and then also to inhibit spreading of tumor cells from the cortical sinus to the medullary sinus. Although the mechanisms functioning in the prevention of metastasis are not clear, an increase of Thy-1 antigen-positive lymphocytes (G. Fujii, unpublished data) and prominent sinus histiocytosis in the regional lymph nodes appeared to be important factors.

It was very interesting that, unlike incomplete Freund's adjuvant, BCG, OK-432, and allogeneic tumor cells described in this study, complete Freund's adjuvant rather enhanced tumor metastasis in the regional lymph nodes. Even incomplete Freund's adjuvant, if used in a large dose, enhanced tumor metastasis. From these findings, it was suggested that NSI resulting in nonimmune and immune cellular reactions rather than exudative ones at the injection area and the regional lymph nodes inhibited tumor metastasis.

The preceding results, obtained in our syngeneic tumor model system, stimulated us to evaluate oral administration of BCG as a local immunotherapy of gastrointestinal cancers. This hazardless method of BCG administration has been studied clinically by Lewis et al. (1976) and Falk et al. (1976). The definite conclusion in regard to the effect of oral administration of BCG on the tumor has not been reported. In animal experiments, Baldwin et al. (1975) and Tokunaga et al. (1979) reported the inhibitory effect of oral BCG on the growth of subcutaneously inoculated tumor cells. Tokunaga indicated from the observation that a significant proportion of viable BCG given orally reached the small intestine and was trapped by Peyer's patches, and only a small amount of BCG passed through the patches and reached the mesenteric lymph nodes. Our observation of the mesenteric lymph nodes in animal experiments and in human biopsy strongly suggested that oral BCG stimulated the lynph nodes to induce cellular reaction such as prominent sinus histiocytosis and follicular hyperplasia. In the lymph nodes, induced and activated macrophages and also T cells reacting with BCG will contribute to the prevention of micrometastasis.

Oral administration of BCG appeared to be a local immunotherapy for only gastrointestinal cancers.

V. SUMMARY

Nonspecific immunostimulators such as BCG and OK-432 (Picibanil), when injected im at the regional sites of tumors, inhibited lymph node metastasis and resulted in prolongation of the host survival time. The metastatic foci were likely to localize in the cortical sinus area and did not spread directly into the medullary sinus in the mice treated by regional injection of NSI.

Oral administration of BCG resulted in lower incidence of lymph node metastasis and localized metastatic foci in the cortical sinus in C3H/He mice presensitized with BCG and inoculated with syngeneic MH134 tumor at the footpad. Activation of macrophages from the peritoneal cavity was shown by chemiluminescence technique in mice given BCG orally.

Oral BCG was given to 42 stomach and colon cancer patients. In 5 of 11 patients who received laparotomy during the period of oral BCG administration, marked sinus histiocytosis was observed in the mesenteric lymph nodes. Oral administration of BCG is likely to stimulate local mesenteric lymph nodes to resist cancer metastasis.

REFERENCES

Baldwin, R. W., Hopper, D. G., and Pimm, M. V. (1976). *Ann. N.Y. Acad. Sci. 277,* 124-134.
Baldwin, R. W., Hopper, D. G., and Pimm, M. V. (1975). *Br. J. Cancer 31,* 124-128.
Eriguchi, M., Fujii, U., Takahashi, T., Hagiwara, T., Mikamo, S., Koishi, T., Miyamoto, Y., Osada, I., Samaru, Y., Sekiguchi, M., and Fujii, G. (1982). *Scand. J. Gastroenterol. 17* (Suppl. 78), 451.
Falk, R. E., MacGregor, A. B., Ambus, U., Landi, S., Langer, B., and Miller, A. B. (1976). *In* "BCG in Cancer Immunotherapy" (G. Lamoureux, R. Turcotte, and V. Portelance, eds.), pp. 217-225. Grune & Stratton, New York.
Lewis, M. G., Jerry, L. M., Rowden, T. M., Phillips, T. M., Shibata, H., and Capek, A. (1976). *In* "BCG in Cancer Immunotherapy" (G. Lamoureux, R. Turcotte, and V. Portelance, eds.), pp. 339-358. Grune & Stratton, New York.
McKneally, M. F., Maver, C. M., and Kausel, H. W. (1976). *Lancet 1,* 377-379.
McKneally, M. F., Maver, C. M., and Kausel, H. W. (1978). *In* "Immunotherapy of Cancer: Present Status of Trials in Man"

(W. D. Terry and D. W. Windhorst, eds.), pp. 161-171. Raven, New York.

Morton, D. L., Eilber, F. R., Holmes, E. C., Hunt, J. S., Ketcham, A. S., Silverstein, M. J., and Sparks, F. C. (1974). *Ann. Surg. 180*, 635-641.

Sakurai, Y., Tsukagoshi, S., Satoh, H., Akiba, T., Suzuki, S., and Takagi, Y. (1972). *Cancer Chemother. Rep. Part 1 56*, 36-43.

Sato, H., Belkin, M., and Essner, E. (1956). *J. Natl. Cancer Inst. (US) 17*, 1-21.

Tokunaga, T., Taguchi, S., Chino, F., and Murohashi, T. (1979). *Jpn. J. Med. Sci. Biol. 32*, 1-18.

Wright, P., Hill, L., Peterson, A., Anderson, R., Bagley, C., Bernstein, I., Ivey, T., Johnson, L., Morgan, E., Ostenson, R., and Pinkham, R. (1979). *In* "Adjuvant Therapy of Cancer II" (S. E. Jones and S. E. Salmon, eds.), pp. 545-552. Grune & Stratton, New York.

Zbar, B., Ribi, E., Kelly, M., Granger, D., Evans, C., and Rapp, H. J. (1976). *Cancer Immunol. Immunother. 1*, 127-137.

DISCUSSION

MATHÉ: Immunizing against BCG may be a way to obtain faster resistance, even nonspecific? Could you verify this hypothesis.

FUJII: In our clinical experience, the more frequent oral BCG administration resulted in the higher rate of marked improvement of PPD skin reaction observed, and swollen mesenteric nodes showed prominent sinus histocytosis. From this experience, we employed presensitization with BCG in animal experiments. I think that sensitized lymphocytes reacted with BCG will release lymphokines that induce more macrophages and activate macrophages and other cells that will attack tumor cells. These are the reasons I want to accept that hypothesis.

YOSHIDA: Your experimental group of mice were preimmunized with an intramuscular injection of BCG, then challenged with oral BCG. Is this a better protocol than to administer oral BCG and then challenge with repeated oral BCG?

FUJII: In the presensitized animals, reaction between sensitized lymphocytes and BCG invading into the nodes will occur and lymphokines will be released. So, I think that presensitization protocol is better.

YOSHIDA: Is the inhibition of lymph node metastasis a result of protection of metastasis or a result of reduction of established metastasis to normal nodes?

FUJII: I think that it is protection against micrometastasis.

CHIHARA: The timing of administration of immunostimulants is es-
            sential. Is an OK-432 injection before surgery the best
            timing? In the case of lentinan, its administration af-
            ter surgery is the best timing.

FUJII: NSI injection before surgery will prevent micrometastatic
            spread due to surgery. Administration of NSI (nonspecific
            immunostimulator) after operation for a long period will
            protect late tumor cell spread into the nodes and local
            recurrence. I think that both pre- and postadministration
            of NSI are needed.

COCHRAN: What changes do you see in the lymphoid tissues of the
            wall of the bowel?

FUJII: I am not sure about that, because there are no cases in
            whom intestine was resected during oral administration of
            BCG. I have not examined the Peyer's patch in the mouse
            experiment.

CHAPTER 13

EFFECTS OF SURGICAL INTERVENTION
AND IMMUNOPOTENTIATORS ON METASTATIC TUMOR
PROLIFERATION AND ITS CELL-MEDIATED IMMUNITY

Hiroaki Miwa
Osamu Hashimoto
Akikazu Hatosaki
Kunzo Orita

Department of Surgery
Okayama University Medical School
Okayama, Japan

BASIC MECHANISMS AND CLINICAL TREATMENT
OF TUMOR METASTASIS

239

I. INTRODUCTION

It is a common experience, both clinically and in animal experiments, to find that a metastatic tumor or tumor tissue remaining in
the cancer-bearing host goes on to proliferate after removal of the
primary tumor. Various possibilities have been put forward to explain this phenomenon, one of which considers changes in the immune
capacity of the host to be important (Milas *et al.*, 1974). In the
present experiment, the role of surgical intervention and effectiveness of immunopotentiators against the proliferation of metastatic
tumors were investigated using autoradiography that followed postoperative changes in the [^{3}H]thymidine-labeling rate of metastatic
tumors in an experimental model of metastasis in mice. In addition,
the effectiveness of administering *Corynebacterium parvum* (Cp)
(Halpern *et al.*, 1964) or OK-432 (Okamoto *et al.*, 1967) and performing a splenectomy (Miwa *et al.*, 1983) was studied in conjunction
with the delayed-type hypersensitivity reaction (DHR).

II. MATERIALS AND METHODS

As the primary tumor, 5×10^5 Lewis lung carcinoma (3LL tumor)
cells in a trypsin-prepared single-cell suspension were implanted
subcutaneously in the right hindleg of female BDF$_1$ mice from 8 to
10 weeks old. The mice were then divided into the following groups:
(1) nonremoval of the primary tumor, (2) removal of the primary tumor, (3) sham operation, (4) administration of Cp before removal of
the primary tumor, and (5) administration of Cp after removal of
the primary tumor. In addition to these five groups, a normal control group and a group in which normal mice underwent amputation
of the right hindleg were added. The following procedures were also
examined: (6) splenectomy on Days 3, 10, and 14 after implantation
of 3LL tumor cells, (7) intratumoral administration of OK-432 at
various doses, and (8) combination therapy with splenectomy, administration of OK-432, and tumor excision (amputation of the right
leg).
The following experiments were performed.
Removal of the primary tumor: On Day 14 after tumor cell implantation in the right hindleg, the right hindleg (groups 2, 4,
and 5) or the left hindleg (group 3) was amputated at the pelvis
under ether anesthesia (Fig. 1).
Administration of Cp: Cp was injected into the abdominal
cavity daily for 5 days beginning on Day 9 in group 4 and on Day
15 in group 5. The dose was 0.4 mg/mouse/day (Fig. 1).
Splenectomy: Mice underwent a splenectomy under ether anesthesia on Days 3, 10, and 14 after 3LL tumor implantation, and were
assessed for length of survival and tumor regression in comparison
with a group subjected to sham operation (laparotomy only) on Day 10
as a control (Fig. 2).

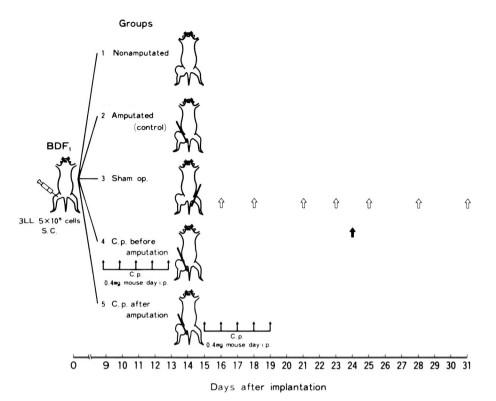

Fig. 1. Schedules of experiment 1. ⇧ Autoradiography using 10 μCi/g of [³H]thymidine intraperitoneally. ↑ Weight of lungs and number of pulmonary metastases were examined.

OK-432 administration: Groups of mice received an intratumoral (it) injection of OK-432 on Day 7 after 3LL tumor cell implantation (Fig. 2).
Autoradiography: [³H]thymidine was given intraperitoneally at a dose of 10 μCi/kg of body weight on Days 16, 18, 21, 23, 25, 28, and 31 for each group as shown in Fig. 1. One hour later, the mice were sacrificed by decapitation. The lungs were removed en bloc, fixed in 10% buffered formalin, embedded in paraffin, and sectioned sequentially. The sections were dipped in Sakura emulsified agent NR-M₂ and developed after 4 weeks exposure at 4°C. Hematoxylin—eosin staining was performed, and more than 3000 tumor cells were counted, about 1000 at three different places along the maximum diameter of the lung metastatic tumor in each specimen. The labeling rate was then calculated.

The macroscopic lung metastatic node number was estimated on Day 24 (see Fig. 1) using the method of Wexler (1966), that is, intratracheal infusion of india ink.

Delayed-type hypersensitivity reaction (Ptak and Asherson, 1969): A 6% solution of picryl chloride in ethanol was painted on the abdominal skin to cause sensitization at the time of tumor im-

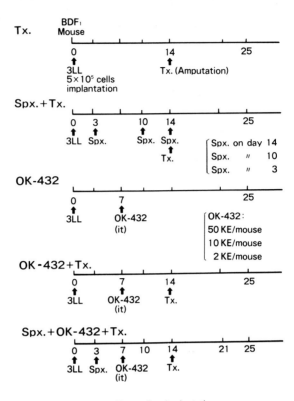

Fig. 2. Schedules of experiment 2. Tx, Amputation of tumor-implanted leg; Spx, splenectomy.

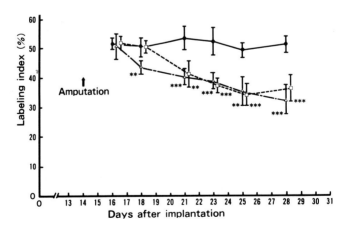

Fig. 3. Labeling indexes of metastatic Lewis lung carcinoma.
●——● Amputated (control) group; Δ———Δ nonamputated group; □———□ sham operation group. **$p < .01$; ***$p < .001$.

plantation and on Days 9 and 18. In each case, a 1% solution of picryl chloride in olive oil was painted on both ears 7 days later; 24 h after this, the thickness of each ear was measured with a dial-thickness gauge. The increase in the thickness of the ear was calculated by subtracting the average background value from the average for the difference in thickness before and after application of the paint.

The data obtained from the preceding experiments were expressed as mean ± SD and compared statistically using Student's t-test.

RESULTS

A. The Effect of Surgical Intervention
    on Proliferation of Metastatic Tumor

Comparison of the labeling rate in the group that had the primary tumor removed with that of the group that did not showed that the former maintained a higher value of around 50% with little variation (Fig. 3). In contrast to this, the nonremoval control group had a value of 50.5% on Day 16 but showed a significantly low value on Day 18, and decreased steadily thereafter to 32.6% on Day 28. However, until the eighteenth day in the sham operation group, the rate was not different from that of the tumor removal group, but was significantly lower from Day 21 onward.

B. The Inhibitory Effect of Cp
    on Proliferation of the Remnant
    Metastatic Tumor

When Cp was administered before operation, the proliferation rate was significantly lower on Day 16 and decreased steadily so that on Day 28 there was a marked inhibition and a rate of 27.6%. However, a value of 36% on Day 31 indicated a weakening in the effect of Cp. In contrast, the group given Cp postoperatively showed no difference until Day 18 but changed to become significantly low from Day 21. However, this value was higher than that of preoperative administration and showed no tendency to decrease (Fig. 4).

C. The Effect of Surgical Intervention and Cp
    on the Number of Pulmonary Metastatic Nodules

The average number of lung metastatic nodules in each group was 8.7 for the nonremoval group, 36.0 for the removal group, 14.4 for the sham operation group, 6.3 for the Cp preoperative administration

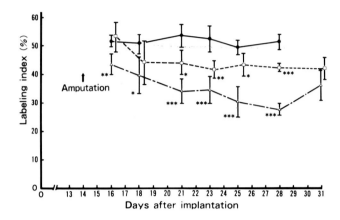

Fig. 4. Labeling indexes of metastatic Lewis lung carcinoma in mice treated with *C. parvum*. ●——● Amputated (control) group; Δ———Δ treated with *C. parvum* before amputation; □----□ treated with *C. parvum* after amputation. *$p < .05$; **$p < .01$; ***$p < .001$.

group, and 8.5 for the postoperative administration group. Removal of the primary tumor caused a significant ($p < .001$) increase in the number of metastatic nodules, but this increase was significantly ($p < .001$) inhibited by preoperative administration of Cp (Table I).

TABLE I

Effects of *C. parvum* on the Pulmonary Metastasis of Lewis Lung Carcinoma (on Day 24 Postimplantation)

Groups	Mean weight of lungs (mg, ± SD)	p	Mean number of pulmonary metastases (± SD)	p
1. Nonamputated	270.3 ± 26.85	< .001	8.7 ± 4.11	< .001
2. Amputated (control)	510.0 ± 46.51	—	36.0 ± 7.46	—
3. Sham operation	249.6 ± 34.89	< .001	14.4 ± 3.20	< .001
4. Cp before amputation	269.2 ± 13.09	< .001	6.3 ± 1.97	< .001
5. Cp after amputation	267.1 ± 42.32	< .001	8.5 ± 4.19	< .001

D. The Effect of Splenectomy
    on Tumor Growth

BDF$_1$ mice underwent a splenectomy on Days 3, 10, and 14 after 3LL tumor implantation, and tumor size was compared with that of the sham operation group. The average tumor sizes 25 days after tumor implantation were 27.6 mm in the sham operation group, 23.7 mm in the Day 3 splenectomy group, 25.4 mm in the Day 10 splenectomy group, and 27.5 mm in the Day 14 splenectomy group. The antitumor effect of splenectomy was significant in the Day 3 ($p < .005$) and Day 10 ($p < .005$) splenectomy groups.

E. The Effect of OK-432 on Tumor
    Regression and Number of Metastatic
    Tumors

The antitumor effect of intratumoral injection of OK-432 was mostly detected when its dosage was 10 KE ($p < .005$) (Fig. 5). The mean tumor size 25 days after the tumor implantation in the 10-KE of OK-432 group was 20.0 mm in contrast to 27.2 mm in the control group. When 10 KE of OK-432 were injected on Day 7 and the excision of the primary tumor (amputation) took place on Day 14 after the tumor implantation, the number (16.3) of metastatic tumors, especially those over 3 mm, was significantly fewer than that (21.6) of the control group ($p < .05$) (Table II).

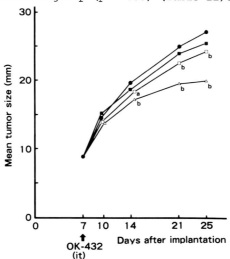

Fig. 5. Antitumor effect of intratumoral injection of OK-432. ●——● Control group; ■——■ administration of OK-432 (50 KE/mouse); △——△ administration of OK-432 (10 KE/mouse); □——□ administration of OK-432 (2 KE/mouse); a, $p < .025$; b, $p < .005$; it, intratumoral injection.

TABLE II

Effects of Splenectomy and OK-432
on the Pulmonary Metastasis Examined by Wexler's Method

Experimental protocol[a]	No. of cases	No. of pulmonary metastases	No. of pulmonary metastases >3 mm
Control	8	21.6 ± 6.9[b]	3.7 ± 1.1[c]
Tx	6	29.5 ± 4.9[b]	6.3 ± 1.4[c]
Spx + Tx	6	21.5 ± 5.4	2.7 ± 1.1[b]
OK-432 + Tx	6	16.3 ± 5.4[b]	2.5 ± 1.0[b]
Spx + OK-432 + Tx	6	14.0 ± 5.2[b]	1.3 ± 1.1[b]

[a] Tx, Amputation; Spx, splenectomy.
[b] $p < .05$.
[c] $p < .005$.

F. The Effect of Splenectomy Combined
    with OK-432 Intratumoral Injection

The groups of animals that underwent a splenectomy on Day 3
after tumor implantation were given an intratumoral injection of
10 KE of OK-432 on Day 7, and were subjected to tumor excision
(amputation) on Day 14 showed the greatest antitumor effect and
reduction in number of metastatic pulmonary lesions, with significantly fewer tumor nodules over 3 mm in diameter (Table II).

G. Survival Rate

The average survival time in days for each group was 31.6 for
the nonremoval group, 30.0 for the removal group, 26.2 for the
sham operation group, 37.5 for the preoperative Cp group, and 34.4
for the postoperative Cp group. Preoperative Cp administration
gave significant ($p < .001$) prolongation of survival (Fig. 6).
Concerning the splenectomy, the mean survival time in days was 30.6
in the Day 3 splenectomy group, 26.5 in the Day 10 splenectomy
group, and 25.0 in the Day 14 splenectomy group, compared to 26.8
in the control group. Splenectomy in early stage of cancer-bearing
mice was significantly effective ($p < .05$). As shown in Fig. 7,
there was a significant prolongation of survival in the 10-KE dose
of OK-432 group with a mean survival of 31.9 days compared to 27.0
in the control group. In addition, the group of animals that underwent a splenectomy on Day 3 after tumor implantation, were gi-

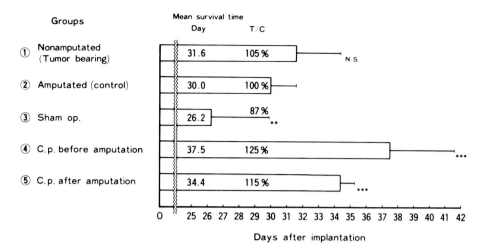

Fig. 6. Effects of *C. parvum* on the survival time. **$p < .02$; ***$p < .001$; N.S., not significant.

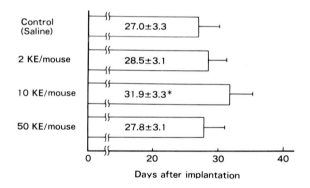

Fig. 7. Effects of intratumoral injection of OK-432 on the survival time. *$p < .005$; days given as mean ± SD ($n = 10$).

ven 10 KE of OK-432 intratumorally on Day 7, and were subjected to tumor excision on Day 14 showed a significantly prolonged survival of 36.1 days compared to 27.5 in the control group (Fig. 8).

H. Delayed-Type Hypersensitivity Reaction (DHR)

The difference in the DHR was not significant in the early cancer-bearing period, although a tendency to be lower than the healthy control group was seen. The DHR on Day 16 was significantly lower than in the healthy group in all of the other groups, and recovery was not seen in the group that had had the primary focus removed. In contrast, there was no increase in DHR in the group of healthy

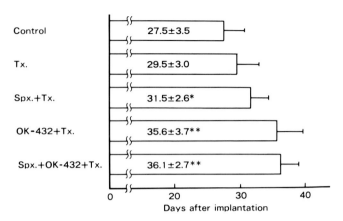

Fig. 8.   Effects of splenectomy and administration of OK-432 on
the survival time.   Tx, Amputation; Spx, splenectomy.
*p < .01; **p < .005.   Days given as mean ± SD days (n = 10).

mice that underwent hindleg amputation. The DHR on the second
postoperative day apparently was not affected by the stress of surgery compared to the DHR in healthy mice. The DHR on Day 25 tended
to be lower in all the groups other than the healthy control group,
and the group given Cp preoperatively had a significantly higher
value than the group with the primary tumor removed (Table III).
A significant enhancement of DHR was evident on Day 25 after tumor
implantation in the group that underwent splenectomy on Day 3.
The effect of intratumoral injection of OK-432 on DHR was observed
on Day 25 in the group given 10 KE of OK-432. The DHR was markedly
enhanced by the administration of OK-432, and this effect of the
immunopotentiator was pronounced in the splenectomy group (Fig. 9).

IV. DISCUSSION

     The reason that metastatic tumors tend to proliferate after
removal of a primary tumor is related to antigenicity of the tumor,
the effect of surgical intervention (Simpson-Herren *et al.*, 1977;
Miwa *et al.*, 1980), and various immunological factors such as the
interaction between primary and metastatic tumor (Sugarbaker *et
al.*, 1977) and the intervention of concomitant immunity (Gorelik
et al., 1978).   In the results of the present experiment, the sham
operation group showed greater proliferation of lung metastasis
over a short postoperative period than the group that did not have
the primary tumor removed. This was probably related to surgical
intervention; however, this tendency was only transitory, and the
presence of the primary tumor inhibited metastatic tumor proliferation thereafter. This result occurred probably because the presence of the primary tumor preserved concomitant immunity, thus in-

TABLE III

Effects of Surgery and C. parvum on the Increase in Ear Thickness

Groups	Increase in ear thickness after implantation[a] ($\times 10^{-3}$ mm)		
	Day 7	Day 16	Day 25
1. Healthy control	2.17 ± 0.624 100% (9)	3.62 ± 0.975 100% (9)	3.83 ± 1.453 100% (9)
2. Healthy + surgery[b]	—	3.75 ± 1.124 ●●●[c] 103.6% (10)	2.95 ± 1.501 ●● 77.0% (10)
3. Nonamputated (tumor bearing)	1.90 ± 0.436 87.6% (10)	1.26 ± 1.089***[d] 34.8% (10)	0.58 ± 0.449*** 15.1% (6)
4. Amputated control[b]	—	1.59 ± 0.821*** 43.9% (11)	1.25 ± 0.968*** 32.6% (11)
5. Sham operation[b]	—	2.05 ± 0.610*** 56.6% (10)	0.50 ± 0.500* 13.1% (2)
6. Cp before amputation[b]	—	2.50 ± 0.640** ●● 69.1% (11)	2.45 ± 1.484 ● 64.0% (10)
7. Cp after amputation[b]	—	1.95 ± 1.036** 53.7% (10)	1.05 ± 1.215*** 27.4% (10)

[a] The numbers of mice are given in parentheses.
[b] Surgical procedures were performed on Day 14 postimplantation.
[c] Experimental group versus amputated control group: ● $p < .05$; ●● $p < .02$; ●●● $p < .001$.
[d] Experimental group versus healthy control group: *$p < .02$; **$p < .01$; ***$p < .001$.

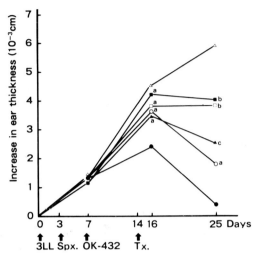

Fig. 9. Effects of splenectomy and administration of OK-432 on the increase in ear thickness. Tx, Amputation; Spx, splenectomy; **a**, $p < .005$ compared to control; **b**, $p < .005$ compared to Tx group; **c**, $p < .05$ compared to Tx group ($n = 5$). ●——●, Control; △——△, healthy mouse; ○——○, Tx; ▲——▲, Spx + Tx; □——□, OK-432 + Tx; ■——■, Spx + OK-432 + Tx.

hibiting metastasis. Immunotherapy using nonspecific immunopotentiators has been suggested as a means of inhibiting metastasis. *Corynebacterium parvum* (Cp) is an immunopotentiator that, given systemically, activates macrophages (Scott, 1974); hence, when given before removal of the primary tumor, it inhibits the continuing proliferation of remnant metastatic tumor. In another attempt to corroborate this hypothesis, we adopted the experimental practice of tumor excision combined with splenectomy and intratumoral injection of the immunopotentiator OK-432.

The spleen is generally believed to be the site for antibody production (Adler, 1965) and for storage of suppressor T cells (Sampson *et al.*, 1975), although much remains to be clarified. Hellström *et al.* (1970) observed depressed production of circulating tumor growth factors in tumor-bearing animals that had undergone a splenectomy prior to tumor implantation. Ferrer and Mihich (1968) reported diminution of blocking factors in mice that had had a splenectomy. A similar antitumor effect has been noted in animals that had their spleens removed in an early stage after tumor implantation, in which case enhancement of cellular immune function was also evident. With respect to cellular immunity, it seems logical to assume that surgical removal of the spleen, the site of suppressor cell storage, would lead to elevation of cellular immune function. The present data demonstrated a prominent antitumor effect in the groups of mice that underwent a splenectomy as early as 3 days after tumor cell implantation, which is

consistent with the reported findings. It is difficult to think
that a splenectomy performed long after tumor implantation would be
effective because of the profound influence of the surgical intervention.

The streptococcal preparation OK-432 acting as an immunopotentiator has the property of enhancing the immune function even in
normal mice, and has been described to be most effective when injected intratumorally. In view of these observations, only intratumoral injection was tested in this study. It is generally recognized that an optimal dosage exists for OK-432, and the present
results indicate it to be 10 KE/mouse, intratumorally, as in reports
by other investigators (Hattori et al., 1976).

Elimination of the immunosuppressive factors combined with appropriate measures to enhance cell-mediated immune function gives
a conspicuous inhibition of tumor growth and prolongation of survival. In the present study, enhancement of cell-mediated immune
function was observed in the form of increased DHR.

The results of the present study indicate that depression of
immune responsiveness arising from surgical intervention and other
factors has great bearing on the growth of metastatic lesions that
occur following surgical excision of the primary tumor. According
to our results, when the immunopotentiator Cp was given before
removal of the primary tumor, the decrease in cell-mediated immunity was inhibited. However, Cp given alone was limited in its
effect of inhibiting metastasis. The results also seem to show
effectiveness of splenectomy and administration of the immunopotentiator in preventing the spread of metastatic lesions.

V. CONCLUSIONS

We examined why the metastatic tumor or residual tumor goes on
to proliferate after the removal of the primary tumor using a model
of BDF$_1$ mice bearing a syngeneic 3LL tumor.

1. In regard to the effect of surgical intervention on the proliferation of metastatic tumor tissue, it was clear that this was
only of importance in the early postoperative period. Thereafter,
the proliferation was gradually inhibited by the presence of the
primary tumor but continued at a high level after removal of the
primary tumor.

2. Administration of Cp, especially preoperative administration
in the group with the primary tumor removed, caused marked inhibition of the proliferation and number of metastases.

3. Early-stage splenectomy in the cancer-bearing mice suppressed tumor growth and prolonged the survival time.

4. The streptococcal preparation of OK-432, one of the immunopotentiators, was injected intratumorally. A significant antitumor
effect and the prolongation of survival were noted at the dose of
10 KE.

5. Early-stage splenectomy and intratumoral injection of 10 KE of OK-432, followed by tumor excision showed the greatest reduction in the number of pulmonary metastases and prolongation of survival.

6. The DHR decreased with the advance of cancer, but this decrease was inhibited by the administration of Cp before removal of the primary tumor and splenectomy combined with intratumoral injection of OK-432.

In conclusion, the proliferation of metastatic tumors after removal of the primary tumor is closely related to immunodeficiency, and immunotherapy using immunopotentiators can reduce the number of metastases and prolong survival of cancer-bearing mice.

REFERENCES

Adler, F. L. (1965). *J. Immunol. 95,* 26–38.
Ferrer, J. F., and Mihich, E. (1968). *Cancer Res. 28,* 1116–1120.
Gorelik, E., Segal, S., and Feldman, M. (1978). *Int. J. Cancer 21,* 617–625.
Halpern, B. N., Prévot, A. R., Biozzi, G., Stiffel, C., Mouton, D., Morard, J. C., Bouthillier, Y., and Decreusefond, C. (1964). *J. Reticuloendothel. Soc. 1,* 77–96.
Hattori, T., Niimoto, M., Yamagata, S., Tohge, T., and Terao, H. (1976). *Gann 67,* 105–110.
Hellström, I., Hellström, K. E., and Sjögren, H. (1970). *Cell. Immunol. 1,* 18–30.
Milas, L., Hunter, N., Mason, K., and Withers, H. R. (1974). *Cancer Res. 34,* 61–71.
Miwa, H., Kawai, T., Nakahara, H., and Orita, K. (1980). *Int. J. Immunopharmacol. 2,* 31–36.
Miwa, H., Kojima, K., Ono, F., Kobayashi, T., Tsurumi, T., Hatosaki, A., Iijima, T., and Orita, K. (1983). *Jpn. J. Surg. 13,* 20–24.
Okamoto, H., Shoin, S., Koshimura, S., and Shimizu, R. (1967). *Jpn. J. Microbiol. 11,* 323–334.
Ptak, W., and Asherson, G. L. (1969). *Immunology 17,* 769–775.
Sampson, D., Grotelueschen, C., and Kauffman, H. M. (1975). *Transplantation 20,* 362–367.
Scott, M. T. (1974). *J. Natl. Cancer Inst. 53,* 855–860.
Simpson-Herren, L., Springer, T. A., Sanford, A. H., and Holmquist, J. P. (1977). *In* "Cancer Invasion and Metastasis: Biologic Mechanism and Therapy" (S. B. Day, W. P. Laird Myers, P. Stansly, S. Garattini, and M. G. Lewis, eds.), pp. 117–133. Raven, New York.
Sugarbaker, E. V., Thornthwaite, J., and Ketcham, A. S. (1977). *In* "Cancer Invasion and Metastasis: Biologic Mechanisms and Therapy" (S. B. Day *et al.,* eds.), pp. 229–240. Raven, New York.
Wexler, H. M. A. (1966). *J. Natl. Cancer Inst. (US) 36,* 641–645.

DISCUSSION

WEISS: How did you determine the labeling indices of 3LL lung metastases?

MIWA: The labeling rates were examined as follows: Mice were injected with 10 μCi/kg [^{3}H]thymidine intraperitoneally; 60 min later, mice were sacrificed and lungs were removed. Thin slices of lung sections were made, and those were exposed to films for 4 weeks at 4°C in the dark box. [^{3}H]thymidine-labeling rates were determined by the number of tumor cells having more than four particles among 3000 tumor cells.

CHAPTER 14

INCREASED IMMUNOGENICITY OF TUMOR CELLS BY INDUCTION
OF COMPLEMENT-ACTIVATING CAPACITY OF CELL MEMBRANE

Hidechika Okada
Hiroko Tanaka

National Cancer Center Research Institute
Tokyo, Japan

Noriko Okada

Department of Bacteriology
The Kitasato Institute
Tokyo, Japan

I. INTRODUCTION

    Since the discovery of the phenomenon called immunological
enhancement of tumor growth by humoral antibodies, the adverse
effect of antibody in the suppression of tumor growth has been
realized (Feldman, 1972). The most simple and clear interpretation of this phenomenon will be that the humoral antibodies
to tumor cells block the antigenic determinants that otherwise

BASIC MECHANISMS AND CLINICAL TREATMENT
OF TUMOR METASTASIS
255

can serve as the sites for the reaction of cytotoxic immune T
lymphocytes.

However, this interpretation could not satisfactorily answer
the question why the antibody could not induce the complement-
mediated cytotoxic reaction in vivo. In this connection, it will
be noteworthy that guinea pig line 10 tumor (GPL10) cells
sensitized with antibody were resistant to complement of homologous guinea pig serum (Ohanian et al., 1973). Furthermore,
neuraminidase-treated erythrocytes never became reactive with
the alternative pathway of homologous complement, although they
usually became reactive with that of heterologous complement
(Fearon, 1979; Okada et al., 1980, 1983a). Again, erythrocytes,
which had adsorbed cobra venom factor (CoVF) (Nelson, 1966) following tannic acid treatment, were highly reactive with
heterologous serum, but their reaction with homologous complement
was extremely limited (Okada and Tanaka, 1981). These evidences
reminded us that some regulatory molecules on the cell membrane
restricted the activation of self-complement. This mechanism
might be playing a role to protect the cell membrane from unde-
sirable complement activation on self-cell membrane.

If this is the case, many tumor cells must also have this regulatory molecules on their cell membranes, and may be able to escape
complement activation even in the presence of antibody reaction
to an extent sufficient to induce complement activation of heterologous serum. However, several tumor cells have been demonstrated
to be able to activate homologous complement via the alternative
pathway (Okada and Baba, 1974; Buzko et al., 1976;
Theofilopoulos and Perrin, 1976; Yoshikawa et al., 1978; Okada
and Okada, 1978; Shimbo et al., 1978). These findings prompted
us to search for some method which allow unreactive tumor cells
to become reactive with homologous complement. If we could make
tumor cells reactive with complement in vivo, polymorphonuclear
leukocytes (PMN) might accumulate around tumor cells as a result
of chemotactic factor (Shin et al., 1968) generated through
complement activation. Since PMN have been demonstrated to
stimulate immune response by releasing an interleukin 1-like
factor (Nakamura et al., 1982; Nakayama et al., 1982; Goto et al.,
1982), the activation of complement on tumor cells might be expected to result in effective immunogenic stimulation of tumor
antigen on the cell membrane to the host immune response system.

II. METHODS TO DETECT COMPLEMENT-ACTIVATING CAPACITY (CAC)

To detect complement-activating capacity of test cells
through the alternative complement pathway (ACP), we stained C3
molecules deposited on test cells as a result of complement activation. Test cells were incubated at 30°C for 30 min with an

equal volume of serum or plasma diluted in Mg-EGTA-GVB (a gelatin veronal-buffered saline containing 2 mM MgCl$_2$ and 10 mM ethylene glycol-bis(β-aminoethyl ether)N,N'-tetraacetate, pH 7.4). In this diluent, only the alternative pathway of complement reacts while the classical pathway is inhibited. After incubation, cells were washed with EDTA-GVB (a gelatin veronal-buffered saline containing 40 mM ethylenediaminetetraacetate, pH 7.4) supplemented with 0.1% sodium azide (EDTA-GVB-NaN$_3$). Precipitates of the washed cells were added with 20 μl of 1 mg/ml of rabbit IgG to block Fc receptors possibly present on test cells and incubated for 10 min at 37°C. After the incubation, 50 μl of antibody to C3 (anti-C3) labeled with fluorescein isothiocyanate (FITC-anti-C3) were added to the treated cells. The mixtures were incubated at 37°C for 20 min and in the cold for 20 min. Then, treated test cells were washed with veronal-buffered saline containing 0.1% sodium azide (VBS-NaN$_3$), and the percentage of cells stained with FITC-anti-C3 was determined by observation under a fluorescence microscope (Okada et al., 1979).

Alternatively, the deposited C3b molecules on test cells as a result of complement activation of test cells in serum (or plasma) in Mg-EGTA-GVB were detected by rosette formation of human erythrocytes (HuE) instead of staining of C3 molecules with FITC-anti-C3. The HuE formed rosettes adhering to C3b molecules deposited on test cells through their C3b receptors. After incubation of test cells with an equal volume of serum in Mg-EGTA-GVB at 30°C for 30 min as described previously, a half-volume of 3 mg/ml of dithiothreitol in EDTA-GVB was added to prevent C3b molecules from inactivation by serum inhibitors (Okada and Nishioka, 1972). The mixtures were shaken well and added with one volume of 1×10^8/ml HuE in EDTA-GVB. After further incubation at 37°C for 1 hr, rosette formation of HuE on test cells was examined microscopically.

To determine the extent of cytotoxic reaction induced by complement activation via the alternative pathway, 100 μl of 5×10^6/ml test cells were treated with an equal volume of serum diluted in Mg-EGTA-GVB. After incubation for 60 min at 37°C, the mixtures were immersed in an ice-water bath, and the cell viability was determined by the trypan blue dye exclusion test after addition of 100 μl of 0.2% trypan blue in phosphate-buffered saline.

III. INDUCTION OF CAC ON TUMOR CELLS BY SENDAI VIRUS INFECTION

Cultured cell lines of Burkitt lymphoma, nasopharyngeal carcinoma, and oat cell lung carcinoma have been demonstrated to activate homologous complement via the alternative pathway, and it was suggested that the CAC might be induced by some viral

agents (Okada and Baba, 1974). McConnell *et al.* (1978) reported
that Epstein-Barr virus could induce CAC on the cells that it
infected. Subsequently, several other viruses were demonstrated
to induce CAC via the alternative pathway on infected cells
(Okada *et al.*, 1979; Sissons *et al.*, 1980; Lambre and Thibon,
1980). Since we found that Sendai virus (SV) had a capacity to
induce the CAC via the alternative pathway on infected cells
even after the irradiation of the virus with ultraviolet light
(UV) (Okada *et al.*, 1979; Okada and Okada, 1981), we used this
virus for induction of CAC on tumor cells. Ultraviolet-irradiated
viruses may not produce progeny viruses. Therefore, UV-irradiated
Sendai virus (UV-SV) would induce CAC on tumor cells without production of progeny viruses, which might cause hazardous effect to
the host.

Guinea pig line 10 (GPL10) tumor cells were infected with
UV-SV, which had been prepared by irradiating Sendai virus strain
Z with 8400 erg/mm^2 of ultraviolet light. After incubation of
GPL10 cells with 10, 3, 1, 0.3, 0.1, or 0.03 PFUeq UV-SV per cell,
the cells were washed with GVB and suspended at 5×10^6/ml in
Mg-EGTA-GVB. Each cell suspension was incubated with an equal
volume of guinea pig serum diluted to 1:10 in Mg-EGTA-GVB. After
the reaction, C3 molecules deposited on the cell membrane as a
result of ACP activation were examined by staining with FITC-
anti-C3 as described previously (Okada *et al.*, 1979). As shown
in Fig. 1, GPL10 cells infected with UV-SV at 0.3 PFUeq/cell or
more showed ACP-activating capacity on homologous complement
(Okada *et al.*, 1983b).

GPL10 cells infected with 10 PFUeq/cell (UV-SV-GPL10 cells)
were incubated at 37°C for 60 min with C4-deficient guinea pig
serum (C4D-GPS), human serum, and rabbit serum diluted 1:10 in
Mg-EGTA-GVB. After incubation, cell viability was determined by
trypan blue exclusion test. UV-SV-GPL10 cells were readily cyto-
lyzed by C4D-GPS in Mg-EGTA-GVB (Okada *et al.*, 1983a). However,
UV-SV-GPL10 cells were not lysed by human serum in Mg-EGTA-GVB,
although they were lysed to some extent by rabbit serum in Mg-
EGTA-GVB (Fig. 2). These results contrasted with the phenomenon
that neuraminidase-treated GPL10 cells as well as neuraminidase-
treated guinea pig erythrocytes were reactive with human serum,
whereas they could not react with the alternative complement
pathway (ACP) of homologous guinea pig serum (Okada *et al.*,
1983b). Induction of complement-activating capacity on GPL10
cells by UV-SV infection would not be due to any neuraminidase
activity that UV-SV had.

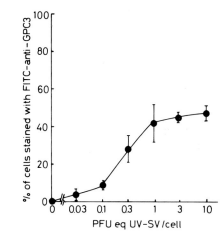

Fig. 1. Complement-activating capacity (CAC) of UV-SV-GPL10 cells determined by staining with FITC-labeled antibody to guinea pig C3 (FITC-anti-GPC3) following incubation of the cells with guinea pig serum (GPS) diluted in Mg-EGTA-GVB, from Okada *et al.* (1983a). GPL10 cells were infected with UV-SV of different doses, and the infected cells were suspended in RPMI-1640 medium supplemented with 10% fetal calf serum (FCS-RPMI). After overnight incubation at $37°C$ in a CO_2 incubator, cells were washed and suspended in GVB at 5×10^6/ml. To examine their reactivity with guinea pig complement via the alternative pathway, the cells were incubated with an equal volume of GPS diluted 1:10 in Mg-EGTA-GVB at $30°C$ for 30 min. Then, treated cells were washed, and C3 deposition on the cell surface as a result of ACP activation was detected by staining with FITC-anti-GPC3. Infection with UV-SV at 0.3 PFUeq/cell or more induced the capacity to activate guinea pig ACP. Vertical bars, SD, triplicate determinations. In control experiments where fresh GPS was replaced by heat-inactivated GPS, or Mg-EGTA-GVB was replaced by EDTA-GVB, no staining of UV-SV-infected GPL10 cells with FITC-anti-GPC3 was observed.

IV. SUPPRESSION OF TUMOR GROWTH BY SENDAI VIRUS-TREATED CELLS

Since UV-SV-GPL10 cells were found to activate the alternative complement pathway (ACP) of GPS and they were cytolysed as a result of the complement activation of homologous serum as described earlier, we examined whether UV-SV-GPL10 cells were readily eliminated *in vivo*. GPL10 cells were infected with different doses of UV-SV, and the cells were washed twice with minimum essential medium (MEM). Thus prepared, UV-SV-GPL10 cells were suspended in MEM at 1×10^6/ml, and 0.1 ml of each cell suspension was inoculated intradermally into strain 2 guinea pigs (St2-GP). When GPL10 cells were infected with 0.1 PFUeq UV-SV/cell or more, no

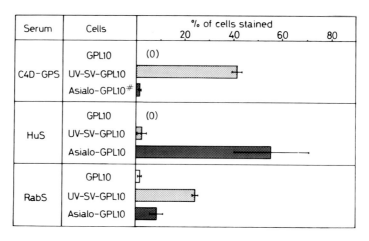

Fig. 2. Staining of GPL10 cells, UV-SV-GPL10 cells, and asiolo-GPL10 cells with FITC-labeled antibody to C3 following treatment with C4D-GPS, human serum (HuS), and rabbit serum (RabS) in Mg-EGTA-GVB. Cells were incubated with C4D-GPS, HuS, or RabS diluted 1:10 in Mg-EGTA-GVB. After incubation at 37°C for 10 min, cells were washed with EDTA-GVB-NaN$_3$ and stained with FITC-anti-GPC3, FITC-anti-human C3, or FITC-anti-rabbit C3, respectively. UV-SV-GPL10 cells incubated with C4D-GPS were stained with FITC-anti-GPC3, indicating that UV-SV-GPL10 cells could activate the ACP of homologous GPS. However, UV-SV-GPL10 cells did not react with human complement. On the other hand, asiolaso-GPL10 cells (treated with neuraminidase) were reactive with heterologous ACP of HuS and RabS, while they did not react with homologous ACP or C4D-GPS. #GPL10 cells treated with neuraminidase.

tumor growth was noted 2 weeks after tumor cell inoculation, whereas after mock infection of GPL10 cells, tumors of more than 10 mm diameter developed at the inoculation site (Okada et al., 1983a). The guinea pigs that eliminated UV-SV-GPL10 cells were found to be resistant to challenge with 1×10^5 intact GPL10 tumor cells 1 month after inoculation of UV-SV-GPL10 cells.

    To demonstrate that the complement reaction in vivo was important in this growth suppression of UV-SV-GPL10 cells, recipient guinea pigs were depleted of complement by cobra venom factor (CoVF) treatment (Nelson, 1966). St2-GP were injected intraperitoneally with 200 units of CoVF 4 hr before intradermal inoculation with 1×10^6 UV-SV-GPL10 (2 PFUeq UV-SV per cell). At 20 hr after CoVF injection, the complement activity of sera of these guinea pigs was less than 6% of the normal level as judged by measuring the hemolytic activity on antibody-sensitized sheep erythrocytes. In two of three St2-GP pretreated with CoVF, tumor growth occurred at the inoculation site of UV-SV-GPL10 cells prepared with 2 PFUeq UV-SV per cell, which was almost 20 times the amount of UV-SV required for suppression of GPL10 growth (Table I). This result indicated that the complement reaction to UV-SV-GPL10 cells in vivo

TABLE I

Growth of UV-SV-GPL10 Cells in Guinea Pigs Depleted
of Serum Complement by Administration of Cobra Venom Factor (CoVF)[a]

Tumor cells[b]	CoVF treatment[c]	Diameter of tumor 40 days after tumor cell inoculation (mm)
GPL10	No	38
		30
		18
UV-SV-GPL10[d]	No	0
		0
		0
UV-SV-GPL10	Yes	17
		10
		0

[a]From Okada et al. (1983a).
[b]1×10^5 GPL10 cells or 1×10^5 UV-SV-GPL10 cells were inoculated intradermally into strain 2 guinea pigs.
[c]Cobra venom factor (200 units) was injected intraperitoneally 4 hr before tumor cell inoculation.
[d]GPL10 cells (2×10^6) were incubated with 4×10^6 PFUeq UV-SV in a volume of 0.2 ml at room temperature for 60 min, washed with minimum essential medium (MEM) and suspended in 2 ml of MEM. This amount (2 PFUeq/cell) of UV-SV was 20 times the amount (0.1 PFUeq/cell) required to sensitize GPL10 cells to be suppressed in vivo.

was essential for suppression of UV-SV-GPL10 cells (Okada et al., 1983a). However, in the experiment, infection with UV-SV might have been incomplete, since 2 PFUeq UV-SV per cell would have left 13.5% of GPL10 cells uninfected. According to the Poisson distribution, if 1 PFUeq is necessary and sufficient for UV-SV infection of a cell, then the negative logarithm of the rate of uninfected cells should be equal to the average number of PFUeq per cell. Therefore, on infection with 2 PFUeq/cell, the rate of uninfected cells could be calculated to be 0.135 from the following equation.

$$2 = -\ln(\text{rate of uninfected cells})$$

The uninfected cells present in the GPL10 cell population treated with 2 PFUeq UV-SV per cell might escape elimination in guinea pigs depleted of complement by treatment with CoVF. Therefore, the growth of tumor cells that escaped the elimination by complement must have been suppressed by some side effects of the complement activation on the cells that were reactive with the

alternative pathway of complement. Complement activation on
UV-SV-GPL10 cells might have stimulated the host immune response
to the tumor cells, since complement activation generates a
chemotactic factor as well as anaphylatoxins that cause inflammation at the reaction site. Since the chemotactic factor brings
about accumulation of polymorphonuclear leukocytes (PMN) at the
site where complement activation occurs, PMN must have accumulated
around UV-SV-GPL10 cells. Since PMN release an interleukin 1-like
mediator that stimulates maturation of pre-T cells (Nakamura *et
al.*, 1982; Nakayama *et al.*, 1982; Goto *et al.*, 1982), PMN accumulated around UV-SV-GPL10 cells as a result of complement activation
might have increased the host immune response to the tumor cells.
If this is the case, UV-SV infection to guinea pig tumor cells
might be useful to increase immunogenicity of tumor cells.

To test this possibility, guinea pigs were inoculated with
UV-SV-GPL10 cells at different sites in addition to inoculation
of intact GPL10 cells. Untreated GPL10 cells (1×10^5 in 0.1 ml)
were inoculated intracutaneously into the flanks of seven guinea
pigs. In addition to the GPL10 cell inoculation, three guinea pigs
were inoculated simultaneously with 1×10^6 UV-SV-GPL10 cells in
0.1 ml into the skin at the other side of the flank. In control
guinea pigs, tumor grew progressively at the site of inoculation.
In contrast, in guinea pigs inoculated with both GPL10 cells and
UV-SV-GPL10 cells in different sites, growth of tumors at the site
of inoculation of untreated GPL10 cells was suppressed as shown in
Fig. 3. This result indicated that the reaction of complement on
UV-SV-GPL10 cells not only suppressed the growth of UV-SV-GPL10
cells, but also induced host immune response so as to suppress the
growth of intact GPL10 cells inoculated simultaneously at different
sites (Okada *et al.*, 1984). Therefore, the tumor antigens on
UV-SV-GPL10 cells probably effectively stimulated the host immune
response in the presence of the interleukin 1-like mediator
released from PMN, which had been accumulated around UV-SV-GPL10
cells as a result of complement activation. It will be noteworthy
that most of the so-called immunopotentiators have a capacity to
activate complement (Okuda *et al.*, 1972; Dukor *et al.*, 1974). If
complement activation *in vivo* has a close relationship to immuno-
potentiating effect, induction of complement-activating capacity
on tumor cells by a UV-irradiated virus such as UV-SV might
qualify tumor cells themselves as a kind of immunoadjuvant.

V. POSSIBLE MECHANISM INVOLVED IN THE INDUCTION OF CAC

The role of the alternative complement pathway (ACP) in the
recognition of microorganisms has been emphasized since the
initial description of the reaction in the name of the properdin
system (Pillemer *et al.*, 1955). Studies on the mechanism of ACP

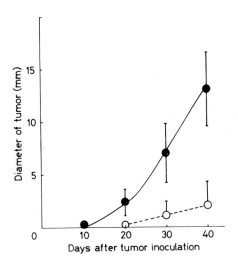

Fig. 3. Suppression of GPL10 tumor by inoculation of UV-SV-GPL10 cells at different sites, from Okada et al. (1984). Tumor diameters at the site of inoculation of 1×10^5 intact GPL10 cells were measured with sliding calipers. Solid circles indicate the mean diameter of tumors in four control guinea pigs, and open circles indicate mean diameter of tumors in three guinea pigs simultaneously inoculated with 1×10^6 UV-SV-GPL10 cells at different sites. Vertical bars, mean ± SD. No tumor growth was noted at the site of inoculation of UV-SV-GPL10 cells.

have revealed that the activation of ACP will be initiated by C3(H_2O)Bb, a C3 convertase generated spontaneously in the fluid phase of serum (Pangburn et al., 1981), which is capable of cleaving C3 to generate C3b. The C3b molecules thus generated are readily inactivated by the regulatory proteins, H (β1H) and I (C3b inactivator) (Nicol and Lachmann, 1973; Whaley and Ruddy, 1976; Weiler et al., 1976). When the nascent C3b happens to encounter a solid surface of a so-called ACP activator, it can escape inactivation by H and I, and subsequently form C3bBb(P), which produces other C3b molecules capable of forming other C3 convertase (Pangburn et al., 1980). These reactions form a positive-feedback circuit, and the generation of C3b is amplified, this process being regarded as activation of ACP. Although the mechanism by which C3b molecules deposited on ACP activators gain the capacity to escape the regulatory reaction by H and I remains to be studied, sheep erythrocytes (ShE), which do not activate human ACP, have been shown to become ACP activators after the removal or destruction of the membrane sialic acids by neuraminidase or potassium peroxide, respectively (Fearon, 1978; Pangburn and Müller-Eberhard, 1978; Okada et al., 1978). However, human erythrocytes (HuE) do not become ACP activators of human complement even after neuraminidase treatment, and Fearon (1979) has demonstrated that a membrane inhibitor with a molecular weight of 205,000 (gp205) extracted from HuE can inhibit

the formation of C3bBb, suggesting that this membrane inhibitor
is responsible for the regulation of the homologous complement
reaction on HuE. The membrane inhibitor gp205 turned out to be
a C3b receptor (Fearon, 1980), and the inhibitory capacity of the
C3b receptor was also demonstrated in the formation of C4b2a,
which is a classical complement pathway (CCP) C3 convertase (Iida
and Nussenzweig, 1981). However, the absence of the C3b receptor
on the surface of erythrocytes of the non-primate species (Nelson,
1963) indicates that regulation of complement activation by C3b
receptors will not occur on those erythrocyte membranes.

It was found that neuraminidase-treated HuE were hemolyzed by
guinea pig serum (GPS) in Mg-EGTA-GVB, whereas they were resistant
to human serum (Okada *et al.*, 1980, 1983b). The results indicated
that the reaction of guinea pig complement was not inhibited by
the C3b receptor, although guinea pig C3b could react with the C3b
receptor (Nishioka and Linscott, 1963). In contrast, neuraminidase-
treated guinea pig erythrocytes (GPE) were hemolyzed by human serum
but not by homologous GPS. Furthermore, neuraminidase-treated
rabbit erythrocytes were also resistant to homologous rabbit serum
(Okada *et al.*, 1980, 1983b). It has been reported that erythrocytes are rather resistant to the membrane attack complexes (MAC)
of homologous complement (Hänsch *et al.*, 1981). Therefore, the
restriction in hemolysis of neuraminidase-treated erythrocytes by
homologous serum might have been due to their resistance to the
homologous MAC. To test this possibility, we examined whether the
neuraminidase-treated erythrocytes consume homologous complement
in Mg-EGTA-GVB and found that the neuraminidase-treated erythrocytes could not activate the homologous ACP, indicating that
inability of complement to hemolyze homologous erythrocytes was
due to lack of complement activation on homologous cells and not
to the resistance of erythrocytes to homologous MAC (Okada *et al.*,
1983b). There may be a mechanism that preferentially inhibits the
activation of the homologous ACP and not the heterologous ACP.

We asked further whether this possible restriction of complement activation on homologous cell membranes could be seen on
nucleated cells. After neuraminidase treatment, HeLa cells of
human origin did not gain a complement-activating capacity on
homologous human ACP, whereas they could activate the guinea pig
ACP. Here again, the neuraminidase treatment of GPL10 cells endowed the cells with the activating capacity on human and rabbit
ACP but not on homologous guinea pig ACP (Fig. 2). These results
suggested that the unreactiveness of ACP on the homologous cell membrane might be a general phenomenon observed on nucleated cells as
well as erythrocytes among different species (Okada *et al.*, 1983b).
Should this be the case, it would indicate that ACP activation *in
vivo* would occur only on infected organisms and accidentally invading extraneous substances, but not on the surface of self-cell
membranes. The mechanism whereby the ACP recognizes homologous
cell membrane remains to be understood. As mentioned earlier, the
C3b receptor may not be responsible for this recognition, as the

C3b receptor does not discriminate between homologous and heterologous C3b. Furthermore, this conclusion is supported by the
finding that HeLa cells that had no detectable C3b receptor could
restrict ACP activation (Okada et al., 1983b). We have found
that sialosylglycoconjugates have a capacity to inhibit the
complement-activating capacity on liposomes incorporated with
trinitrophenylaminocaproyldipalmitoylphosphatidylethanolamine
(Okada et al., 1982a). However, the status of the neuraminidase-
treated erythrocytes and nucleated cells was such that the
function of the sialosylglycoconjugates had been impaired by the
enzyme treatment. Therefore, the unreactiveness of neuraminidase-
treated cell membranes with homologous ACP could not be due to the
inhibition by sialic acid in glycoconjugates of ACP.

Alternatively, natural antibodies to foreign substances may
play a role in the ACP activation of serum on heterologous cell
membrane, since the presence of antibody on cell surfaces enhances
the ACP-activating capacity (Nelson and Ruddy, 1978; Schenkein and
Ruddy, 1981). The natural antibodies may be provided by the
idiotype-anti-idiotype network (Jerne, 1974) of the immune
response system, which may offer any antibody to foreign epitopes.
The antibodies reacting on cell membrane may initiate the ACP activation, and the absence of sialosylglycoconjugates due to the
neuraminidase treatment may permit the amplification reaction of
the ACP. If this is the case, the presence of a putative membrane
inhibitor is not necessarily required in the unresponsiveness of
the ACP on neuraminidase-treated erythrocytes. However,
neuraminidase-treated guinea pig tumor cells and GPE did not gain
activating capacity on homologous ACP following incubation with
heterologous serum in EDTA-GVB to sensitize them with possible
natural antibodies in the heterologous serum (Okada et al., 1983b).

These findings indicate that some particular membrane molecules that inhibit ACP activation with species specificity might
be present on cell membranes. In this connection, glycophorin
fractions from HuE and GPE were found to inhibit hemolytic activity of homologous complement on rabbit erythrocytes, whereas
they could not inhibit hemolytic activity of heterologous complement (Okada and Tanaka, 1983). These findings indicated that
membrane inhibitor that inhibits the activation of self-complement
with a species specificity should exist on cell membranes.
Complement proteins such as C3b may recognize the membrane inhibitor on self-cell membrane with species specificity, and sequentially, the discrimination of the self-cell membrane inhibitor
will result in the recognition of a foreign membrane as "not self."
Thereby, the ACP activation would occur on foreign cell membranes
such as microorganisms and not on self-cell membranes (Fig. 4).
Therefore, the induction of CAC on tumor cells could be regarded
as a change of tumor cell membrane to "not self" phenotype, to
which the ACP as a first line of nonspecific host defense can
react without restriction by the species-specific membrane inhibitor. It could be possible that the species-specific membrane

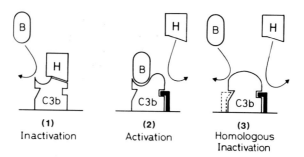

| (1) | (2) | (3) |
| Inactivation | Activation | Homologous Inactivation |

Fig. 4. A schema of a working hypothesis on the mechanism by which cell membranes suppress ACP activation of homologous serum: (1) If no molecules on the cell membrane interacted with C3b molecules deposited on the membrane, binding of H (a serum inhibitor previously called β1H) to the C3b molecules inhibits the formation of C3 convertase (C3bBb) with B; (2) If activator molecules (solid bar) on cell membrane reacted with C3b molecules deposited on the membrane, C3b molecules may lose the site for H and become able to react with B to form C3 convertase (Pangburn et al., 1980); (3) Although activator molecules were available on cell membrane that cause C3b molecules insensitive to H, the activator-reacted C3b molecules might be interacted with membrane inhibitor present on homologous cell surface (bar shown with dotted line) and might lose the reactivity of the C3b molecules with B to form C3 convertase. If the membrane inhibitor has a species specificity in the reaction with C3b, ACP activation on self-cell membrane will be preferentially inhibited. In other words, C3b molecules might recognize foreign membranes as "not self" when C3b molecules could not find the putative species-specific membrane inhibitor. Most tumor cells might have the membrane inhibitor, and if so, induction of ACP-activating capacity on tumor cell membrane should be accompanied with impairment of the membrane inhibitor(s).

inhibitor(s) of the reaction of self-ACP is also playing a role in the discrimination of self-cell surface in cytotoxic reactions by NK cells (Kiessling et al., 1975) and/or activated macrophages (Evans and Alexander, 1972). The membrane inhibitor(s) may protect cells from cell-mediated cytotoxic reactions by self-effector cells. If this is the case, the impairment of the membrane inhibitor(s) that was detected by the induction of ACP-activating capacity could also make the tumor cells sensitive to cytotoxic reaction of NK cells and/or activated macrophages.

ACKNOWLEDGMENTS

The research described was supported by Grants-in-Aid from the Japanese Ministry of Education, Science, and Culture, and from the Adult Disease Clinic Memorial Foundation, and by Public Health Service Grant CA19229.

REFERENCES

Buzko, D. B., Lachmann, P. J., and McConnell, I. (1976). *Cell Immunol.* 22, 98-109.
Evans, R., and Alexander, P. (1972). *Nature (London)* 236, 168-170.
Dukor, P., Schumann, G., Gisler, R. L., Dierich, M., Koning, W., Hadding, U., and Bitter-Suermann, D. (1974). *J. Exp. Med.* 139, 337-354.
Fearon, D. T. (1978). *Proc. Natl. Acad. Sci. USA* 75, 1971-1975.
Fearon, D. T. (1979). *Proc. Natl. Acad. Sci. USA* 76, 5867-5871.
Fearon, D. T. (1980). *J. Exp. Med.* 152, 20-30.
Feldman, J. D. (1972). *Adv. Immunol.* 15, 167-214.
Goto, F., Nakamura, S., Goto, K., and Yoshinaga, M. (1982). *Proc. Jpn. Soc. Immunol.* 12, 398-399.
Hänsch, G. M., Hammer, C. H., Vanguri, P., and Shin, M. L. (1981). *Proc. Natl. Acad. Sci. USA* 78, 5118-5121.
Hugli, T. E., and Müller-Eberhard, H. J. (1978). *Adv. Immunol.* 26, 1-53.
Iida, K., and Nussenzweig, V. (1981). *J. Exp. Med.* 153, 1138-1150.
Jerne, N. K. (1974). *Ann. Immunol. (Paris)* 125c, 373-388.
Kiessling, R., Klein, E., and Wigzell, H. (1975). *Eur. J. Immunol.* 5, 112-117.
Lambré, C., and Thibon, M. (1980). *Ann. Immunol. (Inst. Pasteur)* 131c, 213-221.
McConnell, I., Klein, G., Lint, T. E., and Lachmann, P. J. (1978). *Eur. J. Immunol.* 8, 453-458.
Nakamura, S., Goto, F., Goto, K., and Yoshinaga, M. (1982). *J. Immunol.* 128, 2614-2621.
Nakayama, S., Rodriguez-Pinzon, J., Nakamura, S., and Yoshinaga, M. (1982). *Immunology* 45, 669-677.
Nelson, B., and Ruddy, S. (1978). *J. Immunol.* 122, 1994-1999.
Nelson, D. S. (1963). *Adv. Immunol.* 3, 131-180.
Nelson, R. A., Jr. (1966). *Surv. Ophthalmol.* 11, 498-505.
Nicol, P. A. E., and Lachmann, P. J. (1973). *Immunology* 24, 259-275.
Nishioka, K., and Linscott, W. D. (1963). *J. Exp. Med.* 118, 767-793.
Ohanian, H., Borsos, T., and Rapp, H. J. (1973). *J. Natl. Cancer Inst. (US)* 50, 1313-1320.

Okada, H., and Baba, T. (1974). *Nature (London) 248*, 521-522.

Okada, H., and Nishioka, K. (1972). *In* "Biological Activities of Complement" (D. G. Ingram, ed.), pp. 229-238. Karger, Basel.

Okada, H., and Okada, N. (1981). *Immunology 43*, 337-344.

Okada, H., and Tanaka, H. (1981). *J. Immunol. Methods 46*, 85-95.

Okada, H., and Tanaka, H. (1983). *Mol. Immunol. 20*, 1233-1236.

Okada, H., Tanaka, H., Yokota, M., Ohtani, T., and Okada, N. (1980). *Proc. Jpn. Soc. Immunol. 10*, 629-630.

Okada, H., Tanaka, H., and Okada, N. (1983a). *Immunology 49*, 29-35

Okada, H., Tanaka, H., and Okada, N. (1983b). *Eur. J. Immunol. 13*, 340-344.

Okada, H., Okada, N., Tanaka, H., Kohno, K., and Kuroiwa, A. (1984) *Med. Bull. Fukuoka Univ. 11*, 15-17.

Okada, N., and Okada, H. (1978). *Int. J. Cancer 22*, 282-287.

Okada, N., Anemiya, F., and Okada, H. (1978). *Proc. Jpn. Soc. Immunol. 8*, 446.

Okada, N., Shibuta, H., and Okada, H. (1979). *Microbiol. Immunol. 23*, 689-692.

Okada, N., Yasuda, T., and Okada, H. (1982a). *Nature (London) 299*, 261-263.

Okada, N., Yasuda, T., Tsumita, T., Shinomiya, H., Utsumi, S., and Okada, H. (1982b). *Biochem. Biophys. Res. Commun. 108*, 770-775.

Okuda, T., Yoshioka, Y., Ikekawa, T., Chihara, G., and Nishioka, K. (1972). *Nature (London) New Biol. 238*, 59-60.

Pangburn, M. K., and Müller-Eberhard, H. J. (1978). *Proc. Natl. Acad. Sci. USA 75*, 2416-2420.

Pangburn, M. K., Morrison, D. C., Schreiber, R. D., and Müller-Eberhard, H. J. (1980). *J. Immunol. 124*, 977-982.

Pangburn, M. K., Schreiber, R. D., and Müller-Eberhard, H. J. (1981). *J. Exp. Med. 154*, 856-867.

Pillemer, L., Schoenberg, M. D., and Wurg, L. (1955). *Science (Washington, D.C.) 122*, 545-549.

Rapp, H. J., Churchill, W. H., Jr., Kronman, B. S., Rolley, R. T., Hammond, W. G., and Borsos, T. (1968). *J. Natl. Cancer Inst. (US) 41*, 1-12.

Schenkein, N. K., and Ruddy, S. (1981). *J. Immunol. 126*, 7-10.

Shimbo, T., Yata, J., and Okada, H. (1978). *Int. J. Cancer 22*, 422-425.

Shin, H. S., Snyderman, R., Friedman, E., Mellors, A., and Mayer, M. M. (1968). *Science (Washington, D.C.) 162*, 361-363.

Sissons, J. G. P., Oldstone, M. B. A., and Schreiber, R. D. (1980). *Proc. Natl. Acad. Sci. USA 77*, 559-562.

Theofilopoulos, A. N., and Perrin, L. H. (1976). *J. Exp. Med. 142*, 271-289.

Weiler, J. M., Daha, M. R., Austen, K. F., and Fearon, D. T. (1976). *Proc. Natl. Acad. Sci. USA 73*, 3268-3272.

Whaley, K., and Ruddy, S. (1976). *J. Exp. Med. 144*, 1147-1163.

Yoshikawa, Y., Yamanouchi, K., Hishiyama, M., and Kobune, K. (1978) *Int. J. Cancer 21*, 658-666.

Zbar, B., Bernstein, I. D., and Rapp, H. J. (1971). *J. Natl. Cancer Inst. (US) 46*, 831-839.

DISCUSSION

GOLUB: How do you think the complement system interacts with
            interleukin 1?

OKADA: Complement activation generates a chemotactic factor
            (C5a), which attracts polymorphonuclear leukocytes to
            the site where complement activation occurred.
            Yoshinaga *et al.* have clearly demonstrated that poly-
            morphonuclear leukocytes generate a release interleukin
            1-like mediator, which has a capacity to differentiate
            immature T cells to competent T cells. Therefore,
            complement activation could be able to stimulate immune
            response.

MIYATA: Cytotoxicity (homologous complement) was also observed
            on guinea pig leukocytes after Sendai virus infection?

OKADA: Peripheral lymphocytes of guinea pig became reactive
            with homologous complement via the alternative pathway
            after treatment with UV-irradiated Sendai virus. We
            observed this phenomenon by staining with FITC-anti-C3
            following incubation with guinea pig serum of UV-Sendai
            virus-treated lymphocytes. Therefore, we have not
            tested cytotoxic reaction of UV-Sendai virus-infected
            lymphocytes by homologous complement. However, I think
            the lymphocytes could be cytolysed by homologous com-
            plement.

KONDO: Can you find complement-activating capacity on human
            cancer? If it is the case, the tumor cell is lysed by
            the spontaneous activation of complement in virus?

OKADA: Some tumor cells such as nasopharyngeal carcinoma and
            Burkitt lymphoma have been demonstrated to activate
            the alternative complement pathway as we have reported
            (Okada and Baba, 1974). However, those tumor cells are
            resistant to cytotoxic attack of complement, thereby
            they could become malignant tumor cells. They must
            have acquired a resistive mechanism against complement
            attack to survive selection by host defense in the
            course of carcinogenesis. On the other hand, AKR leu-
            kemia cells are sensitive to complement attack, which
            they can activate via the alternative pathway. However,
            they could become leukemia because the host AKR mice
            are genetically deficient in C5, fifth component of
            complement, which is required to form membrane attack
            complement complex.

KOBAYASHI: I wonder if you have any data showing the increased immunogenicity of tumor cells as you described in the program by the *in vivo*-transplantation immunity?

OKADA: We have not done quantitative *in vivo* analysis, yet.

PART III

The Effects of Soluble Mediators on Tumor Cell Metastasis

Chairpersons

Stanley Cohen
Takeru Ishikawa

CHAPTER 15

NONCYTOTOXIC EFFECTS OF LYMPHOKINES ON TUMOR CELLS*

Stanley Cohen
William Munger
Marion C. Cohen
Takeshi Yoshida

Department of Pathology
University of Connecticut Health Center
Farmington, Connecticut

I. INTRODUCTION

Immunologic recognition involves not only foreign substances but also abnormalities within the organism itself. The best example of this latter situation involves malignant transformation. Thus, it is not surprising that the immune system is thought capable of playing an important role in the control of neoplastic disease. Under normal conditions, however, this role must be limited or circumvented to some extent, since cancer is unfortunately a relatively common occurrence in humans. This does not negate the importance of studying mechanisms of tumor immunity, since it is only through such understanding that we can devise ways of enhancing this form of immune response for beneficial therapeutic effects.

Supported by NIH Grant Number AI-12477.

BASIC MECHANISMS AND CLINICAL TREATMENT
OF TUMOR METASTASIS
273

TABLE I

Cytotoxic Effects on Tumor Cells by the Immune System

Non-cell mediated	Cell mediated
Complement Lymphotoxin	Natural killer (NK) cells T cell-dependent cytolysis (CTL) Antibody-dependent (ADCC) lymphocytes, neutrophils, macrophages, fetal liver, platelets Lymphokine-activated macrophages

The involvement of the immune system in the destruction of tumor cells has been suspected for many years. This concept received support in the rare but documented phenomenon of spontaneous tumor regression. It found additional support in the discovery of a wide variety of tumor-specific antigens and the development of a number of animal models in which immunization against such antigens modified the behavior of transplanted, induced, or spontaneous neoplasms. A large amount of clinical data has accumulated as well.

In all this work, attention has been focused on the destruction of tumor cells by immune mechanisms. Such mechanisms fall predominantly into two categories: those that involve cells as effector agents and those that involve antibodies or other soluble mediators. A summary of various kinds of immunologic killing mechanisms is shown in Table I. As can be seen, the pathways involving cells far outnumber those that are not cell dependent. This is an important generalization; although all of the known forms of immunologic reactivity may play a role in tumor immunity, cell-mediated immunity seems to be of central importance in many cases, especially those involving solid tumors. This, however, does not mean that only mononuclear cells are important. Various other inflammatory cells and, in unusual situations, certain non-inflammatory cells, can participate in these reactions.

As just indicated, most studies of cell-mediated immunity in neoplastic diseases focus on cytotoxic mechanisms. We will consider here two examples of these, both involving the effects of lymphokines. One example involves a direct effect of lymphokines (lymphotoxin), and the other an indirect effect, via macrophages (macrophage activation factor, MAF).

Evidence to support a role of lymphotoxins in lymphocyte-mediated cell killing in tumor immunity has been obtained in many laboratories. This topic has been critically reviewed by Granger (1979). It has been shown that lymphotoxins produced by lymphocytes stimulated with specific antigen or with nonspecific mitogens could kill or at least damage various cell lines in culture. Like other lymphokines, lymphotoxins, although induced by specific immunologic or mitogenic stimuli, are themselves capable of acting in a nonspecific manner. Although lymphotoxins are thus usually cytotoxic to a variety of both normal and malignant cultured cells, a few reports show that tumor cells are more susceptible to lymphotoxins than normal cells. For example, Meltzer and Bartlett (1972) have shown that supernatants obtained from PPD-stimulated spleen cells of BCG-immunized mice could destroy tumor cell monolayers but not normal cell monolayers. Weedon et al. (1973) have shown that lymphotoxins obtained by mitogenic stimulation of human lymphocytes could be cytotoxic to various tumor cells as well as their normal counterparts, and that the tumor cells (glioma) were more susceptible than normal nervous tissue. Although studies by other investigators in addition to those mentioned earlier confirm the nonspecific tumor cell destruction by lymphotoxins, which are produced by reacting lymphocytes with a variety of antigens (or mitogens), there are almost no data available on the production of lymphotoxins by immune lymphocytes stimulated with tumor-associated antigen.

It should be noted that most studies on lymphocyte-mediated cytotoxicity for tumor cells seem to have excluded the possibility of involving nonspecific soluble factors (such as lymphotoxins) in the mechanism of cytotoxicity. Thus, the majority of results suggest that cytotoxic effects of lymphocytes are highly specific and that adjacent nonspecific target cells remain intact. As stated previously, close contact between attacking and target cells is necessary for the effect. However, some studies have demonstrated that innocent bystander cells can also be affected by a specific interaction between immune lymphocytes and target cells.

In any event, it has been almost impossible to recover cell-free lymphotoxins after the specific reactions between immune lymphocytes and target cells. Therefore, one has to assume that lymphotoxins, if generated by such interactions, must be in smaller quantity than that usually generated by antigen- or mitogen-stimulated lymphocytes or that the production and consumption of lymphotoxin must occur at the limited area adjacent to the area of contact.

In contrast to this situation, when macrophages engage in tumor cell killing, they do so following activation by lymphokine. For example, Piessens et al. (1975) and Churchill et al. (1975) have shown that supernatants from cultures of lymphocytes stimulated by an antigen (O-chlorobenzoyl-bovine γ-globulin, OCB-BGG) activate normal macrophages, either as monolayers or in suspension culture. The responsible lymphokine was called "macrophage activating factor" (MAF). These "activated" macrophages exhibit enhanced cytotoxic capacity against syngeneic strain 2 hepatoma and MCA-25 sarcoma cells. Thus, MAF may be induced by unrelated antigens, and it enhances the cytotoxicity of macrophages in the absence of the specific eliciting antigen.

The importance of these results is underscored by studies of
the role of macrophages *in vivo*. Russel and Cochrane (1974)
investigated the relationship between the progressive or
regressive behavior of a murine (Moloney) tumor, and the extent
and nature of the inflammatory infiltrate. Tumors were induced
in adult and neonatal mice by intramuscular injections of a
cultured Moloney sarcoma line. In adults with tumors that regressed, a macrophage-rich infiltrate extended throughout the
neoplastic tissue, whereas in progressive tumors, the mononuclear
infiltrate remained confined to peripheral portions of the tumor
and later disappeared. In either progressing or regressing
tumors, neoplastic cells in close association with mononuclear
cells often showed evidence of damage. Tumors in neonates, which
almost always progressed, never developed an appreciable mononuclear infiltrate. These *in vivo* studies, although pointing to
an important role for macrophages, have yet to be extended to
systems in which one can examine lymphokine-dependent activation.

The preceding examples underscore the fact that experimental
work dealing with mechanisms of tumor immunity have focused on
cell killing. Other effects of the immune system on tumor cells
have not been explored in as great detail. Candidates for such
effects include modification of cell mobility, cell adhesion, and
cell migration properties. It has been thought for many years
that the mobility of individual tumor cells may be important in
local tumor spread and in the establishment of metastases. It
has, however, proved difficult to examine the mobility of tumor
cells in *in vitro* systems.

In this article, we will describe our studies demonstrating
that products of the immune system can influence tumor cell migration, as well as interaction between tumor cells and other cell
types. We will focus entirely on mechanisms of cell-mediated
immunity involving lymphokines. Before doing so, it is necessary
to review the known properties of lymphokines.

II. PROPERTIES OF LYMPHOKINES

Lymphokines are secreted products of antigen- or mitogen-
activated lymphocytes. They are protein or glycoprotein in nature,
and have molecular weights ranging from approximately 10,000 to
70,000. They participate in both the afferent (induction of immunity) arm and the efferent (effector functions) arm of the immune
response. Afferent lymphokines may be antigen specific or nonspecific and may show histocompatibility restriction. In contrast,
efferent lymphokines are, in general, antigen nonspecific and are
not histocompatibility restricted. Many of the efferent and some
of the afferent lymphokines can cross species barriers.

Lymphokines can affect essentially all aspects of cellular
function. For convenience, these can be grouped into effects on

cell growth and proliferation, cell movement, cell differentiation, and cell activation. Targets for lymphokine effects are equally diverse. Target cells include lymphocytes themselves (especially for the afferent lymphokines), monocytes and granulocytes, fibroblasts, smooth muscle, and endothelium, as well as specialized cells such as osteoclasts, and abnormal cells such as tumor cells.

Given the almost overwhelming variety of effects that lymphokines can exert on cells, it is surprising that attention has been almost exclusively focused on cytotoxicity in tumor immunity. We therefore initiated studies to explore the range of lymphokine effects on tumor cells. Our first investigations have been concerned with tumor cell movement.

III. TUMOR MIGRATION INHIBITION FACTOR (TMIF)

Initially, we determined that an ascites tumor, the P815 mastocytoma maintained in DBA/2 mice, was capable of migrating from capillary tubes in the presence of RPMI-1640 medium supplemented with heat-inactivated normal guinea pig serum (Cohen et al., 1975). The pattern was analogous to that observed when inflammatory cells migrate from capillary tubes. This was further extended to other ascites tumors including Ehrlich ascites, Hepatoma 129 and Sarcoma 37, which are of murine origin, and Walker carcinosarcoma, which is of rat origin (Cohen et al., 1978). This provided an assay system for the analysis of an effect of lymphokines on tumor cell movement. Supernatants with known macrophage migration inhibitory (MIF) activity for macrophages were prepared from antigen- or mitogen-activated lymphocytes or from long-term lymphoblastoid T and B cell lines, as described by Yoshida et al. (1976). Those of human or murine origin were found to inhibit tumor cell migration. Migration inhibition was not due to cytotoxicity, since the effect was reversible. This was confirmed by trypan blue exclusion studies. Of particular interest was that guinea pig MIF-containing supernatants did not inhibit tumor cell migration.

Our initial hypothesis was that the inhibition of tumor cell migration that we were observing was due to conventional MIF. However, data obtained from Diaflo ultrafiltration studies indicated that this was not the case. Supernatants prepared from RPMI-8392, one of the long-term lymphoblastoid cell lines, were passed sequentially through PM 30, PM 10, and DM 5 membranes, and the retentates concentrated threefold. When tested against guinea pig macrophages, the inhibitory activity was found in the PM 10 retentate demonstrating a molecular weight greater than 10,000. However, inhibitory activity for mastocytoma cells was found in the DM 5 retentate, indicating a molecular weight between 5000 and 10,000.

This result strongly suggested that the tumor migration-inhibitory lymphokine was distinct from MIF. This was consistent with the finding, indicated earlier, that the guinea pig lymphocytes could make MIF but not the tumor-affecting factor. Also, we have previously reported that lymphocytes from C57BL/6 mice cannot generate MIF activity in the absence of serum. Under such conditions, they can still generate the tumor-affecting factor. For these reasons, we felt that this represented a new lymphokine, and we therefore named it "tumor migration inhibition factor," or TMIF.

Our next series of experiments were designed to characterize TMIF further (Cohen et al., 1982). Specifically, we wished to compare it to the other lymphokines known to affect cell migration. These consist of mediators whose target cells are inflammatory cells. In addition, during the course of these studies, we demonstrated a lymphokine that could inhibit endothelial cell migration (Cohen, 1982), and showed that this also was different than TMIF. This other new mediator activity will be described in a later section.

Since none of the efferent lymphokines have been purified to homogeneity, it is necessary to use indirect means to determine whether two factors are the same or different. A single procedure that inhibits one but not the other is not adequate, as the observed results could be due to differences in assay sensitivity. Thus, it is necessary to find reciprocal conditions, such that one experimental procedure destroys one activity without affecting the other, and another experimental procedure does the opposite. We have already indicated one such reciprocal situation, where guinea pig-derived lymphokine preparations have MIF but not TMIF activity, and serum-free C57BL/6 mouse-derived lymphokine preparations have TMIF but not MIF activity. Also, the Amicon ultrafiltration studies gave rise to one fraction with MIF and no TMIF, and another with TMIF and no MIF. We next studied a variety of other characterization procedures. For example, it is known that MIF is inhibited by fucose and rhamnose. We found that under conditions in which MIF is inhibited by these sugars, TMIF is not. We also studied the effect of protease inhibitors. We found that diisopropylfluorophosphate (DFP) inhibited TMIF but had no effect on MIF. This establishes another reciprocal pair involving suppression of MIF and TMIF. In this regard, it should be noted that DFP can also inhibit leukocyte inhibition factor (LIF), which can inhibit the migration of neutrophils. However, LIF has a molecular weight of approximately 68,000. Also, LIF is inhibited by N-acetyl-D-galactosamine, whereas TMIF is not. Thus, TMIF is also distinct from LIF, as well as MIF.

The properties of TMIF described previously are summarized in Table II, which also includes data that TMIF is sensitive to trypsin but not to treatment with Trasylol or soybean trypsin inhibitor (SBTI).

TABLE II

Some Properties of TMIF

Criteria	Property
Sources	
Human	Yes
Guinea pig	No
Mouse	Yes
Molecular weight	5,000-10,000
Inhibition profile	
Trypsin	Inhibits
Neuraminidase	No effect
Protease inhibitors	
SBTI	No effect
Trasylol	No effect
DFP	Inhibits
Monosaccharides	No effect

IV. ENDOTHELIAL CELL MIGRATION

As indicated earlier, TMIF can inhibit the migration of a variety of tumor cells. Because of difficulties in obtaining samples of normal cells that migrate well in either the capillary or agarose assay systems, it has not yet been possible to study systematically normal and neoplastic cells that are matched as to cell type--for example, fibrosarcomas and fibroblasts. Thus, it is not yet clear whether TMIF activity is uniquely confined to tumor cells. Even if this were not the case, one would expect a differential effect on tumor cells by TMIF *in vivo*, since under most circumstances, normal cells do not demonstrate local invasiveness or distant dissemination.

In spite of this caveat, we wanted to study at least one non-neoplastic cell type other than an inflammatory cell. For this purpose we chose endothelium (Cohen *et al.*, 1982). Endothelial cells were obtained from calf pulmonary arteries and cultured according to standard procedures. Their identity as endothelial cells was established by the detection of factor VIII antigen by indirect immunofluorescence. Migration was studied using the agarose microdroplet technique. Using lymphokine preparations from human lymphoblastoid lines, we found that we could inhibit endothelial cell migration reversibly, but that this activity tracked with MIF activity through the various characterization

procedures. Preparations purified by Amicon ultrafiltration that
had TMIF activity, but were devoid of other lymphokine activities,
were without effect on endothelial cell migration.

To summarize the results on non-neoplastic cells thus far,
TMIF has no effect on neutrophils, macrophages, or endothelial
cells. In unpublished observations, we have shown that TMIF has
no effect on fibroblast migration either.

V. ATTACHMENT OF TUMOR CELLS TO ENDOTHELIUM

The property of TMIF that we have described, namely, its
ability to inhibit the migration of a variety of tumor cells, is
demonstrable *in vitro*. Nevertheless, it represents a good candidate for a protective role *in vivo*, as TMIF could inhibit either
local invasiveness or metastasis. Since the latter involves passage of tumor cells across endothelium, and the first step in
such passage must involve attachment, we wished to determine
whether TMIF-containing supernatants could influence interaction
between tumor cells and endothelium *in vitro*. For these experiments, endothelial cell monolayers were prepared in 12-well tissue
culture plates. Tumor cells, of the various types described
previously, were prepared as suspensions containing 50,000 cells/ml
Tumor cells and endothelium were incubated at 37°C for 30 min to
1 h in the presence of lymphokine or control, followed by three
washes in tissue culture medium. Tumor cell attachment was quantitated either by direct enumeration of adherent cells by light
microscopy or by the use of tumor cells labeled with radioactive
chromium. By either technique, we were able to demonstrate that
in control preparations, approximately 30-50% of the tumor cells
formed tight attachments to the endothelium. The TMIF-containing
supernatants reduced such binding by approximately 50%. Since un-
fractionated supernatants were used, it is not possible to say
whether the effect was due to TMIF itself or a different lymphokine. However, several preparations that had lost TMIF activity
(but that retained MIF and other activities) had no effect on tumor cell attachment, suggesting that TMIF itself was the responsible factor. In any event, these results point to yet another
effect involving tumor cells that can be ascribed to lymphokines.

VI. SUMMARY AND CONCLUSIONS

We have demonstrated that human and murine, but not guinea pig
lymphokine preparations contain a factor (TMIF) that can reversibly
inhibit the *in vitro* migration of a variety of tumor cell types.

Furthermore, TMIF is distinct from other lymphokines affecting cell migration, such as MIF, LIF, and factors inhibiting endothelial and fibroblast movement. Unlike lymphotoxin, TMIF does not exert a cytotoxic effect, as determined by dye exclusion studies and radiolabel release (as well as reversibility of effect). Additionally, we have shown that TMIF-containing supernatants can partially inhibit the *in vitro* attachment of tumor cells to endothelial cells. These noncytotoxic properties of lymphokines could serve important *in vivo* functions. For example, TMIF could immobilize tumor cells at sites where specific or nonspecific killing mechanisms are operative. Also, it could directly interfere with local invasiveness and/or metastasis. Even if endogenously produced TMIF is not efficient in these roles, the possibility remains that exogenously prepared TMIF, when administered in an appropriate manner, could have a therapeutic effect. Studies that will be described in Chapter 16 by Yoshida *et al.*, demonstrating TMIF production *in vivo* and its biologic effect in an intraperitoneal setting, support this possibility.

REFERENCES

Churchill, W. H., Jr., Piessens, W. F., Sulis, C. A., and David, J. R. (1975). *J. Immunol.* *115*, 781-786.
Cohen, M. C. (1982). *Cancer Res.* *42*, 2135-2138.
Cohen, M. C., Zeschke, R., Bigazzi, P. E., Yoshida, T., and Cohen, S. (1975). *J. Immunol.* *114*, 1641-1643.
Cohen, M. C., Goss, A., Yoshida, T., and Cohen, S. (1978). *J. Immunol.* *121*, 840-843.
Cohen, M. C., Picciano, P. T., Douglas, W. J., Yoshida, T., Kreutzer, D. L., and Cohen, S. (1982). *Science (Washington, D.C.)* *215*, 301-303.
Granger, G. A. (1979). *In* "Biology of the Lymphokines" (S. Cohen, E. Pick, and J. J. Oppenheim, eds.), pp. 141-162. Academic Press, New York.
Meltzer, M. S., and Bartlett, G. L. (1972). *J. Natl. Cancer Inst. (US)* *49*, 1439-1443.
Piessens, W. F., Churchill, W. H., Jr., and David, J. R. (1975). *J. Immunol.* *114*, 293-299.
Russel, S. W., and Cochrane, C. G. (1974). *Int. J. Cancer 13*, 54-63.
Weedon, D. D., DeMeester, L. J., Elveback, L. R., and Shorter, R. G. (1973). *Mayo Clinic Proc.* *48*, 556-559.
Yoshida, T., Kuratsuji, T., Takada, A., Takada, Y., Minowada, J., and Cohen, S. (1976). *J. Immunol.* *117*, 548-554.

DISCUSSION

LIOTTA: Regarding the mechanism of effect of TMIF on tumor cell
            adhesion to endothelium, does the TMIF inhibit attach-
            ment to plastic or extracellular matrix? Is it a sub-
            strate or cell effect? What happens if you preincubate
            tumor cells or endothelium with the factor?

COHEN: I've presented preliminary results. We must do pre-
            and postincubation experiments to determine (1) the cell
            target of the effect and (2) whether the effect is
            exerted via potentiation of attachment or enhancement of
            dissociation. I predict that TMIF affects the tumor cell
            and that another lymphokine affects the endothelium, and
            the observed results represent a summation of both. TMIF
            may well affect substrate attachment as well. Analysis
            of receptor sites for TMIF on cells or biologic sub-
            strates represents another approach to these issues, but
            such studies await the production of purified and radio-
            labeled TMIF.

MATHÉ: If I understand you well, contrary to interferons, which
            are species specific, MIF is not?

COHEN: Yes, an important generalization is that afferent lympho-
            kines (those involved in immunologic help suppression
            and regulation) are often species specific, whereas ef-
            ferent lymphokines usually are not. There are sporadic
            reports of species specificity in some interferon studies
            that deal with nonviral effects, and this may reflect the
            fact that "interferon" is a family of biologically active
            macromolecules rather than a single mediator.

WEISS: It is of interest that the end result of cytotoxic
            interactions--necrotic materials--generally enhance
            cancer cell movements in vitro by chemokinetic mechanisms
            Also, we found that when the effects of necrotic material
            on cancer cell migration were assessed by capillary tube
            assays, we sometimes obtained different results from
            transmembrane migration experiments.

COHEN: The movement of tumor cells in vivo depends on many fac-
            tors including their own intrinsic capacity, the physical
            structure of their microenvironment, and a variety of
            physiologically active mediators to which they are ex-
            posed. This latter must include chemotactic and/or
            chemokinetic factors as well as migration-inhibitory fac-
            tors. Interestingly, we have been unable to find
            lymphocyte-derived chemotactic factors for tumor cells.

COCHRAN: We previously studied capillary migration of tumor cells and found that those derived from lymphoid cells moved while carcinomas did not. What is your experience with this? Does TMIF selectively inhibit lymphoid tumors or do you also see an effect on carcinoma cells, the main sources of metastatic disease?

COHEN: TMIF affects a variety of tumors, including hepatoma and carcinosarcoma as well as those derived from cells such as basophils. In humans, it has effects on adenocarcinomas derived from various organs, as Dr. Yoshida will describe in the next presentation. As you have also found, it is difficult to obtain good migration of some of these cell types out of capillary tubes, making analysis difficult. This is a limitation of the assay system, rather than an intrinsic biologic property; using the agarose microdroplet technique allows for good migration and good migration inhibition.

VAAGE: (1) With reference to my observation that the mammary carcinoma used in my *in vivo* experiments described yesterday is rapidly invasive in syngeneic nude mice, but is contained in normal mice, have you looked at the production of MIF and TMIF in nude mice? (2) Have you observed differences in susceptibility to TMIF among different tumors? (3) I find it very interesting that you have anticipated in your *in vitro* studies that TMIF may function to contain tumors where cytotoxic factors may not be available. I believe this is exactly what I am observing *in vivo*.

COHEN: I think that it is indeed possible that TMIF may play a role in your model system. We have not yet studied complex systems, but rather have focused on simple models to demonstrate *in vivo* effects, without regard to protective function. The next step will involve models of invasion and metastasis, and I think we will include the nude mouse in these. Another plan for the future is to compare response to TMIF of a variety of human tumors in an attempt to find correlations with *in vivo* clinical behavior.

CHAPTER 16

IN VIVO EFFECTS OF LYMPHOKINES ON TUMOR CELLS

Takeshi Yoshida
Helen D'Silva
Marion C. Cohen
Mark Donskoy
Stanley Cohen

Department of Pathology
University of Connecticut Health Center
Farmington, Connecticut

I. INTRODUCTION

Lymphokines affecting the *in vitro* functions of tumor cells
have been described by many investigators as discussed in
Chapter 15 (Cohen *et al.*). However, the actual *in vivo* role, if
any, played by such lymphokines has been unclear, although only
a few reports are available discussing this question to any

extent. In this presentation, therefore, discussion will focus
mostly on the data obtained from our recent unpublished studies.
Whenever they are relevant, some results from other investigators will be included for discussion. First, by directly
extending the previous *in vitro* studies on a tumor migration inhibition factor (TMIF), the data will be presented to show that
not only ascites-type tumor cells but also the cells from human
solid tumors can be inhibited of their *in vitro* migratory capacity. This result indicates the significance of TMIF activity in
real human primary tumors rather than that in the *in vitro*-
adjusted murine tumor cell lines. Second, it will be shown that
TMIF is detectable in the serum of animals preimmunized with tumor
cells and also in sera of tumor-bearing mice. This will be discussed together with the findings reported by us and others on
serum lymphokine activities in cancer patients. Finally, the *in
vivo* behavior of TMIF-treated ascites tumor cells will be
discussed.

II. MIGRATION INHIBITION OF THE CELLS OBTAINED FROM HUMAN
     SOLID TUMORS

     Almost a decade ago, three or four laboratories including
ours independently found that the motility of tumor cells can be
measured *in vitro*, and this could be inhibited by lymphokine
preparations (reviewed in D'Silva and Yoshida, 1981). As discussed in the preceding chapter (Cohen *et al.*, Chapter 15, this
volume), the factor responsible for this phenomenon is now called
TMIF. Most of these studies, however, have been performed by the
use of tumor cell lines adapted *in vitro* or the cells from the
ascites. Previously, there was a report by Cochran *et al.* (1973)
describing the migration inhibition of primary Burkitt lymphoma
cells, and leukemia cells by sera from patients with Burkitt
lymphomas. Although the nature of this inhibitory factor has not
been well characterized, some biochemical characteristics reported
by them seem to be different from those of the known lymphokines
such as MIF or TMIF. To confirm and extend that human solid tumor
cells can migrate *in vitro* and that they can be inhibited by a
migration-inhibitory factor, particularly by TMIF, we have studied
20 pathology specimens from various cancer patients. In many
cases, recovery of viable tumor cells was not so easy, since most
portions of the specimens were either necrotic or contained more
normal tissue cells than tumor cells. Table I summarizes the eight
cases that showed good random migration of tumor cells in the
complete medium. As shown in the table, such migration was inhibited significantly, except in one case, in the presence of TMIF.
This result clearly indicates that human solid tumor cells can
migrate *in vitro* and that the migration is inhibitable by TMIF,
which is a distinct molecule from MIF. One case not inhibitable

TABLE I

Migration Inhibition of Primary Human Tumor Cells by TMIF

Organ	Type	Migration inhibition
Ovary	Undifferentiated	25.4 ± 4.6
Lung	Squamous cell carcinoma (inflammatory cells)	1.4 ± 5.1[a]
Stomach	Adenocarcinoma	56.0 ± 4.3
Breast	Medullary carcinoma	52.9 ± 5.0
Ovary	Endometrial carcinoma	23.2 ± 8.5
Ovary	Endometrial adenocarcinoma	28.6 ± 8.1
Stomach	Adenocarcinoma	51.9 ± 3.1
Breast	Ductal carcinoma	35.7 ± 7.9

[a]*Not significant.*

by TMIF (squamous cell carcinoma) contained numerous inflammatory cells. This may be the reason that the TMIF preparation, lacking MIF activity, could not inhibit the migration.

III. DETECTION OF TMIF *IN VIVO*

To explore the *in vivo* role of TMIF, we posed a question whether or not TMIF can be detected *in vivo*. First, we have attempted to induce TMIF by the procedure that is known to induce lymphokines such as MIF *in vivo*. Mice were immunized with BCG and challenged with intravenous injection of PPD 2 weeks later. Serum was collected at various time intervals thereafter and assayed for migration-inhibitory activity against murine macrophages and two tumor cell preparations, P815 mastocytoma and Ehrlich ascites tumor (EAT). Inhibitory activity against murine macrophages (MIF) activity was first detected at 6 h and reached maximum at 24 h. Although the tumor cells showed some inhibition of migration in sera obtained from 6 to 48 h after PPD challenge, the activity level was not greater than 20% inhibition.

Next, we attempted to induce TMIF by injecting KCl extract of EAT into mice that were immunized by transplanting 1 million cells of EAT. A week later, the palpable tumor nodule was surgically removed. Sera collected at 6, 24, and 48 h had detectable inhibitory activity against murine macrophages (MIF activity) and TMIF activity against mastocytoma cells as well as EAT cells. Serum from immunized animals without challenge, or from nonimmunized animals challenged with EAT extract, did not show either

MIF or TMIF activity. In all these sera, the migration inhibition was reversible after 48 h of incubation, indicating the noncytotoxicity of the responsible factor.

IV. CHARACTERIZATION OF SERUM TMIF

The serum samples containing MIF and TMIF were subjected to Diaflo membrane ultrafiltration. The serum obtained from EAT-immune mice at 6 h after the challenge by EAT extract had MIF activity in a fraction with a molecular weight (MW) between 10,000 and 50,000. In contrast, TMIF activity for EAT was found to be between 5000 and 10,000 MW. This is in agreement with the previous findings for TMIF obtained from *in vitro* sources (Cohen *et al.*, 1978, Chapter 15, this volume). From BCG-immune animals, strong MIF activity was also recovered in the fraction with a MW between 10,000 and 50,000, although only weak activity of TMIF was found in the fraction between 5000 and 10,000.

Serum TMIF activity was not inhibited by the presence of L-fucose or rhamnose, in contrast to MIF activity, which is inhibitable with these monosaccharides. This is again in agreement with the previous finding for TMIF obtained from *in vitro* sources.

V. SERUM TMIF IN TUMOR-BEARING MICE

Mice were inoculated with 10 million EAT cells and sacrificed on various days until Day 13 postinoculation. Serum MIF and TMIF activities appeared by Day 7 and persisted until the end of the experiment (animals survive for at least 2 weeks in this type of transplantation of tumor cells). Both of these activities reached relatively high levels (more than 50% migration inhibition), in contrast to 20 to 30% inhibition reached in the EAT-immune animals challenged with EAT extract as mentioned before. This may reflect the intensity of interaction between immune lymphocytes and tumor antigens.

Since it was previously reported by Granger *et al.* (1978) that plasma of randomly selected patients with various types of neoplasia frequently (in more than 70% of the cases) had lymphotoxin activity. Therefore, we have tested the cytotoxic activity of the sera containing TMIF activity. Both conventional lymphotoxin assay with L cells (Kuratsuji *et al.*, 1976) and trypan blue exclusion viability test failed to show any cytotoxic activity in such sera, indicating that the inhibition of tumor cell migration is not due to simple cytotoxicity of the serum.

VI. SERUM LYMPHOKINE ACTIVITIES IN CANCER PATIENTS

As alluded to before, some lymphokines other than TMIF have been detected in the serum of cancer patients. For example, it was first reported that the MIF activity was demonstrated in the sera of patients suffering from lymphoproliferative disorders such as chronic lymphocytic leukemia, multiple myeloma, lymphomas, Hodgkin's disease (Cohen *et al.*, 1974), and Sezary syndrome (Yoshida *et al.*, 1975). Subsequently, several workers have reported MIF or LIF activity in the sera of patients with various neoplastic diseases (reviewed in D'Silva and Yoshida, 1981).

The role of these circulating lymphokine or lymphokine-like activities in cancer patients is still largely unknown. There are some controversial results reported on the correlation between the positive lymphokine activity and the stage or severity of neoplastic diseases (Kjaer, 1976; McCoy *et al.*, 1977). From our studies on desensitization of delayed-type hypersensitivity (DTH) in guinea pigs, we have speculated that circulating lymphokines such as MIF may be suppressing the expression of the DTH through a feedback mechanism (Yoshida and Cohen, 1982). Thus, the detection of some lymphokine activities in cancer patients may have a profound implication in the regulatory mechanism of the cell-mediated immunity in such patients.

In this context, the present finding of TMIF activity in the sera of tumor-bearing animals is intriguing, since a noncytotoxic lymphokine seems to be playing a role directly affecting tumor cells.

VII. EFFECTS OF TMIF ON TUMOR CELLS *IN VIVO*

The effect of TMIF on tumor cells *in vivo* was studied using an experimental procedure similar to that of macrophage disappearance reaction (MDR) (Sonozaki and Cohen, 1972). The TMIF preparation was mixed with 10 million EAT cells and injected intraperitoneally into normal mice. When the peritoneal cavity was washed with medium immediately after the injection, 5.9 million cells were recovered, and this was not significantly different from the number of cells (6.0 million) recovered from control animals that received MIF with EAT, or EAT in culture medium. Three hours after the injection of EAT with TMIF, only 1.1 million cells were recovered, while control groups of animals yielded 4.1-6.2 million tumor cells. By 24 h, however, the number of cells recoverable from the peritoneal cavity did not differ among those groups. This result strongly indicates that TMIF seems to show *in vivo* migration-inhibitory activity for EAT cells, as in the case of MIF, which could show MDR *in vivo* (Yoshida and Cohen, 1974).

TABLE II

Evidence to Support *in vivo* Significance of TMIF

---

1. The mobility of the cells from human primary tumors was
   inhibited by TMIF *in vitro*.
2. TMIF activity was detectable in serum from tumor-immune mice.
   (Only weak activity was found in BCG-immune mice.)
3. TMIF was found in tumor-bearing, nonimmune mice.
4. Exogenous TMIF could temporarily affect the distribution of
   tumor cells in the peritoneal cavity in a manner analogous to
   MDR.
5. On most occasions, TMIF appears *in vivo* concomitantly with
   MIF, but factors are distinct on the basis of their physico
   chemical natures as well as functional behaviors.

VIII. *IN VIVO* EFFECTS OF LYMPHOKINES ON TUMORS

A number of reports are now available to indicate that
lymphokine-containing preparations are able to induce tumor regression *in vivo* when they are injected locally (reviewed in
D'Silva and Yoshida, 1981). At the present time, however, it is
still unclear which of many lymphokines in such preparations is
responsible for that effect. Furthermore, most of the effects
described so far represent only the cytotoxic activity. It is
sometimes difficult to distinguish the lymphokine-dependent cytotoxic activity from nonspecific toxic cell metabolites.

Several lymphokines have been implied to affect the fate of
tumor cells through their effects on such cells as macrophages.
For example, these factors may include macrophage-activating factor (MAF), specific macrophage-arming factor (SMAF), and interferons. Liposomes containing encapsulated lymphokines (MAF),
when injected intravenously, produce significant destruction of
established lung and lymph node metastases from a subcutaneous
highly metastatic melanoma (Fidler *et al.*, 1982). This result
suggests that the augmented host defense against pulmonary and
lymph node metastases is mediated via activated cytotoxic macrophages. Unfortunately, the MAF preparation may not represent a
single entity but a mixture of the factors.

In this context, TMIF as just discussed may represent an
interesting factor, directly affecting the behavior of tumor
cells but not cytotoxic. Thus, TMIF could be relevant to host
resistance against tumor growth, perhaps affecting the tumor's
spread and metastasis.

IX.   CONCLUSIONS

In this presentation, we have focused our discussion on the *in vivo* role in TMIF, an intriguing noncytotoxic lymphokine directly affecting tumor cells. As summarized in Table II, evidence to support an *in vivo* role of TMIF has been accumulated. Thus, TMIF, which is distinct from a conventional migration-inhibitory factor (MIF), is now shown to be present in the serum of tumor antigen-treated immune mice as well as tumor-bearing mice. More importantly, it was shown that TMIF could modify the fate of tumor cells *in vivo*, specifically their ability to move and adhere. More importantly, however, it is yet to be examined if this factor could modify the metastatic character of tumor cells in general.

REFERENCES

Cochran, A. J., Klein, G., Kiessling, R., and Gunven, P. (1973). *J. Natl. Cancer Inst. (US) 51*, 1431-1436.

Cohen, M. C., Goss, A., Yoshida, T., and Cohen, S. (1978). *J. Immunol. 121*, 840-843.

Cohen, S., Fisher, B., Yoshida, T., and Bettigole, R. (1974). *N. Engl. J. Med. 290*, 882-886.

D'Silva, H., and Yoshida, T. (1981). *In* "Handbook of Cancer Immunology" (H. Waters, ed.), Vol. 6, pp. 215-250. Garland STPM Press, New York.

D'Silva, H., Cohen, M. C., Yoshida, T., and Cohen, S. (1982). *Clin. Immunol. Immunopathol. 23*, 77-85.

Fidler, I. J., Barnes, Z., Fogler, W. E., Kirsh, R., Bugelski, P., and Poste, G. (1982). *Cancer Res. 42*, 496-501.

Granger, G. A., Shimizu, I., Harris, L., Anderson, J., and Horn, P. (1978). *Clin. Immunol. Immunopathol. 10*, 104-115.

Kjaer, M. (1976). *Eur. J. Cancer 12*, 889-898.

Kuratsuji, T., Yoshida, T., and Cohen, S. (1976). *J. Immunol. 117*, 1985-1991.

McCoy, J. M., Jerome, L. F., Cannon, G. B., Weese, J. L., and Herberman, R. B. (1977). *J. Natl. Cancer Inst. (US) 59*, 1413-1418.

Sonozaki, H., and Cohen, S. (1972). *Cell. Immunol. 2*, 341-350.

Yoshida, T., and Cohen, S. (1974). *In* "Mechanisms of Cell-Mediated Immunity" (R. T. McCluskey and S. Cohen, eds.), pp. 43-66. Wiley, New York.

Yoshida, T., and Cohen, S. (1982). *Fed. Proc. Fed. Am. Soc. Exp. Biol. 41*, 2480-2483.

Yoshida, T., Edelson, R., Cohen, S., and Green, I. (1975). *J. Immunol. 114*, 915-918.

DISCUSSION

VAAGE: Dr. Yoshida, you mentioned in your second from the last slide that the effects of TMIF was transient in normal mice. Have you studied the activity of TMIF in presensitized mice?

YOSHIDA: We have not. In such experiments, it might be difficult to see the direct effect of TMIF. Rather, I suspect that you may see the rapid and continuous decrease of the number of tumor cells due to cytotoxic factors as well as cytotoxic T cells and macrophages.

VAAGE: In your last slide, you called mice carrying large tumors nonimmune. Why?

YOSHIDA: I have called a group of mice that received 10 million EAT cells the nonimmune group, in contrast to the immune group inoculated with 1 million of the cells that were removed 2 weeks later. This is because the former group of animals dies after around 2 weeks, while the latter not only survives but also can overcome the second challenge of 10 million tumor cells. I know that the former group certainly should have developed some immunity within a couple of weeks, but that might have been too late to cope with a large number of tumor cells. So I agree, it is not a nonimmune state, but for convenience we called it so.

LIOTTA: What information do you have about receptors for TMIF or half-life (turnover) of TMIF?

YOSHIDA: We would like to know this information, but we do not have it, since TMIF is not yet purified to an extent that would permit such a study in a meaningful manner.

GOLUB: Have you or Dr. Cohen succeeded in preparing an antiserum to TMIF?

YOSHIDA: Unfortunately not, although we are working hard to prepare monoclonal antibodies to this factor.

HEPPNER: In your human tumor experiments, did you attempt to remove the infiltrating inflammatory cells from the samples prior to assay?

YOSHIDA: Yes, we did by Ficoll-Hypaque gradient centrifugation.

CHAPTER 17

INDUCTION OF HUMAN SPECIFIC KILLER T CELL
AGAINST AUTOLOGOUS CANCER CELLS
AND ITS PROPAGATION BY T CELL GROWTH FACTOR

Takeru Ishikawa
Tsutomu Ikawa
Yukinori Ichino
Mikio Toya

Department of Otolaryngology
Kumamoto University School of Medicine
Kumamoto, Japan

I. INTRODUCTION

    The direct evidence for the generation of cytotoxic cells to
lyse human autologous tumor cells is obviously valuable in
analyzing the immunologic mechanism for protection against naturally developed tumor and in investigating a possibility of

adoptive immune therapy for cancer (Cheever *et al.*, 1981, 1982; Greenberg *et al.*, 1981b). There has been much excellent work concerned with the generation of cytotoxic lymphoid cells in the human autologous system, by means of various methods and materials (Hellström and Hellström, 1969; Hellström *et al.*, 1971; Baldwin *et al.*, 1973; Martin-Chandon *et al.*, 1975; Golub, 1977; Hirshberg *et al.*, 1977; Vánky *et al.*, 1978, 1979; Vose *et al.*, 1978a; Zarling *et al.*, 1979; Vose and Moore, 1981).

We have also tried to induce human cytotoxic lymphoid cells (CL) against squamous cell carcinoma cell line and fresh osteosarcoma cells, and to propagate the CL with interleukin 2 (TCGF) *in vitro* (Morgan *et al.*, 1976; Gillis and Smith, 1977; Baker *et al.*, 1979; Mills and Paetkau, 1980; Mills *et al.*, 1980; Gillis and Watson, 1981). Cytotoxic activities of the propagated CL to allogeneic tumor have also been investigated.

In this article, our experimental results will be discussed in comparison with previously reported results of other investigators.

II. INDUCTION OF CYTOTOXIC LYMPHOID CELLS AGAINST SQUAMOUS CELL
     CARCINOMA CELL LINE

Surgically obtained maxillary cancer tissue from a patient (65-year-old male) was prepared for cell culture. The cell line was successfully established and named KOIMC-011. Population-doubling time and chromosome analysis of the cell line indicate 22 hr, hyperdiploid type, and 52 as the average chromosome number. Additionally, light- and electron-microscopic findings (Seman and Demochowski, 1975) show the cell line originated as squamous cell carcinoma.

The patient donor of the cell line has supplied his own peripheral blood lymphocytes (PBL) for the experimental work. The lymphoid cell fraction was cocultured with the mitomycin C (MMC)-treated cell line in an effector:target ratio (E:T) of 20:1 for 5 days.

The autologous mixed lymphocyte tumor cell culture (MLTC) induced higher activity of CL than control lymphoid cells without tumor cell stimulation (Fig. 1), but no killing activity of autologous PHA blastoid lymphocytes. Sheep red blood cell (SRBC) rosette-formed lymphocyte fraction was well stimulated by MMC-treated tumor cells and killed the targets. The percentage specific release of ^{51}Cr in the tumor-activated T-rich fraction was 21.2 ± 1.2, but that in non-T cell fraction was 8.2 ± 1.5 (Table I). The cytotoxic activity was blocked by anti-Leu-2a antiserum (Evans *et al.*, 1978; Ledbetter *et al.*, 1981) and complement (Table II), but not by human or rabbit aggregated IgG (Table III) or cold K562 cell line (Table IV). Additionally, the CL activity was restricted by HLA Cw3 in this case (Table V), and

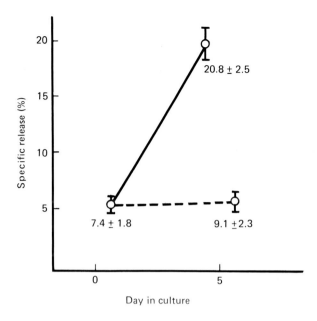

Fig. 1.   Autologous lymphocytotoxicity induced by specific tumor cell stimulation.   o——o Specific stimulation with MMC-treated KOIMC-011; o---o control (lymphocyte only).   The autologous lymphocytotoxicity was significantly induced by 5 days coculture of the PBL and MMC-treated autologous tumor cells (*p* < .001).

TABLE I

Comparison of Cytotoxicity between T and Non-T Cell Fraction

Effector cells	Specific ^{51}Cr release (%)	
	Culture Day 0	Culture Day 5
T cell fraction	11.7 ± 2.1[a]	21.2 ± 1.2 Stimulated
		12.5 ± 2.5 Unstimulated
Non-T cell fraction	4.1 ± 1.8	8.2 ± 1.5 Stimulated
		3.9 ± 0.8 Unstimulated

[a]Mean ± SE.

TABLE II

Blocking Assay by Monoclonal Anti-Human Leu-2a

Anti-human Leu-2a concentration	Specific ^{51}Cr release (%)
None	22.8 ± 2.3[a]
0.2 µg/1 × 10^6	11.7 ± 1.7
1.0 µg/1 × 10^6	10.3 ± 1.4
5.0 µg/1 × 10^6	10.8 ± 1.2

[a]Mean ± SE.

TABLE III

Cytotoxicity after Treatment of Lymphocytes
with Aggregated Human or Rabbit IgG

Aggregated IgG concentration	Specific ^{51}Cr release (%)	
	Human	Rabbit
7 mg/3 × 10^6	17.6 ± 1.4[a]	18.1 ± 1.2
700 µg/3 × 10^6	18.4 ± 1.7	18.2 ± 1.5
70 µg/3 × 10^6	19.2 ± 2.1	18.7 ± 1.9
None	20.3 ± 2.2	

[a]Mean ± SE.

TABLE IV

Cold K562 Target Inhibition Test

Labeled KOIMC-011:cold K562	Specific ^{51}Cr release (%)
1:1	21.7 ± 1.6[a]
1:2	21.2 ± 2.3
1:10	18.7 ± 1.9
1:0	22.7 ± 2.6

[a]Mean ± SE.

TABLE V

Treatment of Lymphocyte with Anti-HLA Serum[a]

Anti-HLA serum	Specific ^{51}Cr release (%)
A2	22.1 ± 1.9
B7	23.7 ± 2.1
Cw3	13.2 ± 1.8
None	24.3 ± 2.6

[a]HLA typing: host lymphocyte, A2,11, B5,7, Cw3; KOIMC-011, A2, B7, Cw3.
[b]Mean ± SE.

TABLE VI

Effect on Cytotoxic Activity of Cryopreservation and Thawing

Effector cell	Specific ^{51}Cr release (%)
Fresh	24.7 ± 2.4[a]
Frozen	22.3 ± 1.9

[a]Mean ± SE.

induction of the CL was not affected by cryopreservation with 10% dimethyl sulfoxide (DMSO) and thawing procedure (Table VI).

These data probably support the concept that the autologous MLTC mainly induces the cytotoxic T cell.

III. INDUCTION OF CYTOTOXIC LYMPHOID CELLS AGAINST AUTOLOGOUS FRESH OSTEOSARCOMA CELLS

In other cases, we also could induce the cytotoxic lymphoid cells by autologous fresh tumor cell stimulation *in vitro*. A 14-year-old female was suffering from osteosarcoma originating in the right mandibula. The histologic diagnosis was chondromatous osteosarcoma. Surgically obtained tumor mass was treated with

TABLE VII

Lysis of Autologous Fresh Osteosarcoma and PHA Blastoid Lymphocytes
by MLTC-Sensitized Effectors[a]

Agent of effector sensitization	Treatment	Target	Cytotoxicity (%)
None	None	Auto OS	10.5 ± 6.0
Auto OS	None	Auto OS	20.4 ± 2.6
Auto OS	Leu-2a + C'	Auto OS	12.2 ± 5.4
None	None	Auto PHA blast	1.9 ± 2.4
Auto OS	None	Auto PHA blast	-0.5 ± 2.1

[a]Auto OS, autologous fresh osteosarcoma cell; Auto PHA blast, autologous PHA blastoid lymphocyte; C', complement.
[b]Nonsensitized effector cells were cultured with medium alone.
[c]Determined in 10-hr ^{51}Cr-release assays at 20:1 effector:target ratio as described in the text.

Dispase, and the cell suspension was cryopreserved in a nitrogen storage tank until use (Ichino *et al.*, 1982).

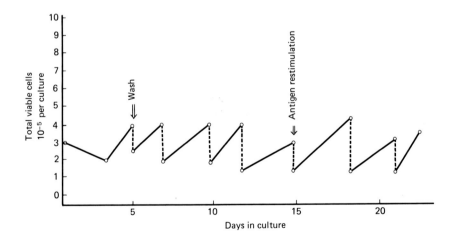

Fig. 2.   Growth profile of lymphoid cell number cultured with TCGF.   Cytotoxic T cells against autologous tumor cell line (KOIMC-011) were cultured in the TCGF medium.   Cell number markedly increased during TCGF culture.   Doubling time of the lymphocyte number was 2.1 days.

Peripheral blood lymphocytes were obtained from the patient and used for MLTC. Lymphoid cells sensitized with MMC-treated autologous osteosarcoma cells for 5 days produced higher cytotoxicity against autologous osteosarcoma cells than nonsensitized lymphoid cells cultured with medium alone (Table VII). The CL were active against autologous tumor but not autologous PHA blastoid lymphocytes. Treatment of sensitized lymphoid cells with anti-Leu-2a reduced the cytotoxicity against autologous osteosarcoma cells.

As described by several authors (Zielske and Golub, 1976; Golub et al., 1979), fetal calf serum (FCS) may induce blastogenesis and cytotoxicity of peripheral blood lymphocytes. As indicated in our report, however, lymphocytes cultured with medium containing only 10% FCS lysed autologous tumor cells to a lesser degree. The lower cytotoxicity may be partly due to the effects of FCS, but the cytotoxic activity induced by MLTC markedly exceeded that of lymphocytes cultured with medium containing FCS only. Additionally, cold-target inhibition and Leu-2a blocking test also indicated that the results of nonspecific cytotoxicity induced by FCS was scarcely reflected in our data.

IV. EFFECT OF CYTOTOXIC LYMPHOID CELLS INDUCED BY AUTOLOGOUS
     TUMOR CELLS AND PROPAGATED BY T CELL GROWTH FACTOR (TCGF)
     (OR INTERLEUKIN 2, IL-2) ON ALLOGENEIC TUMOR CELLS

The cytotoxic lymphoid cells induced by both squamous cell carcinoma cell line and fresh osteosarcoma cells were propagated with TCGF obtained from tonsil lymphocytes according to the method described by Alvarez et al. (1979). Tonsil lymphocytes were isolated by Ficoll-Hypaque density gradient method. Tonsil lymphocytes (2×10^6) were cultured with 1% PHA-M in culture medium. The supernatant was filtered through a 0.45-μm membrane filter, and no further purification was performed. The optimal concentration of TCGF was 50%, and thus we used TCGF at a concentration of 50% in all tests.

Figures 2 and 3 show the increasing curve of autologous cytotoxicity and cell number induced by MLTC using the KOIMC-011, when cultured in culture medium containing 50% TCGF.

Treatment of the induced cytotoxic lymphoid cells with anti-Leu-2a and complement inhibits the cytotoxicity against autologous tumor cell line (Table VIII). The effect of anti-Leu-2a on the killing activity became the more significant with longer cultivation of the cytotoxic lymphocytes with TCGF. This fact may indicate that short-term TCGF culture of the CL mostly induces propagation of T cells. Table VIII and Fig. 4 further demonstrate the results of the cold-target inhibition test of whether the cytotoxicity induced by autologous tumor cell stimulation and TCGF is effective on the allogeneic tumor cell line. The most

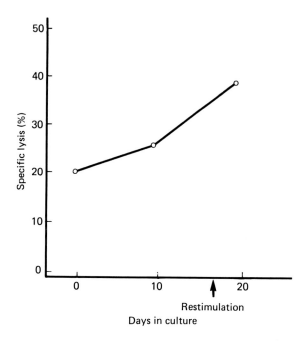

Fig. 3. Cytotoxicity of specific killer T cells cultured with TCGF. Target: effector ratio, 1:20. TCGF culture induced the enhancement of the cytotoxic activity, as well as the increase of cell number. Specific tumor cell restimulation (antigen pulse) might be necessary to maintain or increase lymphocytotoxicity.

significant inhibition of cytotoxicity was seen when the cold KB was added in hot:cold ratio of either 1:5 or 1:20. Hep-2 or HeLa inhibited the cytotoxicity 30-50%. However, K562 and fresh fibrosarcoma cells have almost no effect in inhibiting cytotoxicity. The results may tell us that there is some cross-reactivity between the cell lines originated from the squamous cell carcinoma. HLA was still detectable on the cell surface of KOIMC-011, but not on the other cell lines. Therefore, participation of common HLA in the allogeneic tumor killing was not investigated (Greenbert *et al.*, 1981b). We have no further data explaining whether the cross-reactivity was based on the common antigenic recognition or on populations other than tumor-specific killer T cells.

Figure 5 shows the growth curve of autologous CL induced by MLTC using fresh osteosarcoma cells, when cultured in the TCGF. Cells seeded at a concentration of 2×10^5 cells/ml reached a saturation density of approximately 1×10^6 cells/ml after 3 or 4 days in culture. The exponential growth pattern was repeated over the next 3 days. Cytotoxic lymphoid cells increased in cell number about 30-fold over 12 days, and the duplication time of the TCGF cultures was 2.4 days.

TABLE VIII

Cold-Target Inhibition Test with Allogeneic Tumor Cell Line[a]

Days grown in IL-2[b]	Specific cytotoxicity (%)	Hot:cold ratio	Cold-target inhibition (%)						Leu-2a + complement inhibition (%)
			Hep-2	KB	HeLa	Fibro-sarcoma	K562	KOIMC-011	
0	20.9	1:5	42.8	80.8	42.8	0	14.2	n.d.	61.9
10	25.9	1:5	27.0	69.3	53.8	7.7	n.d.[c]	n.d.	
		1:20	57.4	82.9	56.0	14.8	24.5	87.5	75.0
20	39.1	1:5	43.6	76.9	33.3	0	n.d.	79.5	
		1:20	45.5	73.6	47.9	18.7	26.2	84.3	84.6

[a]Effector: target ratio, 20:1.
[b]On Day 17, antigen restimulation was added.
[c]n.d., Not determined.

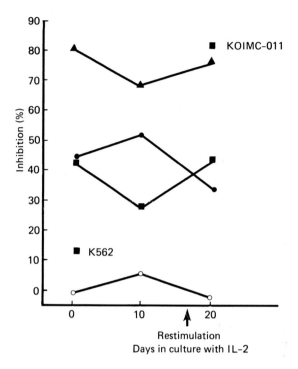

Fig. 4.   Cold-target inhibition test.   Hot target:cold target
ratio, 1:5.   Autologous Tc against the cell line (KOIMC-011) were
propagated by the culture in TCGF (IL-2) medium.   The activity of
the propagated tumor-specific Tc was almost completely inhibited
by addition of cold autologous KOIMC-011 or KB (▲).   Partial inhibition was observed by addition of cold Hep-2 (■) or HeLa (●).
However, K562 or fibrosarcoma (o) did not inhibit the activities
at all.

     TCGF-CL showed higher cytotoxicity (22.7%) for autologous
osteosarcoma than CL before TCGF culture.   No lysis of autologous
PHA blasts was observed at all (Table IX).   TCGF-CL also killed
the K562 to a small extent (11.6%), but this cytotoxicity was much
lower than that of fresh normal lymphocytes against K562 (40-60%
in our data).
     Surface markers (Evans et al., 1978; Ledbetter et al., 1981)
of TCGF-CL against autologous osteosarcoma was inhibited more than
80% by the treatment of Leu-2a plus complement.   The treatment of
Leu-3a plus complement, however, did not reduce the cytotoxicity
of TCGF-CL (Table X).   The cytotoxicity of TCGF-CL was not affected
by complement alone.   Therefore, it was confirmed that almost all
lymphoid cells cytotoxic against autologous osteosarcoma were
Leu-2a-positive and Leu-3a-negative cytotoxic T lymphocytes.

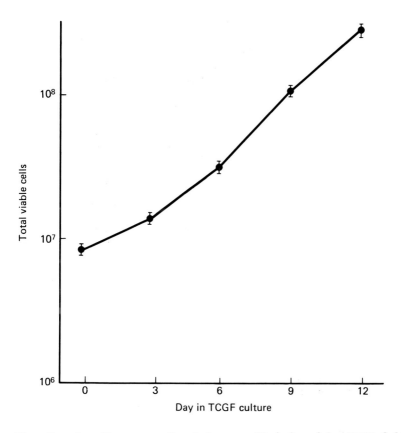

Fig. 5. Growth curve of autologous CL induced by MLTC followed by TCGF culture. Autologous Tc against fresh osteosarcoma cells induced by autologous MLTC were propagated by the culture in the TCGF medium. Doubling time of the cell number was 2.4 days.

Table XI shows the results of cold-target inhibition of cyto-toxicity of TCGF-CL against autologous osteosarcoma cells. Cold target cells were derived from autologous tumor cells and fresh allogeneic tumor cells of five cancer patients (different sites and different histologies). Cytolysis of labeled autologous tumor cells was inhibited by the same cold target, but not by allogeneic cold tumor cells except tumor C, squamous cell carcinoma (SSC) of the larynx. Although the donor patients of tumor A and tumor C had a common HLA-A2 with the patient of osteosarcoma, we could not find any evidence that HLA regulates allogeneic cytotoxicity.

Such an adoptive immunotherapy as to reinject cytotoxic lympho-cytes against autologous tumor into the donor patient is probably one of the most effective cancer immunotherapies. In mouse syn-geneic systems, Gillis (Gillis and Smith, 1977) and Cheever *et al.*

TABLE IX

Lysis of Autologous Fresh Osteosarcoma,
PHA Blastoid Lymphocytes, and K562 by Cytotoxic
Lymphoid Cells Propagated with T Cell Growth Factor[a]

Effector	Target	Cytotoxicity[b] (%)
TCGF-CL	Auto OS	22.7 ± 1.1
TCGF-CL	Auto PHA blast	6.4 ± 1.1
TCGF-CL	K562	11.6 ± 0.9

[a]Abbreviations: TCGF-CL, cytotoxic lymphoid cells propagated with T cell growth factor; Auto OS, autologous fresh osteosarcoma; Auto PHA blast, autologous PHA blastoid lymphocytes.
[b]Assessed in 10-hr ^{51}Cr-release assays at 20:1 effector:target ratios as described in the text. The data are presented as the mean ± SD of quadruplicate determinations.

TABLE X

Serologic Profile of Cytotoxic Lymphoid
Cells Propagated with T Cell Growth Factor[a]

Treatment of TCGF-CL	Target	Cytotoxicity[b] (%)
--	Auto OS	22.7 ± 1.1
Leu-2a + C	Auto OS	4.7 ± 2.2
Leu-3a + C	Auto OS	19.6 ± 4.9

[a]Abbreviations: TCGF, T cell growth factor; Auto OS, autologous fresh osteosarcoma; Leu-2a, anti-Leu-2a antibody; Leu-3a, anti-Leu-3a antibody; C, complement.
[b]Determined in 10-hr ^{51}Cr-release assays at 20:1 effector:target ratios as described in the text. Data presented are the means of quadruplicate determinations ± SD.

(1981) and Mills and Paetkau (1980) have tried to inject cytotoxic T lymphocytes obtained by mixed culture with syngeneic tumor cells into mice.

TABLE XI

Cold-Target Inhibition of Autologous Osteosarcoma
Lysis by Cytotoxic Lymphoid Cells Propagated with TCGF (TCGF-CL)

Effector	Cold target	HLA of donor patients of cold targets	Labeled target	Cytotoxicity[a] (%)
TCGF-CL	None		Auto OS	18.0 ± 5.6
TCGF-CL	Auto OS	A2/10,B40/W54,Cw3/-	Auto OS	6.3 ± 0.2 (65.0%)
TCGF-CL	Tumor A (SCC, maxilla)	A2/w24,B5 or 35/-,Cw1/-	Auto OS	20.5 ± 0.4 (-13.8%)
TCGF-CL	Tumor B (SCC, maxilla)	A11/w24,B5 or 35/w54,C-/-	Auto OS	21.9 ± 4.0 (-21.7%)
TCGF-CL	Tumor C (SCC, larynx)	A2/-,B5/15,Cw4/-	Auto OS	6.0 ± 2.4 (66.7%)
TCGF-CL	Tumor D (adenocarcinoma, thyroid)	A11/w24,B5 or 35/-,C-/-	Auto OS	22.0 ± 0.3 (-22.2%)
TCGF-CL	Tumor E (adenocarcinoma, parotid)	A10/-,B15/35,C-/0	Auto OS	17.6 ± 2.4 (0.3%)

Percentages in parentheses are inhibition of % cytotoxicity in comparison with control (the first row 18.0 ± 5.6).

In human autologous systems, three different ways to generate
cytotoxic lymphocytes against autologous tumor cells have been
reported. One of these described by several investigators
(Ortaldo et al., 1977; Seeley and Golub, 1978; Seeley et al.,
1979; Strausser and Rosenberg, 1978; Strausser et al., 1981;
Zarling and Bach, 1980; Zarling et al., 1976, 1978) was that
mixed lymphocyte culture (MLC) with allogeneic lymphocytes induced
cytotoxic lymphocytes against autologous and allogeneic tumor
cells. Second, Lotze and Grimm (Lotze et al., 1980, 1981)
reported that peripheral blood lymphocytes from cancer patients
could be activated by culture in preparations of TCGF without in
vitro stimulation of autologous tumor cells, resulting in the
development of effector cells cytotoxic to autologous fresh solid
tumor cells. The effector cells activated were different from
cytotoxic T cells generated by MLTC or MLC-induced cytotoxic
lymphocytes. Third, Vose et al. (Vose, 1980; Vose and Bonnard,
1982; Vose et al., 1977, 1978a,b) and Vánky et al. (1978, 1979,
1981, 1982) described that cytotoxic T lymphocytes generated by
autologous MLTC were propagated with TCGF and had much higher
cytotoxicity against autologous fresh tumor cells.

Following the facts proven, the important question of whether
the induced and propagated CL are specifically effective to the
autologous tumor cells has been asked (Masucci et al., 1980).
Vose et al. found that cross reactions against allogeneic tumors
were observed only in 2 out of 31 cross tests by target and
effector cells from 10 cancer patients. In our experimental
results, the cytotoxicity of TCGF-CL against autologous osteosarcoma was not inhibited by fresh allogeneic unlabeled tumor cells
except those from a laryngeal cancer patient; however, those
against KOIMC cell line were inhibited by other squamous cell
carcinoma cell line.

The cytotoxicity generated by allogeneic MLC, however, was effective to allogeneic tumor cells as autologous tumor cells. In
addition, Grimm et al. (1982) found that allogeneic normal lymphokine activating killer (LAK) cells were capable of lysing fresh
autologous and allogeneic tumor cells. Knuth et al. (1981) wrote
that long-term culture of cytotoxic lymphocytes with TCGF had also
resulted to react with a wider range of targets also had been determined by direct tests and competitive-inhibition tests.
Regarding the adoptive immunotherapeutic purpose, it may be a considerable problem that this expansion of cytotoxic effects to
other targets than autologous tumor cells may attack normal tissue. Autologous MLTC-induced CL followed by relatively short-term
propagation with TCGF are considered to be reliable to use for the
adoptive therapy.

The adoptive immunotherapy with tumor-specific CL, however,
still presents problems that should be resolved before application
to patients in vivo. We considered that it was of importance to
assure that TCGF-CL did not become a tumor. Fujimoto and Takata
(Fujimoto and Takata, 1982) reported that TCGF-dependent cytotoxic
T cell line could change into a functional T cell tumor that had

grown independent of TCGF. Electron-microscopic findings showed that TCGF-CL were larger in size and blastoid lymphocytes but were not tumorous. The mode of chromosome number was 46 and normal. In addition to this, the TCGF-CL never grew without TCGF. These facts indicate that TCGF-CL did not change into a tumor.

Another question that should be made clear is whether or not the biologically detectable antigenicity of metastatic tumor cells is the same as that of primary tumor. This question has not yet been resolved; however, it may be the most important problem for application of specific immune therapy to micrometastasis.

REFERENCES

Alvarez, J. M., Silva, A., and de Landazuri, M. O. (1979). *J. Immunol.* *123*, 977-983.
Baker, P. E., Gillis, S., and Smith, K. A. (1979). *J. Exp. Med.* *149*, 273-278.
Baldwin, R. W., Embleton, M. J., Jones, J. S. P. I., and Langman, M. J. S. (1973). *Int. J. Cancer 12*, 73-83.
Cheever, M. A., Greenberg, P. D., and Fefer, A. (1981). *J. Immunol.* *126*, 1318-1322.
Cheever, M. A., Greenberg, P. D., Fefer, A., and Gil lis, S. (1982). *J. Exp. Med. 155*, 968-980.
Evans, R. L., Lazarus, H., Penta, A. C., and Schlossman, S. F. (1978). *J. Immunol. 120*, 1423-1428.
Fujimoto, S., and Takata, M. (1983). *UCLA Forum Med. Sci. 24*, 319-334.
Gillis, S., and Smith, K. A. (1977). *Nature (London) 268*, 154-156.
Gillis, S., and Watson, J. (1981). *Immunol. Rev. 54*, 81-109.
Golub, S. H. (1977). *Cell. Immunol. 28*, 379-389.
Golub, S. H., Golightly, M. G., and Zielske, J. V. (1979). *Int. J. Cancer 24*, 273-283.
Greenberg, P. D., Cheever, M. A., and Fefer, A. (1981a). *J. Exp. Med. 154*, 952-963.
Greenberg, P. D., Cheever, M. A., and Fefer, A. (1981b). *J. Immunol. 126*, 2100-2103.
Grimm, E. A., Mazumder, A., Zhang, H. Z., and Rosenberg, S. A. (1982). *J. Exp. Med. 155*, 1823-1841.
Hellström, I., Hellström, K. E., Sjogren, H. O., and Warner, G. A. (1971). *Int. J. Cancer 7*, 1-16.
Hellström, K. E., and Hellström, I. (1969). *Adv. Cancer Res. 12*, 167-223.
Hirshberg, H., Skare, H., and Thorby, E. (1977). *J. Immunol. Methods 16*, 131-141.
Ichino, Y., Ikawa, T., and Ishikawa, T. (1982). *Rinsho Meneki (Clin. Immunol.) 14* (Suppl. 5), 161-175.
Knuth, A., Shiku, H., Oettgen, H. F., and Old, L. J. (1981). *Proc. Am. Assoc. Res. 22*, 316.

Ledbetter, J. A., Evans, R. L., Lipinski, M., Cunningham-Rundles, C., Good, R. A., and Herzenberg, L. A. (1981). *J. Exp. Med. 153*, 310-328.

Lotze, M. T., Line, B. R., Mathisen, D. J., and Rosenberg, S. A. (1980). *J. Immunol. 125*, 1487-1493.

Lotze, M. T., Grimm, E. A., Mazumder, A., Strausser, J. L., and Rosenberg, S. A. (1981). *Cancer Res. 41*, 4420-4425.

Martin-Chandon, M. R., Vanky, F., Carnaud, C., and Klein, E. (1975). *Int. J. Cancer 15*, 342-350.

Masucci, M. G., Klein, E., and Argov, S. (1980). *J. Immunol. 124*, 2458-2463.

Mills, G. B., and Paetkau, V. (1980). *J. Immunol. 125*, 1897-1903.

Mills, G. B., Carlson, G., and Paetkau, V. (1980). *J. Immunol. 125*, 1904-1909.

Morgan, D. A., Ruscetti, F. W., and Gallo, R. (1976). *Science (Washington, D.C.) 193*, 1007-1008.

Ortaldo, J. R., Bonnard, G. D., and Herberman, R. B. (1977). *J. Immunol. 119*, 1351-1357.

Seeley, J. K., and Golub, S. H. (1978). *J. Immunol. 120*, 1415-1422.

Seeley, J. K., Masucci, G., Poros, A., Klein, E., and Golub, S. H. (1979). *J. Immunol. 123*, 1303-1311.

Seman, G., and Demochowski, L. (1975). *In* "Human Tumor Cells *in vitro*" (J. Fogh, ed.), pp. 395-399. Plenum, New York and London.

Strausser, J. L., and Rosenberg, S. A. (1978). *J. Immunol. 121*, 1491-1495.

Strausser, J. L., Mazumder, A., Grimm, E. A., Lotze, M. T., and Rosenberg, S. A. (1981). *J. Immunol. 127*, 266-271.

Vánky, F., Klein, E., Stjernswärd, J., Nilsonne, U., Rodriguez, L., and Péterffy, Á. (1978). *Cancer Immunol. Immunother. 5*, 63-69.

Vánky, F., Vose, B. M., Fopp, M., and Klein, E. (1979). *J. Natl. Cancer Inst. (US) 62*, 1407-1413.

Vánky, F., Argov, S., and Klein, E. (1981). *Int. J. Cancer 27*, 273-280.

Vánky, F., Gorsky, T., Gorsky, Y., Masucci, M. G., and Klein, E. (1982). *J. Exp. Med. 155*, 83-95.

Vose, B. M. (1980). *Cell. Immunol. 55*, 12-19.

Vose, B. M., and Bonnard, G. D. (1982). *Int. J. Cancer 29*, 33-39.

Vose, B. M., and Moore, M. (1981). *Immunol. Lett. 3*, 237-241.

Vose, B. M., Vánky, F., and Klein, E. (1977). *Int. J. Cancer 20*, 512-519.

Vose, B. M., Vánky, F., Fopp, M., and Klein, E. (1978a). *Br. J. Cancer 38*, 375-381.

Vose, B. M., Vánky, F., Fopp, M., and Klein, E. (1978b). *Int. J. Cancer 21*, 588-593.

Zarling, J. M., and Bach, F. H. (1979). *Nature (London) 280*, 685-688.

Zarling, J. M., and Bach, F. H. (1980). *Transplant. Proc. 12*, 164-166.

Zarling, J. M., Raich, P. C., Mckeough, M., and Bach, F. H. (1976). *Nature (London) 262*, 691-693.

Zarling, J. M., Robins, H. I., Raich, P. C., Bach, F. H., and
  Bach, M. L. (1978). *Nature (London) 274*, 269-271.
Zielske, J. V., and Golub, S. H. (1976). *Cancer Res. 36*, 3842-
  3846.

DISCUSSION

HOSHINO: In both the cell line and fresh cell studies, you incu-
            bated effector cells with target for 5 to 7 days.
            (1) Is there any difference between your autologous
            cytotoxicity and so-called culture-induced cytotoxicity?
            (2) No inhibition of cytotoxicity was seen after IgG
            treatment to effector cells. Does it mean that the
            IgG-Fc receptor does not relate to cytotoxicity?

ISHIKAWA: (1) As mentioned in the presentation, FCS may be respon-
            sible of inducing slight cytotoxic activity by culture
            in medium only without tumor cell stimulation. However,
            this slight cytotoxicity is mostly negligible, when
            compared with the cytotoxicity of the tumor cell induced
            by specific stimulation. (2) I can say, at least, that
            the cytotoxicity observed in our autologous system is
            not expressed through Fc receptor on the lymphocyte.

GOLUB: This is a most interesting study. (1) Do you think it
            is necessary to have specific T cell cytotoxicity in
            order to augment it in culture? (2) Are the markers,
            like Leu-2a, stable on the TCGF-grown cells?

ISHIKAWA: (1) Lymphoid cells from the patient with cancer have
            other populations that have cytotoxic activity other
            than tumor-specific killer T cells. These populations
            may be augmented by culture. However, as far as short-
            term culture with autologous tumor cells followed by
            culture in TCGF is concerned, T cells, mainly Tc, were
            propagated. (2) We don't have data on the detection of
            Leu-2a marker in long-term propagation of the Tc. How-
            ever, as far as a short-term culture with TCGF is
            concerned, Leu-2a can be detected on the propagated
            lymphocytes.

OCHAI: Thank you very much for the beautiful presentation. My
            question is, what is your explanation of possible
            mechanisms of blocking of CML with anti-HLA C3 anti-
            body?

ISHIKAWA: It has been reported that killing activity of tumor-
            specific killer T cell is restricted by H-2 D and K in

the mouse.   We examined whether induced autologous CL
could be restricted by HLA.   Although HLA-A,B may
reasonably be responsible for the dual recognition,
only anti-Cw3 blocked the cytotoxicity.   Therefore, at
least a phenotype of HLA (Cw3 in our case) was closely
related to express the cytotoxicity of autologous
tumor-specific killer T cell.

CHAPTER 18

PROSTAGLANDINS IN TUMOR CELL METASTASIS

Kenneth V. Honn

Departments of Radiology, Radiation Oncology,
and Biological Sciences
Wayne State University
Detroit, Michigan

Bonnie F. Sloane

Departments of Pharmacology and Radiation Oncology
Wayne State University School of Medicine
Detroit, Michigan

BASIC MECHANISMS AND CLINICAL TREATMENT
OF TUMOR METASTASIS

311

I.   ARACHIDONIC ACID (20:4) METABOLISM TO CYCLOOXYGENASE AND
     LIPOXYGENASE PRODUCTS

     The oxidative metabolites of 20:4 are formed via two major
pathways that require the incorporation of one or two molecules
of molecular O_2 into the carbon framework of 20:4. Prostaglandin
endoperoxide synthase (PES) catalyzes the bis-dioxygenation of
20:4 to a hydroperoxy endoperoxide called PGG_2 and the subsequent
reduction of PGG_2 to the hydroxy endoperoxide called PGH_2 (Fig. 1;
Hamberg and Samuelsson, 1973; Nugteren and Hazelhof, 1973;
Miyamoto et al., 1976). PGH_2 is converted by metabolizing
enzymes to classical prostaglandins (PGD_2, PGE_2, $PGF_{2\alpha}$), prostacyclin (PGI_2), thromboxane A_2 (TXA_2), and malonaldehyde (MDA;
Fig. 1). Each of these metabolites has a unique set of biological
activities that are exerted at low concentrations. The profile of
PGH_2-metabolizing enzymes is tissue specific, so that different
tissues elaborate a different pattern of metabolites via this
pathway. Virtually all mammalian tissues display some PES
activity, although the absolute levels vary considerably from tissue to tissue (Christ and Van Dorp, 1972). Many nonsteroidal
anti-inflammatory agents inhibit PES activity (Vane, 1971). The
most widely used compounds are the irreversible inhibitors aspirin
(which acetylates PES), indomethacin, and the substrate analog
5,8,11,14-eicosatetraynoic acid (ETYA). These compounds inhibit
the oxygenation of 20:4 to PGG_2 but do not inhibit the reduction
of PGG_2 to PGH_2 (Fig. 1). No specific inhibitors of the reduction
of PGG_2 to PGH_2 have been described. Likewise, no compounds have
been described that specifically inhibit the isomerization of PGH_2
to the classical prostaglandins PGD_2, PGE_2, and $PGF_{2\alpha}$. In contrast, many compounds, including substituted imidazoles, substituted pyridines, and endoperoxide analogs, inhibit the conversion
of PGH_2 to TXA_2 and to MDA (Gorman et al., 1977; Needleman et al.,
1977; Tai and Yuan, 1978; Randall et al., 1981). Since TXA_2 is a
potent aggregator of platelets, many of these compounds have significant antithrombotic activity (Gorman et al., 1977).
     One year following the discovery of TXA_2 (Hamberg and
Samuelsson, 1973), Vane and co-workers discovered that PGI_2 was
the major transformation product formed from prostaglandin endo-
peroxides by a microsomal fraction of pig aorta. Prostacyclin is
produced by vascular tissue of all species so far tested (Moncada
and Vane, 1980) and is the main product of arachidonic acid
metabolism in isolated vascular tissue. Prostacyclin is the most
potent endogenous inhibitor of platelet aggregation yet discovered,
being 30-40 times more potent than PGE_1 (Moncada and Vane, 1977)
and 1000 times more potent than adenosine (Mullane et al., 1979).
In addition, PGI_2 can reverse secondary platelet aggregation in
vitro (Moncada et al., 1976a) and in circulation in humans
(Szczeklik et al., 1978). It has been suggested that PGI_2 and
TXA_2 play an antagonistic and pivotal role in the control of
thrombosis centered on their bidirectional (PGI_2 increases, TXA_2

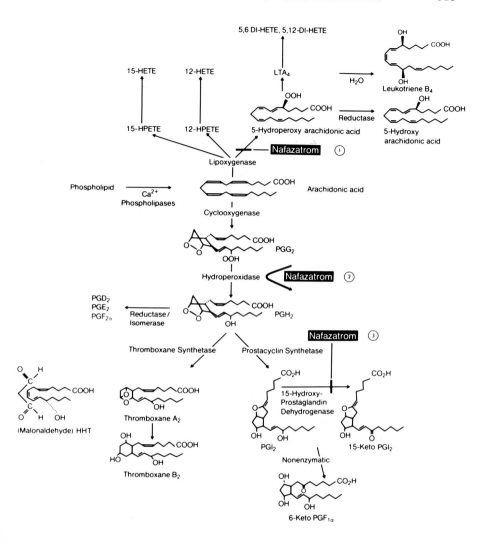

Fig. 1. Arachidonic acid metabolism via the lipoxygenase pathway resulting in hydroperoxy fatty acids and leukotrienes and via the prostaglandin endoperoxide synthase (cyclooxygenase + hydroperoxidase) pathway resulting in prostaglandins (including prostacyclin) and thromboxanes. Possible sites of action of nafazatrom include (1) inhibition of lipoxygenase activity, (2) reducing cofactor for the hydroperoxidase of prostaglandin endoperoxide synthase, and (3) inhibition of prostacyclin (PGI$_2$) degradation by 15-hydroxy-prostaglandin dehydrogenase.

decreases) effect on platelet cAMP levels. The conversion of
PGH$_2$ to PGI$_2$ is potently inhibited by hydroperoxy fatty acids
($K_i \sim 10^{-7}$ M; Moncada et al., 1976a). Little structural
specificity is evident in the inhibition, since a number of
isomeric hydroperoxides are equally effective (Moncada et al.,
1976b).

In 1974, Hamberg and Samuelsson described a monoxygenation
of 20:4 to 12-hydroperoxyeicosatetraenoic acid (12-HPETE) that
was catalyzed by a lipoxygenase in human platelets (Fig. 1).
Until that time, it had been generally believed that lipoxygenases
were solely of plant origin. It is now known that different tissues convert 20:4 to all the conceivable HPETE isomers, 5-, 8-,
9-, 11-, 12-, and 15-HPETE (Moncada et al., 1976b); 6- and
14-HPETEs are unlikely for steric reasons. The biological activities have not been completely explored, but individual HPETEs and
their reduction products, hydroxyeicosatetraenoic acids (HETEs),
are potent chemotactic agents and the HPETEs also appear to have
inhibitor effects on platelet and lymphocyte function (Moncada et
al., 1976b).

Studies of 20:4 metabolism in leukocytes have resulted in the
discovery of a new group of biologically active compounds, the
leukotrienes (Borgeat and Samuelsson, 1979; Fig. 1). This family
of compounds is initially derived from the 5-lipoxygenation of
20:4 (Fig. 1) and consists of leukotriene A$_4$ (LTA$_4$), LTB$_4$, LTC$_4$,
LTD$_4$, and LTE$_4$ (Piper, 1981). Leukotrienes C$_4$ and D$_4$ are broncho-
constrictors and increase the permeability of microvasculature.
Leukotriene B$_4$ is a potent chemotactic agent. Many PES inhibitors,
such as aspirin and indomethacin, do not inhibit lipoxygenases
(Hamberg and Samuelsson, 1974). However, phenidone, BW755C, and
ETYA inhibit both PES and lipoxygenases at comparable concentrations (Hamberg and Samuelsson, 1974). Certain substrate analogs
and HETEs selectively inhibit lipoxygenase but not PES (Hammerstrom, 1977).

II. PLATELET-TUMOR CELL INTERACTIONS AND METASTASIS

The relationship between altered platelet function, blood
coagulability, and malignant disease is a well-recognized but
poorly understood phenomenon, although there are considerable
clinical data to support such a relationship. It has been suggested that tumor cell interaction with host platelets facilitates
metastasis, and this has prompted the use of antiplatelet and
anticoagulant therapy for treatment of metastatic disease. Limited
success has been achieved by the VA Cooperative Study Group in use
of warfarin (Zacharski et al., 1979; Zacharski, 1982). Current
clinical trials with the antiplatelet agent RA233 are planned.

We have proposed that tumor cells disrupt the balance between
PGI$_2$ (produced by the vascular wall) and TXA$_2$ (formed by the

platelet) in favor of thrombosis. We have demonstrated that PGI_2
(Honn *et al.*, 1981), agents that stimulate endogenous PGI_2
production (Honn *et al.*, 1982b), and TX synthase inhibitors (Honn,
1983) are all antimetastatic agents.

Gasic and co-workers (1968) were the first to provide direct
experimental evidence for a role of platelets in tumor cell
metastasis. They had noted that pretreatment of mice with neuraminidase resulted in formation of fewer lung colonies following
injection of TA3 ascites tumor cells. These results were found to
be attributable to neuraminidase induction of thrombocytopenia in
the host (Gasic *et al.*, 1968). Similar antimetastatic effects
were observed when thrombocytopenia was induced with antiplatelet
antiserum. Additional evidence was provided by the fact that the
antimetastatic effects of neuraminidase could be reversed by
platelet infusion. Several other laboratories have confirmed the
in vitro aggregation of platelets by both animal and human tumor
cells and the induction of thrombocytopenia following iv injection
of some tumor lines (Hilgard, 1973; Gastpar *et al.*, 1977; Paschen
et al., 1979; Hara *et al.*, 1980; Pearlstein *et al.*, 1980, 1981;
Skolnik *et al.*, 1980; Bastida *et al.*, 1981). However, most of
these studies only provide circumstantial evidence that host
platelets facilitate hematogenous metastasis.

Studies by Pearlstein *et al.* (1980) provide more direct evidence that a causal relationship exists. Using 10 cell lines
derived from the polyoma-induced PW20 Wister-Firth rat renal sarcoma, they examined the correlation between the ability of the
tumor cells to metastasize spontaneously from subcutaneous sites
in syngeneic hosts and their platelet-aggregating activity *in
vitro*. Platelet aggregation was measured in response to a plasma
membrane material extracted with 1 *M* urea (Pearlstein *et al.*,
1979). A significant correlation between platelet aggregability
and spontaneous metastasis was observed. These workers also correlated sialic acid levels of cell surface glycoproteins with the
ability of these 10 lines to (1) aggregate platelets and (2)
spontaneously metastasize. A high degree of correlation was found
between these parameters, suggesting that the sialic acid content
of tumor cell surface glycoproteins may affect initial adhesiveness to platelets prior to stimulation of platelet aggregation or
may affect arrest in the microvasculature.

Despite the preceding findings, the mechanism by which
platelets enhance metastasis remains to be definitively established.
Several suggestions appear in the literature and include (1) protection against destruction by shear forces and host cytotoxic
macrophages, since tumor cells are physically shielded within the
emboli, and (2) increased ability of tumor platelet emboli to arrest in the microvasculature with possible occlusion of a pre-
capillary sphincter.

III.   PROSTACYCLIN, THROMBOXANES, AND TUMOR CELL METASTASIS

Honn (1982) and Honn *et al.* (1981, 1983) proposed the working hypothesis that the primary tumor, tumor cell-shed vesicles, and/or circulating tumor cells disrupt the intravascular balance between PGI_2 and TXA_2 in favor of platelet aggregation. Based on the assumptions that platelet-tumor cell and/or platelet-tumor cell-vessel wall interactions are important for tumor cell metastasis, they proposed that (1) PGI_2 and TXA_2 synthase inhibitors would inhibit tumor cell-induced platelet aggregation (TCIPA) and platelet release reaction (TCIPR); (2) the exogenous administration of PGI_2 should reduce lung colony formation by tail vein-injected tumor cells; (3) a therapeutic synergism should result from the use of PGI_2 with a phosphodiesterase inhibitor (Since the effect of PGI_2 is mediated by increasing concentrations of cAMP in platelets, it follows that phosphodiesterase inhibitors, by slowing the breakdown of cAMP, should potentiate the antithrombogenic action of PGI_2 and thus its antimetastatic action); (4) prostacyclin acts as a natural deterrent to tumor cell metastasis, therefore, an inhibitor of endogenous PGI_2 biosynthesis should enhance metastasis; (5) agents that augment PGI_2 biosynthesis or activity *in vivo* should function as antimetastatic agents; and (6) thromboxane synthase inhibitors should also possess antimetastatic activity.

We now further propose that platelets facilitate metastasis by increasing tumor cell adhesiveness to other tumor cells (homotypic aggregation), endothelial cells (heterotypic aggregation), and the basal lamina. The nature of this critical increase in adhesion is unknown. However, we have demonstrated that during TCIPA, platelet-derived fibronectin coats tumor cells and may partially account for their increased adhesiveness (Turner et al., 1983). Prostacyclin not only prevents TCIPA but also decreases tumor cell adhesion to substrate (see later).

A.   Prostacyclin Effects on TCIPA

Numerous investigators have demonstrated that a variety of human and animal tumor cells induce platelet aggregation (for review see Jamieson, 1982). All of these studies have utilized whole dispersates (mechanical or enzymatic) of solid tumors or tissue-cultured cells. We have utilized tumor cells purified by centrifugal elutriation from a collagenase-derived dispersate of a solid tumor or from an ascites tumor. Elutriated B16 amelanotic melanoma (B16a), Lewis lung carcinoma (3LL), 15091A mammary adenocarcinoma, and Walker 256 carcinosarcoma (W256) cells induced aggregation of human platelet-rich plasma (PRP) following a short lag time (Figs. 2 and 3). The aggregation of human PRP by tumor cells occurred concomitantly with the generation of TXA_2 (Menter

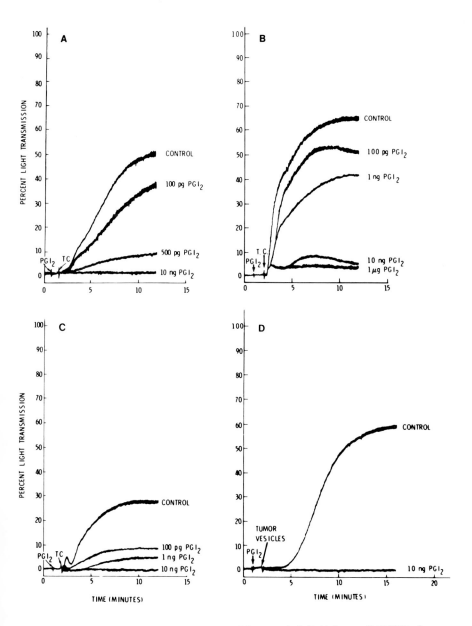

Fig. 2. Effects of prostacyclin on inhibition of TCIPA by (A) B16a (amelanotic melanoma) cells, (B) 3LL (Lewis lung carcinoma) cells, (C) 15091A (mammary adenocarcinoma) cells, and (D) 15091A tumor vesicles. TC, Addition of tumor cells.

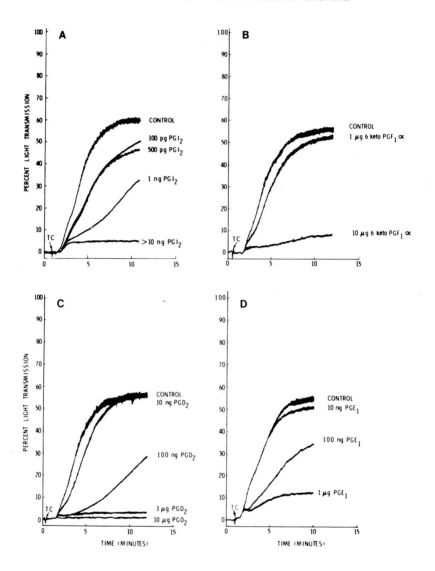

Fig. 3. Comparison of the effects of (A) PGI_2, (B) 6-keto-$PGF_{1\alpha}$, (C) PGD_2, and (D) PGE_1 on Walker 256 carcinosarcoma TCIPA.

et al., 1982). The addition of PGI_2 to platelets 1 min prior to tumor cell addition results in a dose-dependent inhibition of TCIPA (Figs. 2 and 3). The inhibitory effect of PGI_2 on W256 TCIPA was greater than the inhibitory effect of two additional PGs (PGE_1 and PGD_2), which also have been shown to inhibit platelet aggregation (Fig. 3C and D). Prostacyclin (PGI_2) was approximately 100 times more effective than either PGE_1 or PGD_2

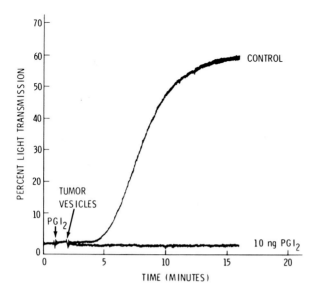

Fig. 4.   Effects of PGI_2 on 15091A tumor cell membrane vesicle-induced platelet aggregation.

(Fig. 3A, C, and D).   The stable metabolite of PGI_2, 6-keto-$PGF_{1\alpha}$, was only effective at supraphysiological doses (Fig. 3B).   In contrast, PGE_2, which competes for the PGI_2 platelet receptor, did not block TCIPA, and PGE_2, when added prior to PGI_2, prevented the PGI_2 inhibition of TCIPA.

Prostacyclin, in addition to its effects on TCIPA, blocked platelet aggregation induced by spontaneously shed membrane vesicles of the 15091A mammary adenocarcinoma (Fig. 4).   Homotypic aggregation of W256 cells was also completely blocked by PGI_2 (10 ng).   It therefore appears that PGI_2 is a universal inhibitor of various tumor cell homotypic and heterotypic interactions.

B.   Prostacyclin Effects on TCIPR

During the release reaction, materials stored in platelet granules (dense granules, α granules, and lysosomes) are released from the platelet.   Not all stimuli provoke release from all three granule compartments (Holmsen and Day, 1970).   The dense granules contain high concentrations of amines (serotonin), adenine nucleotides, and divalent cations.   The α granules contain a variety of proteins, among which are heparin-neutralizing protein (PF4), β-thromboglobulin, fibrinogen, fibronectin, and platelet-derived growth factors (Kaplan, 1981).   Lysosomes contain acid phosphatase, β-N-acetylglucosaminidase (β-NAG), β-glucuronidase, cathepsins D and E, collagenase, and others (Gordon, 1975; Holmsen and Weiss, 1979). Several of the platelet-derived factors could conceivably aid in tumor metastasis. Dense-granule serotonin is a potent vasoconstrictor and can stimulate further platelet aggregation (Kaplan, 1981). α Granule-derived β-thromboglobulin inhibits production of PGI_2, which has demonstrated antimetastatic activity (Honn et al., 1981), by the vascular endothelium (Hope et al., 1979), whereas platelet-derived fibronectin could coat tumor cells and increase adhesiveness as discussed earlier. In addition, platelet-derived fibrinogen could contribute to tumor cell-associated fibrin (Gasic et al., 1976). Finally, platelet-derived growth factors have been demonstrated to be mitogenic for several animal (Lipton et al., 1982) and human tumor cells (Cowan and Graham, 1982).

A variety of human and animal tumor cells have been demonstrated to evoke the release of platelet dense granules (Gasic et al., 1976). We have shown (Honn et al., 1983b) that prostacyclin inhibits the release of dense granules during TCIPA. In addition, we found that PGI_2 caused a dose-dependent decrease in platelet α granule release (measured as β-thromboglobulin release) induced by W256 cells (Table I).

C. Prostacyclin Effects on Platelet-Induced Tumor Cell Adhesion in Vitro

Fantone et al. (1982) have demonstrated that the adherence of W256 cells to plastic plates or nylon fibers can be stimulated by the tumor promoter phorbol myristate acetate and the chemotactic peptide f-Met-Leu-Phe. Prostacyclin directly inhibited this increased adhesion. Tumor cells will not induce aggregation of washed platelets in the absence of a small amount of platelet-poor plasma (PPP; Hara et al., 1980). Therefore, we explored the

TABLE I

Walker 256 Carcinosarcoma-Induced β-Thromboglobulin Release

Dose of Prostacyclin	% Control β-thromboglobulin release	% Control platelet aggregation
100 ng	3.5 ± 3.5[a]	10.7 ± 1.7
10 ng	8.5 ± 4.3	12.5 ± 2.7
1 ng	58.9 ± 36.6	64.2 ± 14.2
100 pg	87.2 ± 19.3	92.5 ± 16.0

[a]Mean ± SEM; $n = 3$.

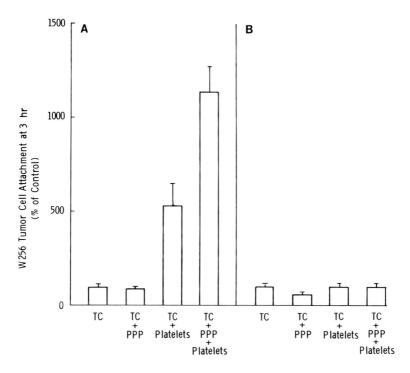

Fig. 5.   Effects of PGI_2 on platelet-enhanced adhesion of W256 cells to plastic.   (A) Untreated; (B) PGI_2 treated.

possibility that platelets would enhance adhesion of W256 cells under nonaggregatory (no PPP) and aggregatory (5% PPP) conditions.

The adhesion of W256 cells to plastic plates was increased in the presence of washed rat platelets (Fig. 5).   This increase was variable with platelet preparation but ranged from 100 to 400%. An even larger increase (300-1400%) was observed if tumor cells were allowed to induce aggregation (addition of 5% PPP) of platelets (Fig. 5A).   This adhesion increased with time and reached a maximum at 1 hr.   The addition of PGI_2 (30 µg/ml) completely prevented the increased adhesion at 1 hr under both aggregatory and nonaggregatory conditions.   The PGI_2 effect was dose dependent both in the presence and absence of PPP, with a 40% decrease observed at 1 µg PGI_2/ml.   Prostacyclin had no effect on basal (unstimulated) W256 cell attachment (Fig. 5B).

D.   Arachidonic Acid Metabolites and Tumor Cell Metastasis

We have previously reported that bolus iv injection of PGI_2 into mice reduced lung colony formation from tail vein-injected B16a cells by greater than 70% (Honn et al., 1981). The combination of PGI_2 with a phosphodiesterase inhibitor (theophylline) inhibited metastasis by >93% (Honn et al., 1981). Prostaglandins E_2, $F_{2\alpha}$, and the stable hydrolysis product of PGI_2, 6-keto-$PGF_{1\alpha}$, were ineffective (Honn et al., 1981). Prostaglandin D_2 is also antimetastatic as reported by Stringfellow and Fitzpatrick (1979); however, we found PGD_2 to be less than one-third as effective as PGI_2 (Honn et al., 1981). The antimetastatic effects of PGI_2 are not due to its pulmonary vasodilatory effects (Honn, 1983). In this regard, PGI_2 does not significantly alter tumor cell distribution patterns. Using $[^{125}I]$deoxyuridine-labeled tumor cells, we demonstrated (Honn, 1983) that, although some alteration of cell distribution may occur, these cells once released from the lung are not retained in the organ of secondary arrest (liver, spleen, etc.). In addition, there is no effect of PGI_2 on the initial entrapment of tumor cells in the lung following iv injection (Honn, 1983), which might be expected if the PGI_2 effect were due to vasodilation. The lack of a PGI_2 effect on initial tumor cell arrest raises the question whether TCIPA occurs while the tumor cell is in circulation or, alternatively, whether the critical aggregation event occurs on arrest and attachment to the endothelium. It is clear from our studies that PGI_2 significantly increases organ clearance of tumor cells (Honn, 1983). Marcum et al. (1980) utilized rabbit aortic segments in a standard Baumgartner perfusion chamber to study tumor cell (HUT 20)-platelet-endothelial interactions. Tumor cells and platelets were perfused in the presence of PGE_1 (30 µg/ml) or PGI_2 (50 ng/ml). Both agents totally inhibited TCIPA and the deposition of both tumor cells and platelets on the vascular surface. Although the preceding studies demonstrate a role for platelets in metastasis, the question whether the critical platelet aggregation occurs prior to or after tumor cell arrest has not been definitively answered.

The time frame for PGI_2 effectiveness is not limited to events immediately preceding or coincident with tumor cell arrest (Honn, 1983). We examined the effects of administration of PGI_2 post-tumor cell injection on the retention of $[^{125}I]$deoxyuridine-labeled B16a cells. Prostacyclin was administered either 15 min prior to tumor cell injection or 1 hr after tumor cell injection. Animals were then sacrificed 3, 8, and 20 hr after tumor cell injection and the lungs removed and tumor colonies counted. Both treatment regimens were equally effective in reducing tumor cell retention in the lung and subsequent tumor colony formation (Honn, 1983), indicating that arrested intravascular tumor cells can be dislodged by PGI_2 presumably, but possibly not exclusively, as a result of disaggregation of adherent platelet-tumor cell thrombi.

The preceding results with exogenous PGI_2 demonstrate its efficacy as an antimetastatic agent. We have also proposed that the production of PGI_2 by the vascular endothelium is a natural deterrent to metastasis (Honn et al., 1981). To test this hypothesis we perfused mice with a lipoxygenase product of arachidonic acid (15-HPETE) prior to tail vein injection of B16a tumor cells. Hydroperoxy fatty acids in general are potent inhibitors of prostacyclin synthase (Salmon et al., 1978). Mice pretreated with 15-HPETE develop 300-500% more metastatic lesions than untreated mice (Honn et al., 1981). The administration of PGI_2 following 15-HPETE treatment reduces metastatic tumor colony formation (Honn et al., 1981). Collectively, these results suggest a role for endogenous PGI_2 production in the inhibition of tumor metastasis.

A new proposal for the prevention of tumor metastasis by PGI_2 is the use of agents that stimulate endogenous PGI_2 biosynthesis or prolong its half-life. One such compound that may represent the prototype of such a new class of pharmacologically active agents is nafazatrom (BAY g 6575; 2,4-dihydro-5-methyl-2-[2-(2-napthyloxy)ethyl]-3H-pyrazol-3-one; L. J. Marnett, P. H. Siedlik, R. Ochs, K. V. Honn, R. Warnock, B. Tainer, and T. E. Eling, unpublished observations; Honn et al., 1982b). Nafazatrom has been reported to possess significant antithrombotic activity in model systems of experimental thrombosis (Seuter et al., 1979). Nafazatrom stimulates the biosynthesis of PGI_2 from arachidonic acid by ram seminal vesicle microsomes (Eling et al., 1982), cultured porcine endothelial cells, and B16a tumor cells (K. V. Honn, L. J. Marnett, and T. E. Eling, unpublished observations). It is unlikely that the actions of nafazatrom are due to a single biochemical effect, since this compound has been found to have multiple effects on arachidonic acid metabolism (Fig. 1). Nafazatrom has been found to inhibit the cytosolic lipoxygenase of B16a cells (Honn and Dunn, 1982), as well as that of human and rabbit neutrophils (Busse et al., 1982). Inhibition of lipoxygenase-produced HPETEs could contribute to protection of PGI_2 synthase (Fig. 1). Nafazatrom also functions as a reducing cofactor for the hydroperoxidase activity of prostaglandin endoperoxide synthase and stimulates PGI_2 biosynthesis by reduction of hydroperoxy fatty acids such as PGG_2 (Fig. 1; Eling et al., 1982; L. J. Marnett, P. H. Siedlik, R. Ochs, K. V. Honn, R. Warnock; B. Tainer, and T. E. Eling, unpublished observations). Finally, nafazatrom has been found to inhibit the 15-hydroxy-prostaglandin dehydrogenase-catalyzed inactivation of PGI_2 (Fig. 1; Wong et al.. 1982).

Nafazatrom has been evaluated for its antimetastatic activity against tail vein-injected elutriated B16a and 3LL tumor cells, and found to inhibit lung colony formation by >80% (Honn et al., 1982b). In addition, this compound significantly reduces spontaneous pulmonary metastasis from subcutaneous B16a and 3LL tumors (Honn et al., 1982b, 1983). These results point to significant antimetastatic properties of this PGI_2-enhancing agent.

Finally, we have proposed that alteration of platelet thromboxane levels with selective TX synthase inhibitors would prevent tumor cell metastasis. We have reported that a series of endoperoxide analogs (Fitzpatrick *et al.*, 1979) were effective in reducing metastasis from tail vein-injected elutriated B16a cells (Honn, 1983). In addition, it was determined that these antimetastatic effects were not peculiar to the endoperoxide structure. A structurally unrelated TX synthase inhibitor also prevented metastasis (Honn, 1983). Unlike PGI_2, TX synthase inhibitors are not effective when administered after tumor cell injection (Honn, 1983). In general, the TX synthase inhibitors were not as effective as PGI_2 in preventing tumor cell metastasis, and this could be related to their inability to block tumor cell-induced platelet aggregation completely.

IV.   ROLE OF TUMOR CELL CATHEPSIN B-LIKE PROTEINASE IN TCIPA
      AND METASTASIS

Tumor cells have been shown to induce aggregation of platelets *in vitro*. However, the mechanism(s) for induction of aggregation by tumor cells is not yet completely elucidated. Gasic and coworkers (1978) have demonstrated that TCIPA can be mimicked by membrane vesicles spontaneously shed (SSMV) from the tumor cells in culture. Karpatkin *et al.* (1980) and Pearlstein *et al.* (1979) have urea-extracted a membrane-derived component from tumor cells that will induce platelet aggregation and whose proaggregatory activity correlates with tumor metastasis. Platelet aggregation can also be induced *in vitro* by addition of exogenous proteinases such as trypsin or the plant cysteine proteinase, papain (Alexander *et al.*, 1962), suggesting that a proteinase present in the membrane of tumor cells may be responsible for TCIPA. Tumor cells possess, in addition to proaggregatory activity, procoagulant activity. Dvorak *et al.* (1981) have shown that tumor SSMV possess procoagulant activity, and Gordon and Cross (1981) have identified one tumor cell procoagulant as a cysteine proteinase. These lines of evidence have led us to speculate that tumor cell proaggregatory and procoagulant activity may be due to a cathepsin B-like cysteine proteinase.

We have previously demonstrated that increased activity of a cathepsin B-like proteinase in murine B16 melanoma cells correlates with increased lung colonization potential of the B16F1, B16F10 melanoma variants (Sloane *et al.*, 1981, 1982a). Cathepsin B-like activity was three to four times higher in the B16F10 tumor cells than in the B16F1 (Sloane *et al.*, 1981, 1982a). Activity in the lysosomal (light mitochondrial) fractions of the B16F10 cells was sevenfold higher than in the B16F1 (Sloane *et al.*, 1981). However, these lines were selected by tail vein injection (Fidler, 1978) and may only represent phenotypic characteristics necessary for successful completion of the latter half of the metastatic cascade, that is, once the tumor cells have entered the circulatory system. Therefore, we developed variants of murine Bl6a and 3LL by sequential passaging of spontaneous pulmonary metastases formed from subcutaneous tumors. We tested the variants for metastatic potential from a subcutaneous tumor and selected two of each for assay of cathepsin B. In these selected variants, cathepsin B-like activity correlated with metastatic potential and with survival of the tumor-bearing animals (B. F. Sloane, J. G. Sadler, and K. V. Honn, unpublished observations).

Of particular relevance to metastasis is the increasing body of literature on release of a cathepsin B-like enzyme from human and animal tumors. Poole and co-workers have shown that up to 11 times more of a cathepsin B-like proteinase is released from malignant human breast tumors than from normal breast tissue or nonmalignant tumors (Poole et al., 1978; Recklies et al., 1980). Other laboratories have reported elevated levels of cathepsin B-like activity in pancreatic fluid of patients with pancreatic cancer (Rinderknecht and Renner, 1980) and in serum of women with diverse invasive neoplastic diseases including vaginal adenocarcinomas (Pietras et al., 1978, 1979, 1981). Recklies et al. (1980) have hypothesized that the tumor cathepsin B is released from viable tumor cells, since a gradient of cathepsin B-like activity within explants of breast tumors suggests that the enzyme is released from the growing and invading tumor periphery, and since protein synthesis is required for enzyme release. Pietras et al. (1981) have shown that neoplastic cervical cells in culture release cathepsin B-like activity into the culture medium and that elevated release appears to correlate with rapid growth in agar. In our laboratories we have found that when the Bl6Fl, Fl0 variants are placed in tissue culture, cathepsin B-like activity can be measured in the medium with time in culture (Sloane et al., 1982a). Bl6a cells (Sloane et al., 1982b) and 15091A mammary adenocarcinoma cells (Cavanaugh et al., 1983) in culture also release cathepsin B-like activity into the medium. In the cases of 15091A cells and the Bl6a cells, the cathepsin B-like activity in the medium was associated with SSMV.

Although cathepsin B-like activity had been indirectly linked to the tumor cell by the preceding studies, no definitive proof existed that cathepsin B-like activity in tumors in vivo was a property of viable tumor cells and not of host cells or necrotic tumor cells. Therefore, we used the technique of centrifugal elutriation to separate viable tumor cells from nonviable tumor cells, macrophages, lymphocytes, and others dispersed from solid subcutaneous tumors (Sloane et al., 1981, 1982a). In variants of the Bl6 melanoma, 80% of the cathepsin B activity was associated with viable tumor cells (β fraction) in the Bl6Fl (low lung colonization potential) and 92% in the Bl6Fl0 (high lung colonization potential) (Sloane et al., 1981). In Bl6a, 3LL, and W256, >95% of cathepsin B activity was associated with the β fraction. Of the cells in the β

fraction, >97% are tumor cells, <2% lymphocytes, <1% monocytes, and <1% PMN.

In order to determine whether tumor cell-derived cathepsin B might be one tumor cell principle responsible for inducing platelet aggregation, we tested a series of proteinase inhibitors of varying specificity for cysteine and serine proteinases against B16a TCIPA using tumor cells purified by centrifugal elutriation (Honn *et al.*, 1982a). The most effective inhibitors were leupeptin and antipain and the specific cysteine proteinase inhibitors iodoacetic acid (IAA) and *p*-hydroxymercuriphenylsulfonate (PHMS). These same inhibitors inhibited the proteolytic activity measured, using a highly selective substrate for cathepsin B (Barrett, 1980), in homogenates of elutriated B16a tumor cells. We further established the identity of our B16a cysteine proteinase as cathepsin B-like by using organic soluble proteinase inhibitors, diazomethyl ketones, which selectively inhibit the cysteine proteinases, cathepsins B and L (Kirschke and Shaw, 1981), and by lack of substantive activity of a cathepsin H-like cysteine proteinase in the tumor cell homogenates (Honn *et al.*, 1982a).

Papain and cathepsin B have substantial sequence homologies and are identical at the active-site grooves (Takio *et al.*, 1980). Thus, we used papain to mimic the action of cathepsin B. Papain-induced aggregation of washed human platelets was inhibited most effectively by leupeptin, antipain, IAA, and PHMS (Honn *et al.*, 1982a). The cysteine proteinase activity of papain measured in the assay for cathepsin B was blocked by these same inhibitors. Platelet aggregation initiated by papain occurred concomitantly with generation of TXA_2 (P. G. Cavanaugh, B. F. Sloane, and K. V. Honn, unpublished observation), and could be blocked by PGI_2 (Honn *et al.*, 1982b) and a TX synthase inhibitor (P. G. Cavanaugh, B. F. Sloane, and K. V. Honn, unpublished observation). In subsequent work we have been able to demonstrate concomitant inhibition of B16a-induced platelet aggregation and of B16a-induced TXA_2 production by leupeptin.

We have also shown that tumor cells and SSMV of line 15091A mammary adenocarcinoma induce platelet aggregation that can be inhibited by the same spectrum of proteinase inhibitors as B16a-induced aggregation (Cavanaugh *et al.*, 1983). Cathepsin B-like activity in 15091A tumor cells and in their SSMV was also inhibited by leupeptin, antipain, and IAA (Cavanaugh *et al.*, 1983). PGI_2 prevented platelet aggregation by 15091A cells or shed vesicles (Figs. 2 and 4).

Mort *et al.* (1980) had reported that the cathepsin B-like proteinase released from human mammary tumors has greater stability at neutral and alkaline pH than human liver cathepsin B. In order for cathepsin B released from tumor cells to play a role in platelet aggregation, one would expect that tumor cathepsin B is not inactivated at neutral pH. Therefore, we investigated the pH dependency of cathepsin B-like activity and its pH stability to alkaline pH in four tumors routinely used in our laboratory (murine

B16a, 3LL, and 15091A, and rat W256; B. F. Sloane, C. Evens, and
K. V. Honn, unpublished observation).

Using a highly specific blocked di-Arg substrate for cathepsin
B, we measured cathepsin B activity at pH values from 3.5 to 8.5.
Cathepsin B-like activity in subcutaneous tumors of 3LL, B16a, and
15091A exhibited a pH optimum of 6.0, similar to that for liver
cathepsin B (Barrett, 1973). The pH optimum curve for W256 was
broader and shifted to the right with an optimum between 6.5 and
7.0. For elutriated tumor cells the pH optimum for cathepsin
B-like activity was shifted toward more neutral pH. The pH optimum for cathepsin B-like activity in cultured cells of 15091A and
B16a was 6.0. Cathepsin B-like activity in both 15091A culture
medium and SSMV exhibited pH-dependence curves with two peaks, a
lower optimum of 4.0 to 4.5 and a higher optimum of 5.5 to 6.0.
In the culture medium the curve for cathepsin B-like activity was
very broad, exhibiting substantial activity from pH 4.0 to 7.0.
Double peaks for pH dependence of cathepsin B-like activity were
not unique to the 15091A tumor line. In 40 to 50% of B16a subcutaneous tumors and tumor cell cultures tested, the pH-dependence
curves had double optima at pH 5.5 and 6.5, with significantly
less activity at pH 6.0.

We tested the effect of exposure to alkaline pH on tumor
cathepsin B-like activity. Samples of tumor homogenates or of
culture media were incubated in the absence of dithiothreitol for
60 min at pH 8.0 and 37°C. Aliquots of these were used to assay
for cathepsin B-like activity stable above neutral pH. Less than
5% of the initial tumor cell cathepsin B-like activity in both
B16a tumors and 15091A tumors was stable after exposure to pH 8.0.
In contrast, the cathepsin B-like activity present in the culture
medium of B16a and 15091A cells retained activity at pH 8.0. At
the pH optimum of 6.0, cathepsin B-like activity in the culture
medium was ∿65% of the initial activity before exposure to pH 8.0.
Cathepsin B-like activity in 15091A SSMV was ∿70% resistant to
alkaline pH and in addition was resistant to high temperature
(56°C for 30 min).

Although the pH optimum for cathepsin B-like activity in tumor
lines does not differ from that in liver, two forms of cathepsin B
may be present within the cells and may be released from the cells.
In contrast to liver cathepsin B, cathepsin B-like activity in
15091A SSMV and culture medium and B16a culture medium is resistant
to inactivation by alkaline pH. We have purified a cathepsin
B-like enzyme from B16a tumor cells that appears to be similar to
cathepsin B isolated from a number of tissues including bovine
spleen (Bajkowski and Frankfater, 1983). This enzyme retained 95%
of its activity on exposure to pH 8.0 for 15 min in the presence
of dithiothreitol and EDTA. Collectively our studies suggest that
the cathepsin B-like enzyme released from tumor cells has activity
at neutral pH and thus may act outside the lysosome and outside
the tumor cell. We hypothesize that the tumor cell cathepsin
B-like enzyme may play a role in metastasis via its proaggregatory
activity and via its possible procoagulant activity.

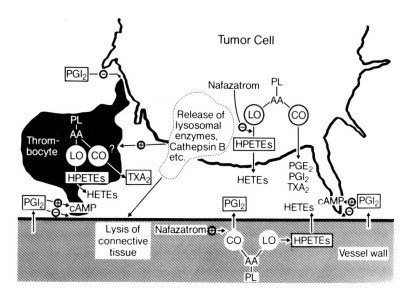

Fig. 6.   Interactions among tumor cells, platelets (thrombo-
cytes), and blood vessel wall. Direct interactions are possible
between the platelet and the vessel wall, the tumor cell and
vessel wall, and the platelet(s) and tumor cell(s). Any one or
all of the preceding may enhance tumor cell arrest and metastasis.
Prostacyclin may prevent attachment of tumor cell(s) to platelet(s)
or to vessel wall. Abbreviations: PL, phospholipids; AA, arachidonic acid; CO, cyclooxygenase; LO, lipoxygenase; HPETEs, hydro-
peroxyeicosatetraenoic acids; HETEs, hydroxyeicosatetraenoic acids;
PGI_2, prostacyclin; and TXA_2, thromboxane A_2.

V.   SUMMARY

It is intuitive that for hematogenous metastasis to occur the
tumor cell must arrest in the microvasculature and attach to the
vessel wall prior to extravasation and growth into a metastatic
focus. Considerable yet indirect evidence supports the concept
that tumor cells interact with platelets during this process as
discussed earlier. We propose that the metabolism of arachidonic
acid in the tumor cell, the platelet, and the vessel wall plays an
essential role in the sum total of these interactions (Fig. 6).
For example, the production of PGI_2 by the vessel wall and of TXA_2
by the platelet is thought to play a key (although possibly not an
exclusive) role in thrombosis.
We propose that exogenous PGI_2 functions as an antimetastatic
agent by inhibiting the association of the tumor cell with the
platelet (thrombocyte), of the platelet with the vessel wall,

and/or of the tumor cell with the vessel wall (Fig. 6). The interactions between the vessel wall and tumor cells or platelets may be inhibited by exogenous PGI_2 stimulation of platelet cAMP or tumor cell cAMP. Similarly, vessel wall PGI_2 serves as a natural deterrent to metastasis by inhibiting these interactions (Fig. 6). Compounds that have the ability to stimulate endogenous PGI_2 production and/or prolong the half-life of PGI_2 (e.g., nafazatrom) are proposed as a new class of antimetastatic agents.

We further postulate that one tumor cell platelet-aggregating principle is an isozyme of the cysteine proteinase cathepsin B. A possible problem with the hypothesis that a tumor cell-derived cathepsin B-like enzyme plays a role in tumor cell-induced platelet aggregation is the pH optimum and stability of cathepsin B. Mort *et al.* (1980) found that tumor-derived cathepsin B is a higher molecular weight isozyme of liver cathepsin B, which retains activity at alkaline pH. We have shown that the cathepsin B-like enzyme released from tumor cells into the culture medium in membrane vesicles is resistant to inactivation by alkaline pH and by heat. The sites of action of cathepsin B are still unknown, but our results suggest that tumor cell cathepsin B can induce aggregation of washed human platelets by a mechanism dependent on generation of TXA_2 and inhibited by selective TX synthase inhibitors, PGI_2, leupeptin, and IAA. The preceding hypotheses (and results) suggest that selective manipulation of the arachidonic acid cascade could be one site used in the control of hematogenous tumor metastasis.

Acknowledgments

Original work in the authors' laboratories has been supported by National Institutes of Health Grants HL 27860, CA 29405, and CA 29997; American Cancer Society Grant BC-356; Miles Institute for Preclinical Pharmacology; and Bayer AG.

REFERENCES

Alexander, B., Pechet, L., and Kliman, A. (1962). *Circulation 26*, 596-611.
Bajkowski, A. S., and Frankfater, A. (1983). *J. Biol. Chem. 258*, 1645-1649.
Barrett, A. J. (1973). *Biochem. J. 131*, 809-822.
Barrett, A. J. (1980). *Biochem. J. 187*, 909-912.
Bastida, E., Ordinas, A., and Jamieson, G. A. (1981). *Nature (London) 291*, 661-662.
Borgeat, P., and Samuelsson, B. (1979). *Proc. Natl. Acad. Sci. USA 76*, 3213-3217.

Busse, W. D., Mardin, M., Grutzmann, R., Dunn, J. R., Theodoreau, M., Sloane, B. F., and Honn, K. V. (1982). *Fed. Proc. Fed. Am. Soc. Exp. Biol. 41*, 1717.

Cavanaugh, P. G., Sloane, B. F., Bajkowski, A. S., Gasic, G. J., Gasic, T. B., and Honn, K. V. (1983). *Clin. Exp. Metastasis 1*, 297-307.

Christ, E. J., and Van Dorp, D. A. (1972). *Biochim. Biophys. Acta 270*, 537-545.

Cowan, D. H., and Graham, J. (1982). *In* "Interactions of Platelets and Tumor Cells" (G. A. Jamieson, ed.), pp. 249-268. Liss, New York.

Dvorak, H. F., Quay, S. C., Orenstein, N. S., Dvorak, A. M., Hahn, P., Bitzer, A. M., and Carvalho, A. C. (1981). *Science (Washington, D.C.) 212*, 923-924.

Eling, T. E., Honn, K. V., Busse, W. D., Seuter, F., and Marnett, L. J. (1982). *In* "Prostaglandins and Cancer" (T. J. Powles, R. S. Bockman, K. V. Honn, and P. W. Ramwell, eds.), pp. 783-787. Liss, New York.

Fantone, J., Kunkel, S., and Varani, J. (1982). *In* "Prostaglandins and Cancer" (T. J. Powles, R. S. Bockman, K. V. Honn, and P. W. Ramwell, eds.), pp. 673-677. Liss, New York.

Fidler, I. J. (1978). *Methods Cancer Res. 25*, 399-439.

Fitzpatrick, F. A., Bundy, G. L., Gorman, R. R., Honahan, R., McGuire, J., and Sun, F. (1979). *Biochim. Biophys. Acta 573*, 238-244.

Gasic, G. J., Gasic, T. B., and Stewart, C. C. (1968). *Proc. Natl. Acad. Sci. USA 61*, 46-52.

Gasic, G. J., Koch, P. A. G., Hsu, B., Gasic, T. B., and Niewiarowski, S. (1976). *Z. Krebsforsch 86*, 263-277.

Gasic, G. J., Boettiger, D., Catalfamo, J. L., Gasic, T. B., and Stewart, C. C. (1978). *Cancer Res. 38*, 2950-2955.

Gastpar, H., Ambrus, J., and Thurber, L. E. (1977). *J. Med. 8*, 53-56.

Gordon, J. L. (1976). *In* "Lysosomes in Biology and Pathology" (J. T. Dingle and R. T. Dean, eds.), Vol. 4, pp. 3-31. Elsevier-North Holland, Amsterdam.

Gordon, S. G., and Cross, B. A. (1981). *J. Clin. Invest. 67*, 1665-1671.

Gorman, R. R., Bundy, G. L., Peterson, D. C., Sun, F. F., Miller, O. V., and Fitzpatrick, F. A. (1977). *Proc. Natl. Acad. Sci. USA 74*, 4007-4011.

Hamberg, M., and Samuelsson, B. (1973). *Proc. Natl. Acad. Sci. USA 70*, 899-904.

Hamberg, M., and Samuelsson, B. (1974). *Proc. Natl. Acad. Sci. USA 71*, 3400-3404.

Hammerstrom, S. (1977). *Biochim. Biophys. Acta 487*, 517-519.

Hara, Y., Steiner, M., and Baldini, M. G. (1980). *Cancer Res. 40*, 1217-1222.

Hilgard, P. (1973). *Br. J. Cancer 28*, 429-435.

Holmsen, H., and Day, H. J. (1970). *J. Lab. Clin. Med. 75*, 841-855.

Holmsen, H., and Weiss, H. J. (1979). *Annu. Rev. Med. 30*, 119-134.

Honn, K. V. (1982). *In* "Prostaglandins and Cancer" (T. J. Powles, R. S. Bockman, K. V. Honn, and P. W. Ramwell, eds.), pp. 733-752. Liss, New York.

Honn, K. V. (1983). *Clin. Exp. Metastasis 1*, 103-114.

Honn, K. V., and Dunn, J. R. (1982). *Fed. Eur. Biochem. Soc. Lett. 139*, 65-68.

Honn, K. V., Cicone, B., and Skoff, A. (1981). *Science (Washington, D.C.) 212*, 1270-1272.

Honn, K. V., Cavanaugh, P., Evens, C., Taylor, J. D., and Sloane, B. F. (1982a). *Science (Washington, D.C.) 217*, 540-542.

Honn, K. V., Meyer, J., Neagos, G., Henderson, T., Westley, C., and Ratanatharathorn, V. (1982b). *In* "Interactions of Platelets and Tumor Cells" (G. A. Jamieson, ed.), pp. 295-331. Liss, New York.

Honn, K. V., Busse, W. D., and Sloane, B. F. (1983a). *Biochem. Pharmacol. 32*, 1-11.

Honn, K. V., Menter, D., Moilanen, D., Cavanaugh, P. G., Taylor, J. D., and Sloane, B. F. (1983b). *In* "Protective Agents in Cancer" (D. C. H. McBrien and T. F. Slater, eds.), pp. 57-79. Academic Press, New York.

Hope, W., Martin, T. J., Chesterman, C. N., and Morgan, F. J. (1979). *Nature (London) 282*, 210-212.

Jamieson, G. A. (ed.) (1982). "Interaction of Platelets and Tumor Cells." Liss, New York.

Kaplan, K. L. (1981). *In* "Platelets in Biology and Pathology" (J. L. Gordon, ed.), Vol. 2, pp. 77-90. Elsevier-North Holland, Amsterdam.

Karpatkin, S., Smerling, A., and Pearlstein, E. (1980). *J. Lab. Clin. Med. 96*, 994-1001.

Kirschke, H., and Shaw, E. (1981). *Biochem. Biophys. Res. Commun. 101*, 454-458.

Lipton, A., Kepner, N., Roger, C., Witkowski, E., and Leitzel, K. (1982). *In* "Interactions of Platelets and Tumor Cells" (G. A. Jamieson, ed.), pp. 233-248. Liss, New York.

Marcum, J. M., McGill, M., Bastida, E., Ordinas, A., and Jamieson, G. A. (1980). *J. Lab. Clin. Med. 96*, 1048-1053.

Menter, D., Neagos, G., Dunn, J., Palazzo, R., Tchen, T. T., Taylor, J. D., and Honn, K. V. (1982). *In* "Prostaglandins and Cancer" (T. J. Powles, R. S. Bockman, K. V. Honn, and P. W. Ramwell, eds.), pp. 809-813. Liss, New York.

Miyamoto, T., Ogino, N., Yamamoto, S., and Hayaishi, O. (1976). *J. Biol. Chem. 251*, 2629-2633.

Moncada, S., and Vane, J. R. (1977). *In* "Biochemical Aspects of Prostaglandins and Thromboxanes" (N. Kharasch and J. Fried, eds.), pp. 155-177. Academic Press, New York.

Moncada, S., and Vane, J. R. (1980). *In* "Advances in Prostaglandin and Thromboxane Research" (B. Samuelsson, P. W. Ramwell, and R. Paoletti, eds.), Vol. 6, pp. 43-60. Raven, New York.

Moncada, S., Gryglewski, R. J., Bunting, S., and Vane, J. R. (1976a). *Nature (London) 263*, 663-665.

Moncada, S., Gryglewski, R. J., Bunting, S., and Vane, J. R. (1976b). *Prostaglandins 12*, 715-733.
Mort, J. S., Recklies, A. D., and Poole, A. R. (1980). *Biochim. Biophys. Acta 614*, 134-143.
Mullane, K. M., Dusting, G. J., Salmon, J. A., Moncada, S., and Vane, J. R. (1979). *Eur. J. Pharmacol. 54*, 217-228.
Needleman, P., Raz, A., Ferrendelli, J. A., and Minkes, M. (1977). *Proc. Natl. Acad. Sci. USA 74*, 1716-1720.
Nugteren, D. H., and Hazelhof, E. (1973). *Biochim. Biophys. Acta 326*, 448-461.
Paschen, W., Patschcke, H., and Worner, P. (1979). *Blut 38*, 17-24.
Pearlstein, E., Cooper, L. B., and Karpatkin, S. (1979). *J. Lab. Clin. Med. 93*, 332-344.
Pearlstein, E., Salk, P. L., Yogeeswaran, G., and Karpatkin, S. (1980). *Proc. Natl. Acad. Sci. USA 77*, 4336-4339.
Pearlstein, E., Ambrogio, C., Gasic, G., and Karpatkin, S. (1981). *Cancer Res. 41*, 4535-4539.
Pietras, R. J., Szego, C. M., Mangan, C. E., Seeler, B. J., Burtnett, M. M., and Orevi, M. (1978). *Obstet. Gynecol. (N.Y.) 52*, 321-327.
Pietras, R. J., Szego, C. M., Mangan, C. E., Seeler, B. J., and Burtnett, M. M. (1979). *Gynecol. Oncol. 7*, 1-17.
Pietras, R. J., Szego, C. M., Roberts, J. A., and Seeler, B. J. (1981). *J. Histochem. Cytochem. 29*, 440-450.
Piper, P. J. (1981). "SRS-A and Leukotrienes." Wiley, New York.
Poole, A. R., Tiltman, K. J., Recklies, A. D., and Stoker, T. A. M. (1978). *Nature (London) 273*, 545-547.
Randall, M. J., Parry, M. J., Hawkeswouk, E., Cross, P. E., and Dickinson, R. P. (1981). *Thromb. Res. 23*, 145-162.
Recklies, A. D., Tiltman, K. J., Stoker, T. A. M., and Poole, A. R. (1980). *Cancer Res. 40*, 550-556.
Rinderknecht, J., and Renner, I. G. (1980). *N. Engl. J. Med. 303*, 462-463.
Salmon, J. A., Smith, D. R., Flower, R. S., Moncada, S., and Vane, J. R. (1978). *Biochim. Biophys. Acta 523*, 250-262.
Seuter, F., Busse, W. D., Meng, K., Hofmeister, F., Moller, E., and Horstmann, H. (1979). *Arzneim. Forsch. 29*, 54-59.
Skolnik, G., Alpsten, M., and Ivarsson, L. (1980). *J. Cancer Res. Clin. Oncol. 97*, 249-256.
Sloane, B. F., Dunn, J. R., and Honn, K. V. (1981). *Science (Washington, D.C.) 212*, 1151-1153.
Sloane, B. F., Honn, K. V., Sadler, J. G., Turner, W. A., Kimpson, J. J., and Taylor, J. D. (1982a). *Cancer Res. 42*, 980-986.
Sloane, B. F., Makim, S., Dunn, J. R., Lacoste, R., Theodorou, M., Battista, J., Alex, R., and Honn, K. V. (1982b). *In* "Prostaglandins and Cancer" (T. J. Powles, R. S. Bockman, K. V. Honn, and P. W. Ramwell, eds.), pp. 789-792. Liss, New York.
Stringfellow, D. A., and Fitzpatrick, F. A. (1979). *Nature (London) 282*, 76-78.

Szczeklik, A., Gryglewski, R. J., Nizankowski, R., Musial, J., Pieton, R., and Mruk, J. (1978). *Pharmacol. Res. Commun. 10*, 545-556.
Tai, H. H., and Yuan, B. (1978). *Biochem. Biophys. Res. Commun. 80*, 236-242.
Takio, K., Towatari, T., Katunuma, N., and Titani, K. (1980). *Biochem. Biophys. Res. Commun. 97*, 340-346.
Turner, W. A., Menter, D. G., Honn, K. V., and Taylor, J. D. (1983). *Proc. Am. Assoc. Cancer Res. 24*, 25.
Vane, J. R. (1971). *Nature (London) New Biol. 231*, 232-235.
Wong, P. Y.-K., Chao, P. H.-W., and McGiff, J. C. (1982). *J. Pharmacol. Exp. Ther. 223*, 757-760.
Zacharski, L. R. (1982). *In* "Interaction of Platelets and Tumor Cells" (G. A. Jamieson, ed.), pp. 113-129. Liss, New York.
Zacharski, L. R., Henderson, W. G., Rickles, F. R., Forman, W. B., Cornell, C. J., Jr., Forcier, R. J., Harrower, H. W., and Johnson, R. O. (1979). *Cancer (Philadelphia) 44*, 732-741.

DISCUSSION

HOSHINO: In some cases of cancer, especially in an advanced case, we could observe thrombocytosis. Do you think this increase of platelets is due to feedback of platelets? Does the increase in platelets potentiate the occurrence of metastasis?

HONN: I am aware of the appearance of thrombocytopenia in patients with advanced disease; however, I was not aware of an increase in platelet production. I think your suggestion that it may be due to some compensatory feedback mechanism is correct. Whether or not this increased platelet production would facilitate further metastasis is unclear. However, as you well know, experimentally induced thrombocytopenia does decrease metastatic tumor formation in experimental animal systems. Therefore, it is reasonable to expect that an increase in platelet numbers may facilitate further metastasis from preexisting metastatic lesions.

COHEN: Do anticoagulants such as heparin or dicumarol influence the platelet's prostaglandin metabolism? In addition to the postulated effect on fibrin meshes around tumor cells, these agents are potent inhibitors of delayed hypersensitivity, and could be harmful. I wonder if they have a third effect, related to the system you describe.

HONN: Heparin has been reported to sensitize platelet thromboxane synthase to external stimuli. High doses of

heparin are required for this effect; however, these
are the kinds of doses used for anticoagulation of
cancer patients.   I do not know of any information
regarding the effects of coumarin derivatives on
arachidonate metabolism.

WEISS: Could you explain the antimetastatic effects of
              prostacyclin without invoking platelets?

HONN: Prostacyclin, most definitely, can have effects directly
              on the tumor cell itself. As I demonstrated with the
              scanning electron micrographs and also the attachment
              data, it is rather obvious that prostacyclin is having
              dramatic effects on the tumor cell. In this regard
              prostacyclin limits the attachment of tumor cells to
              artificial substrata such as plastic and nylon fibers,
              and biologically relevant substrata such as endothelial
              cells and type IV collagen. However, I do not think
              that we are ready to discard the platelet hypothesis
              altogether. It is my feeling that the mechanism of
              platelet enhancement of tumor cell metastasis via the
              formation of large thrombi that arrest in the micro-
              vasculature may be an oversimplified approach to the
              problem. It is our belief that platelets are facilitat-
              ing the attachment of tumor cells to the endothelium.
              By facilitated attachment I do not necessarily mean the
              initial arrest but rather the formation of more perma-
              nent cellular adhesions with the endothelium. The
              mechanism for this facilitated attachment is currently
              unknown.

KONDO: What will happen if you treat animals with cancer as-
              cites by prostacyclin?

HONN: As prostacyclin does prevent homotypic tumor cell aggre-
              gation, I believe that prostacyclin would maintain an
              ascites tumor. However, we have recently published the
              effects of prostacyclin and thromboxanes on tumor cell
              proliferation. It so happens that prostacyclin in-
              hibits tumor cell proliferation. This is not a cyto-
              toxic effect but a cytostatic effect. Therefore, I feel
              that prostacyclin would limit the proliferation of an
              ascites tumor.

PART IV

Immunological Aspects of Metastatic Tumors

Chairpersons

Reiko F. Irie
Takehiko Tachibana

CHAPTER 19

CLINICOPATHOLOGICAL AND IMMUNOLOGICAL ASPECTS
OF METASTATIC MALIGNANT MELANOMA IN MAN

Alistair J. Cochran

Division of Surgical Oncology
John Wayne Clinic and Armand Hammer Laboratory
Departments of Pathology and Surgery
University of California at Los Angeles School of Medicine
Center for the Health Sciences
Los Angeles, California

Duan-Ren Wen

Division of Surgical Oncology
Department of Surgery
University of California at Los Angeles School of Medicine
Center for the Health Sciences
Los Angeles, California

BASIC MECHANISMS AND CLINICAL TREATMENT
OF TUMOR METASTASIS

I. INTRODUCTION

    Cutaneous malignant melanoma arises from melanocytes, melanin-
synthesizing dendritic cells that derive from the neural crest
during embryogenesis, and migrate to occupy a definitive position
in the basal layer of the epidermis, approximately one cell in 10
of the stratum basale being a melanocyte, intercalated between
basal keratinocytes (Cochran, 1970) (Fig. 1A). During the
development of a majority of malignant melanomas (malignant
melanoma with an adjacent component of superficial spreading type,
malignant melanoma with an adjacent component of lentigo maligna
type, and malignant melanoma with an adjacent component of acral
or mucosal lentigenous type), it is possible to recognize a series
of steps that are due to phenotypic alterations in some of the
tumor cells and are clinically relevant. The melanocytes first
acquire the capacity to proliferate within the body compartment
that is their normal location (melanoma *in situ*, horizontal growth
phase of melanoma) (Fig. 1B). Following a period of such growth
in situ, which may be as short as 1 or 2 years in the case of
superficial spreading melanoma or as long as 20 years in lentigo
maligna melanoma, some cells acquire the capacity to invade the
dermis. Initially, most such presumptious cells appear to be
destroyed by the body's defense mechanisms (Fig. 1C), as evidenced
by the presence of dermal fibrosis, telangiectasis, free pigment,
pigment in macrophages, and a variable lymphohistiocytic infiltrate. Subsequently, however, tumor cells arise that are able to
survive in the dermis (Fig. 1D), presumably because they have
acquired new advantageous characteristics, or have lost those that
mark them as abnormal to the host defense mechanisms. Such cells
initially seem capable only of survival in the dermis and lack
the ability to replicate or grow progressively. The sequence of
events from the intraepidermal growth phase to upper dermal involvement without progressive growth corresponds to the radial
growth phase of Clark and colleagues (Elder *et al.*, 1979). Later,
progressive cohesive growth capacities develop, and such cells
produce invasive tumor (vertical growth phase) (Fig. 1E). This
last step is especially important because the development of
metastases from any stage before it is extremely unlikely.
    Following a period of further locally expansive growth, which
is of variable duration, a population of melanoma cells develops
that can penetrate lymphatic or blood vessel walls, survive the
physically and chemically hostile environment of blood or lymph,
repenetrate the vascular wall, and establish themselves in sites
remote from the primary tumor (Fig. 1F). Malignant melanoma
tumor deposits that have reached the regional lymph nodes, presumably via the lymphatic system, are the first detectable
metastases in the great majority of patients, although some
patients develop hematogenously spread deposits as their first
manifestation of metastatic disease.

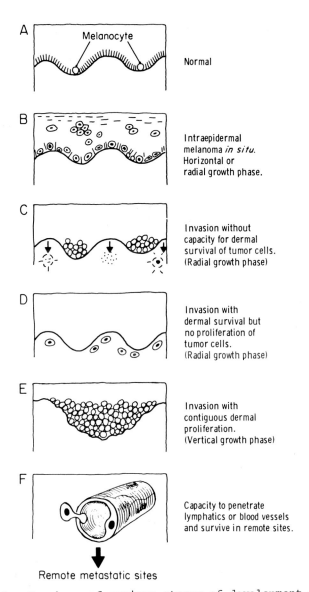

A — Melanocyte — Normal

B — Intraepidermal melanoma *in situ.* Horizontal or radial growth phase.

C — Invasion without capacity for dermal survival of tumor cells. (Radial growth phase)

D — Invasion with dermal survival but no proliferation of tumor cells. (Radial growth phase)

E — Invasion with contiguous dermal proliferation. (Vertical growth phase)

F — Capacity to penetrate lymphatics or blood vessels and survive in remote sites.

Remote metastatic sites

Fig. 1. A schema of various stages of development of malignant melanoma.

The significance of the development of metastases is clearly demonstrated by the survival figures. Patients with primary malignant melanoma have a 5-year survival rate that varies from 75 to 90% (Cochran, 1969; Das Gupta, 1977), and may approach 100% if tumors are identified and treated at an early stage, as assessed by measured tumor thickness (Breslow, 1970) or by depth of penetration relative to standard anatomical landmarks of the dermis (Clark, 1967). The stark contrast is that the 5-year survival rate for patients in whom the disease has spread to the regional lymph nodes may be as low as 14% and

at best may reach 51% (Fortner *et al.*, 1964; Cochran, 1969; Das
Gupta, 1977; Balch *et al.*, 1981; Callery *et al.*, 1982). Survival
rates for patients with blood-spread metastases are even worse,
as few patients are alive even a year after demonstration of their
extended disease.

However dire the survival results are in patients with malignant melanoma spread to the regional nodes, it is apparent that
this group is not homogeneous and the outlook is not uniformly
poor. There are significant numbers of long-term survivors after
therapeutic lymphadenectomy, and identification of those factors
that determine death or survival for the individual seems likely
to provide valuable insights into the nature and mechanisms of
metastatic disease, as well as being of great value in designing
therapeutic strategies.

With this in mind, we recently studied a group of patients
with regionally metastatic malignant melanoma (Callery *et al.*,
1982).

II. PROGNOSTIC FACTORS IN PATIENTS WITH (LYMPH NODE LOCATED)
     REGIONAL SPREAD OF MALIGNANT MELANOMA

Clinical records of all melanoma patients with histologically
proved regional lymph node metastases who were seen at UCLA
between January 1954 and June 1976 were reviewed. Patients were
excluded if unresectable soft tissue invasion was observed at
lymphadenectomy, if they had disseminated melanoma present at the
time of lymphadenectomy, or if they had received prophylactic
immunotherapy or chemotherapy following lymphadenectomy. Patients
who had presented initially with localized melanoma were eligible
if seen subsequently at UCLA when nodal disease developed, provided that nodal disease was diagnosed before systemic involvement.
There were 150 such patients, 90 males and 60 females, aged 14-79
years (median 48 years). The clinical and histological data recorded for each patient and analyzed against survival as being
potentially of prognostic value are given in Table I.

The total number of positive and negative lymph nodes identified in each lymphadenectomy specimen was obtained from the
pathology reports. When slides of the lymph nodes were available,
the actual number of node profiles containing tumor was verified.

Sufficient data were available for valid statistical analysis
of the following: age, sex, parity, site of primary lesion,
presence of satellitosis, clinical status of nodes, number of
histologically positive lymph nodes, and the histological characteristics of the primary lesion. Survival was calculated from
date of lymphadenectomy to last follow-up or death.

Survival curves were calculated using the Kaplan-Meier estimate
(Kaplan and Meier, 1958). The proportional hazards model developed
by Cox (1972) was used to test for differences in the survival of

TABLE I

Clinical and Histological Observations that Were Recorded and
Analyzed against Survival as Being Potentially of Prognostic Value

Clinical observations	Histological Observations
Patient characteristics	Tumor profile
Age	Ulceration
Sex	Presence or absence
Parity	Measured width
Primary tumor characteristics	Histogenetic pattern
Diameter	Level of invasion (Clark)
Site	Tumor thickness (Breslow)
Ulceration	Vascular invasion
Satellitosis	Mitotic rate (McGovern *et*
Treatment	*al.*, 1973).
Local excision	Extent of lymphoreticular
Skin graft	infiltrate
Primary closure	
Lymph nodes	
Clinically palpable	
Clinically impalpable	
Time	
Primary--lymph node disease	
Primary--dissemination	
Lymph node-dissemination	
Complications	
Of primary surgery	
Of lymph node surgery	

patients within different subcategories of each factor. When only
one factor was considered, this procedure was similar to the
Mantel-Haenszel, or log-rank test. This procedure tested differences during the entire period of the survival curve; therefore,
5-year survival rates are given for illustrative purposes only.

Variables such as the number of tumor-containing nodes were
analyzed first as continuous variables, and then by dividing the
overall range into intervals. The effect of the number of tumor-
positive nodes on survival was analyzed by the following subcategories: one node positive versus two to four nodes positive
versus five or more nodes positive, or three or fewer nodes positive versus four or more nodes positive. Subcategories were
revised when analysis suggested that patients in two or more
subcategories could be combined on the basis of similar survival.
The subcategory arrangement that maximally separated the subgroups is reported. The statistical analyses using continuous
factors yielded results similar to those obtained when the factors
were satisfactorily categorized.

Adequate histopathological material was not available for some patients. At each step in the (step-up) Cox analysis, data from all patients with complete information for that step were used. Hence, the total of patients decreased as the number of steps increased. To verify the results of the step-up analysis, all patients with complete data for factors found individually prognostic were selected. Re-analysis of this limited number of patients for whom complete data were available yielded conclusions similar to those of the Cox analysis of the larger, less complete group.

The stepwise procedure included an assessment of the statistical significance of the interaction between factors in the Cox model. The interaction is significant if the effect of a factor on survival is significantly different among patients with varying levels of another factor. For example, the interaction between tumor thickness and number of tumor-positive nodes would be significant if patients with four or more tumor-positive nodes had increased survival when their primary tumor was less than 1 mm thick, but had a decreased survival when their primary tumor was more than 4 mm thick. This was not, in fact, true in the present analysis. A detailed description of the statistical methods and analyses employed will be presented elsewhere (D. J. Roe and A. J. Cochran, unpublished).

III. RESULTS

A. Univariate Analysis

Using a univariate analysis, the following factors were found to be related to survival after lymphadenectomy (Table II). The number of tumor-containing lymph nodes identified microscopically was predictive; patients with three or fewer tumorous nodes survived longer than those with four or more tumor-positive nodes ($p = .026$). The micrometer-measured thickness of the primary tumor also related to survival after lymphadenectomy--patients with thicker tumors survived for shorter periods after lymph node surgery ($p < .001$). The presence or absence of ulceration and the micrometer-measured extent of ulceration in the primary tumor were predictive of survival--patients with nonulcerated tumors survived longest after lymphadenectomy, whereas those with extensively ulcerated primary tumors died quickly ($p = .029$ and $.003$, respectively).

Factors that were not significant in the univariate analysis included patient age, sex, and parity, tumor site, satellitosis, whether the nodes were clinically palpable, whether the tumor was incisionally or excisionally biopsied, the Clark level of invasion, whether the primary tumor had an adjacent component of superficial spreading melanoma type or had no adjacent component

TABLE II

Factors Predictive of Survival after Lymphadenectomy
in Patients with Malignant Melanoma Metastatic to
the Regional Lymph Nodes (Univariate Analysis)

Factor	Subcategory	Number of patients	5-Year survival rate (%)	p [a]
Thickness (mm)	<1.00	13	62	
Breslow	1.00-2.99	46	46	<.001
	3.00-3.99	16	31	
	4.00	12	0	
Ulceration	Yes	49	34	.029
	No	43	47	
Ulceration, width	0	42	49	
	≤6 mm	30	36	.003
	>6 mm	13	0	
Tumor-containing nodes	≤3	95	45	.026
	≥4	27	21	

[a]Continuous variables were tested using a variety of cut-off
points, and only the most significant for each variable is shown.
Statistical significance for each univariate comparison was derived
from the entire Kaplan-Meier life table curve for each factor.
Figures for 5-year survival after lymphadenectomy were derived from
the Kaplan-Meier estimates and are presented for illustrative purposes only.

(nodular melanoma), and the frequency of mitoses in the primary
tumor.

B. Multivariate Analysis

In the multivariate analysis using the Cox procedure, the
thickness of the primary tumor ($p < .001$) and the number of
melanoma-involved lymph nodes ($p = .04$) were statistically significant. The statistical test of the interaction between thickness and number of melanoma-involved lymph nodes (the multipli-
cative effect of these two variables on survival) yielded a
p value of .10. None of the other factors analyzed and found
significant in the univariate analysis achieved significance in
the multivariate analysis. The presence and width of ulceration of the primary lesion were not significant in the multivariate analysis ($p = .21$ and .19, respectively) because of the

strong association between the tumor thickness and the width of
tumor ulceration categories. For example, of the 13 patients
with tumors less than 1 mm thick, 10 (83%) had no ulceration, two
(17%) had a width of ulceration 6 mm or less, and none had a width
of ulceration greater than 6 mm. Conversely, of the 12 patients
with tumors 4 mm thick or thicker, 1 (8%) had no ulceration, 5
(42%) had a width of ulceration 6 mm or less, and 6 (50%) had a
width of ulceration greater than 6 mm. However, this strong association was due largely to our success in choosing subcategories
of thickness and width of ulceration, since the correlation coefficient between these two characteristics (considered as continuous
variables) was .35, mostly a result of the wide scatter of values
observed.

From these data it is clear that one can predict, to a limited
extent, the likely clinical course of groups of patients after
surgical excision of lymph nodes that contain metastatic malignant
melanoma. Thus, patients who had originally thin primary tumors
(<1 mm thick) and who had only a limited number of nodes replaced
by melanoma had a substantial chance (50-60%) of being alive
5 years after lymphadenectomy. By contrast, patients whose primary tumor was thick (>4 mm) or who had many (>4) lymph nodes
replaced by metastatic melanoma had a very high probability of
dying in less than 5 years after lymphadenectomy (80-100%). We
must admit, however, that predictions based on conventional clinical observations and the examinations of routinely stained random
representative sections of lymph nodes are still relatively im-
precise. Predictions of outcome for the individual patient remain
less accurate than one would wish. At least 40% of the "favorable
prognosis" group did badly, dying with melanomatosis less than 5
years after lymphadenectomy, and as many as 20% of the "unfavor-
able prognosis" group survived more than 5 years after node dissection.

Figure 2 depicts the survival of the study group after lymphadenectomy. Three broad groups of survivors may be observed:
Group A consists of 40% of the patients, who died of melanomatosis
within 15 months of nodal surgery; a further 20% (group B) died of
their disease at between 15 months and 4 years after lymphadenectomy; and about 40% (group C) are alive at 4 years and, having
achieved this lengthy survival, most are unlikely to succumb to
their tumor. We believe that these three subgroups are the result
of the interaction of various factors: (1) completeness of the
surgical resection of the tumor, (2) extent and anatomical disposition of residual tumor deposits, (3) tumor characteristics,
including mitotic rate, host-recognizable neoantigenicity, capacity to survive in different body sites remote from the point of
primary origin, and chemosensitivity, and (4) effectiveness of the
various host defense mechanisms against the tumor cells. The
various potential interactions of these factors are shown in
Table III, and the likely outcome of such interactions for each
combination of factors is postulated.

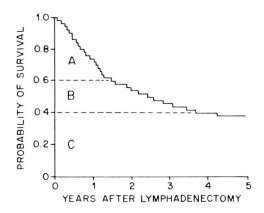

Fig. 2. Probability of survival for 150 stage II melanoma patients (total dead, 92). Group A consists of 40% of patients who died of their disease by 15 months; group B consists of 20% of patients who died of their disease between 15 months and 4 years; group C includes 40% of patients who lived for 4 or more years after lymph node dissection.

TABLE III

Some Potential Combinations of Tumor and Host Factors
and the Likely Clinical Outcome of Such Combinations

Residual tumor	Tumor characteristics	Host defenses	Group	Probable result
Nil	Not relevant	Strong	C	Cure
Minimal	Favorable	Strong	B/C	Cure or late progression
Minimal	Unfavorable	Strong	B	Late progression
Minimal	Unfavorable	Weak	B	Medium progression
Moderate	Favorable	Strong	B	Medium progression
Moderate	Favorable	Weak	B	Early progression
Moderate	Unfavorable	Strong/Weak	B	Early progression
Much	Favorable	Strong	A	Rapid progression
Much	Unfavorable	Weak	A	Very rapid progression

From these considerations, it is apparent that errors in prognosis assessment for the individual melanoma patient could be reduced if we were better able to assess tumor extent, and if significant host defense factors could be identified and assessed. Assessment of residual tumor distribution and extent is probably best undertaken by the recently developed imaging techniques, and

by this type of approach, previously impossible degrees of accuracy
in locating tumor deposits and their extent are becoming attain-
able. This is one of the areas where truly tumor-directed monoclonal antibodies may be applicable. It is also possible that the
identification and quantification of tumor products in blood and
urine may indirectly demonstrate the extent of residual tumor after
lymphadenectomy.

Another approach to this side of the question is to ask
whether our current evaluations of the extent of lymph node involvement by melanoma are accurate. This is a question that we are currently addressing, and our preliminary results are given in Section
IV. It is possible to assess many different aspects of the host
defense mechanisms, especially those relating to the immune system.
Many data have been published on the general immune competence of
cancer patients and allegedly tumor-targeted immune responses (for
a review see Cochran, 1978). Which, if any, of these observations
are most significantly related to tumor progression or regression
remains quite unknown. Most previous studies have concentrated on
the immune system as reflected in the peripheral blood compartment,
whereas studies of those portions of the system most closely linked
to the tumor cells, peritumoral lymphocytes, and tumor-infiltrating
lymphocytes, and the regional lymph nodes that drain the tumor may
be most important. The nature, response, and performance of these
lymphoid cells that are attracted to and influenced by the cells of
a tumor may well give a better indication of the nature of the host
response in a given patient. With this in mind, we are currently
involved in extensive studies of the biology and immunology of the
regional lymph nodes of patients with malignant melanoma. The
final section of this chapter will summarize the nature of these
studies.

IV. AN INVESTIGATION OF THE ACCURACY OF CONVENTIONAL LYMPH NODE
     ASSESSMENT FOR TUMOR PRESENCE

As noted already, the number of lymph nodes found to contain
tumor on microscopic examination is an important predictor of
survival in the patient with melanoma spread to the regional nodes;
in particular, we found that patients who had tumor demonstrable
microscopically in three or fewer lymph nodes had relatively
favorable prognoses, an observation similar to that of others
(Cohen et al., 1977; Balch et al., 1979; Day et al., 1981). Nonetheless, 40% of these patients did badly, and we were concerned
that this might be at least in part a result of our underestimating
the number of tumor-positive lymph nodes, either because of sampling
error or by our missing small numbers of inapparent tumor cells
during examination of conventionally stained sections. We elected
to examine the latter possibility using an antiserum to S-100 protein that we and others have demonstrated to be a useful (although

TABLE IV

S-100 Content of Various Tumors

Tumor type	Number	Positive
Malignant melanoma		
Primary	24	24
Lymph node metastases	21	21
Hematogenous metastases	15	15
All melanomas	60	60
Nevocytic nevi		
Junctional nevi	5	5
Compound nevi	16	16
Intradermal nevi	9	9
Blue nevi	3	3
Epithelial cell nevus	1	1
All nevi	34	34
Nonmelanocytic, nonneural tumors		
Ectodermal	17	1
Mesodermal	21	0
Endodermal	19	0
All	57	1

not absolutely specific) marker for the melanocyte-derived cells of nevi and malignant melanomas (Gaynor et al., 1980, 1981; Nakajima et al., 1981; Clark et al., 1982; Cochran et al., 1982).

S-100 protein is an acidic protein of unknown function; its name derives from its solubility in saturated ammonium sulfate at neutral pH (Moore, 1965). It has been demonstrated in glial cells in the brain (Moore, 1965; Moore and MacGregor, 1965), in the enteric nervous system (Ferri et al., 1982), in Schwann cells of the peripheral nervous system, and in satellite cells in the peripheral ganglia (Eng et al., 1976). More recently, there have been claims that S-100 protein may occur in other tissues including chondrocytes (Stefansson et al., 1982), interdigitating reticulum cells in lymph nodes (Takahashi et al., 1981), and Langerhans cells in the epidermis (Cocchia et al., 1981). It exhibits a strong serological cross-reactivity among a variety of different species (Kessler et al., 1968). The expression of S-100 protein is apparently not correlated with the degree of synthesis of melanin, which makes it suitable for identification of hypomelanotic or amelanotic melanoma cells. S-100 protein persists after formalin fixation and dehydration, and may be sought in conventionally fixed and embedded tissues.

In previous studies, using immunofluorescence of frozen sections (Gaynor et al., 1981) and an indirect immunoperoxidase assay

on formalin-fixed, paraffin-embedded tissues, we found S-100 protein in 60 malignant melanomas tested, regardless of tumor stage
or organ source of the tissues, and in 34 melanocytic nevi of
various kinds. In 57 nonmelanocytic, nonneural tumors tested,
only one, a breast carcinoma, contained S-100 protein (Table IV).

    We are currently attempting to assess whether the antiserum
to S-100 protein can detect small numbers of melanoma cells in
lymph nodes, melanoma cells that had not been detected in conventionally stained tissues during routine assessment. To examine
this, we obtained paraffin blocks containing tissue from lymph
node dissections performed on the patients who comprised the study
population that was the basis of our recent article on prognostic
factors in patients with stage II melanoma (Callery et al., 1982).
Tissue sections were cut at 5 μm and used in an immunoperoxidase
assay (see later). All slides were coded before being read, and
the histological diagnosis (tumor positive or tumor negative) was
not known to the individuals reading the results.

A. Immunoperoxidase Technique

    The slides were deparaffinized by exposure to xylene for
10 min, and washed three times for 3 min in 100% ethyl alcohol.
Slides were then washed in each of the following solutions for
2 min: 95% ethyl alcohol, 75% ethyl alcohol, and distilled water.
Endogenous peroxidases in the tissues were quenched by exposure
to 3% hydrogen peroxidase for 20 min. The slides were then washed
in running tap water for 1 min, dipped in distilled water, and
rinsed three times in a Tris-saline solution. The slides were exposed to 5% egg albumin for 20 min and then rinsed in Tris-saline.
Rabbit antiserum to bovine S-100 protein was applied for 1 hr at
dilutions ranging from 1:50 to 1:200. Negative control slides
were treated with normal rabbit serum at dilutions from 1:20 to
1:100, and the first antibody was omitted. A positive control was
provided by exposing slides containing known reactive melanoma
cells and cutaneous nerves to both antibodies and developer. Absorption of the anti-S-100 protein removed all the activity
against melanoma and nerve. Slides were then washed three times
with Tris buffer. Swine anti-rabbit serum diluted 1:20 (Dako Inc.,
Santa Barbara, California) was applied for 30 min and the slides
then rinsed three times in Tris buffer. A peroxidase antiperoxi-
dase preparation diluted 1:100 (Dako Inc., Santa Barbara, California) was applied for 30 min before the slides were washed in
Tris buffer for 5 min. The slides were then immersed in substrate
solution of 6 ml of aminoethyl carbizole (AEC) developer plus 50 ml
of a 0.02 monosodium acetate buffer, plus 0.4 ml of a 3% solution
of hydrogen peroxide for 10 min. The AEC developer was prepared
by dissolving 167 mg of 3-amino 9-ethyl carbazole and 100 ml of
dimethyl sulfoxide. The slides were cleansed in running tap water,
dipped in distilled water, counterstained by hematoxylin for 3 min,

washed again in tap water, and finally dipped in a saturated
aqueous solution of sodium bicarbonate. The slides were finally
rinsed in distilled water, and a cover glass was applied.

Staining is remarkably durable, but for uniformity we tried
to read the preparations within 24 hr. The advantage of amino-
ethylcarbazole is that it produces a red color that is readily dis-
cernible from the range of browns represented by the melanins.

Antiserum to bovine S-100 protein was prepared against antigen
purified as described previously (Zuckerman et al., 1970). The
serological specificity of the antiserum was shown by double diffusion in agar and by quantitative complement fixation analysis
employing soluble protein extracts of a variety of tissues as
antigen (Gaynor et al., 1980, 1981). Further evidence of
specificity was provided by the extensive immunoperoxidase studies
of a wide range of tumorous and normal tissues described in a recent publication (Cochran et al., 1982).

B. Results

At the present time, material from 18 patients has been
evaluated (Table V). We used the previously described criteria
for assessing likely outcome: Patients with three or fewer lymph
nodes containing tumor were more likely to survive, and those
with four or more positive nodes were more likely to die from
their melanoma. In the group of 12 patients who had three or
fewer nodes positive on H&E staining, eight individuals died of
melanoma, giving an accuracy of prediction of only 33%. In the
group of six patients who had four or more tumorous nodes on H&E
assessment, only one patient survived for 3 years after a lymphadenectomy that yielded six tumor-containing lymph nodes; this was
an accuracy of prediction of 83%.

After staining recut sections as nearly contiguous to the permanent sections as possible with anti-S-100 protein serum, tumor
was identified in an increased number of lymph nodes (relative to
H&E detections) in seven patients. This detection of an increased
number of tumor-positive lymph nodes moved two patients from the
group predicted to have a good prognosis to that regarded as having
a poor prognosis, a move that was apparently appropriate, as both
died of melanoma less than a year after lymphadenectomy. In the
remaining patients, H&E staining had already detected four or more
tumor-positive nodes, and the anti-S-100 protein technique merely
increased the total number of positive nodes detected in those
patients who were already, correctly, regarded as likely to die of
the effects of their tumors.

Staining with anti-S-100 protein serum placed 10 patients in
the good prognosis category ($\leq$3 nodes positive for tumor), and four
died of melanoma after 6, 6, 24, and 48 months, respectively--an
accuracy of prediction of 60%. Similarly, eight patients were
placed in the poor prognosis category ($\geq$4 nodes positive), and of

TABLE V

Accuracy of Predictions of Survival or Death from
Melanoma Based on Detection of Melanoma in Regional
Lymph Nodes by H&E Staining or α-S-100 Protein
Serum Reactivity with Melanoma Cells

Detection technique	Hematoxylin and eosin	Anti-S-100 protein serum
Total patients tested	18	18
≤3 Nodes positive	12	10
Long-term survivors	4	4
Accuracy of prediction of survival (%)	33	40
≥4 Nodes positive	6	8
Melanoma deaths	5	7
Accuracy of prediction of melanoma death (%)	83	88
Overall predictive accuracy (%)	50	61

those only one survived for any length of time, an accuracy of
prediction of 88%.

From these data it is apparent that conventional H&E staining
may underestimate the amount of tumor present in a group of lymph
nodes, particularly if the number of nodes involved is small.
The application of the anti-S-100 protein technique may slightly
improve the accuracy of prognostication by properly placing a few
patients in the high-risk group. Nonetheless, it is clear that
this approach still leaves patients who are inappropriately placed
in the "good" prognosis group, and it is in these individuals that
a more precise assessment of the defense mechanisms seems desirable
It is notable that the accuracy of placement of patients in the
high-risk group is very precise whether by H&E-based assessment of
the nodes or by the application of anti-S-100 serum.

V.   ASSESSMENT OF THE ROLE OF HOST DEFENSE MECHANISMS IN
DETERMINING THE SURVIVAL OF MELANOMA PATIENTS AFTER LYMPHA-
DENECTOMY FOR MALIGNANT MELANOMA SPREAD TO THE REGIONAL
LYMPH NODES

Studies in progress in the Division of Surgical Oncology at
UCLA are designed to examine the manner in which the regional
lymph nodes draining the site of a primary malignant melanoma or

containing metastatic malignant melanoma respond to tumor proximity or presence. We seek to assess whether the node group responds as a whole or whether individual nodes respond differently, perhaps in relation to their proximity to the tumor. To this end, we are examining the distribution of tumor in individual nodes and the nature and extent of lymph node reactions in nodes oriented anatomically in the body and relative to the tumor. The proportions of the different classes and subclasses of lymphocytes and of macrophages are being quantified *in situ* in frozen sections and in cell suspensions, using monoclonal antibodies and immunoperoxidase and rosetting techniques. Tumor-directed sensitization and T, K, and NK cytotoxicity are being investigated (see also Golub *et al.*, Chapter 7, this volume).

It seems likely that truly accurate predictions of survival or death for the individual with malignant melanoma metastatic to nodes will be possible only when immunological and possibly biochemical data (see Morton *et al.*, Chapter 32, this volume) are added to the more conventional observations noted earlier in this chapter.

ACKNOWLEDGMENTS

The studies here described were supported by Public Health Service (PHS) grants CA 29938, CA 12582, CA 29605, and Contract CB 18525 from the National Cancer Institute (NCI).

REFERENCES

Balch, C. M., Murad, T. M., Soong, S. J., *et al.* (1979). *Cancer (Philadelphia) 43*, 883-888.
Balch, C. M., Soong, S. J., Murad, T. M., *et al.* (1981). *Ann. Surg. 193*, 377-388.
Breslow, A. (1970). *Ann. Surg. 172*, 902-908.
Callery, C., Cochran, A. J., Roe, D. J., Rees, W., Nathanson, S. D., Benedetti, J. K., Elashoff, R. M., and Morton, D. L. (1982). *Ann. Surg. 196*, 69-75.
Clark, H. B., Santa Cruz, D., Hartman, B. K., and Moore, B. W. (1982). *Lab. Invest. 46*, 13A (Abstr.).
Clark, W. H., Jr. (1967). *In* "Advances in Biology of Skin" (W. Montagna and F. Hu, eds.), Vol. 8, pp. 621-647. Pergamon, Oxford and New York.
Cocchia, D., Michetti, F., and Donato, R. (1981). *Nature (London) 294*, 85-87.
Cochran, A. J. (1969). *Cancer (Philadelphia) 23*, 1190-1199.
Cochran, A. J. (1970). *J. Invest. Dermatol. 55*, 65-70.

Cochran, A. J. (1978). "Man, Cancer and Immunity." Academic Press, London and New York.

Cochran, A. J., Wen, D.-R., Herschman, H. R., and Gaynor, R. B. (1982). *Int. J. Cancer 30*, 295-297.

Cohen, M. K., Ketcham, A. S., *et al.* (1977). *Ann. Surg. 186*, 635-642.

Cox, D. R. (1972). *J. R. Stat. Soc. B 34*, 187-220.

Das Gupta, T. K. (1977). *Ann. Surg. 186*, 201-209.

Day, C. L., Jr., Sober, A. J., Lew, R. A., *et al.* (1981). *Cancer (Philadelphia) 47*, 955-962.

Elder, D. E., Ainsworth, A. M., and Clark, W. H., Jr. (1979). *In* "Human Malignant Melanoma" (W. H. Clark, Jr., L. I. Goldman, and M. J. Mastrangelo, eds.), pp. 109-124. Grune & Stratton, New York.

Eng, L. F., Kosek, J. C., Forno, L., Deck, J., and Bigbee, J. (1976). *Trans. Am. Soc. Neurochem. 7*, 211.

Ferri, G. L., Probert, L., Cocchia, D., Michetti, F., Marangos, P. J., and Polak, J. M. (1982). *Nature (London) 297*, 409-410.

Fortner, J. G., Booker, R. F., and Pack, G. T. (1964). *Surgery (St. Louis) 55*, 485-494.

Gaynor, R., Irie, R. F., Morton, D. L., and Herschman, H. R. (1980). *Nature (London) 286*, 400-401.

Gaynor, R., Herschman, H. R., Irie, R. F., Jones, P. C., Morton, D. L., and Cochran, A. J. (1981). *Lancet 1*, 869-871.

Kaplan, E. L., and Meier, P. (1958). *J. Am. Stat. Assoc. 53*, 457-481.

Kessler, D., Levine, L., and Fassman, G. (1968). *Biochemistry 7*, 758-764.

McGovern, V. J., Mihm, M. C., Jr., Bailly, C., *et al.* (1973). *Cancer (Philadelphia) 32*, 1446-1457.

Moore, B. W. (1965). *Res. Commun. 19*, 739-747.

Moore, B. W., and MacGregor, D. (1965). *J. Biol. Chem. 240*, 1647-1653.

Nakajima, T., Watanabe, S., Sato, Y., Kameya, T., and Shimosato, Y. (1981). *Gann 72*, 335-336.

Stefansson, K., Wollman, R. L., and Moore, B. W. (1982). *Nature (London) 295*, 63-64.

Takahashi, K., Yamaguchi, H., Ishizeki, J., *et al.* (1981). *Virchows Arch. B 37*, 125-135.

Zuckerman, J., Herschman, H. R., and Levine, L. *J. Neurochem. 17*, 247-251.

DISCUSSION

MATHÉ: (1) Have you searched if S-100 protein is in immune com-
          plexes? (2) What is the proportion of patients who do
          not need BCG reduction?   (3) What is the correlation
          between BCG reduction need and lymph node invasion?

IRIE: S-100 proteins are *not* autoimmunogenic and would not be
          expected to be present complexed with antibody in any
          spontaneous situation.

COCHRAN: In this study 127 patients (84%) did not require reduc-
          tion of BCG dose. We have not yet correlated the need
          for reduction of BCG dose and the number of nodes
          positive by the anti-S-100 protein technique. We will
          certainly undertake this analysis in the future.

POSTE: Is the S-100 protein shed by melanoma cells? If so,
          might it be possible to assay this molecule in the cir-
          culation as a possible marker for occult metastasis at
          extranodal sites?

COCHRAN: We have no information on shedding of S-100 protein,
          although it *will* certainly escape dying cells. We are
          certainly interested in the detection of S-100 protein
          in body fluids, as a marker for the presence of residual
          melanoma. Our initial studies had some difficulties in
          identifying small quantities of S-100 protein in the
          presence of large amounts of other proteins. We will
          examine specific fluids such as ocular fluids, in which
          the probability of success seems relatively high.

LIOTTA: (1) Effects of fixation on immunoreactivity? (2) What
          percentage of tumor cells stain in a given section?

COCHRAN: S-100 protein is remarkably resistant to conventional
          fixation and embedding; however, delay in placing the
          tissue in formalin leads to a reduction in staining in-
          tensity. Formalin fixation is better than glutaralde-
          hyde. In a reactive tumor we would expect virtually all
          tumor cells to show some S-100 protein staining, but
          there would be a range of intensity.

OCHIAI: What is the survival rate of melanoma cancer patients
          if decided by malignancy and host defense mechanism?
          What kinds of factors will decide host defense activity?
          Is it decided by genetic restriction or nutrition?

COCHRAN: All aspects of the immune system seem to have a genetic
          background that will determine the response potential of

the individual. The actual response that results at the
time of a given antigenic challenge will vary according
to the individual's general health status, including nutritional status and immunological preoccupation with
other recent and concomitant antigenic challenges.

KONDO: A basic question concerning S-100 protein. You said the
protein is obtained from aged CNS and not young ones.
Can you stain CNS neoplasms providing immature character?

COCHRAN: Regarding your first point, there are age-related changes
in S-100 protein content, but the age of the bovine (or
other) brain used for extraction of S-100 protein is
probably not critical. Anti S-100 protein is useful in
categorizing gliomas, schwannomas, and, curiously,
granular cell myoblastoma, in addition to malignant
melanomas and nevi.

WEISS: Presumably the increased accuracy in correlation between
survival and lymphnode status is because you can detect
ultramicrometastases. Have you any idea of the upper
limit in number of melanoma cells in a lymph node that
have no prognostic significance? The Fishers consider
that within certain limits, axillary node micrometastases
have no prognostic significance; their assessment was
made on hematoxylin and eosin-stained material.

COCHRAN: We do not yet know the minimum number of tumor cells that
is significant, nor do we know which patterns of intra-
nodal spread are critical. These are subjects of current
study. In contrast to the breast cancer studies, it
looks as though small collections of tumor cells may be
relevant in the prognosis of stage II melanoma patients.
It should be remembered that the present study involves
a marker detection system.

CHAPTER 20

THE PRIMARY IMMUNOREGULATORY ROLE OF REGIONAL LYMPH NODES
ON THE DEVELOPMENT OF LOCAL TUMOR
AND LYMPHATIC METASTASIS

Kikuyoshi Yoshida
Takehiko Tachibana

Department of Immunology
Research Institute for Tuberculosis and Cancer
Tohoku University
Sendai, Japan

BASIC MECHANISMS AND CLINICAL TREATMENT
OF TUMOR METASTASIS

I.   INTRODUCTION

The regional lymph node is the organ that initially recognizes
antigens from the primary tumor. The first immune response to a
tumor antigen in the regional lymph node is an important factor
influencing the subsequent development of the primary tumor and
the secondary spread of the tumor. The immune response to a tumor
results in the generation of effector cell to the tumor, and also
suppressor cells.
   Goldfarb and Hardy (1975) demonstrated the role of the
regional lymph node in the initial processing of tumor antigenic
information, and Barna and Deodhar (1975) reported that the
initial tumor inhibition response is provided by the regional lymph
node cells. When a tumor grows progressively, the reactivity in
the regional lymph node declines, although the intermediate node
and spleen reactivities remain unchanged (Flannery et al., 1973;
Barna and Deodhar, 1975). In the absence of a regional lymph
node, no apparent sinecomitant or concomitant immunity develops
(Fisher and Fisher, 1971). The removal of an immunized node may
diminish the resistance of the host to metastasis (Crile, 1972).
These reports all suggest that the regional lymph node inhibits
tumor growth.
   In contrast, other reports indicate that the immunological responses of the regional lymph node have an adverse effect on the
host. The progressive growth of a tumor evokes a suppressive
activity in the regional lymph node mediated by T cells that produce soluble blocking factors (Barna and Deodhar, 1979) and
suppressor T cells (Hawrylko, 1982).
   In this chapter we study the relationship between immunological
responses and metastasis in the regional lymph node, using transplantable ascitic tumor MM48 cells derived from spontaneous
mammary tumor of C3H mouse, SMC XXIII described by Irie (1971).

TABLE I

Metastatic Capacity of the Original MM48 Tumor
and N10 Tumor Cell Lines

		Metastasis (RIDIT of HDM[a])		
Route	Lymph nodes	Original	N10	Difference
Deep	Popliteal	0.796 ± 0.100	0.545 ± 0.195	n.s.[b]
	Lumbar	0.769 ± 0.105	0.575 ± 0.224	n.s.
	Renal	0.355 ± 0.135	0.260	n.s.
Super-ficial	Popliteal	0.796 ± 0.100	0.656 ± 0.195	n.s.
	Inguinal	0.463 ± 0.146	0.550 ± 0.223	n.s.
	Axillary	0.390 ± 0.145	0.272 ± 0.091	n.s.

[a]The metastases in lymph nodes were histologically examined
20 days after tumor implantation. They were graded from (−) to
(+++): (−), a few tumor cells scattering in the marginal sinus;
(+), tumor cells clustering in the marginal sinus but not in intermediate, medullary sinuses and cortex; (++), tumor cells invading
into the intermediate, medullary sinuses and cortex; (+++), tumor
cells occupying more than half of the total area of a lymph node.
The grades were evaluated according to RIDIT analysis (Bross,
1958). Standard RIDIT values of metastasis grading were as follows: (−) 0.260; (±) 0.530; (+) 0.641; (++) 0.792; (+++) 0.941.
Results show the mean RIDIT value of 10 mice ±95% confidence
limits.
[b]n.s., Not significant.

II. PROPERTIES OF MM48 CELLS METASTASIZED IN THE REGIONAL LYMPH NODE

We initially tried to separate the metastatic tumor cell
variants in the node from the original tumor cell population.
MM48 tumor cells were implanted in the right hind footpad of
specific pathogen-free C3H/He female mice. Approximately 20 days
after implantation, the metastatic popliteal lymph node was removed. Tumor cells recovered from the node were directly implanted
into the footpad of a syngeneic recipient. Metastatic tumor cells
were obtained again from the regional lymph node (N1 cells). The
same procedure was repeated 10 times. Thus, N10 cells were obtained, and they were compared with the original MM48 cells. Significant differences were not found in their metastatic capacity
(Table I). In addition, significant differences were absent in
rate of tumor growth, immunogenicity tested by immunization
challenge assay, and immunosensitivity to MM48-specific antibodies
and cytotoxic T cells. Thus, it is considered that either the

metastatic MM48 tumor cell population is similar to the original
tumor cell population or the MM48 tumor cell line consists of a
rather homogeneous cell population.

III. ROUTES OF LYMPH FLOW AND LYMPHATIC METASTASES

The lymphatic metastasis was investigated systematically using
dye injection methods (Dunn, 1954; Zeidman and Buss, 1954; Fisher
and Fisher, 1967). Brilliant blue in 5% serous solution was injected into the hind footpad; the dye was drained off into lymph
flow and stained the popliteal lymph node rapidly and deeply.
Thereafter, the lymph flow seemed to divide into two routes, that
is, a superficial and deep route.
     The superficial route consisted of a channel connecting the
popliteal-inguinal-axillary lymph nodes, but a bypass from the
footpad to inguinal node might have existed, because there was no
effect on staining the inguinal node on removal of the popliteal
node. This is consistent with the report of Franchi et al. (1972).
Another route is the popliteal-lumbar-renal route. The lymph flow
from the footpad to the lumbar node drains mainly via the popliteal node, because resection of the popliteal node resulted in
almost no staining of the lumbar node. As for the development of
lymphatic metastasis, MM48 tumor cells implanted in the right hind
footpad metastasized into the draining lymph node along the same
route as the lymph flow. No lymphatic metastasis was found in
other ipsi- and contralateral nodes during the 20 days observation
time after tumor implantation.

IV. THE GROWTH OF THE PRIMARY TUMOR AND METASTASIZING TUMOR
    in Vivo

A. Effect of Local Immunization on Local Tumor Growth

In untreated normal mice, 10^6 MM48 tumor cells were implanted
in the right hind footpad. As shown in Fig. 1, the tumor showed
a slow growth around 10 days after tumor implantation. This slow
growth was observed in several repeated experiments. It is
speculated that some tumor immune responses were induced and affected tumor growth.
     The immunological role of the regional lymph node was examined
by immunizing mice with three weekly injections of 5×10^6 or 10^5
X-irradiated (10,000 R) tumor cells and a challenge of 10^6 live
tumor cells into the right hind footpad 10 days after the last immunization.

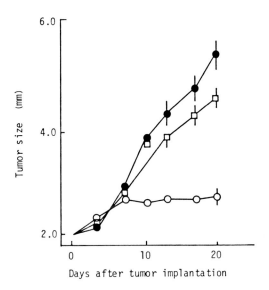

Fig. 1.   Effect of local immunization on the growth of subsequent challenged tumor.   Mice were immunized by three weekly injections of X-irradiated (10,000 R) tumor cells into the right hind footpad.   Ten days later, 10^6 viable tumor cells were challenged at the same site.   The tumor size data represent the mean size of 10 mice.   Vertical bars, SE.   □ , Unimmunized control mice;   ● , mice immunized with 5×10^6 X-irradiated tumor cells in the right hind footpad;   ○ , mice immunized with 10^5 X-irradiated tumor cells in the right hind footpad.

In mice preimmunized in the footpad with larger doses of irradiated tumor cells, subsequent tumor growth was enhanced with no slowed growth, whereas local immunization with smaller doses of irradiated tumor cells inhibited the growth of the local tumor.

B.   Influence of Local Immunization on Metastases

A similar effect was also observed in the development of metastasis in the regional and distant lymph nodes.   Highly immunized mice showed enhanced lymphatic metastasis compared with untreated mice and weakly immunized mice (Fig. 2).

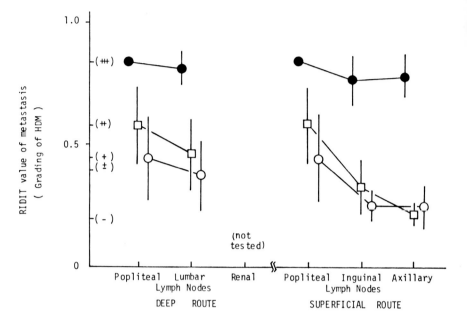

Fig. 2. Effect of local immunization on the development of
lymph node metastases. Metastases were graded by histological
examination of lymph nodes as described in Table I. HDM, histologically detectable metastasis. The ordinate represents mean
RIDIT values of 10 mice. Vertical bars indicate 95% confidence
limits. □ , Unimmunized control mice; ● , mice immunized with
5×10^6 X-irradiated tumor cells in the right hind footpad; ○ ,
mice immunized with 10^5 X-irradiated tumor cells in the right hind
footpad.

V. *In Vitro* ANALYSIS OF THE IMMUNE RESPONSE OF THE REGIONAL LYMPH
    NODE TO TUMOR CELLS

A. No Effector Cell Activity in Regional Lymph Node

The immune response of the regional lymph node to tumor cells
was investigated. The cytotoxic activity of lymphoid cells from
the regional popliteal and other nondraining lymph nodes was determined by ^{51}Cr-release assay *in vitro*. Radiolabeled MM48 cells and
lymphoid cells collected 10 days after tumor implantation were
used. This time corresponded to the period of slow local tumor
growth in untreated mice. No detectable effector activity was
found in even regional lymph node cells of untreated tumor-bearing
mice.

Effector Cell   Regulatory Cell

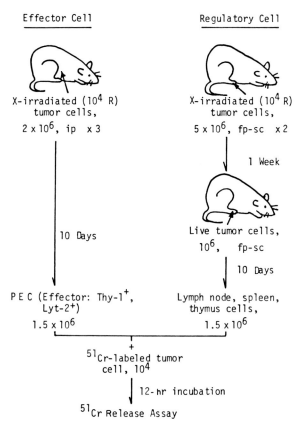

X-irradiated (10^4 R)   X-irradiated (10^4 R)
   tumor cells,   tumor cells,
2×10^6, ip $\times 3$ 5×10^6, fp-sc $\times 2$

                                          1 Week

                                 Live tumor cells,
    10 Days 10^6,   fp-sc

                                          10 Days

PEC (Effector: Thy-1$^+$,   Lymph node, spleen,
         Lyt-2$^+$)   thymus cells,
     1.5×10^6 1.5×10^6

                        +
              ^{51}Cr-labeled tumor
                  cell, 10^4

                        12-hr incubation

              ^{51}Cr Release Assay

Fig. 3. Experimental procedure to assay the activity of
immunoregulatory cells. ^{51}Cr-Labeled target cells (10^4) were
added to a mixture of effector cells and test cells at a target:
effector:regulator ratio of 1:150:150 in a final volume of 0.2 ml
in wells of a microtest plate. The plate was incubated for 12 hr
at 37°C, and the radioactivity released in the supernatant was
measured. PEC, Peritoneal exudate cells; ip, intraperitoneal injection; fp-sc, subcutaneous injection in a hind footpad.

B. Immunoregulatory Activities in the Regional Lymph Node

     As effector activity was not found in the regional node, im-
munoregulatory activity of regional lymph node cells was tested.
Figure 3 gives the experimental procedure for assaying the
activity of immunoregulatory cells. Mice were immunized by three
weekly injections of 2×10^6 X-irradiated tumor cells intraperitoneally (ip) to obtain effector cells. Ten days after the last
immunization, peritoneal exudate cells (PEC) were obtained.
Cytotoxic cells in PEC specific for MM48 cells were Thy-1 and
Lyt-2 positive. Lymphoid cells to be assayed were collected 10
days after tumor implantation. The regulatory activities of the
regional lymph node and other lymphoid tissues were assayed by

TABLE II

Immunoregulatory Activity of Regional Lymph Nodes

Treatment of mice		Lymph node cells	Specific ^{51}Cr release	Regulatory activity
Immunization[a]	Tumor implantation[b]			
−	−	Popliteal	6.3 ± 0.6	Control
−	+	Popliteal	12.4 ± 0.6	Enhancing
		Inguinal	10.0 ± 0.3	Enhancing
		Nondraining	10.1 ± 1.1	Enhancing
+	+	Popliteal	0.8 ± 0.4	Suppressiv
		Inguinal	5.5 ± 0.4	--
		Nondraining	6.1 ± 0.2	--

[a]Mice were twice immunized by two weekly injections of 5×10^6 X-irradiated (10^4 R) tumor cells in the right hind footpad 7 days apart.

[b]Seven days after the last immunization, 10^6 viable tumor cells were challenged at the same site. Ten days after tumor implantation, the lymph nodes were removed and tested for regulatory activities. The "suppressive" or "enhancing" activity showed statistica significance ($p < .05$, Student t-test) in comparison with the control value.

admixing lymphoid cells to the effector-target system for a 12-hr incubation period.

Immunoregulatory activity, that is, killer-enhancing activity, was observed in regional lymph node cells and in distant inguinal and nondraining lymph node cells (Table II), but not in spleen and thymus cells (data not shown) from untreated tumor-bearing mice. In contrast, regional lymph node cells from mice preimmunized with larger doses of tumor cells showed suppressor cell activity, but nont of the other lymph nodes and lymphoid tissues showed such activity. Both regulatory activities resided in Thy-1-positive cells and suppressor cells had Lyt-1^+2^- phenotype (data not shown). The Lyt phenotype of killer-enhancing cells has not been determined yet

C. Influence of Tumor Dose Used in Immunization and Challenge on Induction of Regulatory Cells

Table III summarizes the results. First, implantation of 10^5 tumor cells in untreated mice did not induce the killer-enhancing activity observed with 10^6 tumor cell implantation. Second, implantation of 10^5 tumor cells in mice preimmunized with larger doses of tumor cells induced the killer-enhancing activity. This

TABLE III

Influence of the Tumor Cell Dose Used in Immunization
and Challenge on Induction of Regulatory Cells

Tumor dose in immunization[a]	Tumor dose in challenge[b]	Specific ^{51}Cr release	Regulatory activity
--	--	7.1 ± 1.6	Control
--	10^5	5.0 ± 0.8	--
	10^6	11.6 ± 1.1	Enhancing
10^5	10^5	n.d.	
	10^6	4.7 ± 0.7	--
5×10^6	10^5	12.1 ± 1.4	Enhancing
	10^6	1.6 ± 1.4	Suppressive

[a,b]See footnotes to Table II.

finding contrasted strikingly with the fact that suppressor cell
activity was induced with large tumor loads. Third, a challenge
with a large inocula in mice preimmunized with smaller doses of
tumor cells did not induce a significant regulatory activity compared with the control. These data on the regional lymph node
indicate that the dichotomy of immune regulatory activity was
determined on the stimulation of the regional lymph node with
tumor antigen in a dose-dependent manner. The activity of suppressor cells seemed to be tumor specific. Suppressor cells
generated by immunization and challenge with MM48 cells diminished
MM48-specific killer cell activity, but not specific killer cell
activity against antigenically unrelated MH134 hepatoma cells of
C3H mouse.

D.   Kinetics of Immunoregulatory Activities in Regional Lymph Node

     Regulatory activity in the regional lymph node was tested in
the course of tumor development (Fig. 4). In untreated tumor
bearers, killer-enhancing activity appeared earlier and reached
the highest level at 10 days after tumor implantation, followed
by the appearance and increase of suppressor activity. Finally,
the node was occupied by the tumor to establish metastasis. In
contrast, in tumor-immunized and challenged mice, no killer-
enhancing but suppressor activity appeared earlier and reached the
maximal level at Day 10, followed by metastasis that was noted 2
weeks earlier than in the controls.
     From these results, it is probable that suppressor cell induc-
tion in the regional lymph node is associated with metastasis.

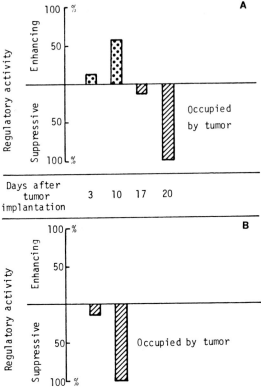

Fig. 4.   Kinetics of regulatory activity in the regional lymph node.   (A) Untreated tumor bearers;   (B) locally immunized mice. The percentage of enhancement or suppression of effector cell activity by regulatory cells was calculated as follows:

$$\% \text{ Regulation} = (1 - \frac{\text{Counts of effector plus test cells}}{\text{Counts of effector plus control cells}}) \times 100$$

VI.   RELATIONSHIP BETWEEN REGULATORY ACTIVITIES AND METASTASIS
      IN THE LYMPH NODE

A.   Measurements of Metastasis in Regional Lymph Node

We examined lymphatic metastases by bioassays and microscopic examinations.

In bioassays, the popliteal lymph node was removed.   The lymphoid cell suspension was injected into the peritoneal cavity of a syngeneic normal host.   The development of tumor ascites in recipients was taken as a tumor-positive lymph node.   A high incidence of tumor cell detection was observed the day after tumor implantation.   At Day 10, the detection rate was lowered to almost 50% (Fig. 5).   This period corresponds to the time observed for the generation of killer-enhancing activity in the node (Fig. 4)

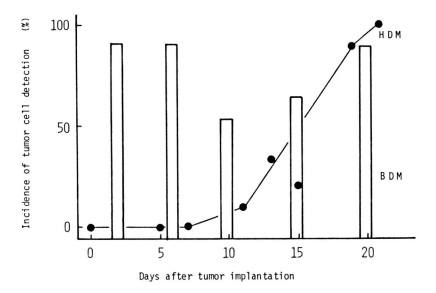

Fig. 5. Kinetics of histologically detectable metastasis
(HDM) and metastasis detected by bioassay (BDM). HDM, Metastases
with grade (+) or over were included; BDM, metastasis was determined by inoculation of test lymph node cells into the peritoneal
cavity of recipient mice. The recipient that died of ascitic
tumor was judged as having lymph node metastasis.

and with slow tumor growth (Fig. 1). In histological examinations,
metastasis was clearly observed after Day 10 and reached 100% after
Day 20. The increase in metastasis detection rate seemed to
parallel the generation of suppressor cells.

B. Effect of Removal of the Regional Lymph Node on Subsequent
    Tumor Growth

It is now clear that in spite of the temporary generation of
killer-enhancing T cells in the regional lymph node in the course
of local tumor development, antigen-specific suppressor T cells
are soon generated and become dominant. Host tumor immunity is
suppressed by suppressor T cells generated in the regional node,
and the tumor thus develops. Thus, the regional lymph node was
resected prior to tumor cell implantation. Mice were adenectomized
3 weeks before implantation. Tumor regression was observed in 4
of 10 adenectomized mice, but in none of all 10 untreated mice
(data not shown).

TABLE IV

Increase in Survival Rate by Resection of the Regional
Lymph Node Together with the Primary Tumor

Day no. of leg amputation	Resection of regional node	Survival rate[a]	Dead mice	
			Rate	Life span (Days ± SE)
7	+	7/10	3/10	55.3 ± 6.7
	−	8/10	3/10	58.3 ± 3.5
14	+	8/10	2/10	46.0 ± 4.0
	−	3/10	7/10	46.2 ± 3.9
21	+	6/8	3/9	47.7 ± 4.7
	−	0.5	5/5	50.6 ± 5.3
No operation		0/5	5/5	54.6 ± 6.7

[a]Mice were observed for 100 days.

C. Immunoregulatory Role of Regional Lymph Node for Host
Antitumor Immunity

The effect of the removal of the regional lymph node together
with the primary tumor was examined on the survival rate of host
animals. A hind leg implanted with the tumor was amputated just
below the knee joint. The regional lymph node was resected by
bluntly excising the content of the popliteal fossa.

In the group of mice amputated on Day 7, a simultaneous
adenectomy was not effective in improving the survival rate
(Table IV). However, on Day 14, adenectomy with the primary tumor
resection remarkably increased survival rate. The same tendency
was also observed in mice operated on Day 21. The cause of death
was a tumor recurrence. The life span of mice dead of tumor ranged
from 45 to 60 days, but no significant difference was observed in
the life span between all the groups of mice operated on different
days.

VII. CONCLUSION

MM48 ascitic mouse mammary tumor cells spread to the regional
lymph node when inoculated subcutaneously. To attempt to select
tumor cell variants with metastatic potential from the original
MM48 tumor cell population, we performed repeated cycling
(10 times) of MM48 tumor cells from the regional lymph node to
directly implanting in a footpad subcutaneously without the trans-

fer to tissue culture in each cycle. However, the selected tumor cells were not different from the original tumor cells in metastatic potential, growth rate, and immunogenic properties. Therefore, it is probable that the MM48 tumor cell line consists of a rather homogeneous cell population. Alternatively, it may be assumed in lymphatic metastasis that the whole tumor cell population is carried to and proliferates in the lymph node, which is quite different from the preferential spread of metastatic variants to a particular organ, such as Fidler (1973) demonstrated in lung metastasis of B16 melanoma cells. This issue should be clarified in further investigations.

Immunoregulatory responses induced in the regional lymph node and the secondary spread of tumor were determined on antigenic stimulation from the primary local MM48 tumor in a dose-dependent manner (K. Yoshida and T. Tachibana, unpublished). As the primary tumor develops, antigenic information becomes optimal for induction of killer-enhancing T cells in the regional lymph node. The cells help effector cells to inhibit the proliferation of both the primary and the secondary spread of tumor cells through the host defense mechanism. As the local tumor continues to grow and further antigenic stimulation is given to the node, however, antigen-specific suppressor T cells emerge and suppress the generation and function of effector cells in local and systemic immunity.

The immune response to a tumor antigen in distant nodes of mice with previous resection of the regional node is also interpreted in terms of antigen doses. A positive regulatory activity is generated in distant lymph nodes by antigen stimulation at higher doses, which induce suppressor T cells in the regional node, because antigen doses are distributed in several nodes, resulting in smaller amounts of antigen stimulation per node. Thus, it is conceivable that the optimal dose for killer-enhancing T-cell induction is very limited in the regional lymph node. Once suppressor cell activity is induced, the local tumor grow, resulting in excess antigenic stimulation to the regional lymph node. Thus, a continuous generation of suppressor T cells in the node on stimulation of excess antigen facilitates the establishment of metastasis and vice versa.

In the MM48 tumor system, it is concluded that the regional lymph node plays an important role in primary regulation of antitumor immunity against the development of local tumor and lymphatic metastasis.

ACKNOWLEDGMENT

This study is in part supported by Grants-in-Aid for Cancer Research from the Ministry of Education, Science, and Culture, Japan.
The authors wish to thank Dr. H. Sato, Dr. M. Suzuki, and Dr. I. Abe of the Department of Oncology of this Institute for valuable advice.

REFERENCES

Barna, B. P., and Deodhar, S. D. (1975). *Cancer Res. 35*, 920-926.
Barna, D. S., and Deodhar, S. D. (1979). *Cancer Res. 39*, 2711-2717.
Bross, I. J. D. (1958). *Biometrics 14*, 18-38.
Crile, G. (1972). *Lymphology 5*, 89-93.
Dunn, T. B. (1954). *J. Natl. Cancer Inst. (US) 14*, 1281-1409.
Fidler, I. J. (1973). *Nature New Biol. 242*, 148-149.
Fisher, B., and Fisher, E. R. (1967). *Cancer (Philadelphia) 20*, 1907-1913.
Fisher, B., and Fisher, E. R. (1971). *Cancer (Philadelphia) 27*, 1001-1004.
Flannery, G. R., Chalmers, P. J., Rolland, J. M., and Mairin, R. C. (1973). *Br. J. Cancer 28*, 118-122.
Franchi, G., Inocenti, I. R., Garattini, S., Affieri, O., Gademartiri, G., and Ottariani, G. (1972). *Lymphology 5*, 31-36.
Goldfarb, P. M., and Hardy, M. A. (1975). *Cancer (Philadelphia) 35*, 778-785.
Hawrylko, E. (1982). *Cell. Immunol. 66*, 121-138.
Irie, R. F. (1971). *Cancer Res. 31*, 1682-1689.
Zeidman, I., and Buss, J. M. (1954). *Cancer Res. 14*, 403-405.

DISCUSSION

GOLUB: Isn't the Lyt-1^+2^- phenotype an unusual phenotype for a suppressor cell?

TACHIBANA: Yes, it is. We do not know, however, the reason why suppressive activity resides in Lyt-1^+ T cells. There are three possibilities to be considered. First, suppressor T cells of mice having Lyt-1.1 allele, such as C3H mouse, seem to have Lyt-1^+ phenotype, in contrast with Lyt-2^+ phenotype of suppressor T cells in mice having Lyt-1.2 allele, such as the C57BL mouse.

Second, Lyt-1$^+$ suppressor T cells may be a suppressor inducing T cells by which suppressor T cells will be induced and regulate effector cell function. Third, peritoneal exudate cells used for cytotoxic assay contain macrophages in addition to Lyt-2$^+$ cytotoxic T cells as effector cells. Therefore, Lyt-1$^+$ cells stimulated with antigen will function to induce suppressive macrophages, which inhibit cytotoxic activity of effector cells nonspecifically.

OKADA: How do you explain the result that unrelated control tumor-bearing mice survived longer than experimental mice whose original tumor had been surgically removed?

TACHIBANA: There is no significant difference statistically between both experimental groups.

CHAPTER 21

ANTIBODIES TO TUMOR-ASSOCIATED GANGLIOSIDES (GM2 AND GD2):
POTENTIAL FOR SUPPRESSION OF MELANOMA RECURRENCE

Reiko F. Irie
Tadashi Tai
Donald L. Morton

Division of Surgical Oncology
John Wayne Clinic and Armand Hammer Laboratories
Jonsson Comprehensive Cancer Center
University of California at Los Angeles School of Medicine
Los Angeles, California

I.   INTRODUCTION

     Methods for augmenting specific immune responses against cancer
in humans have included active immunization with tumor cell vaccine
and passive administration of specific antibodies and cytotoxic
T-cells. In 1973, our group, the Division of Surgical Oncology at
UCLA, embarked on a random trial of active specific immunotherapy
with cultured allogeneic melanoma cells for stage II melanoma patients. Following the establishment of lymphoblastoid cell lines
autologous to the immunizing tumor cell lines used in the vaccine,
it became possible to monitor a patient's specific humoral immune

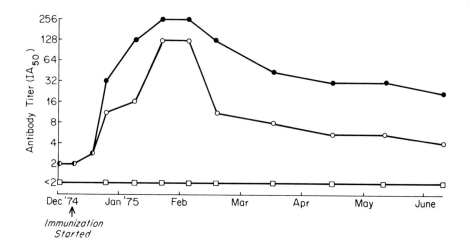

Fig. 1. Antibody responses to melanoma cells in a patient
after active specific immunization with tumor cell vaccine. The
patient received immunization with an equal mixture of three kinds
of cultured melanoma cells (Ml4, M7, and Ml2). The immunization
protocol consists of four sequential schedules. First, 100 million irradiated cells were intradermally injected every week for
4 weeks. For the next 2 weeks, 70 million irradiated cells and
30 million viable cells were given every week. After that, 100
million viable cells were given every week for 2 weeks. Finally,
100 million viable cells were injected every other week continuously. For the purpose of antibody characterization, a serum
sample was obtained every 1-2 weeks. Antibody titer in the sera
were assays by immune adherence (IA) using Ml4 target cells, one
of the lines used in the vaccine. Lymphoblastoid cells derived
from the Ml4 donor were used to absorb alloantibodies from the
sera. ●, Unabsorbed sera; ○, absorbed by lymphoblasts; □,
absorbed by lymphoblasts and fetal brain.

response against the tumor-associated antigens by absorption techniques. The lymphoblastoid cell lines had been shown to express
the same HLA antigens as the paired tumor cells (Saxton *et al.*,
1978). The results presented in Fig. 1 show the levels of antibody induced against melanoma cells in an immunotherapy patient.
Alloantibodies were removed by absorption with paired lymphoblastoid cell lines. The predominant remaining reactivity was removed
by absorption with the second- or third-trimester fetal brain tissues (Irie *et al.*, 1979), but not by adult normal tissues or by
fetal tissues other than brain. However, tumor tissues other than
the melanoma tissues could absorb the antibody. The results indicated that the allogeneic melanoma cell vaccine could induce
humoral immune responses against a tumor-associated membrane
antigen that was shared by melanoma and tumors of other histological types.

To examine the distribution of the antigen in human tumors, we tested 170 tissue specimens obtained from patients with various types of cancer. Melanoma, at 82%, had the highest prevalence of this antigen. Other tumor tissue types having a high prevalence of the antigen included lung (71%), sarcoma (61%), brain (55%), and breast (53%). By comparison, tumors from the gastrointestinal tract, such as colon, stomach, or liver, had little or no antigen expression (Rees et al., 1981). The antigen was named oncofetal antigen-immunogenic (OFA-I). This antigen is unique when compared with other previously described human tumor-associated fetal antigens, because it is immunogenic in cancer patients. The natural anti-OFA-I antibody found in human sera is predominantly of the IgM class, and it is highly cytotoxic to OFA-I-positive tumor cells in the presence of complement in vitro (Sidell et al., 1979a).

II. EFFECT OF ANTI-OFA-I TITER ON SURVIVAL OF MELANOMA PATIENTS

In an effort to evaluate the antitumor effect of anti-OFA-I in vivo, we performed a retrospective analysis of the survival of melanoma patients in relation to levels of IgM anti-OFA-I antibody (Jones et al., 1980). Serum specimens obtained from 112 stage II melanoma patients during 4 months after surgery were tested for the antibody. Patients then were classified into one of three groups: patients with high anti-OFA-I titers, those with intermediate titers, and those with low titers. Survival for each group was monitored for a 5-year period. Patients with high titers of IgM anti-OFA-I had significantly prolonged survival compared to the other two groups. To date, only 2 of 24 patients (8%) with high levels had died from metastatic melanoma, whereas 16 of 20 patients (80%) with low titers died of melanoma within 5 years. Of these 112 patients, 40 received adjuvant immunotherapy with OFA-I-positive tumor cell vaccine, and 14 (35%) developed higher titers of IgM anti-OFA-I antibody. Of the remaining 72 nonvaccinated patients, only 10 (14%) achieved naturally elevated titers. Both of these groups contributed to overall survival rates significantly, particularly because no deaths occurred among the 10 patients.

More recently, 44 patients with stage III melanoma were immunized with the tumor cell vaccine by the intralymphatic route (Ahn et al., 1982). It was our hope that direct contact between tumor antigen and lymphoid tissues might stimulate an increased immune response to tumor antigens. Fourteen patients (32%) had stabilization, regression, or remained free of disease. Median survival was 17 months, compared to 6 months for histological controls ($p < .001$). Association of the better prognosis with the levels of anti-OFA-I antibody was assessed. Of 22 patients (50%) who developed elevated antibody titers within 4 months, 12 (55%)

had no disease progression, in contrast to 20 (91%) who failed to
develop elevated titers and who had disease progression (p < .01).
These data suggested that augmentation of immunity to the OFA-I
may have conferred a measure of immunity against melanoma. This,
finding formed the basis of our new project aimed at the production
of monoclonal anti-OFA-I antibody in vitro.

III. In Vitro PRODUCTION OF HUMAN MONOCLONAL ANTIBODY TO OFA-I

     Specific monoclonal antibodies to tumor-associated antigens
have been passively administered successfully. Miller et al.
(1982) described successful treatment of B-cell lymphoma with
mouse monoclonal antibody. Although no serious side effects or
allergic reactions have been noted in these patients, some potential problems include the induction of anti-mouse immunoglobulin
after the repeated administration of mouse antibody and the
potential reaction of mouse antibody to certain normal tissues.
Clearly, a human monoclonal antibody would be desirable as a
reagent for long-term passive immunotherapy of cancer patients.
While the hybridoma technology is most promising, there is no established method available today for making monoclonal antitumor
antibody by human hybridoma cell lines. As an alternative method,
we are producing human monoclonal antibody in vitro using human
B-lymphoblastoid cells transformed by Epstein-Barr virus (EBV).
     Infection with EBV triggers the transformation of human
B lymphocytes; these B-cell lines then produce specific human antibody. In 1977, Steinitz et al. first produced antibody directed
against the hapten antigen, NNP. Following these studies, several
other groups successfully produced human antibodies to a variety
of different antigenic specificities (Viallat and Kourilsky, 1982).
In 1981, we reported the successful establishment of human B lymphoblasts that produce human antibodies to the tumor-associated
antigen, OFA-I (Irie et al., 1981). Using two of these human
monospecific anti-OFA-I antibodies, we found that OFA-I was composed of at least two antigenic specificities (Irie et al., 1982).
     The method used to establish antibody-producing human B lym-
phoblasts has been described elsewhere (Irie et al., 1981, 1982).
Briefly, 2-5 million viably frozen peripheral blood lymphocytes
(PBL) from melanoma patients were used as the source of B lymphocytes. The EBV suspension was obtained from the spent medium of
a B-95-8 marmoset lymphoid cell culture. After the human lymphocytes were infected with the EBV in vitro, the culture medium was
replaced with the fresh medium every 3-4 days. Anti-OFA-I produced
in the spent medium of each culture was monitored by the immune adherence (IA) assay using an OFA-I-positive melanoma target cell
line, UCLA-SO-M14 (Irie et al., 1976). After antibody was detected
in the spent medium, cells were cloned in microtiter plates with
5 to 20 cells each using the limiting dilution method. Of 232

TABLE I

Production of Antibody to OFA-I by EBV-Transformed
Human Peripheral Blood Lymphocytes (PBL)[a]

Production	Number of PBL cultures tested
Continuous >1 year	1 (L72)
6 months	1 (L55)
2 months	29
None	201

[a]Peripheral blood lymphocytes from patients with melanoma
were injected with EBV *in vitro*. Spent tissue culture media
from each culture were tested every 3-4 days for the production
of antibody to an OFA-I-positive melanoma cell line, Ml4,
using the immune adherence assay.

human PBL samples transformed by EBV, only 31 cultures displayed
detectable anti-Ml4 antibody in the spent medium (Table I). For
reasons we do not understand, in most instances this antibody
production was not permanent. Of the 31 cultures, 29 ceased to
secrete antibody after 1 to several weeks. Only two lines were
established as long-term antibody-producing cultures. One line
(L72) had been continuously producing a consistent titer of anti-
OFA-I for more than 1 year. The other line (L55) produced anti-
OFA-I for 6 months. The kinetics of antibody production by 14 of
the cultures is illustrated in Fig. 2. Initial detection of
antibody occurred within 7 to 22 days after virus infection.
Lines that failed to produce detectable antibody after 3 weeks
rarely started production. To test the specificity of the antibodies, absorption assays were performed with UCLA-SO-L14
lymphoblasts that expressed the same HLA antigens as our target
OFA-I-Ml4. The L14 cells did not decrease the antibody titer,
confirming that the reactivity was not directed against HLA
alloantigens. However, both antibody activities were completely
abolished by absorption with an OFA-I-positive fetal tissue
(fetal brain from a second-trimester fetus). Fetal liver obtained
from the same fetus did not absorb any antibody.
     Antibodies produced by the two long-term cell lines, L55 and
L72, were further studied for their immunological specificities
and immunoglobulin properties. Figure 3 shows antibody reactivity
with a number of malignant melanoma cell lines. Both L55 and L72
antibodies reacted to more than 50% of our melanoma cell lines.
However, the reactivity pattern was clearly different for each of
these antibodies. For example, while our target Ml4 melanoma and
several other lines reacted with both antibodies, other lines
reacted with only one of the antibodies. These results suggested

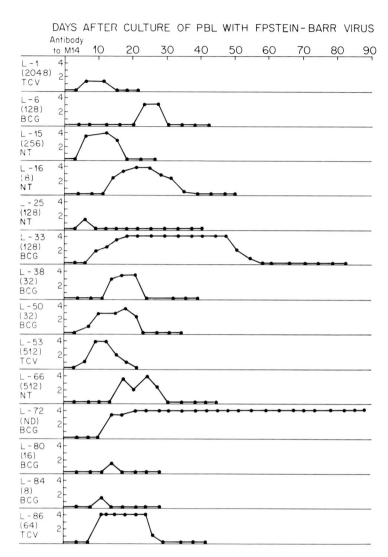

Fig. 2. Monitoring of antibody to Ml4 secreted in spent media of EBV-transformed human lymphoblasts. Vertical axis indicates IA score of antibodies to Ml4. If more than 90% of the OFA-I-positive Ml4 target cells formed rosettes with human erythrocytes in the immune adherence assay, an IA score of 4+ was given. If 50% of Ml4 cells formed rosettes, 2+ was given, and if no cells formed rosettes, 0 was given. Number in parentheses indicates anti-OFA-I titer in the sera of corresponding PBL donors. Patients received tumor cell vaccine (TCV), BCG immunotherapy, or no treatment (NT) after stage II surgery.

that L55 and L72 antibodies detected different antigenic determinants. We then designated these antibodies as anti-OFA-I-1 and anti-OFA-I-2, respectively. Figure 4A shows results of the assay

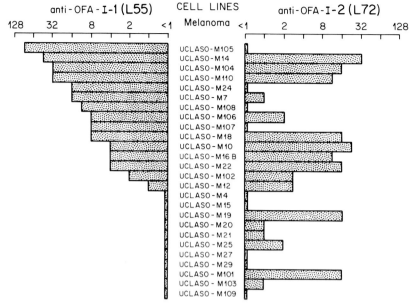

Fig. 3. Spent media of L55 and L72 cultures were tested for antibody reactivity to cultured human melanoma cell lines in the immune adherence assay. Media were each concentrated to adjust their titers to 32 (IA$_{50}$) with M14 target cells. IA$_{50}$ indicates reciprocal dilution of antibody required to obtain an immune adherence score of 2+ (50% of tumor cells form erythrocyte rosettes).

with lymphoid target cell lines autologous to the OFA-I-positive tumors. None were positive with either the anti-OFA-I-1 or anti-OFA-I-2 antibodies. Figure 4B shows antibody reactivity with cultured fibroblasts of skin or muscle. In contrast to the negative results with anti-OFA-I-2, anti-OFA-I-1 reacted to all of the cell lines tested. Because skin or muscle tissues were nonreactive to the antibody before culturing, OFA-I-1 antigen expression probably occurred during transformation process in culture. In our initial description of OFA-I, we reported that the sera of some patients reacted to cultured fibroblasts in a similar manner (Irie et al., 1976). In Fig. 4C, antibody reactivity with biopsied melanoma tissues confirmed that reactivity patterns are different for each antibody. Figure 5A shows that both antibodies reacted against gliomas and neuroblastomas. It is noteworthy that these tumors and melanomas are of neuroectodermal origin. Figure 5B shows a very different reactivity pattern when various carcinomas, sarcomas, and lymphoid tumors were tested. Whereas anti-OFA-I showed positive reactivity to several of these tumors, anti-OFA-I-2 reacted to none. Results of this tissue typing indicated that OFA-I-1 and OFA-I-2 were immunologically distinct and that OFA-I-1

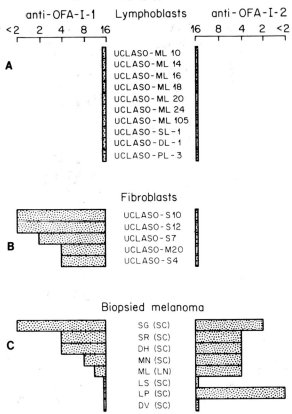

CELL LINES

Fig. 4. Spent media of L55 and L72 cultures were tested for antibody reactivity to (A) cultured B lymphoblasts, (B) skin (S) and muscle (M) fibroblasts, and (C) biopsied melanoma tissues in the IA absorption assay. Titers of nonabsorbed antibody to M14 were each adjusted to 32 (IA_{50}). Packed biopsied melanoma tissue (minced) or cultured cell suspension (2×10^7 lymphoblasts/100 μl antibody and 5×10^6 fibroblasts/100 μl antibody) were admixed with an equal volume of L55 or L72 spent medium and incubated at 4°C overnight. Titers of remaining antibody were assayed by the IA assay with M14 target cells. Biopsied melanomas were obtained from stage III melanoma patients with subcutaneous (SC) or lymph node (LN) metastasis.

was found on various histological types of human cancer cells, whereas OFA-I-2 was restricted to tumors of neuroectodermal origin.

Identification of the immunoglobulin class produced in the L55 and L72 cultures was accomplished by indirect membrane immunofluorescence assays using M14 cells as targets. Anti-OFA-I produced in both cultures was limited to IgM κ class. The amount of IgM in the culture medium of L55 on Day 5 was 4 μg/ml, and that of L72 was

CELL LINES

A

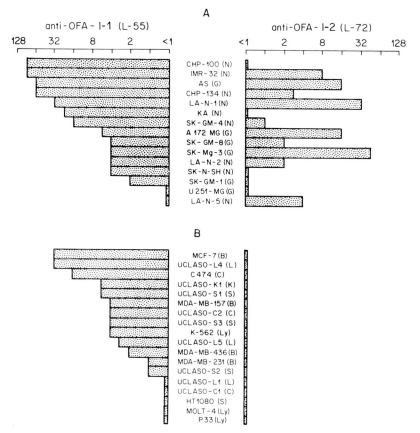

Fig. 5. Spent media of L55 and L72 cultures were tested for antibody reactivity to cultured human tumor cell lines in the immune adherence assay. Media were each concentrated to adjust their titers to 32 (IA_{50}) with Ml4 target cells. A, Reactivity patterns of anti-OFA-I-1 and anti-OFA-I-2 antibodies against gliomas (G) and neuroblastomas (N). B, Reactivity patterns of the same two antibodies against various tumors: (B) Breast carcinoma; (C) colon carcinoma; (K) kidney carcinoma; (L) lung carcinoma; (Ly) lymphoid cancer; (S) sarcoma.

9 µg/ml by a radioimmunoassay (Irie *et al.*, 1982). The IgM was completely absorbed by Ml4 cells. This finding, together with the fetal brain absorption data, indicated that antibodies produced by both the L55 and L72 cultures were only directed against OFA-I specificities on Ml4 cells. Dr. Mitsuo Katano in our group has confirmed the monoclonal character of the anti-OFA-I-2 antibody using agarose isoelectric-focusing techniques (Katano *et al.*, in press). The therapeutic potential of the monoclonal antibody for passive immunization has been assessed using an *in vivo* model system. Our successful suppression of melanoma growth in nude

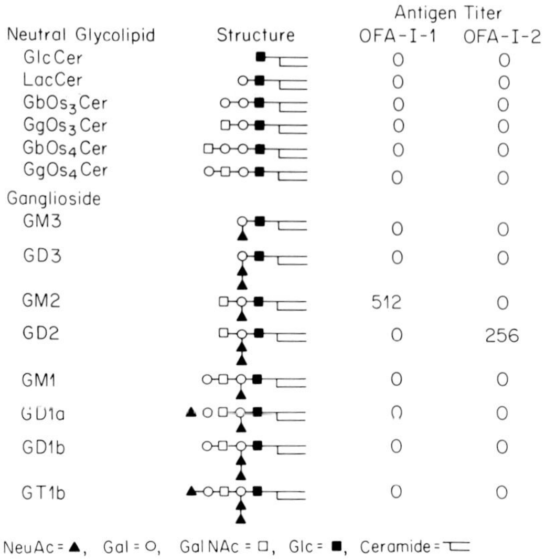

Antigen Titer

Neutral Glycolipid	Structure	OFA-I-1	OFA-I-2
GlcCer		0	0
LacCer		0	0
GbOs$_3$Cer		0	0
GgOs$_3$Cer		0	0
GbOs$_4$Cer		0	0
GgOs$_4$Cer		0	0
Ganglioside			
GM3		0	0
GD3		0	0
GM2		512	0
GD2		0	256
GM1		0	0
GD1a		0	0
GD1b		0	0
GT1b		0	0

NeuAc = ▲, Gal = O, GalNAc = □, Glc = ■, Ceramide = ⊏

Fig. 6. OFA-I-1 and OFA-I-2 antigenicity in authentic glyco-lipids. Glycolipids (6 nmol) were serially diluted in a phosphate-buffered saline and tested for inhibition of monoclonal anti-OFA-I-1 and anti-OFA-I-2 bindings to UCLASO-M14 cells in the immune adher-ence assay. Antigen titer is given as the reciprocal dilution for 50% IA inhibition.

mice by the antibody is described in Katano and Irie, Chapter 28, this volume.

IV. IDENTIFICATION OF THE OFA-I-1 AND OFA-I-2 ANTIGENS
     AS GANGLIOSIDES GM2 AND GD2

     With these monospecific antibodies, the chemical properties of
the OFA-I-1 and OFA-I-2 antigens were identified as follows
(Cahan et al., 1982; Tai et al., 1983): OFA-I-positive melanoma
cells were treated first with various enzymes. The results showed
that sialidase completely abolished the antigenicity of both
OFA-I-1 and OFA-I-2. Although OFA-I-1 antigenicity was not affected by sialidase alone, it could be destroyed by treatment with
sialidase in the presence of a detergent, tauocholate. Trypsin
did not affect the antigenicity of either antigen. These preliminary results indicated that both the OFA-I-1 and OFA-I-2 antigens
contained at least one sialic acid residue in their antigenic
determinants.
     To investigate the possibility that OFA-I antigens were gang-
liosides--that is, glycolipids containing sialic acid--we isolated
the ganglioside fraction of OFA-I-positive M14 melanoma cells or
the spent culture medium by chloroform-methanol-water extraction
followed by DEAE-Sephadex column chromatography (Svennerholm and
Fredman, 1980; Ledeen and Yu, 1982). Using the human monospecific
antibodies to OFA-I-1 and OFA-I-2, we found that both antigens
were detected exclusively in the ganglioside fraction. The ganglioside fraction was then separated into its component gangliosides
by thin-layer chromatography in a solvent composed of chloroform-
methanol-0.22% $CaCl_2$ (55:45:10). Gangliosides from M14 melanoma
cells had four prominent bands corresponding to the standard
gangliosides from top to bottom as follows: GM3, GM2, GD3, and
GD2. Each ganglioside appeared as a doublet. The antigenicity of
each ganglioside fraction was determined by scraping off 2-mm wide
sections and eluting the antigens. The OFA-I-1 antigen activity
was detected in the doublet fraction that comigrated with the GM2
standard, whereas OFA-I-2 antigen activity was detected in the
fraction that comigrated with the GD2 standard. The GM2 fraction
was absolutely negative for OFA-I-2 antigenicity, and the GD2
fraction was similarly completely free of OFA-I-1 activity.
     To confirm that OFA-I-1 and OFA-I-2 were identical to GM2 and
GD2, respectively, we tested the antigenic reactivity of various
authentic glycolipids (Fig. 6). We tested 14 glycolipid analogs,
including neutral glycolipids and gangliosides, for the reactivity
with anti-OFA-I-1 antibody. Only GM2 showed OFA-I-1 activity.
Analog glycolipids that differ by the addition of one galactose
(GM1) or the loss of one N-acetylgalactosamine (GM3), or sialic
acid (asialo GM) were completely devoid of antigenicity. When
these authentic glycolipids were tested for OFA-I-2 antigenicity,
only GD2 synthesized from brain gangliosides showed antigenic activity. The GM2 ganglioside identified by anti-OFA-I-1 antibody
had no OFA-I-2 antigenic activity. Thus, the human tumor antigen,
OFA-I-1, was identified as ganglioside GM2, GalNacβ1 → 4 (NeuAcα2
→ 3) Galβ1 → 4Glc → Cer, and the neuroectodermal tumor antigen,

OFA-I-2, was identified as ganglioside GD2, GalNacβ1 → 4
(NeuAcα2 → 8 NeuAcα2 → 3) Galβ1 → 4Glc → Cer. The difference
between GM2 and GD2 is only one sialic acid residue. Thus, these
two monospecific antibodies clearly can distinguish the difference
of one sialic acid residue in the ganglioside of the OFA-I.

V. PROSPECTS

Currently, we are developing methods to augment anti-OFA-I
responses in humans using the purified GM2 and GD2 antigen. If
the purified OFA-I gangliosides can be coupled with an adjuvant
that is highly immunogenic in humans, active specific immunization
may provide us with a most powerful method for preventing metastatic spread of tumor cells in postoperative cancer patients.

ACKNOWLEDGMENTS

We would like to thank Lan Sze and Estella Farmatiga for their
technical assistance, and E. Jane Shaw for her editorial assist-
ance.
This work was supported by Grants CA00543, CA30647, and
CA12582, awarded by the National Cancer Institute, DHHS. Reiko
F. Irie is a recipient of an NCI Research Career Development Award.

REFERENCES

Ahn, S. S., Irie, R. F., Weisenburger, T. H., Jones, P. C.,
Juillard, G. J. F., Denise, J. R., and Morton, D. L. (1982).
Surgery 92, 362-267.
Cahan, L. D., Irie, R. F., Singh, R., Cassidenti, A., and Paulson,
J. C. (1982). *Proc. Natl. Acad. Sci. USA 79,* 7629-7633.
Irie, R. F., Irie, K., and Morton, D. L. (1976). *Cancer Res. 36,*
3510-3517.
Irie, R. F., Giuliano, A. E., and Morton, D. L. (1979). *J. Natl.
Cancer Inst. (US) 63,* 367-373.
Irie, R. F., Jones, P. C., Morton, D. L., and Sidell, N. (1981).
Br. J. Cancer 44, 262-266.
Irie, R. F., Sze, L. L., and Saxton, R. E. (1982). *Proc. Natl.
Acad. Sci. USA 79,* 5666-5670.
Jones, P. C., Sze, L. L., Morton, D. L., and Irie, R. F. (1980).
J. Natl. Cancer Inst. (US) 66, 249-254.

Katano, M., Saxton, R. E., and Irie, R. F. *J. Clin. Lab. Immunol.*, in press.

Ledeen, R. W., and Yu, R. K. (1982). *Methods Enzymol. 83*, 139-191.

Miller, R. A., Maloney, D. G., Warnke, R., and Levy, R. (1982). *N. Engl. J. Med. 306*, 517-522.

Rees, W. V., Irie, R. F., and Morton, D. L. (1981). *J. Natl. Cancer Inst. (US) 67*, 557-562.

Saxton, R. E., Irie, R. F., Ferrone, S., Pellegrino, M. A., and Morton, D. L. (1978). *Int. J. Cancer 21*, 199-206.

Sidell, N., Irie, R. F., and Morton, D. L. (1979a). *Br. J. Cancer 40*, 950-953.

Sidell, N., Irie, R. F., and Morton, D. L. (1979b). *Cancer Immunol. Immunother. 7*, 151-155.

Steinitz, M., Klein, G., Koskimies, S., and Makel, O. (1977). *Nature (London) 169*, 420-422.

Svennerholm, L., and Fredman, P. (1980). *Biochim. Biophys. Acta 617*, 97-109.

Tai, T., Paulson, J. C., Cahan, L. D., and Irie, R. F. (1983). *Proc. Natl. Acad. Sci. USA 80*, 5392-5396.

Viallat, J. R., and Kourilsky, F. M. (1982). *Pathol. Biol. 30*, 232-242.

DISCUSSION

POSTE: Can OFA-I-1 or OFA-I-2 be modulated on melanoma cells? What was the source of neuraminidase used in your studies on the saccharides in OFA-I-2 and its specificity?

IRIE: When patients' sera containing anti-OFA-I antibodies were preincubated with OFA-I-positive melanoma target cells at 37°C for 30 min, the target cells became insensitive to complement-dependent cytolysis (Sidell et al., 1979b). However, it is unknown which antibody, anti-OFA-I-1 or anti-OFA-I-2, is responsible for the modulation, since the serum samples contained both antibodies. Immunomodulation tests have not been done using the monoclonal antibodies. The source of neuraminidase was *Clostridium perfringens* sialidase (type X; Sigma).

KONDO: Is anti-OFA-I IgM antibody cytotoxic to CNS tissue? I am afraid patients with high titer of antibody may suffer from CNS damage especially in case of cerebral hemorrhage where antibody and complement will be focally supplied.

IRIE: Although we have no direct evidence that anti-OFA-I antibodies may not damage CNS tissues, those patients who had

extremely high titers of IgM anti-OFA-I antibody
in their circulation showed no neurological symptoms or
any other clinically evident changes. Since only minimal OFA-I gangliosides are present on normal adult brain
cells, and the brain is an immunological-privileged
organ, we assume that immunological reactions on brain
cells by the antibody and complement is minimal, if any
are present.

OKADA: Have you some result on cytotoxic T lymphocytes in patients directed to OFA-I? Although the presence of IgM
antibody to OFA-I indicated a good prognosis while IgG
type did not, it might be a reflex of the situation of
the capacity of the cell-mediated immune system against
OFA-I.

IRIE: No, we have not examined T-cell cytotoxic activity
against OFA-I. One method to detect OFA-I-specific
T-cell cytotoxicity will be the blocking assay. Purified OFA-I gangliosides will be utilized to see if
T-cell cytotoxicity against OFA-I-positive tumor target
can be inhibited.

ISHIKAWA: Is there no worry about production of the idiotypic de-
terminant of immunoglobulin by repeated injection of
monoclonal antibody to OFA-I?

IRIE: The possibility that human IgM antibodies to OFA-I-
injected in patients may induce anti-idiotype antibodies
should be tested. We will be able to monitor the anti-
idiotype antibodies for OFA-I specificity by ELISA
using purified monoclonal anti-OFA-I antibody as an
antigen source.

CHAPTER 22

A STUDY OF IMMUNE COMPLEX OF GLOMERULI IN CANCER PATIENTS,
ASSOCIATED WITH IgG-RHEUMATOID FACTOR AND ANTINUCLEAR ANTIBODY

Tetsuzo Sugisaki
Hiroaki Nakajima
Takanori Shibata
Hisashi Kawasumi

Department of Internal Medicine
Showa University School of Medicine
Tokyo, Japan

BASIC MECHANISMS AND CLINICAL TREATMENT
OF TUMOR METASTASIS

I. INTRODUCTION

    The important role of immunological events against malignant
tumors has been recognized in many areas such as tumor antigen,
mechanisms of tumor cell destruction by the host, and host immune
response. In addition, the presence of large amounts of
circulating immune complexes has also been frequently reported in
correlation with tumor metastasis and with subsequent subversion
of other potentially effective host defense mechanisms. The
reports of nephrotic syndrome due to immune complex in glomeruli
have increased in cancer patients. This event is one of the most
interesting areas interrelating tumor progression of metastasis
with host-protective mechanisms.
    The purpose of this chapter is to elucidate components of the
immune complexes in glomeruli obtained from two cases of cancer
patients and to discuss the relationship between the immune complexes in glomeruli and circulating antinuclear antibody (ANA) or
rheumatoid factor (RF).

II. CIRCULATING IMMUNE COMPLEXES IN CANCER PATIENTS

    With the recent availability of highly sensitive assays for
detection of circulating immune complexes, a number of studies
have appeared attempting to relate quantitative levels of complexes
detected with clinical staging, survival, and various peripheral
manifestations of cancer. In the study by Teshima et al. (1977),
^{125}I-labeled Clq deviation tests were performed on 459 sera from
various cancer patients. These workers have reported that more
than 50% of the sera tested showed strong inhibition of Clq
binding, indicating significant levels of circulating immune complexes. Using the same procedure, Rossen et al. (1976) found 82%
of 136 patients with various form of neoplasms to have measurable
levels of soluble complexes. We performed Clq-binding enzyme immunoassay for detection of circulating immune complexes and found
some of the patients with lung cancer and colon cancer to have
the immune complexes, although the number of these cases was very
small (Fig. 1).
    It has been reported by Sjögren et al. (1971), Baldwin et al.
(1972), and Jose and Seshadri (1974) that the circulating immune
complexes may serve as blocking factors, having the capacity to
modulate the immune response by interaction with sensitized lymphocytes, suppressing the cytotoxic potential of these cells. In
fact, Staab et al. (1980) have reported that cancer patients in
whom circulating immune complexes were detected showed statistically poor prognosis. They found that circulating immune complexes
were present in 89 of 363 patients with histologically confirmed

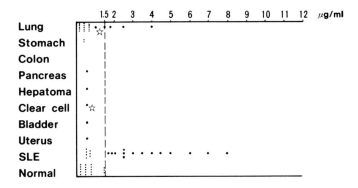

Fig. 1. Immune complexes in sera of patients with various
forms of malignancies. Circulating immune complexes were detected
by Clq-binding enzyme immunoassay. ☆ Cases demonstrated membranous nephropathy.

adenocarcinoma of the gastrointestinal tract before surgery and in
a postoperative follow-up as well. Of these 89 patients with immune complexes, 72 showed already metastatic disease progression.

III. NATURE OF CIRCULATING IMMUNE COMPLEXES IN CANCER PATIENTS

The most important problem is to elucidate the nature of the
antigen(s) present in immune complexes. Many investigators
(Hellström et al., 1971; Sjögren et al., 1971; Jose and Seshadri,
1974; Hellström and Hellstrom, 1974; Baldwin and Price, 1976)
have suggested that the antigens of immune complexes in animal
systems and in humans are often derived from tumor. Among the
various sorts of antigens reported, carcinoembryogenic antigen
(CEA) in carcinoma of the gastrointestinal tract was extensively
investigated by Kapsapoulow-Dominos and Anderer (1979), who found
that the circulating immune complexes were composed of CEA-IgM
and CEA-IgG. It has also been reported that a great number of
cancer patients have circulating immune complexes. However, the
detailed components of the immune complexes have not been elucidated.

IV. NEPHROPATHY IN CANCER PATIENTS

Nephrotic syndrome associated with various cancers has been
recognized in patients with renal complications such as lymphoma-
tous infiltration (Richmond et al., 1962), amyloidosis (Kimball,

1961), and renal vein thrombosis (Swiet and Wells, 1957). In addition, studies of nephrotic syndrome in cancer patients have since suggested that immune complex deposition in glomeruli probably does occur and demonstrate membranous nephropathy characterized by thickening of glomerular basement membrane associated with IgG and C_3 deposits in granular fashion by immunofluorescence. This type of lesion is of particular interest because it has an immunological basis of animal models (Edgington et al., 1968) and in certain other clinical situations such as idiopathic membranous nephropathy.

Lee et al. (1966) further elucidated the problem by studying 11 of 105 cancer patients who had nephrotic syndrome without known causes. They noted that the incidence of cancer in patients with nephrotic syndrome in their series was much higher than that expected for a similar population group without renal disorders. In 8 of their 11 cases, the renal lesion responsible for the nephrotic syndrome was morphologically compatible membranous glomerulonephritis. On the basis of these observations, they discussed the possibility that the renal lesion was produced by circulating antigen-antibody complexes in an immune response to the tumor. This speculation would be supported by considerable evidence that membranous glomerulonephritis is produced in humans by glomerular deposition of soluble immune complexes demonstrable in a granular pattern along glomerular basement membrane by immunofluorescence. Similar observations have been made in cancer of the breast (Loughridge and Lewis, 1971), bronchus (Costa et al., 1974), colon (Couser et al., 1974), and stomach (Wakashin et al., 1980), as well as in Hodgkin's disease (Froom, 1973)--possibly related to the glomerular deposition of antibody to tumor antigen.

Given the interactions just noted between tumor-associated antigens and the host's immune response, it would seem plausible that some patients with tumor would be susceptible to the glomerular deposition of tumor-associated antigen-antibody complexes with the subsequent induction of significant glomerular injury. However, the pathogenesis of the majority of immune complex-mediated glomerulonephritides, not only those associated with cancer but also primary nephropathy, have not been fully elucidated.

V. NATURE OF IMMUNE COMPLEXES IN GLOMERULI IN CANCER PATIENTS

A number of antigens have been documented as components of the immune complexes in glomeruli (Wilson and Dixon, 1981). With regard to antigens in glomeruli in cancer patients, several agents have been documented, such as those associated with tumors, viruses, DNA, and normal tissue. In this section, we would like to discuss involvement of these antigens and also the IgG-IgG

rheumatoid factor system in the membranous nephropathy of our two
cancer patients (one with oat cell carcinoma and one with clear
cell carcinoma).

A. Tumor-Associated Antigen

Although complete information in any single case is not available, individual investigations (Lewis *et al*., 1971; Costanza *et
al*., 1973; Gault, 1973; Weksler *et al*., 1974; Wakashin *et al*.,
1980) have provided supportive evidence showing either tumor-
associated antigens or antibodies to these antigens in glomerular
deposits in several instances of tumor-related membranous
nephropathy. Lewis *et al*. (1971) first described a nephrotic
patient with squamous cell bronchogenic carcinoma, in whom immunoglobulin eluted from the glomeruli reacted specifically with the
tumor cells of the patient but not with his normal lung tissue,
when studied by membrane immunofluorescence and immunodiffusion
techniques. Subsequent articles were focused mainly on the carcinoembryonic antigen (CEA) and antibody system in cancer of the
gastrointestinal tract.
Costanza *et al*. (1973) demonstrated in a patient with colon
cancer using the immunofluorescence technique that the glomerular
deposits contained CEA, a cancer-related antigen. In three cases
of gastric cancer, similarly, the evidence of presence of CEA in
glomeruli in membranous nephropathy was suggested by Wakashin *et
al*. (1980). They demonstrated that fluorescein-conjugated eluate
obtained from the IgG deposited in glomeruli of two of the patients stained the surface of tumor cells as well as the glomerular deposits of the same and other patients. Melanoma-associated
antigen has also been reported as a component of glomerular
immune deposits in the kidney, associated with nephrotic syndrome
in melanoma patients (Weksler *et al*., 1974).

B. Non-Tumor-Associated Antigens

On the other hand, non-tumor-associated antigens such as DNA,
virus, and normal tissue antigen have also been documented.
Higgins *et al*. (1974) reported a case of metastatic oat cell
carcinoma of the lung, associated with nephrotic syndroma and circulating antinuclear antibody. The glomeruli demonstrated the
deposits of the IgG and complements in granular fashion. They
demonstrated the presence of large amounts of extracellular DNA in
necrotic tumor tissue and Feulgen-positive deposits within the
glomerular basement membrane, and they suggested the possibility
that tumor-induced anti-DNA antibody might result in this immune
complex-associated glomerulonephritis with nephrosis.
Viral antigen is also frequently reported as a component in
immune complexes of glomerular deposits. It has been reported

(Hyman *et al.*, 1973; Sutherland and Mardinay, 1973; Oldstone *et al.*, 1974) that the viral antigen-antibody complexes could conceivably lead to the development of immune complex disease in cancer patients. The evidence of various viral antigens in glomeruli includes antigens to Epstein-Barr virus in a case of African Burkitt's lymphoma (Oldstone *et al.*, 1974), onconavirus in a case of acute myelomonocytic leukemia (Sutherland and Mardinay, 1973), and herpes zoster viral antigen in a case of Hodgkin's disease associated with cutaneous herpes zoster (Hyman *et al.*, 1973).

Since Heymann *et al.* (1959) reported that kidney antigen-- later reported as brush border antigen by Edgington *et al.* (1968)-- was the agent, as a normal tissue antigen, responsible for the development of autologous immune complex nephritis in rats, several investigators (Naruse *et al.*, 1974; Strauss *et al.*, 1975) suggested that the brush border antigen of human kidney was also involved in the pathogenesis of some cases of idiopathic membranous nephropathy. The involvement of the brush border antigen has also been reported in membranous nephropathy in some patients, associated with renal cell carcinoma (Ozawa *et al.*, 1975). Another possibility for involvement of normal tissue antigen in glomerular immune complexes is lung tissue antigen. An instance of membranous glomerulopathy in a patient with an epidermoid lung carcinoma supports the evidence that the immune complex disease may be mediated by a tissue-specific antigen-antibody system (Richard-Mendes Da Costa *et al.*, 1974). In this case, renal eluate was shown to react not only with the patient's normal lung tissue and tumor, but also with lung tumor from other patients.

Thus, there are many articles that have demonstrated various components of the immune complexes in glomeruli. However, the pathogenesis of immune complex-mediated glomerulonephritis in cancer patients does not seem to be fully elucidated, because of the small number of cases and limited materials.

C. IgG-IgG Rheumatoid Factor-Type Immune Complexes

In our examination of kidneys obtained at postmortem, 2 of 47 patients were found to have membranous nephropathy characterized by thickening of glomerular basement membrane associated with IgG in granular fashion detected by immunofluorescence (Table I).

Using these kidney materials, we set out to analyze the composition of the immune complexes.

Case Reports

Case 1. A 67-year-old man was admitted because of an abnormal shadow on the X-ray film of his chest taken during a routine examination for elderly people. He appeared well except for a 4-week history of occasional cough. No abnormalities were found in urine.

TABLE I. Percentages of Kidneys with Immune Complexes by Clinical Groups

Clinical group	Number of kidneys examined	Positive for both γ-globulin and complement	
		Number	Percentage
Lung Ca	21	1	4.2
Hepatoma	6	0	0
Stomach Ca	5	0	0
Esophagus Ca	1	0	0
Colon Ca	3	0	0
Rectum Ca	1	0	0
Jejunum Ca	1	0	0
Hodgkin's disease	1	0	0
AML	1	0	0
CML	1	0	0
Myeloma	2	0	0
Breast Ca	1	0	0
Thymoma	1	0	0
Clear cell Ca	1	1	100
Total	46	2[a]	

[a] Two cases are membranous nephropathy.

Normal serum values were obtained for urea nitrogen, creatinine, electrolytes, and cholesterol. The serum concentrations of immune complexes and complements were all within normal range. A rheumatoid factor and an antinuclear factor were negative. A CT scan revealed tumor masses in the right-lung hilus, left lower lobules of the lung, and right kidney. On hospital Day 30, the patient died. Postmortem examination revealed clear cell carcinoma in the tumor masses, which was consistent with the findings revealed by CT scan (Fig. 2). Light-microscopic study of the kidney obtained from this patient showed mild thickening of the glomerular capillary loop (Fig. 3). No abnormalities were found in the interstitial tissue. By immunofluorescence study, the staining for IgG and C_3 was found along the glomerular capillary walls in granular fashion (Fig. 4). Electron microscopy revealed electron-dense deposits on the subepithelial side of the glomerular basement membrane (GBM). The glomerular eluate demonstrated neither antinuclear activity nor anti-brush border activity by indirect immunofluorescence technique, and no rheumatoid factor activity by latex slide test.

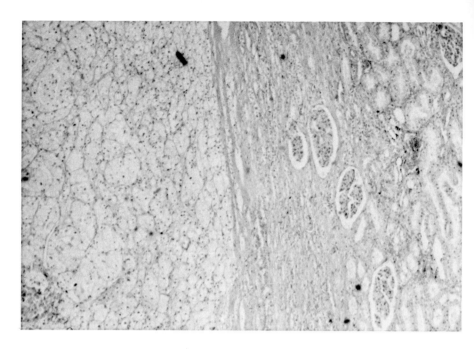

Fig. 2. Kidney section (case 1) obtained at postmortem examination, showing clear cell carcinoma on the left and normal kidney structure on the right (H&E; ×100).

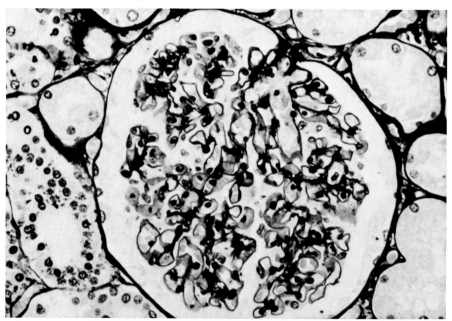

Fig. 3. Kidney section (case 1) obtained at postmortem examination, showing mild thickening of glomerular capillary loops and no glomerular hypercellularity. No cellular infiltration is evident in the interstitial tissue (PAS-methamine; ×400).

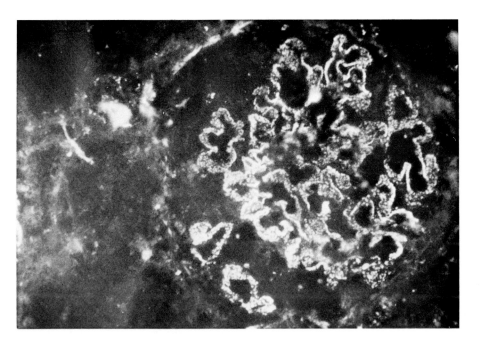

Fig. 4. Frozen kidney section (case 1) obtained at postmortem examination, staining for human IgG in granular fashion along glomerular capillary walls by immunofluorescence (×400).

Case 2. A 72-year-old man was admitted because of cough and facial edema. An X-ray film of his chest showed a mass in the left lung and a pleural effusion. No abnormalities were found in urine. Normal serum values were obtained for urine, urea nitrogen, creatinine, electrolytes, and cholesterol. A rheumatoid factor and an antinuclear factor were negative. The serum concentrations of immune complexes and complements were within normal range. The diagnosis of oat cell carcinoma was made from the biopsy specimen by bronchofiber. Despite radiation treatment and chemotherapy, the patient died on hospital Day 60. Necropsy showed oat cell carcinoma of the right main-stem bronchus and the left lower lobule (Fig. 5).

The kidney specimen from the patient showed membranous nephropathy characterized by thickening of glomerular capillary walls and deposits of IgG and C_3 along glomerular capillary walls in granular fashion by immunofluorescence study. The glomerular eluate demonstrated neither antinuclear antibody or anti-brush border activity with normal human kidney as substrate, and no rheumatoid factor activity by latex slide test.

Using these kidney specimens obtained from two cancer patients, we have set out to elucidate the composition of the immune complexes. Penner *et al.* (1982), Sugisaki *et al.* (1982a), and Kawasumi *et al.* (1982) in our laboratory established a procedure to dissociate the immune complexes deposited in the frozen kidney specimens. Methods of dissociation testing for IgG deposits in

393

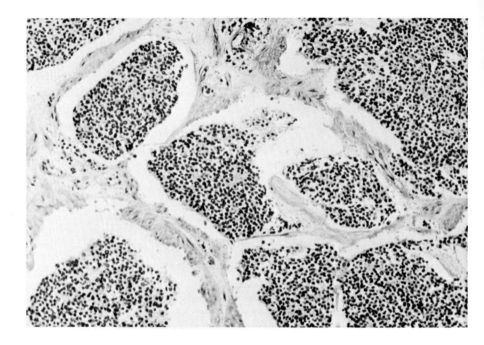

Fig. 5. Lung section (case 2) obtained at postmortem examination, showing clustering of oat cell cancer cells (H&E; ×200).

glomeruli are described in Fig. 6. Many 4-μm thickness frozen sections are made and are washed twice in PBS for 30 min. Then the various materials are mounted on the kidney specimens for 1 hr and washed in PBS. After repeating these procedures six times, the sections are stained with fluorescein-isothiocyanate-conjugated goat anti-human IgG or C3. The materials used in this study are shown in Table II. They are 50 mg/ml human native Cohn fraction II (FrII), 50 mg/ml 63°C heat-aggregated Cohn fraction II,

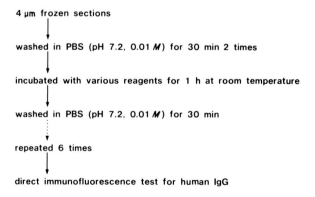

4 μm frozen sections

↓

washed in PBS (pH 7.2, 0.01 *M*) for 30 min 2 times

↓

incubated with various reagents for 1 h at room temperature

↓

washed in PBS (pH 7.2, 0.01 *M*) for 30 min

⋮
↓

repeated 6 times

↓

direct immunofluorescence test for human IgG

Fig. 6. Methods of dissociation test for IgG deposits in glomeruli.

TABLE II. The Various Reagents Used for the Dissociation Test and Results of Immunofluorescence Test for Human IgG

	Concentration (mg/100 ml)	Case 1: clear cell Ca	Case 2: oat cell Ca
Human native aggregated Cohn FrII	50	--	--
		--	--
Human IgG	10	--	--
Rabbit native aggregated Cohn FrII	50	++	++
Rat native aggregated Cohn FrII	50	++	++
Bovine native aggregated Cohn FrII	50	++	++
Human brush border	20	++	++
DNA	1	++	++
nucleohistone	1	++	++
PBS	--	++	++

10 mg/ml human IgG, 50 mg/ml each of rabbit, rat, and bovine fraction II, 20 mg/ml brush border of the human kidney, 1 mg/ml DNA, 1 mg/ml nucleohistone, and PBS. The IgG deposits were completely dissolved by incubation of tissue section with human γ-globulin at the concentration of 50 mg/ml and with human IgG at the concentration of 10 mg/ml (Fig. 7), but the IgG deposits were not affected by incubation with the other materials (refer to Table II). Glomerular immune deposits disappeared after incubation of tissue sections with native or untreated γ-globulin at a concentration of 1 mg/ml, whereas heat-aggregated γ-globulin at a concentration as low as 0.1 mg/ml dissociated the immune deposits completely (Table III).

Thus, these results indicate that human IgG, especially aggregated human IgG, is specific for the dissociation.

To analyze which portion of the IgG is effective for the dissociation, the materials as shown in Table IV were prepared. Although only pepsin-treated IgG, which contains mainly F(ab) fragments, was not effective, the other materials, all of which contain Fc portion, did work very well for this dissociation study (refer to Table IV).

In our laboratory, solubilization of immune complexes by this *in vitro* technique has been achieved in glomeruli of patients

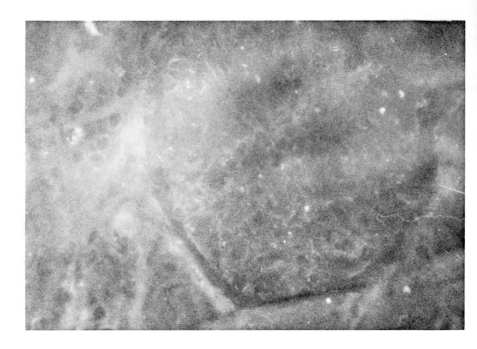

Fig. 7. Frozen kidney section (case 1) obtained at postmortem examination, showing no staining for human IgG in glomerulus following incubation of human IgG at the concentration of 10 mg/ml (×400).

with idiopathic membraneous, lupus, and membranoproliferative glomerulonephritis, IgA nephropathy, and Henoch-Schönlein's purpura by means of incubating kidney sections with human Cohn fraction II, human IgG, DNA, brush border from human kidney, rabbit, rat, and bovine Cohn fraction II. Granular IgG deposits along glomerular capillary loop or in the mesangial area in lupus nephritis, membranous nephropathy, and membranoproliferative glomerulonephritis disappeared completely following incubation with human IgG or Fc portion, but not with F(ab) portion. Whereas IgA deposits in IgA deposit nephropathy were not affected (Kawasumi *et al.*, 1982).

All these data indicated that immune complexes in glomeruli presumably contained the patient's own denatured IgG and IgG rheumatoid factor. This explanation supports the possibility that once IgG rheumatoid factor binds to the IgG, the IgG rheumatoid factor itself becomes an antigen, after which another IgG rheumatoid factor may react, with the result that the immune complexes start growing *in situ*. Therefore, it is not surprising to identify the patient's own IgG as the antigen of the immune complexes deposited in the various glomerulopathies, including membranous nephropathy in cancer patients.

On the basis of these observations, we propose that the structure of the immune complexes in the GBM is somewhat lattice-like in nature.

TABLE III. The Various Concentrations of Human Cohn Fraction II (FrII) for the Dissociation Test and the Results of Immunofluorescence Test for Human IgG

	Case number[a]	Concentration of Cohn FrII (mg/ml)				
		5	1	0.1	0.01	0.001
Native Cohn FrII	1	−	−	±	++	++
	2	−	−	±	++	++
Aggregated Cohn FrII	1	−	−	−	+	++
	2	−	−	−	±	++

[a]Case 1, clear cell Ca; case 2, oat cell Ca.

TABLE IV. The Dissociation Test Using the Various Portions of Human IgG

	Staining for IgG[a]	
	Case 1	Case 2
PBS	++	++
Human IgG	−	−
PEG-treated γ-globulin	−	−
S-sulfonated γ-globulin	−	−
Plasmin-treated γ-globulin	−	−
Pepsin-treated γ-globulin	++	++
Fc portion	−	−

[a]Case 1, clear cell Ca; case 2, oat cell Ca.

VI. SIGNIFICANCE OF IgG RHEUMATOID FACTOR (RF) AND IgG ANTINUCLEAR ANTIBODY (ANA) IN CANCER PATIENTS

Since we postulated the possibility that the components of immune complexes in glomeruli mainly contained IgG and IgG RF, the problem arose how IgG RF was detected in the sera of cancer patients. It is well known that IgM RF is easily detected with the procedure of latex slide test, but IgG RF is fairly difficult to detect by this test. In addition, IgM RF has fairly good reactivity not only with human denatured IgG, but also with the other species' (such as rabbit, rat, and sheep) denatured IgG, whereas IgG RF has reactivity with human denatured IgG but fairly poor reactivity with denatured IgG of other species. Therefore, human IgG has to be used as an antigen for the detection of IgG RF, but, as far as the procedure used in immunoassay, detection of IgG RF may become very difficult, because both antibody and antigen belong to IgG.

In contrast, Hannestad and Stollar (1978) have contributed a very interesting article discussing a certain IgM rheumatoid factor that has reactivity with nuclear antigen of the cells. This article stimulated us very much, because we have postulated the nature of the immune complexes in various nephropathies, even in lupus nephritis, to be composed of IgG and IgG RF. However, we had no convincing explanation for the dissociation phenomenon of IgG from glomeruli in lupus nephritis, because the immune complex in lupus nephritis is generally believed to be composed of DNA and anti-DNA antibody. Moreover, since antinuclear antibody and rheumatoid factor were detected separately, both of the antibodies had been believed to be independent and to have no cross-reactivity.

On the basis of such evidence as the cross-reactivity of IgM RF with nuclear antigen, the characteristics of IgG RF, and the dissociation phenomenon of IgG from glomeruli, we had an idea that antinuclear antibody might have cross-reactivity with human IgG. Shibata *et al.* (1982) in our laboratory performed an inhibition test on the activity of antinuclear antibody obtained from patients with systemic lupus erythematosus (SLE) and rheumatoid arthritis (RA) by incubation with IgG or Fc portion of various species. The materials used for the inhibition test are human Cohn fraction II, aggregated human Cohn fraction II, sulfonated γ-globulin, polyethylene glycol-treated human γ-globulin, human Fc fragments, rabbit Cohn fraction II, rat IgG, native DNA, and phosphate-buffered saline (PBS). The activity of antinuclear IgG antibody obtained from some SLE or RA patients was completely inhibited by incubation with human Cohn fraction II, aggregated Cohn fraction II, and sulfonated γ-globulin, but not with PBS, pepsin-treated γ-globulin, PEG-treated γ-globulin, rabbit Cohn fraction II, rat IgG, or DNA. This finding suggests that a certain IgG antinuclear factor (ANF) is cross-reactive with human IgG, especially Fc portion; in other words, IgG ANF may be partially identical with IgG RF. If this hypothesis is correct, detection of IgG RF become possible by demonstration of IgG ANA by immunofluorescence procedure.

It has been repeatedly confirmed that cancer patients have a high incidence of non-organ-specific autoantibodies including antinuclear factor (Whitehouse and Holborow, 1971; Friou, 1974). Whitehouse and Holborow (1971) found that ANA at a titer of 1:10 were present at an overall incidence of 24%, as compared with none in the control group. The incidence in patients with breast carcinoma was 50%, whereas none with neuroblastoma exhibited ANA. The antibodies detected in the study of Albin and Soanes (1971) were mainly of the IgG class.

TABLE V. Frequency of Rheumatoid Factor (RF) and Antinuclear Antibody (ANA) in Various Forms of Malignancies

Type of malignancy	No. of cases tested	RF	ANA
Lung	19	4	3
Pancreas	1	0	0
Stomach	3	0	0
Colon	1	1	1
Thyroid	1	0	0
Hepatoma	1	0	1
Clear cell Ca.	1	0	0
Bladder	1	0	0
Adenoidal Ca.	1	1	0
Total	29	6 (20%)	5 (17%)

Similarly, we performed indirect immunofluorescence studies on sera obtained from 29 cases of various malignancies (Table V). Using the latex slide test, rheumatoid factors were detectable in 6 (20%) and antinuclear antibodies in 5 (17%) of the 29 cases, indicating that the results were consistent with the articles previously described.

We also performed inhibition tests on the five antinuclear antibody-positive sera using various materials (Table VI). The activity of ANA was completely inhibited following incubation with human IgG, human S-sulfonated γ-globulin, and human Fc portion, but not with human pepsin-treated γ-globulin, or rabbit or rat IgG. These data indicate that ANA in the sera from cancer patients reacts with human IgG, especially Fc portion, suggesting that a certain IgG ANA is identical with IgG RF.

Most recent studies of experimental Heymann type nephritis have suggested the possibility of immune complex formation *in situ*, caused by circulating anti-brush border antibody against glomerular-fixed antigens (Couser *et al.*, 1978). This hypothesis immediately fit in with our hypothesis, because circulating anti-brush border antibody could replace circulating IgG RF-IgG ANA, which could fix to the antigen--presumably tumor-associated, fetal, viral, or normal tissue antigen or denatured IgG previously planted in glomeruli--and cause the immune complex-type nephropathy (such as membranous nephropathy).

TABLE VI. Inhibition Test of Antinuclear Antibody (ANA) Following Incubation with Various Reagents[a]

			Activity of ANA following incubation with			
	PBS	Human IgG	PEG-treated γ-globulin	S-sulfonated γ-globulin	Plasmin-treated γ-globulin	Pepsin-treated γ-globulin Fc portion
ANA-positive sera (n = 5)	5	0	1	0	0	5 0

[a]Certain ANA are cross-reactive with human IgG, mainly the Fc portion.

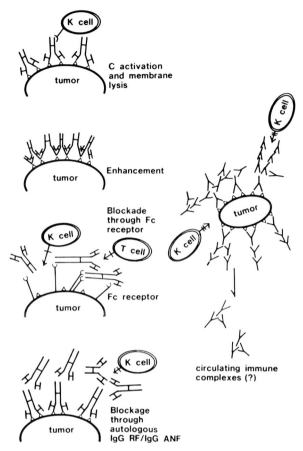

Fig. 8. The hypothesis indicates several possible ways that K cell function may be abrogated by IgG-rheumatoid factor, IgG antinuclear antibody, or circulatory immune complexes.

VII. SUMMARY

These reactions involving IgG rheumatoid factor and/or IgG antinuclear antibody in the glomeruli may occur on the surface of malignant cells that are already fixed by antitumor antibody or immune complexes. Such conglomerate complexes may block the function of K cells (Fig. 8). This hypothesis may be correct, on the basis of a report described by Eagan and Lewis (1977), who indicated that the clinical course of patients with nephrotic syndrome has been grave. Of 44 cancer patients associated with nephrotic syndrome, 34 (77%) died within a relatively short time span. The median survival of the patients (from the onset of their clinical presentation) was 12 months, with only a few surviving for 2 or more years. All of these patients had progressive carcinomatosis as a major contributing factor to their deaths. Therefore, the data described in this chapter suggest that measurement of immune complex, IgG ANA, and RF may be important in evaluating the prognosis of cancer patients.

REFERENCES

Albini, R. J., and Soanes, W. A. (1971). *Ann. Clin. Res. 3*, 226-230.
Baldwin, R. W., and Price, M. R. (1976). *Annu. Rev. Med. 27*, 151-163.
Baldwin, R. W., Price, M. R., and Robins, R. A. (1972). *Nature New Biol. 238*, 185-186.
Costa, C. R. M., Dupont, E., Hamers, R., Hooghe, R., Dupuis, F., and Potvliege, P. (1974). *Clin. Nephrol. 2*, 245-251.
Costanza, M. E., Pinn, V., Schwartz, R. S., and Nathanson, L. (1973). *N. Engl. J. Med. 289*, 520-522.
Couser, W. G., Wagonfeld, J. B., Spargo, B. H., and Lewis, E. J. (1974). *Am. J. Med. 57*, 962-970.
Couser, W. G., Jermanovich, N. B., Belock, S., and Stilmant, . (1978). *J. Clin. Invest. 61*, 561-572.
Eagan, J. W., and Lewis, E. J. (1977). *Kidney Int. 11*, 297-306.
Edgington, T. S., Glassock, R. J., and Dixon, F. J. (1968). *J. Exp. Med. 127*, 555-572.
Friou, G. J. (1974). *Ann. N.Y. Acad. Sci. 230*, 23054.
Froom, D. W. (1973). *Arch. Pathol. 94*, 547-553.
Gault, M. H. (1973). *Proc. Am. Soc. Nephrol. 39* (Abstr.).
Hannestad, K., and Stollar, B. D. (1978). *Nature (London) 275*, 671-673.
Hellström, I., and Hellström, K. E. (1974). *Cancer (Philadelphia) 34*, 1461-1468.
Hellström, I., Hellström, K. E., Sjogren, H. O., and Warner, G. A. (1971). *Int. J. Cancer 8*, 185-191.
Heymann, W., Hackel, D. B., Harwood, S., Wilson, S. G. F., and Hunter, J. L. P. (1950). *Proc. Soc. Exp. Biology Med. 100*, 660-664.
Higgins, M. R., Randall, R. E., and Still, W. J. (1974). *Br. Med. J. 3*, 450-451.
Hyman, L. R., Burkholder, P. M., Joo, P. A., Segar, W. E., Wis, M. (1973). *J. Pediatr. 82*, 207-217.
Jose, D. G., and Seshadri, R. (1974). *Int. J. Cancer 13*, 824-838.
Kapsopoulow-Dominos, K., and Anderer, F. A. (1979). *Clin. Exp. Immunol. 35*, 190-195.
Kawasumi, H., Talase, S., Shibata, T., Saito, K., Uchida, J., Yamamoto, J., Kitazawa, K., Sato, S., Yonekura, M., Ito, S., Shiwachi, S., Kan, K., and Sugisaki, T. (1982). *Jpn. J. Nephrol.*

24, 625-639.
Kimball, K. G. (1961). *Ann. Intern. Med. 55*, 958-974.
Lee, J. C., Yamauchi, H., and Hopper, J. (1966). *Ann. Int. Med. 64*, 41-51.
Lewis, M. G., Loughridge, L. W., and Phillips, T. M. (1971). *Lancet 2*, 134-135.
Louchridge, L. W., and Lewis, M. G. (1971). *Lancet 1*, 256-258.
Naruse, T., Miyakawa, Y., Kitamura, K., and Shibata, S. (1974). *J. Allergy Clin. Immunol. 54*, 311-318.
Oldstone, M. B. A., Theofilopoulos, A. N., Gunven, P., and Klein, G. (1974). *Intervirology 4*, 292-302.
Ozawa, T., Pluss, R., Lacher, J., Boedecker, E., Guggenheim, S., Hammond, W., and McIntosh, R. (1975). *Q. J. Med. 44*, 523-541.
Penner, E., Albini, B., Glurich, Andres, G. A., and Milgrom, F. (1982). *Int. Arch. Allergy Appl. Immunol. 67*, 245-253.
Richard-Mendes Da Costa, C., Dupont, E., Hamers, R., *et al.* (1974). *Clin. Nephrol. 2*, 245-251.
Richmond, J., Sherman, R. S., Diamond, H. D., Craver, L. E. (1962). *Am. J. Med. 32*, 184-207.
Rossen, R. D., Reisberg, M. A., Hersh, E. M., and Gutterman, J. U. (1976). *Clin. Res. 24*, 462A.
Shibata, T., Soeda, K., Takase, S., Saito, K., Kawasumi, H., Uchida, J., Kitazawa, K., Yonekura, M., Shiwachi, S., Kan, K., and Sugisaki, T. (1982). *Arerugi Jpn. J. Allergol. 31*, 773.
Sjögren, H. O., Hellström, I., Bansal, S. C., and Hellström, K. E. (1971). *Proc. Natl. Acad. Sci. USA 68*, 1372-1375.
Staab, H. J., Anderer, F. A., Stumpf, E., and Fischer, R. (1980). *Br. J. Cancer 42*, 26-33.
Strauss, J., and Pardo, V. (1975). *Am. J. Med. 58*, 382-387.
Sugisaki, T., Kano, K., Brentjens, J. R., Anthone, S., Anthone, R., Andres, G. A., and Milgrom, F. (1982a). *Transplantation 34*, 90-94.
Sugisaki, T., Shiwachi, S., Yonekura, M., Kitazawa, K., Yamamoto, J., Uchida, J., Saito, K., Shibata, T., Kawazumi, H., Takase, S., and Soeda, K. (1982b). *Fed. Proc. 41*, 692.
Sutherland, J. C., and Mardinay, M. R. (1973). *J. Natl. Cancer Inst. (US) 50*, 633-644.
Swiet, J., and Wells, A. C. (1957). *Br. Med. J. 2*, 1341-1343.
Teshima, H., Wanebo, H., Pinsky, C., and Day, N. K. (1977). *J. Clin. Invest. 59*, 1134-1142.
Wakashin, M., Wakashin, Y., Iesato, K., Ueda, S., Mori, Y., Tsuchida, H., Shigematsu, H., and Okuda, K. (1980). *Gastroenterology 78*, 749-756.
Weksler, M. E., Carey, T., Day, N., Susin, M., Sherman, R., and Becker, C. (1974). *Kidney Int. 6*, 112A.
Whitehouse, J. M. A., and Holborow, E. J. (1971). *Br. Med. J. 4*, 511-513.
Wilson, C. B., and Dixon, F. J. (1981). "The Kidney." Saunders, Philadelphia.

DISCUSSION

COHEN: Have you been able to show dissociation of complexes
           from tumor cells by your immunofluorescence technique?
           This could be very important in making the tumor cell
           accessible to attack, as you have already indicated.

SUGISAKI: We have not done this yet. We are now planning to do
           this in *in vitro* tests.

COHEN: Is there any evidence for receptors for Fc in glomeruli?
           If so, the Fc-induced dissociation you show could be due
           to competitive inhibition by the Fc as well as the
           solubilization of complexes that you find. In any case,
           the effect is very important because it provides the
           possibility of therapeutic application.

SUGISAKI: There is a single paper that indicates the presence of
           Fc receptor in glomeruli. However, this concept has
           not been generally accepted yet.
              In vitro solubilization of immune complexes by in-
           cubation of human γ-globulin is a very important
           implication for treatment. We have already started
           γ-globulin treatment for the patients with immune
           complex-mediated glomerulonephritis and are getting
           clinical improvement (Sugisaki *et al.*, 1982b).

CHAPTER 23

ANTIBODY THERAPY OF METASTATIC PROLIFERATION OF HUMAN NEOPLASTIC
CELLS HETEROTRANSPLANTED INTO IMMUNODEFICIENT MICE

Emilio A. Machado
David A. Gerard

Laboratory of Experimental and Comparative Pathology
Department of Medical Biology
Memorial Research Center
University of Tennessee College of Medicine
Knoxville, Tennessee

Bismarck B. Lozzio[1]
James R. Mitchell
Elena G. Bamberger

Laboratory of Experimental Hematology and Oncology
University of Tennessee Memorial Research Center
Knoxville, Tennessee

Carmen B. Lozzio

Laboratory of Experimental Hematology and Oncology
and
Laboratory of Medical Genetics
Department of Medical Biology
Center for the Health Sciences
University of Tennessee Memorial Research Center
Knoxville, Tennessee

Carl J. Wust

Department of Microbiology
University of Tennessee
Knoxville, Tennessee

[1]Deceased.

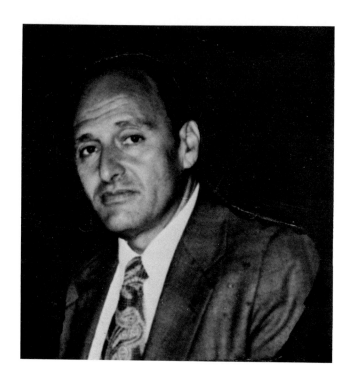

IN MEMORIAM

Dr. Bismarck B. Lozzio died on October 28, 1982. He was a
driving force in our experimental work; Bismarck was an
idealistic and compassionate man, and his scientific endeavors
were characterized by an unusual fervor. For many of us, working
with Bismarck was not something casual, but represented a joint
scientific venture rooted in a friendship that lasted more than
15 years. The continuation of the research programs to which he
dedicated his life is the best respect that our group can pay to
his memory.

                                                              EAM

I. INTRODUCTION

     Metastases may render useless the surgical or clinical treat-
ment of primary tumors and are, therefore, one of the most common
causes of death among cancer patients.
     The many factors involved in the process must be understood
before methods can be developed that will interfere with tumor
cell dissemination or lead to the abrogation of metastases already established. However, the polymorphic characteristics of
neoplastic disease pose difficult problems for the researchers.
First, there are more than 200 different types of tumors that
have been recognized in human pathology; second, tumors of similar
histogenetic type demonstrate changing patterns of evolution in
different patients; and, third, it is not possible to define the
moment of release of neoplastic cells that will successfully proliferate in target organs. Not surprisingly, the advances in the
investigation of the mechanisms of metastases have been slow,
because there is a lack of wholly satisfactory experimental
models (Foulds, 1969).
     During its evolution, a primary tumor liberates an enormous
number of cells, of which only a few develop metastases (Griffiths
and Salsbury, 1963; Crile *et al*., 1971; Salsbury, 1975; Liotta *et
al*., 1976). Many of the neoplastic cells entering the circulation
either are not viable or else undergo cytolysis in the blood or in
the target tissues. The inability to define the length of time
preceding the formation of metastases is a major drawback in
studies of the mechanisms of dissemination. Clinical and histopathological observations reveal that the length of the premeta-
static phase and the number of metastases is variable not only
among various types of tumors but also among individual neoplasias
of similar histogenetic origin. One possible approach to the experimental studies on malignant cell dissemination is the use of

"compromise" models, that is, systems that, while they do not
fulfill all the characteristics of spontaneous metastases, reach
a certain degree of comparability (Weiss, 1976; Day et al., 1977;
Fidler et al., 1978; Grundmann, 1980; Poste and Fidler, 1980).
These experimental models complement rather than exclude each
other. Hence, it is important to analyze the findings realized
with the various model systems, bearing in mind their limitations,
and to compare each with the natural history of "spontaneous"
human neoplasias.

II. EXPERIMENTAL MODELS OF METASTASES

Transplantation of Neoplastic Cell Suspensions

     An experimental model should satisfy at least two requisites:
(1) control over the initiation and evolution of the process, and
(2) reproducibility of the phenomenon under identical conditions.
These requirements are not met by spontaneous tumors, because the
occurrence of cell detachment and the ensuing stages of spread,
arrest, and extravasation cannot be predicted.
     Transplantation of tumorigenic cells into appropriate reci-
pient hosts has become a widely used method because the various
phases of dissemination can be repeatedly examined under controlled
conditions. However, Weiss (1980b) pointed out that neoplastic
cells are not released from a primary tumor, and the events occurring after inoculation might be comparable only to the implantation
phase of metastases.
     Results obtained via the injection of tumor cells may vary
greatly because of the various factors involved, including (1) the
characteristics of the animal hosts, (2) the tumorigenic cells
used, and (3) the route of cell inoculation. This last aspect is
critical, and there are particular problems associated with the
use of either intravenous (iv) or extravascular routes for injecting tumor cells (Fig. 1).
     The incidence and distribution of neoplastic nodules yielded
by iv injection of neoplastic cells are greatly influenced by the
vein into which the cells are inoculated. Since the circulating
neoplastic cells do not "spontaneously select" target organs,
their lodging in particular tissues suggests that the visceral
nodules are the result of a distant transplantation of tumor cells
rather than metastases.
     As noted earlier, primary tumors release various numbers of
cells over an extended period of time, and only some of these
cells give rise to metastases. This process is hardly comparable
with a single iv inoculation of a large number of cells, which may

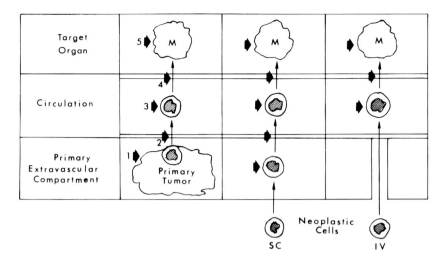

Fig. 1. Comparison between the development of metastases (M) from an autologous primary tumor and the stages of experimental reproduction of the process by subcutaneous (sc) or intravenous (iv) inoculation of neoplastic cells. Thick black arrows indicate the areas in which neoplastic cells may be influenced by the environment: (1) primary tissue, (2) vascular wall (intravasation), (3) circulation of cells carried by lymph and blood, (4) vascular wall (extravasation), and (5) tissue of the target organ.

lead to transient modifications of hemodynamics and blood viscosity. These changes, associated with the terminal branching of the vein into which the tumor cells were inoculated, may account for the distribution of "metastases."

A significant observation on the importance of the route of cell inoculation was made by Weiss (1980a,b), who injected intramuscularly (im), rather than iv, "highly metastatic" clones of melanoma B16 (Fidler and Kripke, 1977) into mice. The im-injected melanoma cells developed large, localized tumors that yielded a low number of pulmonary metastases in contrast to the numerous neoplastic nodules found in the lungs after iv injection.

Platelet adhesion to neoplastic cells has been proposed to be a characteristic phenomenon that could determine the attachment to endothelial surfaces and extravasation of tumor cells (Wood, 1958, 1971; Hiramoto et al., 1960; Gasic et al., 1973; Warren, 1973; Dvorak et al., 1979, 1981; Gaspar, 1980; Hilgard, 1980). Yet, platelet-cell surface interaction is one of the general mechanisms of behavior of blood cells at interfaces (Silberberg, 1977; Vroman et al., 1977). Neoplastic cells maintained in culture media have a "clean" surface to which mouse plasma proteins and, consequently, platelets can adhere after iv injection (Fig. 2). Furthermore, the adherence of platelets and fibrin to iv-injected neoplastic cells could not be reproduced in several experimental systems (Baserga and Saffiotti, 1955; Locker et al.,

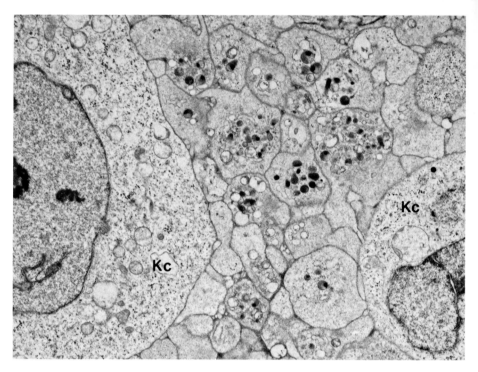

Fig. 2. Aggregate of partially degranulated platelets surrounding K-562 cells (Kc) 5 min after iv injection. The neoplastic
cells show swelling and disruption of mitochondria (×7500). (From
Machado *et al.*, 1982a.)

1970; Chew *et al.*, 1976; Dingemans *et al.*, 1978; Hilgard, 1980;
Machado *et al.*, 1982a). Concerning human pathology, Winterbauer
et al. (1968) found that only 20% of 366 patients with metastases
of various types of malignant tumors also had associated pulmonary
thrombosis and tumor emboli. Although platelets and fibrin may
possibly be involved in the formation of metastases of some tumors,
the experimental data are not conclusive and may result from a
nonspecific interaction with plasma.

Extravascular inoculation could avoid circulatory artifacts
that influence the arrest of the neoplastic cells in the host's
organs. A model of this type can be developed by sc injection of
neoplastic cells into newborn immunodeficient mice. Most malignant cells transplanted into *adult* mice proliferate, forming
tumors that do not metastasize (Shimosato *et al.*, 1976; Stiles *et
al.*, 1974, 1976; Fogh *et al.*, 1977; Sordat *et al.*, 1977;
Giovanella *et al.*, 1978; Machado *et al.*, 1978; Sharkey and Fogh,
1979). However, after injection into *newborn* nude mice, those
cells give rise to multiple visceral neoplastic nodules (Sordat
et al., 1977, 1982; Lozzio *et al.*, 1979; Lozzio and Machado,
1982; Machado *et al.*, 1982a,b,c). This change in the *in vivo*
behavior of malignant cells might be due to a functional deficiency of the natural killer (NK) lymphocytes in nude mice during the

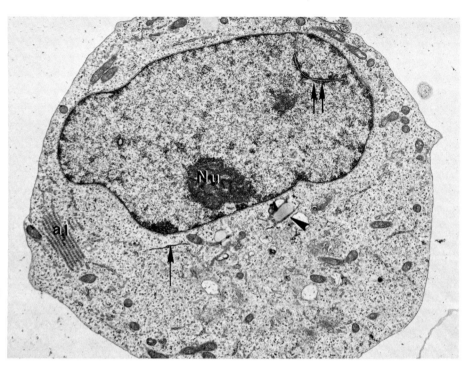

Fig. 3.   Transmission electron micrograph of K-562 cell in
suspension culture.   Double arrows indicate a nuclear cleft:
Nu, nucleoli.   Membranous inclusions (single arrow) and crystal-
loids (arrowhead) are present in the cytoplasm along with an
annulate-lamellae-type inclusion (a*l*) (×6000).

first 3 weeks of life (Herberman *et al.*, 1975; Herberman, 1978;
Fidler *et al.*, 1976), or to nonimmunological systemic factors
(DeWys, 1972).

Most neoplastic cells undergo necrosis after sc injection.
However, some viable cells remain at the site of inoculation and,
after a variable period of time ranging from hours to a few days,
will penetrate into the capillaries of the sc tissue (Machado *et
al.*, 1978).   This stage may permit the cells to attain a certain
degree of "adaptation" to the biological environment.

Vascular penetration of the neoplastic cells is gradual,
and therefore, abrupt changes in the composition and dynamics of
the blood of the host would not occur.   Since the neoplastic
cells reach the systemic circulation through secondary vascular
pathways (rather than by direct entrance into the main circulatory stream as occurs with an iv injection), their arrest in various
organs follows spontaneous patterns.

1. K-562 Cell Line

In our experimental model, we have used the K-562 cell line derived from a patient with chronic myelogenous leukemia (CML) in terminal blast crisis (Fig. 3) (Lozzio and Lozzio, 1975). The cells have been maintained in suspension culture for over 10 years and 554 serial passages. They contain the Philadelphia (Ph^1+) chromosome and a translocation 15;17. The properties of K-562 cells have been reviewed in several publications (Klein et al., 1976; Collins et al., 1977; Andersson et al., 1979; Lozzio and Lozzio, 1979a,b; Maxwell et al., 1979; Fukuda et al., 1981; Lozzio et al., 1981, 1983; Vainchenker et al., 1981; Fuhr et al., 1982).

After transplantation into immunodeficient mice, K-562 cells behave as malignant cells derived from epithelial or mesenchymal solid tumors; they proliferate, forming nodular tumors without modifying the hematopoietic tissues or the peripheral blood of the host. The neoplastic proliferation is consistently reproduced and can be maintained by serial passages in the immunodeficient mice. For all practical purposes, the K-562 line constitutes an excellent tool for investigating the formation of tumors and metastases and for studies on therapy of malignancies.

In our earlier studies, we used athymic-asplenic (lasat) mice (Lozzio et al., 1976; Machado et al., 1976). However, the cells are currently transplanted into athymic (nude) mice with similar results. In adult mice, 5×10^6 viable cells, enmeshed in a fibrin clot, are implanted sc in the dorsal-anterior region. Newborn mice, on the other hand, receive sc an aliquot of 50 μl of culture medium containing 10^7 K-562 cells, also in the dorsal area. In adult mice, the cells developed an sc myelosarcoma at the site of injection, while in the newborn mice, neoplastic growths were produced in the lungs, kidneys, brain, and lymph nodes of the host (Table I).

2. Subcutaneous K-562 Myelosarcomas

After 5 to 7 days from the moment of transplantation of the K-562 cells, an sc nodule appeared and enlarged steadily (Fig. 4). Because the length of the lag period, the rate of tumor growth, and the final volume reached (Fig. 5) varied among different K-562 cell samples, we consistently used cells from selected passages. The neoplastic growth progressed for the next 20-25 days, reaching a fivefold increase over the initial size of the transplant (Machado et al., 1977).

Sequential histological examinations demonstrated multiple capillary sprouts from the mouse sc tissue in the marginal area of the transplant (Fig. 6). The neocapillaries penetrated toward the center of the transplant and were supported by parallel arrays of developing reticulin fibrils (Fig. 7). The transplanted cells proliferated along the fibrovascular arrays and finally formed a

TABLE I. Incidence and Distribution of Metastases Arising from K-562 Cells Injected Neonatally into Nude and Lasat Mice

Mice	Detectable metastases (days[a])	Incidence of metastases[a,b]		Distribution of metastases[a,b]			
		Number	Percentage	Lung	Brain	Kidney	Lymph nodes
BALB/c Nude	10-86	59/97	60.8	52/97	20/97[c]	9/97	3/97[c]
BALB/c Lasat	17-62	24/39	61.6	20/39	16/39[c]	4/39	3/39[c]

[a] As determined on autopsy and microscopic examination.
[b] Ratios are number of mice with metastases/total number of mice.
[c] $\chi^2 = 12.4$ ($p < .001$).

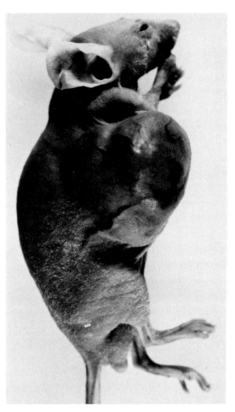

Fig. 4. Subcutaneous myelosarcoma arising from K-562 cells implanted in a fibrin clot in a nude mouse 32 days previously. (From Lozzio and Machado, 1982.)

solid myelosarcoma (Fig. 8). Thirty days after transplantation, either the growth of the vascular network did not match the speed of neoplastic cell proliferation or capillary thrombosis occurred, which led to focal ischemic necrosis. A large part of the tumor, however, retained the mitotic activity and could be serially transplanted.

As in most heterotransplanted malignancies, infiltration of surrounding tissue by the malignant cells was only occasionally observed, but the invasion of the vascular lumen of the tumor capillaries by K-562 cells was a common feature (Fig. 9). Despite the intravascular release of cells, microemboli of cells and/or metastases were not observed in an extensive number of serial histological sections of various organs from early 2000 tumor-bearing nude mice.

The sc myelosarcomas are readily accessible to inspection for assessing the effects of various agents on tumor growth. Since biopsies of the tumors are obtainable, any change can be verified by histopathological examinations. This is important because naked-eye observations are deceptive; modifications of neoplastic volume may result from edema or hemorrhage. Furthermore, subtle,

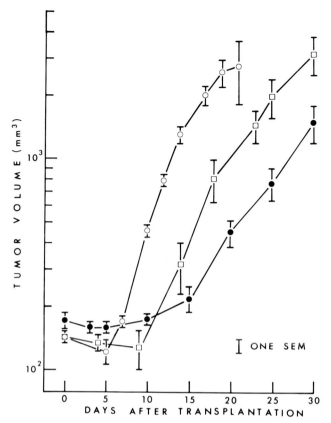

Fig. 5. Growth of three mouse-to-mouse passages of a K-562 myelosarcoma of passage 221 of the cell line. Each point denotes the mean ± 1 SEM of 10 to 15 mice. (From Lozzio and Machado, 1982.) •, 1st mouse passage; □, 10th mouse passage; o, 20th mouse passage.

early cell changes induced by therapeutic agents only be detected by light- and electron-microscopic examinations.

3. *Disseminated K-562 Myelosarcomas*

Lasat and nude mice, within 24 hr of birth, were injected sc in the dorsal area with 50 μl of minimal essential medium containing 10^7 K-562 cells (Lozzio *et al.*, 1979; Machado *et al.*, 1982a,b). No further treatment was given. After the edema was resorbed, mice did not show visible or palpable sc nodules. Autopsies performed at variable periods of time after inoculation revealed multiple neoplastic nodules in the lungs, kidneys, and lymph nodes, and a diffuse infiltration of the meningeal space (Figs. 10-12). About one-third of the mice (27%) also developed sc myelosarcomas at or near the site of injection. These local sc

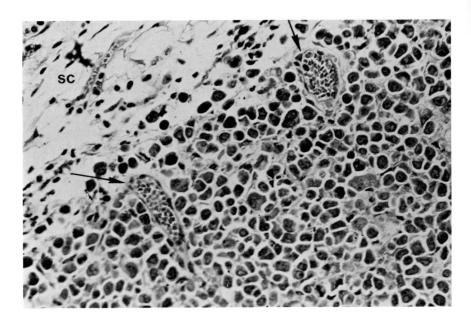

Fig. 6. Early stage (Day 5) of development of a myelosarcoma after sc transplantation of K-562 cells into an adult nude mouse. Capillaries (arrows) advance from the sc tissue of the host amidst the proliferating neoplastic cells (H&E; ×400). (From Machado *et al.*, 1977.)

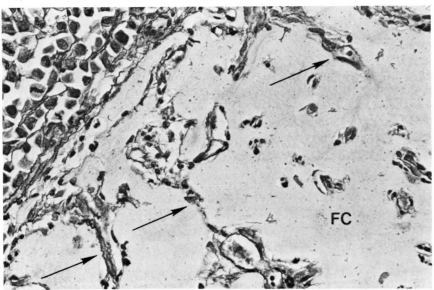

Fig. 7. Capillary outgrowths (arrows) precede the proliferation of K-562 cells toward the center of the transplant formed by necrotic debris and remnants of fibrin (FC) (Gomori's silver method; ×400). (From Machado *et al.*, 1977.)

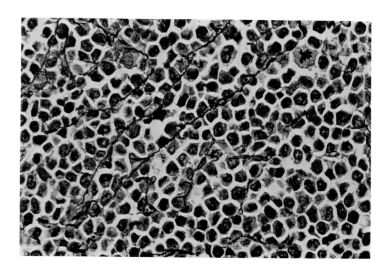

Fig. 8. Fully developed sc K-562 myelosarcoma (Gomori's silver method; ×400).

tumors were preceded by lag periods lasting from 15 to 34 days (as compared to 7 to 9 days when the cells were transplanted into adult nude mice). The sc myelosarcomas developing from neonatally injected K-562 cells induced macrophages and giant multinucleated cell proliferation (Fig. 13). Similar macrophages were not observed around the myelosarcomas grown in adult nude mice.

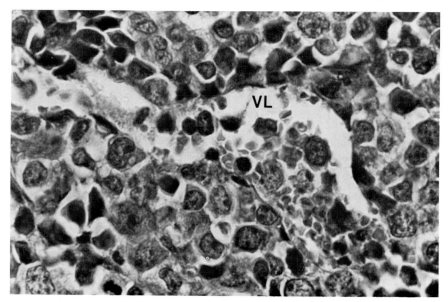

Fig. 9. A capillary of the fibrovascular stroma of an sc K-562 tumor shows discontinuous walls. Tumor cells are exposed to circulation, and some of them appear detached into the vascular lumen (VL) (H&E; ×520). (From Machado *et al.*, 1977.)

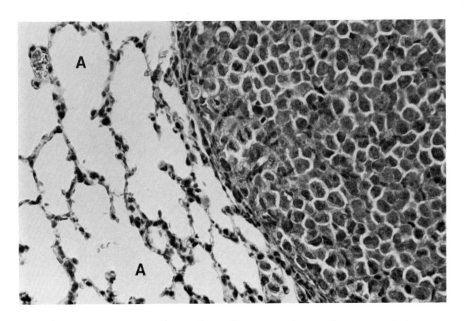

Fig. 10. Neoplastic nodule in lung of a nude mouse injected neonatally with K-562 cells 30 days earlier (A, alveoli) (H&E; ×400).

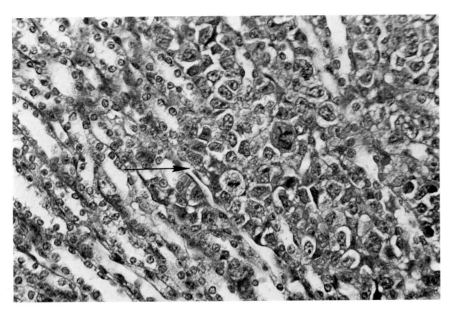

Fig. 11. Same nude mouse as in Fig. 10, showing development of a neoplastic nodule (arrow) formed by K-562 cells in kidney (H&E; ×400).

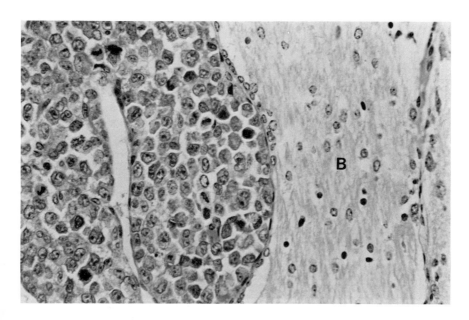

Fig. 12. Same nude mouse as in Fig. 10. The K-563 cells in-filtrate the meningeal space of the brain (B) (H&E; ×400).

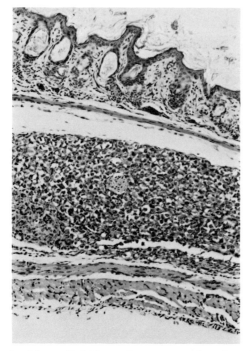

Fig. 13. Small sc K-562 myelosarcoma developed after a long lag period in a nude mouse with disseminated neoplastic growth (H&E; ×75).

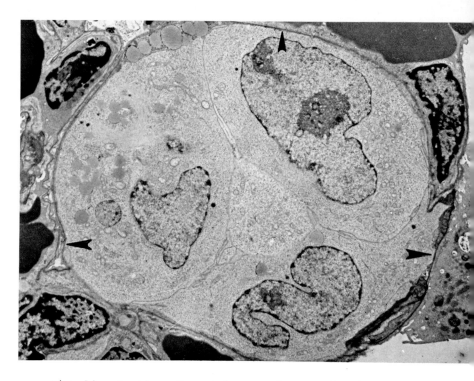

Fig. 14. Section of an intravascular neoplastic nodule showing portions of four cells. Compression of the endothelium as
well as endothelial gaps are observed in this micrograph (arrowheads) (×4000). (From Machado *et al.*, 1982a).

During the early stage (1-6 hr after injection), the K-562
cells penetrated into the capillaries of the sc tissues, and
thereafter, intact K-562 cells were difficult to detect in the
injection area, which contained accumulations of nuclear and cytoplasmic debris. However, a small number of viable K-562 cells
may have remained at the site of injection because, as noted
already in some mice, after a long lag period, they started proliferating. Semiserial sections of tissue from various organs
obtained at sequential periods after injection of the cells were
examined by light and transmission electron microscopy. As early
as 1 to 3 hr after sc inoculation, K-562 cells were found in lung
capillaries. The cells displayed mitotic activity and, after
2 days, formed multiple microemboli distributed throughout the
organ. The neoplastic cells appeared uniformly attached to the
entire endothelial surface and did not extend through the junctions (Fig. 14). Gradually, the endothelium and underlying layers
of the capillary walls were destroyed by the proliferating neoplastic cells, which formed large nodules (Fig. 15). These neoplastic nodules protruded into the alveolar spaces and, after the
capillary wall had disappeared, came in contact with the alveolar
epithelial cells and capillaries (Fig. 16). The metastatic
nodules then acquired a morphological structure similar to that

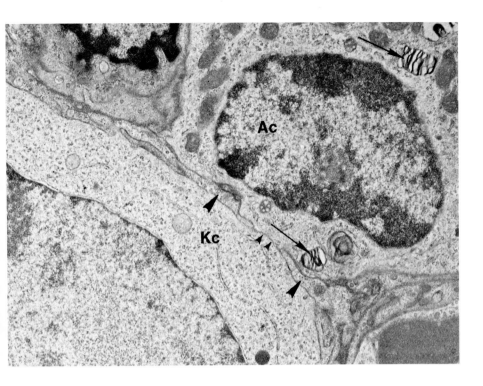

Fig. 15. Micrograph showing a K-562 cell (Kc) in direct contact with an alveolar cell (Ac, small arrowheads). Portions of the endothelium (large arrowheads) can be seen surrounding the area of intercellular contact (×12,000).

observed in sc myelosarcomas (Fig. 17). Platelets were not observed during the neoplastic cell arrest and extravasation.

4. Cyclic Transplantation of K-562 Cells

The permanence of the characteristics of the K-562 cells proliferating as local or metastatic tumors was assessed by cyclic culture and transplantation (Machado *et al.*, 1982c). An aliquot of K-562 cells was inoculated into adult mice (Fig. 18); then cells recovered from sc myelosarcomas were injected into newborn nude mice, producing pulmonary and renal metastases and infiltrating the meningeal space and lymph nodes. This change in the growth pattern of the K-562 cells in nude mice was consistently observed during sequential reculturing and retransplantation of the cells comprising the sc tumors or metastases that had been derived from a single cell passage. The development of local or disseminated myelosarcomas was not associated with morphological, antigenic, or chromosomal changes of the K-562 cells (Machado *et al.*, 1982c).

A remarkable feature of the experimental design is that only one variable and three constant factors influenced the results.

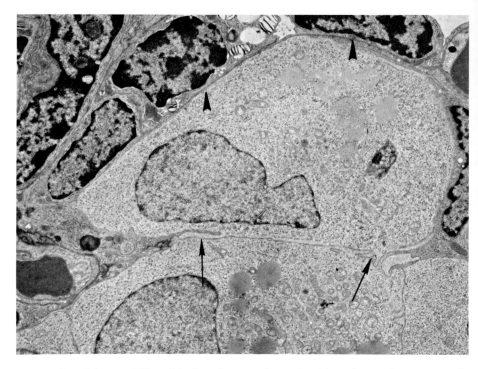

Fig. 16. K-562 cell forming an invagination into the surrounding pulmonary tissue. This protruding cell maintains interdigita-
tions with the adjoining intravascular K-562 cell (arrows).
Despite the pronounced protrusion of the neoplastic cell into normal tissue, the basement membrane (arrowheads) and endothelial
lining remain intact (×4500).

The variable factor was the age of the recipient nude mice. The
three constant factors were (1) a single passage of K-562 cells
grown and recultured under identical conditions, (2) hosts of
identical genetic background kept in the same environment, and
(3) identical procedures of culture and sc inoculation of the
cells in each step. It appears, then, that all or some K-562
cells of the initial aliquot and their descendants had the potential for disseminated growth, which was expressed only under
certain environmental conditions.

5. *Experimental Metastases of Human Melanomas*

Experiments were conducted with a different malignant cell
type to demonstrate whether or not the metastatic process in *newborn* nude mice was a particular property of the K-562 cells or
was conditioned by the host. Thus, human melanomas transplanted
sc were maintained for more than 40 successive passages in *adult*
nude mice. The growth of the sc melanoma was always local;
metastases were not observed by macroscopic or microscopic exami-

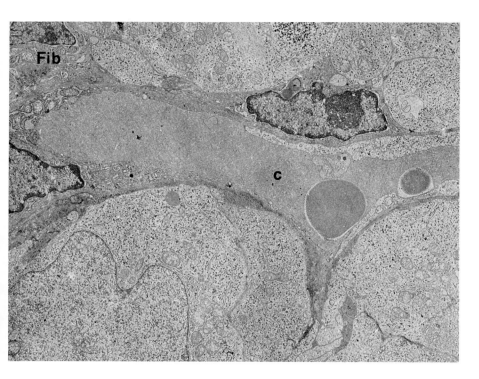

Fib

c

Fig. 17. K-562 cells proliferating in the extravascular pulmonary compartment display a sarcomatous pattern. Newly formed capillaries (c) and fibroblasts (Fib) form the stroma of the neoplastic growth (×4500).

nations. A suspension of cells from an sc melanoma was then injected into *newborn* nude mice, resulting in multiple pulmonary metastases, preserving the cytological features of the original tumor (Lozzio and Machado, 1982).

6. New Models of Disseminated Neoplastic Proliferation

The maintenance in serial passages of a variety of human malignancies transplanted into nude mice is now well documented (Povlsen *et al.*, 1982). The serial heterotransplantation of human malignant hematopoietic cells, however, has been mostly unsuccessful. On the whole, such studies have been restricted to use of the K-562 cell line (Lozzio and Lozzio, 1975, 1979b; Machado *et al.*, 1977), two cell lines derived from the African (Abongo) and American (Ramos) varieties of Burkitt's lymphoma (B. C. Giovanella, personal communication), and, more recently, the T-lymphoblast cell lines JM and MOLT-4 and the promyelocytic cell line HL-60 (Lozzio and Machado, 1982). Other transplanted leukemia and lymphoma cell lines (Epstein *et al.*, 1976; Nilsson *et al.*, 1977; Giovanella *et al.*, 1979; Schaadt *et al.*, 1979) have not been perpetuated in nude mice by serial passage over a long period of time.

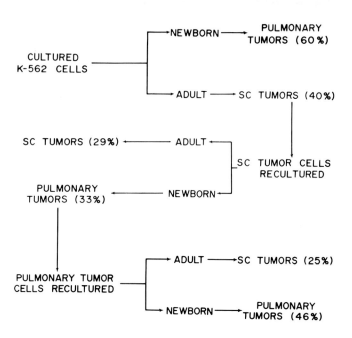

Fig. 18. Subcutaneous and pulmonary myelosarcomas arise from an sc injection of K-562 cells into either adult or newborn nude mice, respectively. The neoplastic cells in these cyclic transplantations and cultures derived from a single initial aliquot. Figures represent percentages of inoculated mice developing tumors. (From Machado *et al.*, 1982c.)

We have developed transplantable myelosarcomas composed of human myeloid leukemia cells such as the KG-1 (Koeffler and Golde, 1978), KG-1a (Koeffler *et al.*, 1980), and HL-60 (Collins *et al.*, 1977). The myeloid cells that were injected sc into newborn nude mice proliferated both at the site of inoculation and in the lungs and kidneys of the hosts (Figs. 19-21). The incidence and distribution of neoplastic growths of human hematogenous cell lines in nude mice appear in Table II, which includes updated figures from our experiments with the K-562 cell line.

III. SPECIFIC IMMUNOTHERAPY

A. Antibody Therapy

The immunological approach to therapy of cancer is still a matter of debate. Many contradictions arising from experimental attempts may be due to the characteristics of the models used and to unwarranted generalizations of the results obtained with a particular system.

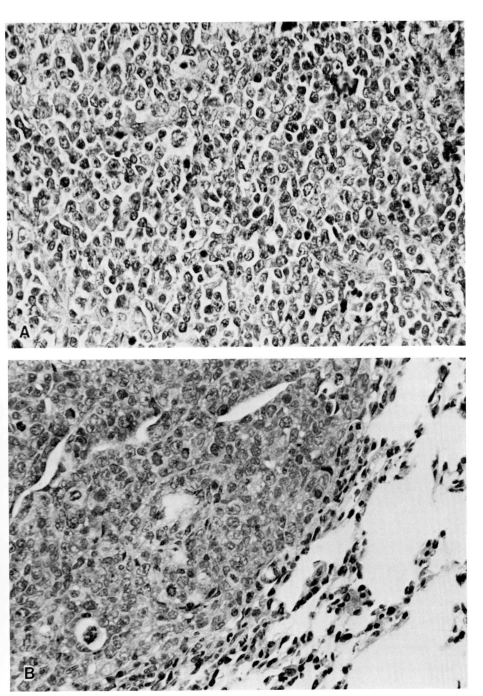

Fig. 19. (A) Subcutaneous KG-1 myelosarcoma. (B) Pulmonary KG-1 myelosarcoma (H&E; ×250).

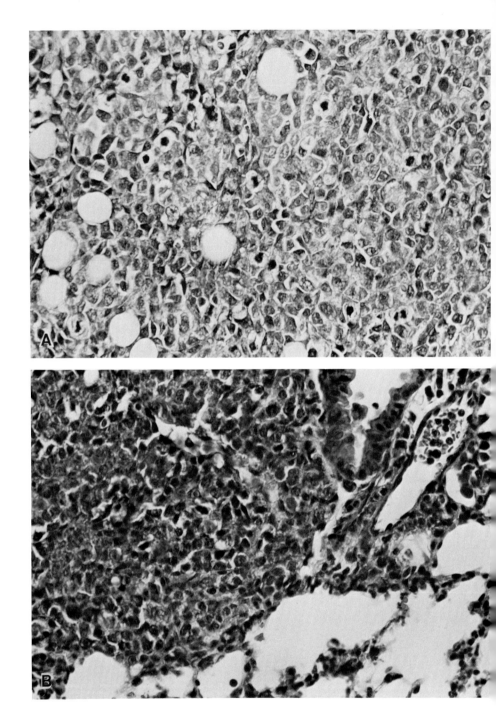

Fig. 20. (A) Subcutaneous KG-1a myelosarcoma. (B) Pulmonary KG-1a myelosarcoma (H&E; ×250).

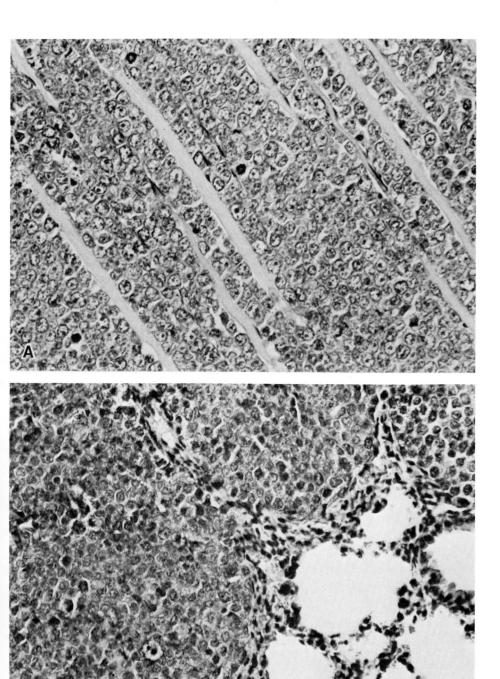

Fig. 21. (A) Subcutaneous HL-60 myelosarcoma. (B) Pulmonary HL-60 myelosarcoma (H&E; ×250).

TABLE II. Incidence and Distribution of Neoplastic Processes Arising from Human Hematopoietic Cells Inoculated Neonatally into Nude Mice

	Nature[a]	Number of mice with neoplastic growth/total number of mice	Number of mice with sc tumors	Number of mice with visceral disseminations						
				Lungs	Kidneys	Brain	Lymph nodes	Bone marrow	Liver	Spleen
62	Pluripotential (CML)	89/136	35	74	15	38	4	0	0	0
1	Myelogenous (AML)	31/39	31	5	1	0	1	0	0	0
1a	Myelogenous (AML)	34/35	34	17	1	0	0	0	0	0
60	Promyelocytic (APL)	2/21	2	2	2	0	0	0	0	0
I	Burkitt's lymphoma (B)	34/50	27	10	14	12	3	3	4	5
T-4	T Lymphoblasts (ALL)	2/12	2	0	0	0	0	0	0	0
	T Lymphoblasts (ALL)	20/48	14	3	5	7	0	0	0	0

[a]CML and AML: chronic and acute myelogenous leukemia; APL and ALL: acute promyelocytic and lymphoblastic kemia; B and T: bone marrow- and thymus-derived cells.

TABLE III. [^{3}H]TdR Uptake by Myelosarcomas Made Up of K-562 Myelogenous Leukemia Cells[a]

Group	Tumor volume (mm^3)	Tumor weight (mg)	Specific [^{3}H]TdR incorporation (10^{-5} µC/mg)	Total [^{3}H]TdR incorporation (10^{-5} µC)
Control	236 ± 39	305 ± 61	10 ± 0.7	3158 ± 704
Preimmune sera[b]	164 ± 34	235 ± 47	9 ± 0.4	2109 ± 448
Immune sera	71 ± 14	64 ± 24	5 ± 1.4	543 ± 307

[a]Numbers are means ± 1 SE of six to eight tumors, rounded to the nearest unit.
[b]Plus guinea pig serum.

Yang and Vas (1972) demonstrated that a specific antibody to leukemia cells can inhibit cell growth and metabolism in the absence of effector cells and complement. It has also since then been observed that a polyclonal antibody to the human cell line K-562 inhibited DNA synthesis (Table III) and resulted in cell death and lysis (Lozzio *et al.*, 1982). These findings are significant for studies on immunotherapy of malignant neoplastic growths of hematopoietic origin and tumors of other histogenetic types as well. To test the ability of the antibody to K-562 cells to abrogate local and metastatic malignant cell proliferation in a biological environment, we used the tumor-mouse systems described in the preceding sections. It must be emphasized that the K-562, KG-1, KG-1a, and HL-60 cells used in these models behave in the mice as do transplanted cells from malignant solid tumors: They form discrete nodular growths and do not affect the bone marrow, spleen, or peripheral blood of the host. The lag phase, logarithmic growth, and appearance of ischemic necrosis of such experimental tumors have been well characterized, and therefore, the changes produced by therapeutic regimens can be readily evaluated.

1. *Immune γ-Globulin*

A specific antibody was developed by im injection into goats of K-562 cells emulsified in complete Freund's adjuvant at a concentration of 2.5×10^6 cells/kg. The injections were given on Days 1, 7, 14, and 21, followed, on Day 28, by an iv injection of cells without adjuvant. On Day 35, goats were bled and the serum was separated. The serum complement was then heat inactivated at $56°C$ for 30 min. Subsequently, the serum was absorbed with human cells for *in vitro* assays and with mouse cell for *in vivo* assays. γ-Globulins were isolated by precipitation with a 37% solution of ammonium sulfate. Protein content was determined by a modification of the Lowry method (Hartree, 1972).

The absolute concentration of IgG was determined in γ-globulin preparations via the radial immunodiffusion technique (Mancini *et al.*, 1965) using monospecific rabbit anti-goat IgG H and L chains (Lot no. 04161, Pel-Freeze Biologicals, Rogers, Arkansas) incorporated in agarose gel, and by rocket immunoelectrophoresis in agarose (Laurell, 1966) containing rabbit anti-goat IgG. The final product, lyophilized in 30-mg aliquots, were kept at $4°C$ until use. Preimmune (normal) γ-globulin was processed as the immune γ-globulin. Quantitative data on the immune IgG were obtained by subtracting the normal value found in preimmune serum from that of the immune serum of each goat.

In vitro tests demonstrated that the anti-K-562 γ-globulin not only bound specifically with K-562 cells but also cross-reacted with several human malignant hematopoietic cell lines (Lozzio *et al.*, 1983). The cell lines tested included T lymphoblasts (JM and MOLT-4), promyelocytes (HL-60), Burkitt's lymphoma cells

(RAJI), and myeloblasts (KG-l and KG-la). When the immune
γ-globulin was absorbed with an equal number of cells from each
of the cell lines assayed, the antibody responsible for cytolysis
of K-562 target cells was diminished but not entirely removed.
Thus, the K-562 cells appear to possess common and specific
antigens that may be only partially expressed on other cell lines
studied (Lozzio and Machado, 1982; Lozzio et al., 1983).

2. Immunotherapy of Experimental Tumors

Since the results of in vitro experiments demonstrated that
the anti-K-562 cells γ-globulin had cytolytic properties on several human hematopoietic malignant cell lines, studies were
initiated to assess the antineoplastic effect of the antibody in
vivo. The tumor-mouse systems used included the local and metastatic K-562 and KG-l myelosarcomas (Lozzio et al., 1979; Lozzio
and Machado, 1982; Machado et al., 1982b), and the JM and MOLT-4
lymphosarcomas. Human carcinomas and melanomas proliferating in
nude mice served as controls.

a. Subcutaneous Tumors

Nude mice bearing serially transplanted tumors were injected
intraperitoneally (ip) with goat γ-globulin against K-562 cells
(Lozzio et al., 1979). Treatment was started 7 days after transplantation during the logarithmic phase of growth when tumors are
already well vascularized, and was continued with ip injections
of 6 mg of γ-globulin given every 3 days for 15 days. Control
groups of mice with sc tumors were either treated with nonimmune
(normal) γ-globulin or did not receive further treatment. The
immune γ-globulin abrogated the growth of both the K-562 and KG-l
myelosarcomas as well as the JM and MOLT-4 lymphosarcomas (Figs.
22 and 23). Sequential histopathological examinations demonstrated
that, during the early phase of treatment, the myelosarcoma cells
underwent hydropic degeneration (swelling) and nuclear pyknosis
(Fig. 24); following this stage, there was massive coagulation
necrosis of the tumor (Fig. 25). In many tumors, hydropic cell
degeneration and necrosis were present simultaneously in adjacent
areas.
    Human prostatic, pulmonary, and mammary gland carcinomas and
melanomas proliferating after sc transplantation into the mice
were not affected by the immunoglobulin treatment (Figs. 26 and
27). In other experiments, adult nude mice were implanted sc with
a K-562 myelosarcoma in one flank and either a prostatic carcinoma
or melanoma in the contralateral side. As in the preceding experiments, the administration of immune γ-globulin was started 7 days
after transplantation when each tumor was well vascularized. The
immune γ-globulin selectively abrogated the proliferation of the

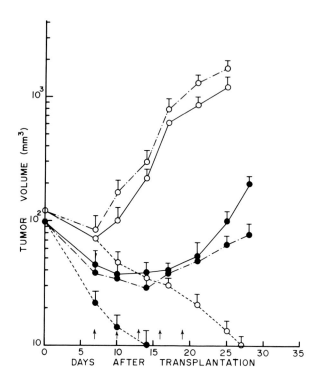

Fig. 22. Therapeutic effect of specific IγG on the growth of sc K-562 (o) and KG-1 (●) myelosarcomas. Controls were treated with nonimmune globulin or did not receive any treatment. In this and following graphics, vertical arrows indicate injection of antibody or nonimmune globulin. Each point represents the mean ± 1 SEM of 5 to 10 mice. —— • ——, Untreated; ————, NγG; ------, IγG.

K-562 myelosarcomas, whereas the prostatic carcinoma and the melanoma proliferated and formed large tumors (Fig. 28). Thus, the suppression of cell proliferation by the immune γ-globulin to K-562 cells was restricted to myelosarcomas and lymphosarcomas.

b. Metastatic Tumors

Two of the models of metastatic proliferation (the K-562 and KG-la myelosarcomas), produced by neonatal injection of the cells into nude mice, have been used for immunotherapeutic trials with the anti-K-562 cells immune γ-globulin. The treatment regimen was identical to that described for serially transplanted sc tumors.

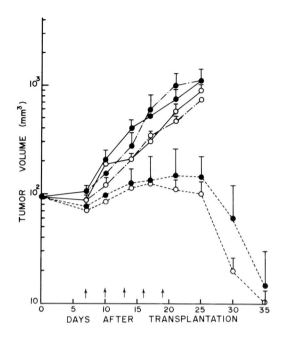

Fig. 23. Therapeutic effect of antibody to K-562 cells on JM
(●) and MOLT (o) sc sarcomas.

c. *K-562 Metastatic Myelosarcomas.* Seven days after receiving sc implantations of 10^7 K-562 cells, newborn mice were
injected with both immune and normal γ-globulin; doses of 250
mg/kg each were repeated every 3 days for a total of five injections. The control groups receiving normal γ-globulin or no
treatment did not modify the overall incidence (≈60%) of pulmonary
metastases. In marked contrast, only 16.7% of the mice treated
with immune γ-globulin had small intravascular emboli of K-562
cells (Table IV and Fig. 29). The cells showed signs of necrosis
and were only detectable after careful light-microscopic examinations of serial sections of the lungs.
    Extravasation of the malignant cells was rare, and, when
present, the K-562 cells displayed signs of necrosis similar to
those described in sc myelosarcomas of mice treated with immune
γ-globulin. The presence of intravascular emboli or metastases
in the kidneys and brain was ruled out by repeated histological
examinations.

d. *KG-la Metastatic Myelosarcomas.* Since it was difficult to
establish the KG-la myelosarcomas as a serially transplantable tumor in adult nude mice, immunoglobulin treatment (as described
previously) was immediately initiated in mice inoculated at birth

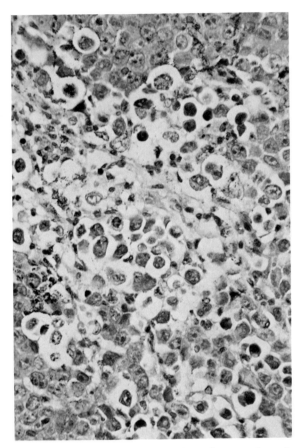

Fig. 24. Cytoplasmic swelling and nuclear pyknosis of cells
of a K-562 myelosarcoma at early stages of antibody treatment
(H&E; ×400).

with 10^7 cells. The ensuing therapeutic protocol was identical to
that described for the K-562 myelosarcomas. Preliminary results
indicated that the anti-K-562 immune γ-globulin has the same cytotoxic effect against the KG-1a cell line as for the other malignant
hematopoietic cell lines. The 35 untreated mice injected sc at
birth with KG-1a cells showing a 48% incidence of lung metastases
and a 97% incidence of sc tumor formation. Eight other mice
treated with normal γ-globulin showed a 38% incidence of lung
metastases and 100% incidence of sc tumor formation. In contrast,
18 mice treated with immune γ-globulin had only a 5.5% incidence
of lung metastases and 11% incidence of sc tumor formation.

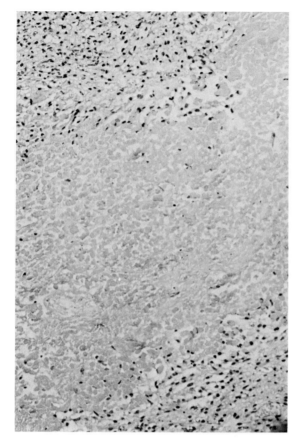

Fig. 25. Massive coagulation necrosis of a K-562 myelosarcoma, advanced stages of treatment (H&E; ×280).

B. Mechanisms of Action of Immune γ-Globulin

    The mechanisms by which a heterologous antibody inhibited the
development of metastases are probably similar to those producing
the suppression of the growth of K-562 myelosarcomas and the
proliferation of other human malignant hematopoietic cells transplanted in nude mice (Latif et al., 1979, 1980; Lozzio, 1979;
Lozzio et al., 1981), and may produce in some ways the mechanism
of lysis of those cells in vitro (Lozzio et al., 1982; Wust et
al., 1982). However, the results indicated that abrogation of
cell proliferation by the antibody is also effective in mice de-
complemented by treatment with cobra venom factor (CoF) (Fig. 30).
Therefore, antibody-dependent, complement-mediated cytotoxicity
(ADCMC) is apparently not the in vivo mechanism. In contrast to
observations for in vitro antibody cytolysis (Lozzio et al.,
1982), it was found that only intact globulin and not the fragment F(ab), was able to restrict tumor growth in mice (Fig. 31).

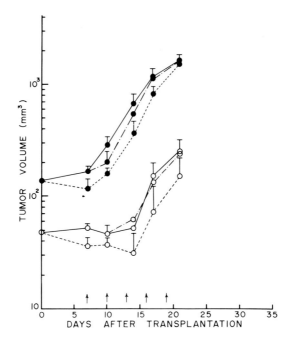

Fig. 26.   The growth of human lung (●) and prostate (o) carcinomas transplanted in nude mice is not influenced by I G to
K-562 cells. —·—, Untreated; ———, NγG; -----, IγG.

    Thus, a probable mechanism of action of the antibody *in vivo*
is direct antibody cytolysis with a secondary cytolysis mediated
by effector cells (ADCC) (Lozzio *et al.*, 1982).   Earlier studies
(Latif *et al.*, 1979) have demonstrated that K-562 cells were
lysed *in vitro* even at very high (1:1000) antibody dilutions if
nude mice spleen cells were added to the system.
    Thus, immune γ-globulin administered to immunodeficient mice
could react with target cells, leading to involvement of macrophages of killer cells in ADCC, which would destroy K-562 cells
transplanted into nude mice.

IV.   SUMMARY

    We have developed models of local and disseminated growth of
human malignant cells in immunodeficient mice.   These tumor-
mouse systems are reproducible, and the morphological, karyotypic,
and antigen features of the neoplastic cells are preserved
through serial transplantation.   These characteristics make the
models suitable for experimental therapeutic testing.   In this

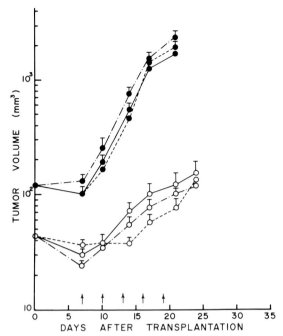

Fig. 27. Human breast carcinoma (●) and melanoma (o) proliferate in nude mice without being affected by the IγG to K-562 cells.
—·—, Untreated; ———, NγG; -----, IγG.

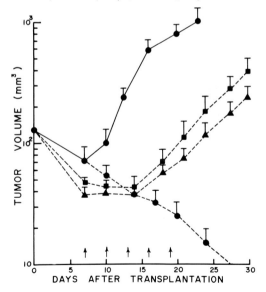

Fig. 28. The antibody abrogates the growth of K-562 myelosarcoma (●) but does not influence human prostate carcinoma (■) or
melanoma (▲) transplanted in the same host. ———, NγG;
-----, IγG.

TABLE IV. Incidence and Distribution of Metastases Arising from K-562 Cells Injected Neonatally into Nude Mice

Group	Detectable metastases (days[a])	Incidence of metastases[a,b]		Distribution of metastases[a,b]			
		Number	Percentage	Lung	Brain	Kidney	Lymph nodes
Untreated	10-102	83/139	59.7	74/139	36/139	13/139	5/139
γ-Globulin							
normal	16-107	31/53	58.5	29/53	2/53	5/53	0/53
immune	21-91	9/54[c]	16.7[c]	9/54[c]	0/54	0/54	0/54

[a] As determined on autopsy and microscopic examination.
[b] Ratios are number of mice with metastases/total number of mice.
[c] One or two emboil (see Fig. 2) of K-562 cells in the lungs. Fully developed metastases were not observed.

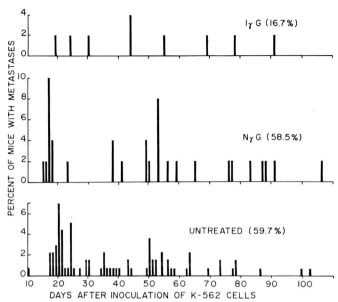

Fig. 29. Graphic representation of (1) abrogation of metastatic growth by immune γ-globulin, (2) incidence of metastatic
growth after a single transplantation of K-562 cells into newborn
nude mice; and (3) lack of influence of normal globulin on the
process. Each bar represents cumulative incidence of metastases
in five to eight mice. Numbers in parentheses correspond to percentage of mice with metastases.

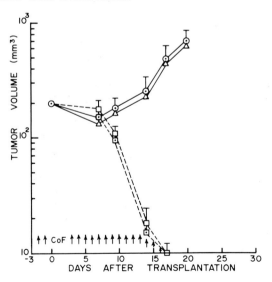

Fig. 30. Decomplementation of mice by cobra venom factor
(CoF) does not influence the therapeutic effect of antibody on
K-562 myelosarcomas. Δ, NγG; □, IγG; ⊡, IγG + CoF; ⊙, CoF.

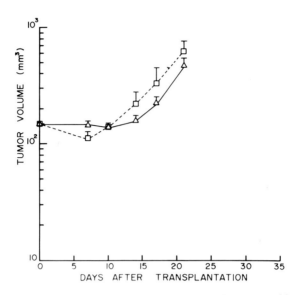

Fig. 31. Immune F(ab) (□) does not show an effect on the growth of K-562 myelosarcomas. Δ, Normal F(ab).

study, a heterologous polyclonal antibody raised against the neoplastic cells has proved to be an effective therapeutic agent that produces massive degeneration in local tumors and abrogates the development of disseminated neoplastic growth in the internal organs of the host. Our current studies are aimed at detecting similar therapeutic effects of monoclonal antibodies developed against the K-562 and other human malignant cell lines as well. Since these experiments are still in the trial stage, our findings are to be reported in the near future.

We are aware of the problems encountered in comparing results gathered from the use of various models in which experimental conditions differ. Furthermore, the extrapolation of findings in experimental systems to the human situation is particularly difficult. Nevertheless, we believe that the observations described here are indicative of the potentials of passive immunotherapy in local and metastatic neoplastic growth by specific antibodies developed against the types of malignant cells involved in the process.

Finally, specific antibodies could also be used as carriers for chemical and radioactive agents in order to achieve a high concentration of the therapeutic compound on the neoplastic cells without affecting normal tissues. This hypothetical use of antibodies is currently being explored in several laboratories, including ours.

ACKNOWLEDGMENTS

We thank Dr. Sandra Bell for her collaboration in the karyo-
typing of heterotransplanted human neoplastic cells, and
Ms. Bobbie Rush for her assistance in histopathological studies.
We also want to thank Ms. Marty Evers for her editorial work and
the skillful secretarial assistance of Ms. Ruth Martin and
Ms. Lucille Simpson.

These investigations were supported by Grants CA 18185 and
CA 17533, awarded by the National Cancer Institute, National
Institutes of Health, Department of Health and Human Services,
and were also aided in part by the Institutional Biomedical
Research Support Grant FR 5541 from the National Institutes of
Health, and by the Physicians Medical Education and Research
Foundation from the University of Tennessee Hospital, Knoxville,
Tennessee.

REFERENCES

Andersson, L. C., Nilsson, K., and Gahmberg, C. G. (1979).
   Int. J. Cancer 23, 143-147.
Baserga, R., and Saffiotti, U. (1955). *AMA Arch. Pathol. 59*,
   26-34.
Chew, E. C., Josephson, R. L., and Wallace, A. C. (1976). *In*
   "Fundamental Aspects of Metastasis" (L. Weiss, ed.), pp. 121-
   150. North-Holland, Amsterdam.
Collins, S. J., Gallo, R. C., and Gallagher, R. E. (1977).
   Nature (London) 270, 347-349.
Crile, G., Jr., Isbister, W., and Deodhar, S. D. (1971). *Cancer
   (Philadelphia) 28*, 655-656.
Day, S. B., Myers, W. P. L., Stansly, P., Garattini, S., and
   Lewis, M. G. (1977). "Cancer Invasion and Metastasis: Biologic
   Mechanisms and Therapy." Raven, New York.
DeWys, W. D. (1972). *Cancer Res. 32*, 374-379.
Dingemans, K. P., Roos, E., van den Bergh Weerman, M. A., and
   van de Pavert, I. V. (1978). *J. Natl. Cancer Inst. (US) 60*,
   583-598.
Dvorak, H. F., Dvorak, A. M., Manseau, E. J., Wiberg, L., and
   Churchill, W. H. (1979). *J. Natl. Cancer Inst. (US) 62*, 1459-
   1472.
Dvorak, H. F., Quay, S. C., Orenstein, N. S., Dvorak, A. M.,
   Hahn, P., Bitzer, A. M., and Carvalho, A. C. (1981). *Science
   (Washington, D.C.) 212*, 923-924.
Epstein, A. L., Herman, M. M., Kim, H., Dorfman, R. F., Path,
   M. R. C., and Kaplan, H. S. (1976). *Cancer (Philadelphia) 37*,
   2158-2176.

Fidler, I. J., and Kripke, M. L. (1977). *Science (Washington, D.C.) 197*, 893-895.

Fidler, I. J., Caines, S., and Dolan, Z. (1976). *Transplantation 22*, 208-212.

Fidler, I. J., Gersten, D. M., and Hart, I. R. (1978). *Adv. Cancer Res. 28*, 149-250.

Fogh, J., Fogh, J. M., and Orfeo, T. (1977). *J. Natl. Cancer Inst. (US) 59*, 221-226.

Foulds, L. (1969). "Neoplastic Development," Vol. 1, pp. 112-114. Academic Press, New York.

Fuhr, J. E., Bamberger, E., Lozzio, C. B., Lozzio, B. B., Felice, A. E., Altay, G., Webber, B. B., Reese, A. L., Mayson, S. M., and Huisman, T. H. J. (1982). *Am. J. Hematol. 12*, 1-12.

Fukuda, M., Fukuda, M. N., Papayannopoulou, T., and Hakomori, S. (1981). *In* "Hemoglobins in Development and Differentiation" (G. Stamatoyannopoulos and A. W. Niehuis, eds.), pp. 433-434. Liss, New York.

Gasic, G. J., Gasic, T. B., Galanti, N., Johnson, T., and Murphy, S. (1973). *Int. J. Cancer 11*, 704-718.

Gaspar, J. (1980). *In* "Metastatic Tumor Growth" (E. Grundmann, ed.), pp. 321-331. Fischer, New York.

Giovanella, B. C., Stehlin, J. S., Jr., Williams, L. J., Jr., Lee, S. S., and Shepard, R. C. (1978). *Cancer (Philadelphia) 42*, 2269-2281.

Giovanella, B., Nilsson, K., Zech, L., Yim, O., Klein, G., and Stehlin, J. S. (1979). *Int. J. Cancer 24*, 103-113.

Griffiths, J. D., and Salsbury, A. J. (1963). *Br. J. Cancer 17*, 546-557.

Grundmann, E. (ed.) (1980). "Metastatic Tumor Growth." Fischer, New York.

Hartree, E. F. (1972). *Anal. Biochem. 48*, 422-427.

Herberman, R. B. (1978). *In* "The Nude Mouse in Experimental and Clinical Research" (J. Fogh and B. C. Giovanella, eds.), Vol. 2, pp. 135-166. Academic Press, New York.

Herberman, R. B., Nunn, M. E., and Lavrin, D. H. (1975). *Int. J. Cancer 16*, 216-229.

Hilgard, P. (1980). *In* "Metastatic Tumor Growth" (E. Grundmann, ed.), pp. 107-116. Fischer, New York.

Hiramoto, R., Bernecky, J., Jurandowski, J., and Pressman, D. (1960). *Cancer Res. 20*, 592-593.

Klein, E., Ben-Bassat, H., Neumann, H., Ralph, P., Zeuthen, J., Polliack, A., and Vánky, F. (1976). *Int. J. Cancer 18*, 421-431.

Koeffler, H. P., and Golde, D. W. (1978). *Science (Washington, D.C.) 200*, 1153-1154.

Koeffler, H. P., Billing, R., Lusis, A. J., Sparkes, R. S., and Golde, D. W. (1980). *Blood 56*, 265-273.

Latif, Z. A., Lozzio, B. B., Lozzio, C. B., Herberman, R. B., and Wust, C. J. (1979). *Leuk, Res. 3*, 371-378.

Latif, Z. A., Lozzio, B. B., Wust, C. J., Krauss, S., Aggio, M. C., and Lozzio, C. B. (1980). *Cancer (Philadelphia) 45*, 1326-1333.

Laurell, C. B. (1966). *Anal. Biochem.* *15*, 45–52.
Liotta, L. A., Kleinerman, J., and Saidel, G. M. (1976). *Cancer Res.* *36*, 889–894.
Locker, J., Goldblatt, P. J., and Leighton, J. (1970). *Cancer Res.* *30*, 1632–1644.
Lozzio, B. B. (1979). *Adv. Med. Oncol. Res. Educ. 1*, 97–108.
Lozzio, B. B., and Lozzio, C. B. (1979a). *Int. J. Cancer 24*, 513.
Lozzio, B. B., and Lozzio, C. B. (1979b). *Leuk. Res. 3*, 363–370.
Lozzio, B. B., and Machado, E. A. (1982). *In* "The Nude Mouse in Experimental and Clinical Research" (J. Fogh and B. C. Giovanella, eds.), Vol. 2, pp. 521–567. Academic Press, New York.
Lozzio, B. B., Machado, E. A., Lozzio, C. B., and Lair, S. (1976). *J. Exp. Med. 143*, 225–231.
Lozzio, B. B., Machado, E. A., Lair, S. V., and Lozzio, C. B. (1979). *J. Natl. Cancer Inst. (US) 63*, 295–299.
Lozzio, B. B., Lozzio, C. B., Bamberger, E. G., and Feliu, A. S. (1981). *Proc. Soc. Exp. Biol. Med. 166*, 546–550.
Lozzio, B. B., Machado, E. A., Lozzio, C. B., Mitchell, J., and Wust, C. J. (1982). *Cancer Immunol. Immunother. 12*, 135–140.
Lozzio, B. B., Machado, E. A., Mitchell, J., Lozzio, C. B., Wust, C. J., and Golde, D. W. (1983). *Blood 61*, 1045–1053.
Lozzio, C. B., and Lozzio, B. B. (1975). *Blood 45*, 321–334.
Machado, E. A., Lozzio, B. B., and Lair, S. V. (1976). *In* "Immuno-Aspects of the Spleen" (J. R. Battisto and J. W. Streilein, eds.), pp. 215–226. North-Holland, Amsterdam.
Machado, E. A., Lozzio, B. B., Lozzio, C. B., Lair, S. V., and Aggio, M. C. (1977). *Cancer Res. 37*, 3995–4002.
Machado, E. A., Lozzio, B. B., Lozzio, C. B., and Aggio, M. C. (1978). *In* "Advances in Comparative Leukemia Research 1977" (P. Bentvelzen, J. Hilgers, and D. S. Yohn, eds.), pp. 418–421. Elsevier/North-Holland, Amsterdam.
Machado, E. A., Gerard, D. A., Mitchell, J. R., Lozzio, B. B., and Lozzio, C. B. (1982a). *Virchows Arch. A 396*, 73–89.
Machado, E. A., Lozzio, B. B., Lozzio, C. B., Lair, S. V., and Maxwell, P. A. (1982b). *In* "Proceedings of the Third International Workshop on Nude Mice" (N. D. Reed, ed.), pp. 391–402. Fischer, New York.
Machado, E. A., Mitchell, J. E., Lozzio, B. B., Lozzio, C. B., and Gerard, D. A. (1982c). *Br. J. Cancer 46*, 383–391.
Mancini, G., Carbonara, A. O., and Heremans, J. F. (1965). *Int. J. Immunochem. 2*, 235–254.
Maxwell, P. A., Machado, E. A., Lozzio, C. B., and Lozzio, B. B. (1979). *Annu. Proc. Electron Microsc. Soc. Amer. 37th*, pp. 234–235.
Nilsson, K., Giovanella, B. C., Stehlin, J. S., and Klein, G. (1977). *Int. J. Cancer 19*, 337–344.
Poste, G., and Fidler, I. J. (1980). *Nature (London) 283*, 139–146.
Povlsen, C., Rygaard, J., and Fogh, J. (1982). *In* "The Nude Mouse in Experimental and Clinical Research (J. Fogh and B. C. Giovanella, eds.), Vol. 2, pp. 79–93. Academic Press, New York.

Salsbury, A. J. (1975). *Cancer Treat. Rev. 2*, 55-72.

Schaadt, M., Kirchner, H., Fonatsch, C., and Diehl, V. (1979). *Int. J. Cancer 23*, 751-761.

Sharkey, F. E., and Fogh, J. (1979). *Int. J. Cancer 24*, 733-738.

Shimosato, Y., Kaemya, T., Nagai, K., Hirohashi, S., Koide, T., Hayashi, H., and Nomura, T. (1976). *J. Natl. Cancer Inst. (US) 56*, 1251-1260.

Silberberg, A. (1977). *Ann. N.Y. Acad. Sci. 283*, 553-556.

Sordat, B., Merenda, C., and Carrel, S. (1977). *In* "Proceedings of the Second International Workshop on Nude Mice" (T. Nomura, N. Ohsawa, N. Tamaoki, and E. Fujiwara, eds.), pp. 313-326. Fischer, New York.

Sordat, B., Yeyama, Y., and Fogh, J. (1982). *In* "The Nude Mouse in Experimental and Clinical Research" (J. Fogh and B. C. Giovanella, eds.), Vol. 2, pp. 95-147. Academic Press, New York.

Stiles, C. D., Roberts, P. E., Saier, M. H., Jr., and Sato, G. (1974). *In* "Modern Trends in Human Leukemia. Biological, Biochemical and Virological Aspects" (R. Neth, R. C. Gallo, S. Spiegelman, and F. Stohlman, Jr., eds.), pp. 185-194. Grune & Stratton, New York.

Stiles, C. D., Roberts, P. E., Saier, M. H., Jr., and Sato, G. (1976). *Haematol. Bluttransfus. 19*, 185-194.

Vainchenker, W., Guerasio, A., Testa, U., Titeux, M., Guichard, J., Beuzard, Y., Rosa, J., and Breton-Gorius, J. (1981). *In* "Hemoglobins in Development and Differentiation" (G. Stamatoyannopoulos and A. W. Niehuis, eds.), p. 507. Liss, New York.

Vroman, L., Adams, A. L., Klings, M., Fischer, G. C., Munoz, P. C., and Solensky, R. P. (1977). *Ann. N.Y. Acad. Sci. 283*, 65-76.

Warren, B. A. (1973). *In* "Thrombosis: Pathogenesis and Clinical Trials" (E. Deutsch, K. M. Brinkhous, and K. Lechner, eds.), pp. 139-148. Springer-Verlag, Stuttgart.

Weiss, L. (1976). "Fundamental Aspects of Metastasis." Elsevier/North-Holland, New York.

Weiss, L. (1980a). *Pathobiol. Ann. 10*, 51-81.

Weiss, L. (1980b). *In* "Metastatic Tumor Growth" (E. Grundmann, ed.), pp. 53-84. Fischer, New York.

Winterbauer, R. J., Elfenbein, I. B., and Ball, W. C., Jr. (1968). *Am. J. Med. 45*, 271-290.

Wood, S., Jr. (1958). *AMA Arch. Pathol. 66*, 550-568.

Wood, S., Jr. (1971). *Pathobiol. Ann. 1*, 281-308.

Wust, C. J., Green, M., Lozzio, C. B., and Lozzio, B. B. (1982). *Blood 59*, 133-140.

Yang, T. J., and Vas, S. I. (1972). *Can. J. Microbiol. 18*, 83-86.

DISCUSSION

VAAGE: You stated that the nude mice had to be less than 48 hr
            old to permit disseminated growth of the tumor. When
            did the young nude mice develop the full adult charac-
            teristic of not permitting any metastatic growth?

MACHADO: Nude mice lack NK cells during approximately the first
            3 weeks. During that period, and particularly during
            the first 2 days of age, injected cells disseminate.

COCHRAN: Have you considered that a vasculo-occlusive mechanism
            would be involved, leading to tumor infraction? For
            example, have you looked for antibody attachment to the
            tumor vascular endothelium and/or evidence of diffuse
            intravascular coagulation?

MACHADO: From our extended experience examining K-562 myelosar-
            comas, we feel confident about distinguishing the
            zonal (ischemic) necrosis that even spontaneously oc-
            curs after 30 days of transplantation from the diffuse
            coagulative necrosis induced by the IgG at early stages
            of evolution. However, we have not examined antibody
            attachment to the vascular endothelium. It seems an
            excellent idea. Nevertheless, it should be noted that
            vascular alterations were not found in the nonnecrotic
            areas of treated tumors. Still, your point is good and
            should be examined.

HEPPNER: Does the pattern of cross-reactivity of your anti-K562
            antibody with other tumor cells in the immunotherapy
            experiments correlate with the sensitivity of these
            cells to NK killing?

MACHADO: Yes, there is a fair correlation of sensitivity of cells
            that cross-react with the IgG.

KONDO: By the experiment using CoF, you mentioned that comple-
            ment is not important for the killing of tumor by
            immune γ-globulin. Have you checked complement level?
            If you use small amounts of γ-globulin, it is possible
            to demonstrate the requirement of complement?

MACHADO: The levels of complement were markedly decreased. How-
            ever, your point is valid regarding the amounts of IgG.
            We cannot rule out participation of complement in the
            in vivo process.

EMBLETON: Lymphoreticular tumors are known to be more susceptible
            to killing by antibody than solid tumors; did the solid

tumors that were resistant to the antibody react with
it *in vivo*, and could you comment on the relative susceptibility of solid and lymphoreticular tumors in
view of your *inference* that antibody therapy could be
used clinically?

MACHADO: The human solid tumors transplanted in the mice and used
as controls did not react *in vitro* with the antibody,
since this was specific for myeloid and lymphoid cells.
Similar antibodies should have to be raised against
epithelial tumors. The K-562 myelosarcoma is a compact
tumor. Therefore, the activity of the antibody *in vivo*
is not a matter of structure but rather one of
specificity.

PART VA

Clinical and Experimental New Approaches to Cancer Treatment

Chairpersons

G. Mathé
Motoharu Kondo

CHAPTER 24

EFFECT OF INTRAPLEURAL INSTILLATION OF *NOCARDIA RUBRA* CELL
WALL SKELETON ON LUNG CANCER

Kosei Yasumoto
Kiyoshi Inokuchi

Second Department of Surgery
Kyushu University School of Medicine
Fukuoka, Japan

Kikuo Nomoto

Department of Immunology
Institute for Bioregulation
Kyushu University
Fukuoka, Japan

Ichiro Azuma

Institute of Immunological Science
Hokkaido University
Sapporo, Japan

Yuichi Yamamura

Osaka University
Osaka, Japan

BASIC MECHANISMS AND CLINICAL TREATMENT
OF TUMOR METASTASIS

449

I. INTRODUCTION

Previously, we have reported that the cell wall skeleton of *Mycobacterium bovis* BCG (BCG-CWS) was as active as live BCG for various kinds of experimental tumor systems (Azuma *et al.*, 1974; Meyer *et al.*, 1974; Yoshimoto *et al.*, 1976). The BCG-CWS treatment was applied to lung cancer patients, and a remarkable effect was observed especially in stages I and II of lung cancer (Yasumoto *et al.*, 1976, 1978, 1979). However, some limitations of the effect of the BCG-CWS treatment have also been revealed in advanced stages of lung cancer.

The antitumor activity of cell wall skeleton of *Nocardia rubra* (N-CWS) has been compared with that of BCG-CWS (Yamamura *et al.*, 1981). Such experimental mouse tumors as MH-134 hepatoma, B16 melanoma, EL-4 leukemia, Br-1 mammary adenocarcinoma, and MCA fibrosarcoma were more effectively suppressed by the treatment with N-CWS than with BCG-CWS. Furthermore, intrapleural injections of N-CWS were more effective against malignant pleurisy than intrapleural injections of BCG-CWS.

Therefore, we have applied intrapleural instillation of the N-CWS followed by intradermal injections in patients with lung cancer since 1977 in a randomized fashion. The present chapter will introduce the trial and the results.

II. MATERIALS AND METHODS

A. Patients

The trial of the N-CWS immunotherapy against lung cancer had been started in November 1977 and was closed for patient entry in June 1981. Ambulatory patients who had histologically or cyto-logically proved lung cancer and were under 75 years of age were eligible. A total of 190 patients were entered into this trial.

B. Stratification and Randomization of Patients

   Patients were stratified by five prognostic factors including sex, age, operability, stage of the disease, and histological type of disease, and randomly assigned to the control of the N-CWS groups by use of the modified envelope method.

C. Treatment Other than the Immunotherapy

   Before the randomization, all patients were given the following treatments according to operability and curability.

   1. Resectable patients
       a. Curative and relatively curative resection: standard resection with mediastinal node dissection followed by chemotherapy
       b. Noncurative resection; palliative resection followed by radiotherapy and chemotherapy
   2. Nonresectable and localized inoperable patients: radiation to the primary tumor and mediastinum (5000-6000 rad) followed by chemotherapy
   3. Disseminated inoperable patients: chemotherapy alone

   The chemotherapeutic regimen was decided by histological type of lung cancer as follows:

   1. Squamous cell carcinoma and adenosquamous cell carcinoma

Mitomycin C	4 mg	
Cyclophosphamide	100 mg	twice weekly × 4 weeks
Thio-TEPA	0.5 mg	
Chromomycin A3	5 mg	

   2. Adenocarcinoma and large cell carcinoma

Mitomycin C	4 mg	
5-Fluorouracil	500 mg	twice weekly × 4 weeks
Cytosine arabinoside	20 mg	

   3. Small cell carcinoma

Vincristine	1 mg/week	4 weeks
Cyclophosphamide	100 mg	
Mitomycin C	4 mg	twice weekly × 4 weeks
Chromomycin A3	5 mg	

D.   Procedure for N-CWS Administration

Oil-attached form of 300 μg of N-CWS suspended in 10 ml of
saline was instilled into the affected side of the intrapleural
space at the first injection as an induction therapy by use of a
19-gauge injection needle.   Thereafter, 200 μg of N-CWS were injected id into the forearm as a maintenance therapy.   The interval between injections was 2 weeks until 20 weeks, and thereafter
it was 4 weeks.
     The control group was given no further treatment until recur-
rence.

E.   Follow-up of Patients and Evaluation of Effect of N-CWS
     Treatment

Each patient was evaluated monthly by physical examinations,
chest roentgenograms, complete blood counts, liver function tests,
and serum levels of carcinoembryonic antigen.   Whenever indicated
for evaluation of metastasis, RI scanning of bone and CT scanning
of the liver and the brain were employed.
     In this trial, survival time and remission duration were
settled as evaluation end points.   Relapse was diagnosed by the
appearance of new metastatic lesions or by increase in size of
tumor that had been treated previously.
     The survival and remission rates were calculated by the
Kaplan-Meier method (Kaplan and Meier, 1958).   The statistical
analysis was carried out by the generalized Wilcoxon test (Gehan,
1965).

F.   Evaluable Patients

Among 190 patients entered, 119 were operable and 71 were inoperable.   The operable patients were randomly assigned to the
control group (64 patients) and the N-CWS group (55 patients).
However, the evaluable patients were 62 in the control group and
49 in the N-CWS group, for the reasons listed in Table I.   Among
71 inoperable patients, 32 were assigned to the control and 39 to
the N-CWS group.   Four of the control and seven of the N-CWS
group were dropped out from the study for the reasons listed in
Table I.

TABLE I. Analysis of Patients in this Study

Patient Status	Operable		Inoperable	
	Control ($n = 64$)	N-CWS ($n = 55$)	Control ($n = 32$)	N-CWS ($n = 39$)
Causes of dropouts				
Refusal	0	1	0	0
Failure of intra-pleural injection	--	2	--	0
N-CWS injection less than 3 months	--	3	--	3
Death within 3 months	2	0	4	4
Total number of dropouts	2	6	4	7
Total number of evaluable patients[a]	62	49	28	32

[a] n - Total number of dropouts.

III. RESULTS

A. Comparability of Patients in Each Group

1. Operable Patients

Comparability of operable patients was assessed by five prognostic factors including histological type of the disease, pathological stage, curability of operation, sex, and age. As shown in Table II, no statistically significant difference was observed between the control and the N-CWS groups.

2. Inoperable Patients

Comparability of inoperable patients was assessed by four factors including histological disease type, clinical stage, sex, and age. As shown in Table III, there was no statistically significant difference between the two groups.

TABLE II. Characteristic of Evaluable (Operable) Patients[a]

Characteristic	Control	N-CWS	χ^2-Test
Histological disease type			
Squamous cell carcinoma	22 (35.5)	20 (40.8)	
Adenocarcinoma	30 (48.4)	20 (40.8)	n.s.[b]
Small cell carcinoma	5 (8.1)	2 (4.1)	
Large cell carcinoma	3 (4.8)	6 (12.2)	
Adenosquamous cell carcinoma	2 (3.2)	1 (2.0)	
Pathological stage			
I	30 (48.4)	24 (49.0)	
II	7 (11.3)	6 (12.2)	n.s.
III	19 (30.6)	18 (36.7)	
IV	6 (9.7)	1 (2.0)	
Curability of operation			
Curative	23 (37.1)	20 (40.8)	
Relatively curative	21 (33.9)	14 (28.6)	n.s.
Noncurative	8 (12.9)	10 (20.4)	
Exploratory thoracotomy	10 (16.1)	5 (10.2)	
Sex			
Male	44 (71.0)	32 (65.3)	n.s.
Female	18 (29.0)	17 (34.7)	
Age (years)			
36-49	8 (12.9)	4 (8.2)	
50-64	33 (53.2)	28 (57.1)	n.s.
65-75	21 (33.9)	17 (34.7)	

[a]Number of patients in each category is given. Numbers in parentheses are percentages of total.
[b]Not significant.

B. Effect of N-CWS Treatment in Operable Patients

1. *Prolongation of Survival*

Figure 1 shows the survival curves of operable patients. Four-year survival rate of the control group was 54.0%; it was 57.2% in the N-CWS group. Seventy-five percent survival periods were 19 months in the control and 31 in the N-CWS group ($p < .10$). These operable patients were divided into curative + relatively curative resection group (C + RC) and noncurative resection + exploratory thoracotomy group (N + E). Figure 2 shows the survival curves of the C + RC group. Four-year survival rates were 63.0% in the control and 82.3% in the N-CWS group. The difference

TABLE III. Characteristics of Evaluable (Inoperable) Patients[a]

Characteristic	Control	N-CWS	χ^2-Test
Histological disease type			
Squamous cell carcinoma	14 (50.0)	8 (25.0)	
Adenocarcinoma	5 (17.9)	12 (37.5)	
Small cell carcinoma	4 (14.3)	8 (25.0)	n.s.[b]
Large cell carcinoma	4 (14.3)	4 (12.5)	
Adenosquamous cell carcinoma	1 (3.6)	0	
Clinical stage			
I	1 (3.6)	1 (3.1)	
II	1 (3.6)	4 (12.5)	n.s.
III	11 (39.3)	13 (40.6)	
IV	15 (53.6)	14 (43.8)	
Sex			
Male	24 (85.7)	27 (84.4)	n.s.[c]
Female	4 (14.3)	5 (15.6)	
Age			
36-49	1 (3.6)	2 (6.3)	
50-64	11 (39.3)	19 (59.4)	n.s.
65-75	16 (57.1)	11 (34.4)	

[a,b]Same as footnotes to Table I.
[c]Fisher test.

was statistically significant ($p < .05$). On the other hand, no statistically significant difference was observed in the N + E group, as shown in Fig. 3.

2. Prolongation of Remission Duration

Figure 4 indicates the remission curves of operable patients. Four-year remission rates were 29.7% in the control group and 53.7% in the N-CWS group. The difference was statistically significant ($p < .05$). Figure 5 shows the remission curves of the C + RC group. Four-year remission rates were 35.0 and 76.8%, respectively, in the control and the N-CWS groups ($p < .01$). Figure 6 shows the remission curves of the N + E group. The duration of 50% remission for the control group was 5 months. In contrast, it was 10 months in the N-CWS group ($p < .10$).

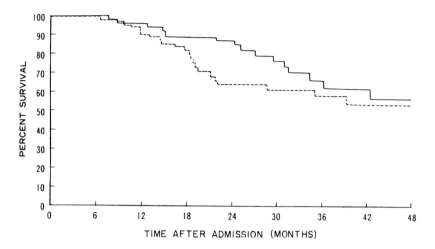

Fig. 1. Survival curves of operable lung cancer patients
($p < .10$, $z = 1.661$). (————) N-CWS, $n = 49$; (----) control,
$n = 62$.

C. Effect of N-CWS Treatment in Inoperable Patients

Figure 7 shows the survival curves of inoperable patients.
Survival rates at 47 months were 11.6 and 21.3% in the control and
the N-CWS groups, respectively. However, no significant difference was observed. Figure 8 shows the remission curves of
inoperable patients. Durations of 50% remissions were 3 months
in the control group and 6 months in the N-CWS group. The
difference was statistically significant ($p < .01$).

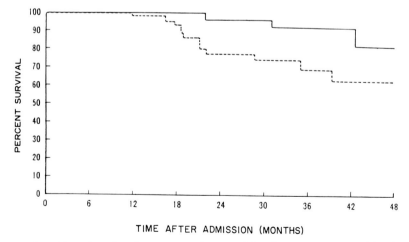

Fig. 2. Survival curves of operable lung cancer patients,
curative + relatively curative resection groups ($p < .05$, $z =
2.369$). (————) N-CWS, $n = 34$; (----) controls, $n = 44$.

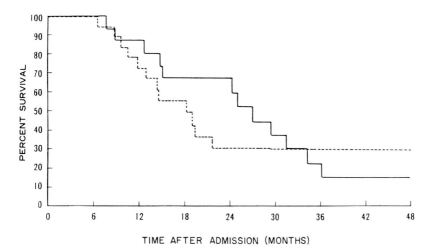

Fig. 3. Survival curves of operable lung cancer patients, noncurative resection + exploratory thoracotomy groups (z = .926). (———) N-CWS, n = 15; (----) control, n = 18.

D. Comparison of Mode of Recurrence

Mode of recurrence was classified as local recurrence (including metastasis to ipsilateral mediastinal lymph nodes) and distant metastasis. The difference of mode of recurrence in the C + RC group is summarized in Table IV. In the control group, recurrence was observed in 21 of 44 patients (47.7%). The 21 recurrences included local recurrence in 6 patients (13.6%) and distant metastasis in 15 patients (34.1%). In contrast,

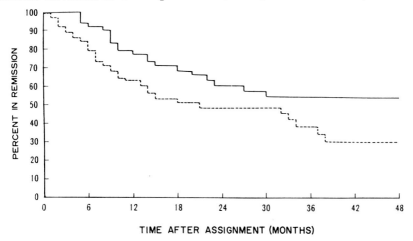

Fig. 4. Prolongation of remission duration by N-CWS treatment in operable lung cancer patients (p < .05, z = 2.159). (———) N-CWS, n = 49; (----) control, n = 62.

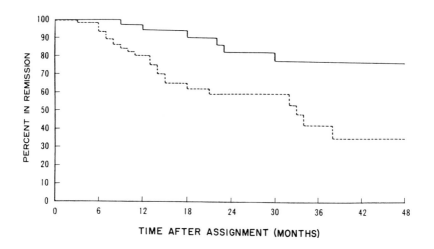

Fig. 5. Prolongation of disease-free survival by N-CWS treatment in operable lung cancer, curative + relatively curative
resection groups ($p < .01$, $z = 2.931$). (———) N-CWS, $n = 34$;
(----) control, $n = 44$.

recurrence was observed in only 6 of 34 patients (17.6%) in the
N-CWS group. All of the six recurrences in the N-CWS group were
distant metastases. No local recurrence was detected in the
N-CWS group. Such a difference in mode of recurrence could not
be obtained in the N + E group or in inoperable patients.

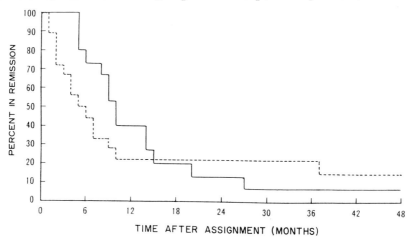

Fig. 6. Prolongation of remission duration by N-CWS treatment in operable lung cancer patients, noncurative resection
+ exploratory thoracotomy groups ($p < .10$, $z = 1.832$). (———)
N-CWS, $n = 15$; (----) control, $n = 18$.

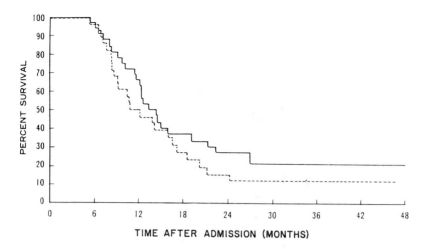

Fig. 7. Survival curves of inoperable lung cancer patients
(z = 1.022). (———) N-CWS, n = 32; (----) control, n = 28.

E.   Side Effects of N-CWS Treatment

   The chief common side effects of the N-CWS treatment were
fever and skin reaction at the site of id injection of N-CWS.
Fever as high as 40°C (average 38.0-39.0°C) was encountered in 74
of 93 patients by intrapleural instillation of N-CWS with a fever
duration of 1 to 3 days. However, only 4 of 91 patients were
febrile after id injection. Skin reaction at the site of id

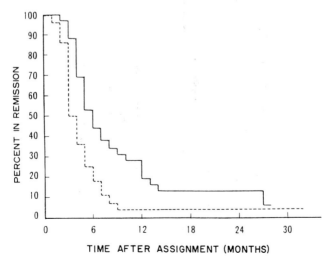

Fig. 8. Prolongation of remission duration by N-CWS treatment
in inoperable lung cancer patients (p < .01, z = 3.179). (———)
N-CWS, n = 32; (----) control, n = 28.

Table IV. Mode of Recurrence in Cases with Curative or Relatively Curative Resection [a]

Experimental group	Number of patients	Site of recurrence		Number of patients in remission
		Local	Distant	
Control	44	6 (13.6)	15 (34.1)	23 (52.3)
N-CWS	34	0[b]	6 (17.6)	28 (82.4)[c]

[a]Same as footnote a in Table II.
[b]Significantly low incidence in local recurrence ($p < .05$; Fisher's direct calculation method).
[c]Significantly high rate in remission ($p < .05$; χ^2 test).

injection included redness, induration, and ulceration. However, ulceration was experienced in only 9 of 91 patients. No serious side effect was experienced in the present study.

IV. DISCUSSION

Immunotherapies for cancer are classified as specific and non-specific. The latter comprise about 90% of all immunotherapy trials. Live BCG has been utilized as the most popular immuno-stimulant for human malignant tumors among nonspecific immuno-therapies. However, the problems inherent in the production and testing of any biological preparation are significant (Gutterman *et al.*, 1978).

As an alternative to live BCG, we have extracted the cell wall skeleton of BCG (BCG-CWS) from live BCG and reported its adjuvant activity on immune response (Azuma *et al.*, 1975, 1978a; Yasumoto *et al.*, 1976), mitogenic activity on lymphocytes (Azuma *et al.*, 1976), and antitumor activity in experimental tumor systems (Azuma *et al.*, 1974; Meyer *et al.*, 1974; Yoshimoto *et al.*, 1976). Furthermore, we applied the BCG-CWS immunotherapy in patients with lung cancer and reported the effect of the BCG-CWS (Yasumoto *et al.*, 1976, 1978, 1979). In that article, intradermal injections of BCG-CWS brought favorable effects in prolonged survival periods for patients with lung cancer.

However, some limitations have also been revealed, especially in patients at such advanced stages as III and IV. Therefore, we began to search for more potent and less toxic antitumor adjuvants. Results of previous experiments using 11 species of nonpathogenic *Nocardia* have shown that the cell wall skeleton of *Nocardia rubra* (N-CWS) has induced the most potent antitumor effect against many syngeneic murine tumors (Azuma *et al.*, 1978b). Moreover, the antitumor activity induced by N-CWS was more potent than the ac-tivity induced by BCG-CWS in many experimental systems (Yamamura *et al.*, 1981).

On the basis of these experimental data, we have applied intra-pleural injections of BCG-CWS and N-CWS in patients with malignant pleurisy as a pilot study, and compared the results (Yamamura *et al.*, 1981). Disappearance of malignant cells from pleural effusion was observed in 11 of 18 patients (61.8%) treated with BCG-CWS. In contrast, 17 of 24 patients (70.0%) showed disappearance of malignant cells by the treatment with N-CWS.

These data encouraged us to apply the intrapleural N-CWS treatment in lung cancer patients without malignant pleurisy. The N-CWS was instilled into the pleural space at the first administra-tion as an induction therapy and thereafter was injected intra-dermally with an interval of 2 to 4 weeks as a maintenance therapy. The intrapleural induction therapy may be the most important point of this trial, because favorable antitumor effects were induced by a direct contact between N-CWS and tumors in all experiments mentioned previously. The data obtained indicated that the N-CWS treatment is effective in all patients with lung cancer, whether they are operable or inoperable, in a sense of improvement of remission rate. However, improvement of survival rate was effected only in operable patients, and especially in the curative or relatively curative resection group. Further analysis of our data according to stages of the disease revealed that the N-CWS treatment improved only the survival rate of stage I and II patients significantly. This is consistent with McKneally's data (McKneally et al., 1981), in which single intrapleural injection of live BCG (Tice strain) was effective only in stage I lung cancer.

The N-CWS treatment could not improve survival rate of patients with more advanced lung cancer, that is, the noncurative resection + exploratory thoracotomy group and the inoperable group, or stages III and IV. In order to obtain improvement of survival rate in such advanced lung cancer patients, the second new N-CWS trial--in which N-CWS is injected intramediastinally at the time of operation, followed by two intrapleural injections and serial intradermal injections--has been ongoing since August 1981.

On comparing the difference of mode of recurrence between the control and the N-CWS groups, local recurrence and distant metastasis were suppressed in the curative + relatively curative resection group given the N-CWS treatment. Such a suppression of recurrence could not be observed in other groups. This may be explained by postulating that the N-CWS treatment can eradicate only minimal residual cancer cells. Suppression effects of regional N-CWS on local recurrence and distant metastasis have also been elucidated in experimental autochthonous murine tumor systems in our laboratory (Nagano et al., 1982; Ichinose et al., 1983).

REFERENCES

Azuma, I., Taniyama, T., Hirao, F., and Yamamura, Y. (1974). Gann 65, 493-505.
Azuma, I., Kanetsuna, F., Taniyama, T., Yamamura, Y., Hori, M., and Tanaka, Y. (1975). Biken J. 18, 1-13.
Azuma, I., Taniyama, T., Sugimura, K., Aladin, A. A., and Yamamura, Y. (1976). Jpn. J. Microbiol. 20, 263-271.
Azuma, I., Yamawaki, M., Ogura, T., Yoshimoto, T., Tokuzen, R., Hirao, F., and Yamamura, Y. (1978a). Gann Monogr. Cancer Res. 21, 73-86.
Azuma, I., Yamawaki, M., Yasumoto, K., and Yamamura, Y. (1978b). Cancer Immunol. Immunother. 4, 95-100.
Gehan, E. A. (1965). Biometrika 52, 203-223.

Gutterman, J. U., Mavligit, G. H., Schwarz, M. A., and Hersh,
E. M. (1978). *In* "Immunological Aspects of Cancer" (J. E.
Castro, ed.), pp. 415-470. MTP Press, Lancaster, England.
Ichinose, Y., Yasumoto, K., Tanaka, K., Yaita, H., and Nomoto, K.
(1983). *Gann 74*, 143-147.
Kaplan, E. L., and Meier, P. (1958). *J. Am. Stat. Assoc. 53*, 457.
McKneally, M. F., Maver, C., Lininger, L., Kausel, H. W.,
McIlduff, J. B., Older, T. M., Foster, E. D., and Alley, R. D.
(1981). *J. Thorac. Cardiovasc. Surg. 81*, 485-492.
Meyer, T. J., Ribi, E. E., Azuma, I., and Zbar, B. (1974). *J.
Natl. Cancer Inst. (US) 52*, 103-111.
Nagano, N., Yasumoto, K., Tanaka, K., Ichinose, Y., Yaita, H.,
and Nomoto, K. (1982). *Gann 73*, 613-617.
Yamamura, Y., Yasumoto, K., Ogura, T., and Azuma, I. (1981).
In "Augmenting Agents in Cancer Therapy" (E. M. Hersh, ed.),
pp. 71-90. Raven, New York.
Yasumoto, K., Manabe, H., Ueno, M., Ohta, M., Ueda, H., Iida, A.,
Nomoto, K., Azuma, I., and Yamamura, Y. (1976). *Gann 67*, 787-
795.
Yasumoto, K., Manabe, H., Ohta, M., Nomoto, K., Azuma, I., and
Yamamura, Y. (1978). *Gann Monogr. Cancer Res. 21*, 129-141.
Yasumoto, K., Manabe, H., Yanagawa, E., Nagano, N., Ueda, H.,
Hirota, N., Ohta, M., Nomoto, K., Azuma, I., and Yamamura, Y.
(1979). *Cancer Res. 39*, 3262-3267.
Yoshimoto, T., Azuma, I., Nishikawa, H., Sakatani, M., Ogura, T.,
and Yamamura, Y. (1976). *Gann 67*, 737-740.

DISCUSSION

MORTON: How was the cell wall *Nocardia* preparation instilled
            into the pleural space, considering the postoperative
            adhesions between the visceral and parietal pleura?

YASUMOTO: It is sometimes very difficult; however, most of the
            postoperative patients have dead space in the pleural
            cavity that can be detected by chest roentgenograms.
            In such cases, intrapleural injection is easy. In pa-
            tients with tight adhesion between visceral and
            parietal pleura, we have failed intrapleural injection
            in two patients, and about 7% of patients suffered
            from pneumothorax following intrapleural injection of
            N-CWS.

WEISS: Does it matter whether the N-CWS is injected into any
            particular region of the pleura, even allowing for ad-
            hesions and locculation?

YASUMOTO: It does not matter in most of the cases. However, in
             2 of 91 patients, we failed in intrapleural injection.

TORISU: Have you checked the changes of cell population after
             N-CWS injection into malignant pleurisy? What kind of
             cell was attracted by destruction of tumor cells?

YASUMOTO: Intrapleural injection of N-CWS in patients with malig-
             nant pleurisy causes PMN-cell accumulation at the first
             1 to 3 days, followed by accumulation of mesothelial
             cells and lymphocytes.

TORISU: This phenomenon was no different whether N-CWS or
             BCG-CWS was injected into the pleural space? Is that
             correct?

YASUMOTO: Principally, there was no difference.

MATHÉ: Did you stratify in three groups--adenocarcinoma,
             squamous cell, or small cell tumor--before immunization?

YASUMOTO: We stratified our patients by five factors including
             histological type, stage of the disease, operability,
             sex, and age. In the case of histological type, adeno-
             carcinoma, squamous cell carcinoma, large cell
             carcinoma, adenosquamous cell carcinoma, and small cell
             carcinoma are subfactors. On comparing these factors
             between the control and the N-CWS group, there was no
             significant difference.

CHAPTER 25

NONSPECIFIC IMMUNOTHERAPY ON GASTRIC CANCER

Takenori Ochiai
Hiroshi Sato

Second Department of Surgery
Chiba University School of Medicine
Chiba, Japan

BASIC MECHANISMS AND CLINICAL TREATMENT
OF TUMOR METASTASIS

I. INTRODUCTION

Nonspecific immunotherapy has received much attention as a
new modality of treatment of cancer in the last decade (Mathé et
al., 1969; Eilber et al., 1976). This enthusiasm seems to have
disappeared in the United States; however, nonspecific immunotherapy has been very widely applied clinically in Japan. In
order to answer a crucial question whether or not nonspecific
immunotherapy actually exists, we have performed two series of
randomized clinical trials of nonspecific immunotherapy (Ochiai
et al., 1983). Gastric cancer was chosen as a disease of our
study because it exists among a larger proportion of people in
Japan, and therefore, its clinicopathological features, definition of the cancer stage, and patients' prognoses have been well
studied by the Japanese Research Society for Gastric Cancer (1981).
In both protocols, all the subjects of the study received distal,
proximal, or total gastrectomy with or without combined dissection of the spleen, pancreas, or lower esophagus. The operative
technique that may influence radicality of cancer was performed,
with closely similar procedures in all cases under the same
practical principles (Nakayama, 1968).

Immunotherapy was initiated within the first postoperative
week, and it was combined with chemotherapy. The effectiveness
of immunotherapy on postoperative patient survival rate was
evaluated comparing the chemotherapy group with the chemotherapy
plus immunotherapy group. The same regimen of chemotherapy was
given in both groups. We used BCG cell wall skeleton (BCG-CWS)
for the first protocol and Nocardia rubra cell wall skeleton
(N-CWS) for the second protocol as immunotherapeutic agents.
These substances were prepared and their nature of antitumor,
adjuvant, and mitogenic activity elucidated by Yamamura and
Azuma (Azuma et al., 1974, 1978).

II. THE FIRST PROTOCOL: RANDOMIZED CLINICAL TRIAL WITH BCG-CWS

A. Subjects and Methods

The subjects of the first study were 140 gastric cancer patients who underwent gastrectomy at Chiba University Hospital
during a period from January 1976 through December 1978.

All the patients who received gastrectomy during that period
were enrolled in this study, but two patients were later excluded
because they died in surgery. The remaining 138 patients
received relevant treatment and were subjected to evaluation of
the treatment to which they were assigned.

Postoperative randomization of the patients was accomplished by the so-called envelope method. The envelope contained the direction of treatment and the assignment of patients to any of the three treatment groups, that is, control (neither chemotherapy nor immunotherapy), chemotherapy only, and chemotherapy plus immunotherapy (referred to hereinafter as immunotherapy) groups. The immunotherapeutic agent used in the first protocol, BCG-CWS, was injected intradermally into the upper arm in a dose of 400 µg. The BCG-CWS therapy was begun within the first postoperative week and was given weekly during the first 2 months. Subsequently, the patient received monthly injections for as long a period as was practicable. The patients who received injections of BCG-CWS during the first 2 months were categorized as having received immunotherapy and became qualified to receive such treatment. Actually, however, all patients received immunotherapy for more than 2 months, and accordingly, they were considered as part of the immunotherapy group.

Chemotherapy was initiated 1 week after surgery to both experimental groups. The dosage schedule consisted of 10 weekly injections of a combination of 2 mg mitomycin C, 250 mg of 5-fluorouracil, and 20 mg of cytosine arabinoside, which is called MFC therapy in Japan. It was subsequently accompanied by daily oral administration of 600 to 800 mg of Tegafur as long as the patients survived.

Laboratory tests were periodically repeated during treatment. If and when the liver function or bone marrow function was depressed, chemotherapy was interrupted forthwith until the function was recovered. Chemotherapy was considered as completed when 10 weekly doses of MFC had been given. All the patients in the chemotherapy or immunotherapy group received 10 weekly doses of MFC therapy.

B. Results

A survey of the subjects with regard to survival periods was conducted in January 1982, when all surviving patients had completed a full 3 years or more after radical operation. The postoperative survival rate curves of all patients in each treatment group, as calculated by the Kaplan-Meier life table method (Kaplan and Meier, 1958) are shown in Fig. 1, demonstrating statistically significant differences between the control and immunotherapy groups ($p < .01$) and also between the chemotherapy and immunotherapy groups ($p < .05$) by the generalized Wilcoxon test (Gehan, 1965).

In order to ensure the validity of comparison of survival rate curves, patient background factors in terms of age, sex, operative procedure, and histological stage of cancer were analyzed statistically for eventual biases between the groups (Table I). Distribution of the stages of cancer was compared by

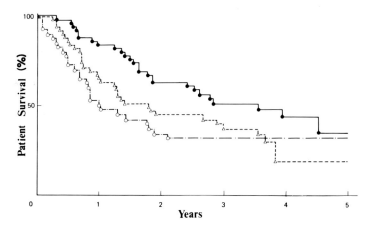

Fig. 1. Survival rate curves of the control (○, $n - 40$),
chemotherapy (△, $n = 49$), and immunotherapy (●, $n = 49$) groups.
Statistically significant difference was seen between the
immunotherapy and control groups ($p < .01$), and the immunotherapy
and chemotherapy groups ($p < .05$).

the U test of Mann-Whitney, and no significant difference was
detected between the groups. Also, no significant difference
was detected in age by the U test of Mann-Whitney, or in
operative procedures by the χ^2 test. A statistically significant
difference was seen only in sex between the control and immunotherapy groups ($p < .05$). The clinical result indicated that
nonspecific immunotherapy with BCG-CWS on postoperative gastric
cancer patients was effective.

III. THE SECOND PROTOCOL: RANDOMIZED CLINICAL TRIAL WITH N-CWS

A. Subjects and Methods

The second clinical trial was carried out at the Second
Department of Surgery, Chiba University School of Medicine, and
the surgical departments of its 14 affiliated hospitals. All
surgeons at all the participating institutions were trained at
the Second Department of Surgery, Chiba University, and operate
under the same practical principles with closely similar procedures (Nakayama, 1968). The study was directed by an independent controller who was responsible for random allocation of
therapy regimens, sealing of the randomly allocated key codes in
envelopes, preservation of the key codes, and integrity in
determining patient eligibility for inclusion in the analysis of
data and for treatment of data.

TABLE I. Statistical Analysis of Patients' Background Factors

Background factor	Number of patients			Significance test[b]	
	Control	Chemo-therapy	Immuno-therapy	Control versus immunotherapy	Chemotherapy versus immunotherapy
Stage					
I	5	7	8		
II	6	3	4	n.s.	n.s.
III	13	25	27	($z = 1.191$)	($z = .865$)
IV	16	14	10		
Sex					
Male	29	28	23	$p < .05$	n.s.
Female	11	21	26	($\chi^2 = 4.918$)	($\chi^2 = 0.654$)
Age					
20-29	0	2	2		
30-39	1	6	3		
40-49	4	5	13	n.s.	n.s.
50-59	15	14	12	($z = 1.926$)	($z = 0.783$)
60-69	13	13	13		
70-79	7	8	6		
80-89	0	1	0		
Operative procedure[a]					
D	20	25	20		
P	5	7	7	n.s.	n.s.
T	15	17	22	($\chi^2 = 1.438$)	($\chi^2 = 1.231$)

[a]D, Distal; P, proximal; T, total gastrectomy.
[b]z, Mann-Whitney U test; χ^2, Chi-square test; n.s., not significant.

The subjects were consecutive patients with gastric carcinoma undergoing gastrectomy at the participant institutions during the 19-month period from September 1, 1979 until March 31, 1981. After the patients received gastrectomy, they were classified into 12 strata, from macroscopic stage of gastric cancer and degree of surgical curability at the time of operation, according to the General Rules for Gastric Cancer Study of the Japanese Research Society for Gastric Cancer (1981). They were randomly allocated in the stratum to the chemotherapy or the immunotherapy group according to the randomization of therapy regimens arranged in advance by the controller.

After the specimen was examined microscopically, the patients were classified by histological stage of cancer and radicality of

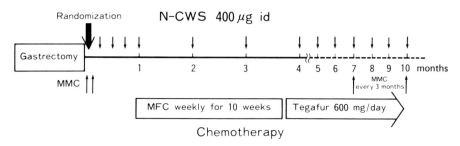

Fig. 2. Schedule of immunotherapy and chemotherapy in the N-CWS controlled trial.

surgical intervention into curative and noncurative resection cases. The effect of immunotherapy was assessed between the groups on the basis of histological curability.

The immunotherapeutic agent used in this study, N-CWS, was suspended in physiological saline and injected intradermally into the upper arm in a dose of 400 μg. The N-CWS therapy was begun within the first postoperative week as a rule, and given weekly for the first month. Subsequently, the patient received monthly injections for as long a period as practicable (Fig. 2).

The dosage regimen employed for anticancer chemotherapy in this study is also illustrated in Fig. 2. The patient received intravenous injections of mitomycin-C (MMC) during surgery and on the following day. The patient was then given MFC chemotherapy for 10 weeks, beginning 1 month after surgery. Immediately after completion of the MFC therapy, oral Tegafur was instituted in a daily dose of 600 mg. A single iv injection of MMC 10 mg was combined with Tegafur therapy trimonthly during the first year and at 6-month intervals thereafter.

B. Results

A total of 302 patients were registered in the study--143 for the chemotherapy group and 159 for the immunotherapy group. Of these, 258 subjects were analyzed, consisting of 118 for the chemotherapy group and 140 for the immunotherapy group. The criteria for treatment of the enrolled subjects had been determined in advance by the controller (Table II). There were 44 exclusions, 25 from the chemotherapy group and 19 from the immunotherapy group. Nine dropouts excluded from analysis were three from the chemotherapy group and six from the immunotherapy group.

After histological examination of the specimens, 90 patients from the chemotherapy group and 97 patients from the immunotherapy group were designated as curative resection cases, and 28 of the chemotherapy and 43 of the immunotherapy group were designated as noncurative resection cases, respectively.

TABLE II. Criteria for Treatment of Enrolled Subjects and the Number of Patients Excluded or Dropped out from Analysis of Efficacy

Criteria for treatment of enrolled subjects	Number of patients		
	Chemo-therapy group	Immuno-therapy group	Total
Exclusions			
Infringement against allocation of therapy regimens	0	1	1
Early stage of gastric cancer	13	7	20
Malignancies other than gastric cancer	1	2	3
No surgical resection	1	1	2
Simultaneous multicarcinogenesis	0	1	1
Died within 30 days after operation	2	0	2
Serious complications existing prior to operation	2	1	3
Study treatment impracticable due to postoperative complications	1	1	2
Over 76 years of age at operation	2	3	5
Histologically unevaluable	0	1	1
Carcinoma other than common type of adenocarcinoma	3	1	4
Total	25	19	44
Dropouts			
Usage of other immunotherapy before completion of study treatment	2	5	7
Died of other disease (cardiac failure, pneumonia)	1	1	2
Total	3	6	9

The curative and noncurative resection cases in both groups were analyzed with respect to various background factors to test intergroup statistical differences. No significant difference was noted between the chemotherapy and immunotherapy groups with respect to the various factors listed in Table III.

The frequency of N-CWS injections was distributed from 2 to 35 times in 140 patients of the immunotherapy group. The mean frequency was 16.5.

The patients enrolled in the study were surveyed for survival as of December 31, 1981. The mean duration of observation from the day of operation until the time of the survival survey was

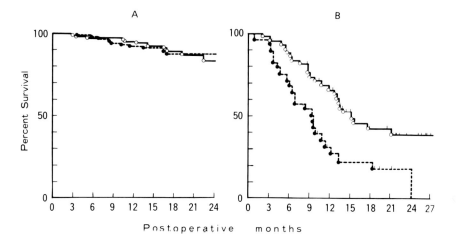

Fig. 3. Survival rate in patients with (A) curative and (B) noncurative resection of gastric cancer. (A) Chemotherapy (●), $n = 90$; chemoimmunotherapy (○), $n = 97$. (B) Chemotherapy (●), $n = 28$; chemoimmunotherapy (○), $n = 43$. In (B) there was a statistically significant difference between the two treatment groups ($p < .01$, $z = 2.792$).

593 days in the total of 258 patients inclusive for analysis. The curative and noncurative resection patients in these two groups were compared for survival rate curves on the similar patient background factors, including actual practice of chemotherapy (Fig. 3). In the curative resection cases (Fig. 3A), both treatment groups showed a survival rate of better than 80% by the time of the survival survey. No significant intergroup difference was noted.

In the noncurative resection cases (Fig. 3B), there was a significant difference in the survival rate curves between the two treatment groups ($p < .01$). These findings indicate that postoperative immunotherapy with N-CWS was effective in the patients with noncurative resection for gastric carcinoma.

IV. ASSOCIATION OF HLA DR4 WITH LONG-TERM SURVIVORS OF
    GASTRIC CANCER

HLA typing was performed in long-term survivors of stage III gastric cancer patients of the first protocol. Trays for HLA typing were imported from the Terasaki's laboratory (Los Angeles, California). The HLA DR4 phenotype frequency of the long-term (more than 3 years) survivors among stage III postoperative gastric cancer patients, who received both chemotherapy and BCG-CWS immunotherapy postoperatively according to the protocol,

TABLE III.   Background Factors Analyzed between the Chemotherapy and N-CWS Immunotherapy Groups

---

Sex
Age
Extent of resection
Concomitant resection
Grade of lymph node removal
Grade of liver metastasis
Grade of disseminating peritoneal metastasis
Grade of lymph node metastasis
Depth of cancerous invasion
Cancer infiltration at the resection margin
Growth pattern of cancer
Histological pattern of cancer
Actual practice of chemotherapy

---

was 70.6%. Frequencies of the HLA DR4 phenotype among all gastric
cancer patients and among stage III gastric cancer patients tested
for HLA on admission were 30.6% and 28.6%, respectively. Frequency
of the DR4 phenotype among 64 healthy Japanese was 29.7% in our
laboratory. A statistically significant increase in DR4 frequency
was observed among long-term survivors of a group of stage III
postoperative gastric cancer patients (Table IV).

V. DISCUSSION

There is a discrepancy in evaluation of the clinical effectiveness of nonspecific immunotherapy between the United States and
Japan. From the results of our series of randomized clinical
trials, we have concluded that nonspecific immunotherapy on postoperative gastric cancer patients is effective if an appropriate
immunotherapeutic agent is applied. Several possible explanations
may be offered for our positive results, the first of which is that
we chose gastric cancer as our disease of study. Gastric cancer
has a poorer prognosis than cancers of other organs. A poor prognostic cancer in advanced stages seems to be a good choice to see
an effect of immunotherapy. The second explanation for our positive results is the schedule of postoperative adjuvant therapy in
our trial. Immunotherapy was combined with chemotherapy in our
trial, and the chemotherapeutic regimen was sufficient as anticancer treatment. Combination of immunotherapy with sufficient
chemotherapy seems to be good schedule for better survival.
   The most important factor in our positive results is the
choice of immunotherapeutic agents. On the basis of a full under-

TABLE IV. HLA DR Phenotype Frequency (%) of Gastric Cancer Patients

HLA Phenotype	Healthy (n = 64)	Gastric cancer (n = 36)	Gastric cancer stage III (n = 14)	Gastric cancer long-term survivor stage III (n = 17)
DR1	9.4	16.7	21.4	11.8
DR2	37.5	30.6	21.4	23.5
DR3	--	2.8	7.1	--
DR4[a]	29.7*	30.6	28.6**	70.6***
DR5	6.3	5.6	--	--
W6	6.3	--	--	--
W7	--	--	--	--
W8	26.6	25.0	21.4	23.5
W9	29.7	13.9	21.4	17.6
Cy6	20.3	22.2	21.4	23.5

[a]Between * and ***, $p < .0025$; between ** and ***, $p < .02$; between * and **, not significant.

standing of the immunological mechanisms of BCG-CWS and N-CWS, we were able to bring about positive results with them.

Recent advances of immunology revealed to us the association between immune responsiveness and histocompatibility antigen (Buell, 1973), and between susceptibility to oncogenic virus and histocompatibility antigen (MacMahon, 1971). It was reported that certain HLA types were associated with long-term survival in patients with acute lymphocytic leukemia (Hester *et al.*, 1977) and lung cancer (Weiss *et al.*, 1980). Although an association with HLA frequency was not found in gastric cancer patients, long-term survivors among stage III gastric cancer patients did show a high frequency of the HLA DR4 phenotype. This fact indicates a possible involvement of an immunological response gene in effectiveness of immunotherapy.

In conclusion, nonspecific immunotherapy with BCG-CWS and N-CWS was effective on postoperative gastric cancer patients.

REFERENCES

Azuma, I., Taniyama, T., Hirao, F., and Yamamura, Y. (1974). *Gann* 65, 493-505.

Azuma, I., Yamawaki, M., Yasumoto, K., and Yamamura, Y. (1978). *Cancer Immunol. Immunother.* 4, 95-100.

Buell, P. (1973). *J. Natl. Cancer Inst. (US) 51*, 1479-1483.
Eilber, F. R., Morton, D. L., Holmes, E. C., Sparks, F. C., and Ramming, K. P. (1976). *N. Engl. J. Med. 294*, 237-240.
Gehan, E. A. (1965). *Biometrika 52*, 203-223.
Hester, J. P., Rossen, R. D., Templeto, J. W., McCredie, K. B., and Freireich, E. J. (1977). *In* "HLA and Malignancy" (G. P. Murphy, ed.), pp. 71-79. Liss, New York.
Kajitani, T. (1981). *Jpn. J. Surg. 11*, 127-145.
Kaplan, E. L., and Meier, P. (1958). *J. Am. Stat. Assoc. 53*, 457-481.
MacMahon, B. (1971). *Lancet 2*, 900-902.
Mathé, G., Amiel, J. L., Schwarzenberg, L., Schneider, M., Cattan, A., Schlumberger, J. R., Hayat, M., and De Vassal, F. (1969). *Lancer 1*, 697-699.
Nakayama, K. (1968). Atlas of Gastrointestinal Surgery, pp. 235-382. Igaku-Shoin, Tokyo.
Ochiai, T., Sato, H., Hayashi, R., Asano, T., Sato, H., and Yamamura, Y. (1983). *Cancer Immunol. Immunother. 14*, 167-171.
Weiss, G. B., Nawrocki, L. B., and Daniel, J. C. (1980). *Cancer (Philadelphia) 46*, 38-40.

CHAPTER 26

SUPERIORITY OF AVCF (ADRIAMYCIN, VINCRISTINE, CYCLOPHOSPHAMIDE,
AND 5-FLUOROURACIL) OVER CMF (CYCLOPHOSPHAMIDE, METHOTREXATE,
AND 5-FLUOROURACIL) AS ADJUVANT CHEMOTHERAPY FOR BREAST CANCER:
A PHASE III TRIAL OF ASSOCIATION ONCOFRANCE

G. Mathé
J. L. Misset
R. Plagne
D. Belpomme
J. Guerrin
P. Fumoleau
R. Metz
M. Delgado

Institut de Cancérologie et d'Immunogenetique (INSERM, CNRS)
et Service des Maladies Sanguines et Tumorales
Groupe Hospitalier Paul-Brousse
Villejuif, France

I. INTRODUCTION

It was with lymph node-positive breast cancer patients that
Nissen-Meyer *et al.* (1978) using small doses of cyclophosphamide
(CPM), Fisher and Redmond (1974) using phenylalanin mustard
(L-PAM), and Rossi *et al.* (1981) using a combination of cyclo-
phosphamide, methotrexate, and fluorouracil (CMF), showed that

their adjuvant chemotherapies significantly increased disease-free survival as well as overall survival.

As one of us obtained good results (Gouveia et al., 1978) in advanced mammary carcinoma with the combined application of Adriamycin (doxorubicin) (ADM), vincristine (VCR), cyclophosphamide (CPM), and 5-fluorouracil (5-FU) (AVCF), and as Hammond et al. (1977), with ADM and CPM and ourselves with AVCF (Pagne et al., 1982) obtained apparently better results than Rossi et al. with CMF in adjuvant phase II trials, our group decided to compare the AVCF combination to CMF in a randomized trial. We are reporting here the preliminary results of this trial.

II. PATIENTS AND METHODS

Only patients after primary surgery with axillary node dissection were eligible for the trial. They were stratified according to the following categories: T2N-MP (premenopausal), T2N-MP+ (postmenopausal), T1T2N+MP-, T1T2N+MP+, T3T4N-MP-, T3T4N+MP+, T3T4N+MP-, T3T3N+MP+. Adjuvant postoperative radiotherapy was optional and happened to be performed in 50.8% of the patients according to the standards of participating centers.

A total of 329 patients from eight French cancer centers entered the trial between May 1978 and May 1981.

After registration, patients were randomized within each stratification subgroup just described to receive 12 monthly cycles of adjuvant chemotherapy, either with CMF according to Bonadonna's schedule (Rossi et al., 1981) or in the following combination: Adriamycin 30 g/m^2 iv on Day 1 (omitted in N-patients), vincristine 1 mg/m^2 iv on day 2, cyclophosphamide 300 mg/m^2, and 5-fluorouracil 400 g/m^2 iv or im on Days 3-6 (AVCF).

The next cycle begins on Day 29 if hematological recovery is satisfactory.

Disease-free survival and survival curves were drawn according to the Kaplan-Meier life table analysis, and comparisons were made with the log rank test.

III. RESULTS

A. Tolerance

One patient in the AVCF group died during chemotherapy from a cause unrelated to the disease or its treatment. Another 51 of the patients did not complete their 1-year program: 29 in the

TABLE I.   Stratification of the Patients

	Total	VCF	AVCF	CMF
N+	251	3	135	113
N-	78	36	--	42
	329	39	135	155
MP-	170	19	74	77
MP+	159	20	61	78
	329	39	135	155

CMF group and 22 in the AVCF group. More patients relapsed during chemotherapy in the CMF group; refusal and discontinuation for poor tolerance (mainly hematological) were balanced in the two treatment groups.

We studied the percentage of protocol dose of each drug received during the whole treatment on a sample of 129 N+ patients. The results are presented in Table I, and it appears that patients treated with CMF received significantly lower doses than those prescribed by the protocol (72%), while AVCF patients were less underdosed (88%). The difference between percentages is significant, and underdosage appears comparable in pre- and postmenopausal patients. The same percentage of patients in each group was submitted to radiotherapy before the beginning of chemotherapy.

No toxic death occurred and no cardiac abnormality attributable to adriamycin was recorded among the 116 patients who received the drug at the total dosage of 360 mg/m^2 over 1 year.

B.   Prognostic Factors

1.   Nodal Involvement

Seventy-eight node-negative patients were entered in the trial. Only one patient in this group died from disease progression, but 18% have relapsed at 3 years follow-up, despite adjuvant chemotherapy, confirming that this group of patients may not have an excellent prognosis. The difference is statistically significant in favor of the N- patients for survival (p = .02), but only borderline significance for disease-free survival (p = .059).

2. Hormonal Status

Surprisingly, no difference could be detected in disease-free
survival or in survival between pre- and postmenopausal women.

3. Performance of Radiotherapy

This trial was not designed to evaluate the effect of adjuvant
radiotherapy, which was performed optionally according to the
standards of participating centers. Analyses of the populations
submitted to radiotherapy showed that the choice was far more
doctor-determined than patient-determined, some participants
giving radiation to all patients (even N-), others to none.
Overall, 50.8% of the patients received adjuvant radiotherapy,
and disease-free survival as well as survival were identical in
the groups of irradiated and nonirradiated patients. This result
merely allows us to conclude that, in this setting, radiotherapy
is not detrimental to patients as has been claimed (Stjernsward,
1974), even through delay in the onset of adjuvant chemotherapy
(Nissen-Meyer *et al.*, 1978), and that no bias was introduced in
our chemotherapy trial through this optional performance of adjuvant radiotherapy.

C. Results According to Treatment

If the entire group of patients is considered, a highly significant difference is seen in favor of the AVCF-VCF group over
the CMF group, with a *p* value adjusted for nodal status of .005
for disease-free survival and .03 for survival. In N- patients
the difference is in favor of the VCF group, but it is not statistically significant (*p* = .27 for disease-free survival).
In the 246 N+ patients, the difference is highly significant
in disease-free survival (*p* = .01) and in survival (*p* = .01), in
favor of AVCF over CMF. Three-year disease-free survival is 68%
for AVCF and 57% for CMF.
Premenopausal N+ patients have a 3-year disease-free survival
of 77% after AVCF and 48% after CMF. According to the log rank
test, the difference between the two curves is highly significant
in disease-free survival (*p* = .006) and survival (*p* = .02). Among
postmenopausal N+ patients, the differences, although in favor of
AVCF, are not statistically significant (Fig. 1). Dose-effect
relationship was studied using the same method as Bonadonna and
Valagussa (1981), and no correlation was found between dose administered and efficacy of treatment. However, this part of the
study was performed on a limited number of patients, and as can
be seen in Table I, few patients received low doses of chemotherapy.

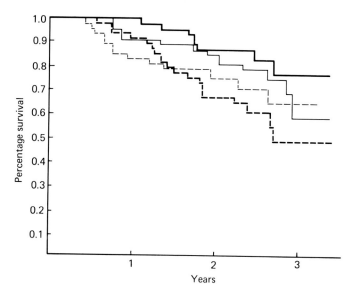

Fig. 1. Disease-free survival in node-positive patients according to treatment and menopausal status. Premenopausal: (———) AVCF, $n = 73$; (━━━━) CMF, $n = 57$; $p = .006$. Postmenopausal: (———) AVCF, $n = 63$; (-----) CMF, $n = 53$; $p = .39$.

IV. DISCUSSION

This study clearly demonstrates the superiority of AVCF over CMF as adjuvant chemotherapy for surgically treated breast cancer, whether irradiated or not. The difference is more striking in premenopausal N+ patients, but it is in favor of AVCF in any subgroup studied. Although Adriamycin has already been included in adjuvant regimens by several groups (Hammond et al., 1977; Plagne et al., 1982), no randomized study had so far shown the superiority of such a regimen over other forms of adjuvant treatment, mainly CMF. Our result was expected, since Adriamycin is one of the most active drugs in breast cancer treatment (Mathé and Kenis, 1975). Vinca alkaloids are active in 20% of advanced breast cancers; moreover, they may prevent invasion of normal tissue by tumor cells (Marcel and De Brabander, 1978; Storme et al., 1981) and thus prevent the establishment of micrometastases. The results of our CMF group seem less good than in the Milan study. This can be explained by the higher percentage of patients with 4+ nodes included in our trial, compared with the distribution in Milan.

Adriamycin is potentially cardiotoxic. Although the drug has been given at doses far under the potential cardiotoxic dose over the whole year of therapy (360 mg/m^2) in patients carefully monitored with no cardiac toxicity attributable to the drug, so far we obviously cannot rule out potential late adverse effects of

this regimen in this respect. Patients will have to be carefully
followed. Despite this potential drawback, the policy of avoiding
the use of Adriamycin in the adjuvant situation and keeping it
"in case of relapse" is in our opinion unwarranted, since we know
no curative treatment of relapsed breast cancer (except for a very
small number of patients), and therefore, definitive cure at the
time of primary treatment must be the goal of the therapist.
Furthermore, we may soon have available new anthracycline derivatives as active as Adriamycin and much less cardiotoxic (Dantchev
et al., 1980).

The results regarding hormonal status are unexpected and not
clearly explained. Bonadonna and Valagussa (1981) attributed the
lower efficacy of CMF in postmenopausal women to underdosage of
these patients. In our hands, as earlier discussed, underdosage
has been similar in pre- and postmenopause, and we could not observe any dose-response relationship. Furthermore, postmenopausal
CMF patients did slightly better than premenopausal ones (Fig. 1),
so that for the whole population results were identical in pre-
and postmenopause. Further analyses of prognostic factors may be
necessary to obtain a satisfactory explanation of these observations. Subsequent to the initiation of this trial, hormone receptor status has been proven to be a major prognostic factor,
independent of others, mainly nodal status. Unfortunately too few
of our patients have been assessed for this parameter to obtain
meaningful results.

The optimal length of adjuvant chemotherapy has been ques-
tioned (Tancini et al., 1979) and may well be shorter than the 12
monthly cycles used in this study. In fact, in our current
study, patients receive only 6 months of AVCF, which is given to
node-negative patients only if the tumor is devoid of hormone
receptors.

Finally, some have argued that an early advantage in disease-
free survival may not be confirmed by longer follow-up and final
survival.

The Milan study has now over 5 years of follow-up, and survival advantage has been confirmed at each analysis. At 3 years
only, our study already shows a highly significant survival advantage for the AVCF group. Benefit due to CMF over controls is
an increment of 22% of disease-free expectancy at 5 years of
premenopausal women. We add a 29% increment of disease-free
expectancy at 3 years and may well hope that this reflects a real
increase of cure rate.

REFERENCES

Bonadonna, G., and Valagussa, P. (1981). *New Engl. J. Med. 304*, 10-15.
Dantchev, D., Slioussartchouk, V., Paintrand, M., Bourut, C., Hayat, M., and Mathé, G. (1980). *In* "Cancer Chemo- and Immunopharmacology" (G. Mathé and F. M. Muggia, eds.), Vol. 1, pp. 223-249. Springer, Heidelberg and New York.
Fisher, B., and Redmond, C. (1979). *In* "Adjuvant Therapy Cancer II" (S. E. Jones and S. E. Salmon, eds.), pp. 215-226. Grune & Stratton, New York.
Gouveia, J., Misset, J. L., Bayssas, M., Belpomme, D., De Vassal, F., Delgado, R., Gil, M., Hayat, M., Jasmin, C., Machover, D., Musset, M., Pico, J. L., Ribaud, P., Schwarzenberg, L., and Mathé, G. (1979). *Med. Oncol. 4*, 13 (Abstr. 49).
Hammond, N., Jones, S. E., Salmon, S. E., Giordano, G., Jackson, R., Miller, R., and Heusinkveld, R. (1977). *In* "Adjuvant Therapy of Cancer" (S. E. Salmon and S. E. Jones, eds.), pp. 153-160. North-Holland, Amsterdam.
Mareel, M., and De Brabander, M. (1978). *J. Natl. Cancer Inst. (US) 61*, 787-791.
Mathé, G., and Kenis, Y. (1975). "La chimiothérapie des cancers: leucémies, hématosarcomes et tumeurs solides," 3rd ed. Expansion Scientifique Française, Paris.
Nissen-Meyer, R., Kjellegren, K., Malmia, K., Manssen, B., and Narin, T. (1978). *Cancer 41*, 2088-2098.
Plagne, R., Misset, J. L., Belpomme, D., Guerrin, J., Le Mevel, B., Metz, R., Chollet, P., Delgado, M., Fargeot, P., Fumoleau, P., Jeanne, C., Ferrière, P., Schneider, M., De Vassal, F., Jasmin, C., Schwarzenberg, L., Hayat, M., Machover, D., Ribaud, P., Dorval, T., and Mathé, G. (1982). *Proc. Am. Assoc. Cancer Res. 23*, 157 (Abstr. 617).
Rossi, A., Bonadonna, G., Valagussa, P., and Veronesi, U. (1981). *Br. Med. J. 282*, 1427-1431.
Stjernsward, J. (1974). *Lancet 2*, 1285-1286.
Storme, G., Mareel, M., de Bruyne, G., and van Cauwenberge, R. (1981). *Proc. Int. Vinca Alkaloid Symp. Vindesine*, pp. 7-15.
Tancini, G., Bajetta, E., Marchini, S., Valagussa, P., Bonadonna, G., and Veronesi, U. (1979). *Cancer Clin. Trials 2*, 285-292.

DISCUSSION

KOBAYASHI: With regard to the high efficacy of AVCF treatment, I wonder if you could involve any immunological aspects on that, for example, inhibiting suppressor cell activity by such Adriamycin?

MATHÉ: Adriamycin is not known as being very efficient in re-
                gard to suppressor cells, while among the tetracyclines,
                aclacinomycin is.

ADDENDUM

    At the time of proof correction, the survival of the AVCF group
is not any more statistically significant for the overall patients,
and even for the premenopausal women.

CHAPTER 27

MONOCLONAL ANTIBODIES FOR TUMOR DETECTION
AND TARGETING OF ANTITUMOR AGENTS

M. J. Embleton
M. V. Pimm
R. W. Baldwin

Cancer Research Campaign Laboratories
University of Nottingham
Nottingham, England

I. INTRODUCTION

    The therapy of metastatic cancer could be materially advanced
if it were possible to direct therapeutic agents specifically to
the site of the tumor. In comparison with conventional systemic
chemotherapy, this would result in a reduction of toxicity to the
cancer patient while concentrating the effect of anticancer agents
at the tumor site. It could also considerably improve therapy
with biological response modifiers (BRM), which when administered
systemically, augment natural killer (NK) cell and macrophage activity (Lederer, 1980; Berthold et al., 1981). To have any
influence on tumor development, these effector cells have to
travel to tumors and infiltrate them to gain intercellular contact,

and it has been shown experimentally that introduction of BRM to
the tumor site gives an enhanced response. For example, intrapleural treatment with BCG has been shown to be an effective
measure against pleural effusions (Pimm et al., 1976), and
Nocardia rubra cell wall skeleton suppresses lung metastases when
targeted to alveolar macrophages by encapsulation within appropriately sized liposomes (Sone and Fidler, 1982).

The idea of using antibodies for targeting diagnostic or
therapeutic agents to tumors is not a new one (Arnon, 1979), but
it has received a renewed stimulus following the introduction of
techniques for producing monoclonal antibodies by constructing
somatic cell hybrids (Köhler and Milstein, 1975). The sources of
antibodies hitherto available were xenogenic antisera raised
against tumors and absorbed with normal cells, and to a lesser
extent sera from cancer patients, but neither of these are sufficiently specific for targeting to be a practical proposition.
In practice, xenoantisera are extremely difficult to render
"tumor specific," since antigens expressed at the surface of
tumor cells are predominantly the normal antigens of the host.
Absorption extensive enough to remove antibodies to normal components therefore leaves little or no reactivity against tumor
cells, and conversely, more limited absorption results in
unacceptably high levels of cross-reactive antibodies. Despite
many claims to the contrary, sera from cancer patients only rarely have antibodies directed toward tumor cells, as indicated by
the work of Old and colleagues (Old, 1981). The advent of monoclonal antibodies, however, has overcome these problems.

Most hybridoma antibodies are produced following appropriate
immunization of a xenogeneic species (usually mouse), but in this
case the clonal derivation of cell lines producing a single immu-
noglobin means that the antibody can be fully characterized, and
that reagents with the required affinity and specificity for a
particular tumor can be selected. This approach has led to the
production of monoclonal antibodies to a wide range of human
tumors. Some of these antibodies appear to detect antigens
associated with a particular tumor type, others being cross-
reactive among several different tumors (Baldwin et al., 1981).
A few monoclonal antibodies have direct tumor-suppressive action
on xenografts in vivo, but this is not a universal property, and
therefore they are being exploited predominantly for their
tumor-localizing properties.

Initially, monoclonal antibodies have been used to target
radioisotopes, this serving a twofold purpose. First, concentration of radiolabeled antibody at the tumor site provides a
demonstration that the antibody is indeed able to localize
specifically on tumors, and second, the external detection of
localized radiolabeled antibody may serve to aid detection of
distant metastases or otherwise occult tumors. Goldenberg et al.
(1980) have previously used radiolabeled polyclonal antibodies to
carcinoembryonic antigen (CEA) for this purpose, and Mach et al.
(1981) have reported the localization of an ^{131}I-labeled monoclonal

anti-CEA antibody in colorectal tumors. Radioiodinated monoclonal antibodies to cell surface antigen of a human osteogenic sarcoma cell line (Farrands *et al.*, 1981) and to milk fat globule membrane (Epenetos *et al.*, 1982a) have also been used to demonstrate primary and metastatic tumor deposits in human patients by external scanning.

The use of monoclonal antibodies to target cytotoxic agents to tumors is an obvious application of their localizing properties and is currently the most widely investigated approach with respect to antibody therapy. Cytotoxic agents amenable to antibody coupling include plant and bacterial toxins and conventional chemotherapeutic drugs. Toxins, modified from their native form by blocking their sugar-binding site or removal of the B chain of the molecule, have perhaps received the most attention. A number of groups have shown that the A chains of ricin and diphtheria toxin conjugated with monoclonal antibodies can exert cytotoxic effects on target cells that bind the antibody, comparable to the effects of the native toxin (Gilliland *et al.*, 1980; Trowbridge and Domingo, 1981). Effects on cell lines that do not react with the antibody are usually minimal, comparable with the A chain alone, which is relatively nontoxic because it has no inherent cell-binding potential. Conventional cytotoxic drugs can also be conjugated to monoclonal antibodies, and Pimm *et al.* (1982b) have shown that Adriamycin linked to specific monoclonal antibody by a dextran bridge had therapeutic properties against a spontaneously arising mammary carcinoma of an inbred rat strain.

In this chapter we describe the derivation of a monoclonal antibody to a human osteogenic sarcoma and its application for detecting tumor deposits by localization of radioactive iodine, and also the development of cytotoxic drug and BRM conjugates using the antibody as a specific carrier.

II. MONOCLONAL ANTIBODIES TO HUMAN OSTEOGENIC SARCOMA

A number of past reports have indicated that patients with sarcomas may have a humoral antibody response to their tumor (Morton and Malmgren, 1968; Moore and Hughes, 1973). However, the early studies were not well controlled, and it has since been established that much of the serum reactivity formerly observed was due to antibodies to non-tumor-related antigens such as blood group antigens, fetal antigens, and even tissue culture artifacts such as adsorbed bovine serum (Bloom *et al.*, 1973; Irie and Morton, 1974; Thorpe *et al.*, 1977). Partly in an attempt to overcome these problems, several groups have prepared monoclonal antibodies to sarcoma cells. Deng *et al.* (1981) reported a cytotoxic monoclonal antibody prepared against freshly prepared leiomyosarcoma cells that was nonreactive with a variety of normal cell types and a small range of unrelated tumor cells, although it was

reactive against a T-cell leukemia line. Monoclonal antibodies
have also been raised against freshly isolated osteogenic sarcoma
cells (Hosoi *et al.*, 1982). Three antibodies were found to be
preferentially reactive with osteogenic sarcoma and chondrosarcoma
when tested by immunofluorescence on cryostat sections of various
tumors and normal tissues, but there was also weak reactivity
with normal chondrocytes. Although this lack of complete tumor
specificity is at first sight disappointing, it seems to be a
frequent feature of murine monoclonal antibodies, and there are
other examples where apparently tumor-specific monoclonal antibodies have been shown to react with differentiation antigens
expressed on normal cell lineages (Greaves *et al.*, 1980; Old,
1981).

In our laboratory we have prepared two monoclonal antibodies
against an osteogenic sarcoma cell line, designated 791T, and these
also show patterns of reactivity not restricted entirely to the
immunizing tumor type (Embleton *et al.*, 1981a,b). Hybridomas
were prepared by fusing spleen cells from a mouse immunized
against cultured 791T cells with the P3-NS1 mouse myeloma. Two
of the hybridoma supernatants contained IgG2b antibodies reacting
with 791T cells in ^{125}I-labeled protein A-binding tests, and
these hybridomas (791T/36 and 791T/48) were cloned. Both monoclonal antibodies reacted strongly with cells of 791T and a
second osteogenic sarcoma, 788T, but were negative with cultured
fibroblasts from the tumor donors. More extensive specificity
testing revealed that 791T/36 bound to 7/13 osteogenic sarcoma
cell lines and 6 of 26 unrelated tumors, but not to a range of
normal fibroblasts, blood mononuclear cells or erythrocytes. The
791T/48 antibody, in contrast, was more restricted and reacted
against only 3 of 10 osteogenic sarcomas and one unrelated tumor.
The differing patterns of reactivity suggested that the two
antibodies were reacting against different epitopes shared by the
791T and 788T cell lines, and this was confirmed by the fact that
binding of ^{125}I-labeled 791T/36 antibody could be inhibited by
competition or blocking with cold 791T/36 but not by cold 791T/48,
and vice versa (Price *et al.*, 1982). The availability of
multiple cell lines with known binding reactivity makes these
antibodies suitable as models for targeting studies, and for this
purpose we have selected 791T/36 in particular because of its
wider range of activity. Its reactivity against a selected series
of target cells is summarized in Table I. These data illustrate
that in addition to reacting with a significant proportion of
osteogenic sarcomas, 791T/36 binds to cells of three in five
colon carcinomas tested, as well as individual examples of other
tumor types. Only a limited number of the cell lines that fail
to bind 791T/36 are listed in the table, sufficient to make the
point that the cross-reactions with unrelated tumors tend to be
sporadic rather than always related to certain tumor types (e.g.,
two of three lung carcinomas were negative).

Biochemical data have shown that the 791T/36 monoclonal antibody precipitates a glycoprotein with a molecular weight of

TABLE I.   Reactivity of 791T/36 Monoclonal Antibody with
Cultured Tumor Target Cells: ^{125}I-Labeled Protein A Assay[a]

Cell lines giving positive reaction	Cell lines giving negative reaction
Osteogenic sarcomas 791T 788T 2 OS T278 393T 805T 845T	Colon carcinomas HCT8 HRT18
	Lung carcinomas 9812 A427
Colon carcinomas HT29 LS174T HCLo	Melanomas RPMI 5966 Mel-57
Prostate carcinoma EB33	Bladder carcinoma T24
Cervix carcinoma Hela	Ovarian carcinoma PA-1
Lung carcinoma A549	

[a]Reactivity of 791T/36 antibody was determined by indirect
^{125}I-labeled protein A assay, by binding of ^{125}I-labeled 791T/36,
and by binding of fluorescein isothiocyanate (FITC)-labeled
791T/36.

72,000 from solubilized homogenates of 791T osteogenic sarcoma
cells. This glycoprotein is referred to as gp72, and it is shared
by all of the cell lines that react with antibody 791T/36, indicating that they share a common antigenic molecule rather than
different molecules with a common 791T/36-reactive epitope. This
molecule, however, is expressed to differing degrees on different
lines. On the most reactive sarcomas (791T and 788T), there are
2.2×10^6 antibody-binding sites per cell and on other tumors
there are 5×10^5 or fewer binding sites per cell (Price et al.,
1982).

III.   LOCALIZATION OF ANTI-OSTEOGENIC SARCOMA MONOCLONAL ANTIBODY

A.   Tumor Xenografts

1.   *Organ Distribution*

     To evaluate the tumor-localizing properties of monoclonal
antibody 791T/36, it was first purified by affinity chromatography
and labeled with radioiodine (^{125}I or ^{131}I); its reactivity was
confirmed by its ability to bind specifically to the positive cell
lines listed in Table I. Tumor xenografts were established in CBA
mice rendered immunodeficient by thymectomy, cytosine arabinoside
treatment, and whole-body irradiation (Pimm *et al.*, 1982a). The
subcutaneous (sc) inoculation of 10^6 human tumor cells resulted in
progressively growing tumors in more than 90% of immune-deprived
mice. Three days following injection of labeled 791T/36 antibody
into tumor-bearing mice, the distribution of radioactivity in
various organs was measured, the assessment of isotope uptake being
carried out by calculating tissue:blood ratios (mean counts per
minute per gram of tissue, divided by mean counts per minute per
gram of blood). The tissue:blood ratio was in all cases markedly
higher for 791T xenografts than for normal tissues (Fig. 1A). To
prove that the apparent localization in the xenograft was not
merely due to increased vascularity of the tumor, mice were treated
simultaneously with ^{125}I-labeled normal Ig2b and ^{131}I-labeled
791T/36 antibody. Normal immunoglobulin accumulated in all normal
tissues at a low level comparable with that of the antibody, and
did not show any increased association with the tumor compared
with the normal tissues. Moreover, the 791T/36 antibody was subsequently found to localize in xenografts of other osteogenic
sarcomas that bind 791T/36 (788T and 2 OS), but not in tumors
that do not react with the antibody (colon carcinoma HCT8 and
bladder carcinoma T24) (Fig. 1B). These studies conclusively
demonstrate that the radiolabeled 791T/36 monoclonal antibody
was specifically taken up by appropriate target tumors, and con-
firmation of this was obtained in images obtained by external
scanning of 791T xenografts (Fig. 2). The figure depicts gamma
camera images obtained with two mice treated with ^{131}I-labeled
791T/36, before and after enhancement by computerized subtraction
of blood pool images following injection of $[^{113m}I]$indium
chloride or $[^{99m}Tc]$pertechnetate. In both cases the subcutaneous
tumor clearly showed accumulation of ^{131}I over and above background levels.

2.   *Factors Influencing Localization of Xenografts*

     Tumor localization of antibody is influenced by a complex in-
terplay of factors, and xenografts provide a convenient model for
the analysis of the processes resulting in the eventual homing of

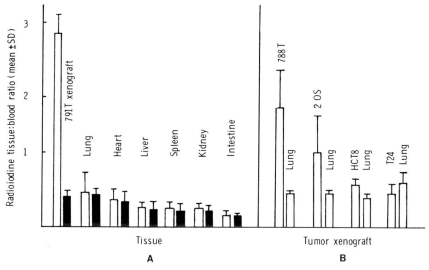

Fig. 1. (A) *In vivo* distribution of radiolabeled 791T/36
monoclonal antibody (white bars) compared with normal immunoglobulin (black bars) in athymic mice bearing xenografts of osteogenic sarcoma 791T. Mice bearing 791T tumors were inoculated
with ^{131}I-labeled 791T/36 and ^{125}I-labeled normal mouse Ig2b
simultaneously. Three days later, tissue:blood ratios of radioactivity were calculated as:

$$\frac{\text{Mean \% radioactivity in tissue}}{\text{Mean \% radioactivity in blood}}$$

(B) Localization of radiolabeled 791T/36 monoclonal antibody in
other tumors. Tumor-bearing mice were treated ip with [125]I-
labeled 791T/36, and 3 days later tissue:blood ratios were calculated as in (A). 788T and 2 OS are osteogenic sarcomas that
react with 791T/36 antibody *in vitro*. Bladder carcinoma T24 and
colon carcinoma HCT8 are nonreactors.

the antibody to its target tissue. One of the first problems involves the kinetics of antibody uptake, posing the question when
is the optimum time to acquire an external image. Experiments
shown in Fig. 3 were designed to compare the relative uptake of
[131]I-labeled 791T/36 and ^{125}I-labeled normal mouse Ig in mice
bearing 791T xenografts over a time course of 7 days. Antibody
was detectable in the tumor within 24 h, reaching peak levels
2-4 days after injection. Normal Ig, in contrast, showed little
variation within the tumor over the 7-day time course. The total
body loss of labeled antibody over the first 24 h was 66%, and
this was followed by a constant further decline. As a result,
the specific uptake of antibody by the tumor appears to be greatly
increased from 2 days onward. If the antibody uptake is calculated with respect to the uptake of normal Ig, it is possible to
derive a "localization index" that increases from 2.16 on Day 1
to 6.48 on Day 7.

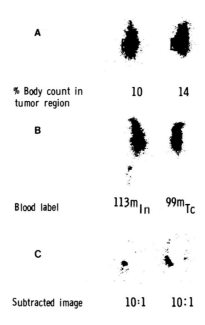

A

% Body count in   10   14
tumor region

B

Blood label ^{113m}In ^{99m}Tc

C

Subtracted image   10:1   10:1

Fig. 2. Demonstration of localization of 791T/36 monoclonal antibody in 791T xenografts by gamma scintigraphy. Athymic mice bearing 791T xenografts were treated ip with ^{131}I-labeled 791T/36, and 3 days later they were scanned on a gamma camera. Intravenous [^{99m}Tc]pertechnetate or [^{113m}In]indium chloride were used to acquire an image caused by the blood pool. (A) Image acquired with ^{131}I-labeled 791T/36. (B) Image acquired with blood label. (C) Computerized subtraction showing enhanced image of subcutaneously growing tumor. The area delineated in (A) is the region of the tumor.

Further useful information can be gained by calculating the proportion of injected radioactivity present within the tumor, and here it is necessary to determine the relationship between the dose of injected antibody and the amount taken up into the tumor. As shown in Fig. 4, over a dosage range of 2 to 50 µg of antibody protein per mouse, the amount of accumulated antibody is proportional to the dose administered. No plateau was reached, but at the highest dose (50 µg/mouse, equivalent to 2 mg/kg body weight), the tumor tissue contained 9 µg antibody per gram of tissue. At an injected dose of 40 µg/mouse or greater, normal Ig began to accumulate in normal tissues. Thus, while it may be possible to increase the proportion of antibody taken up into the tumor by giving larger doses of antibody, this may concomitantly result in higher background levels with no overall gain in resolution.

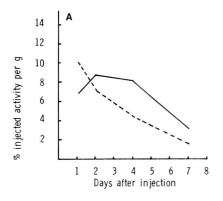 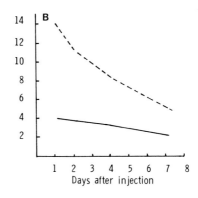

Fig. 3. Kinetics of uptake of radiolabeled 791T/36 (A) and normal Ig (B) into 791T xenografts and survival in blood. Mice were injected simultaneously with ^{131}I-labeled 791T/36 and ^{125}I-labeled normal Ig2b. At Day 1 the tumor:blood (T:B) ratio of radioactivity for 791T/36 was 0.67, and for normal Ig it was 0.31. At Day 7 the T:B ratios were 2.79 and 0.43, respectively. The localization index (calculated as T:B ratio for 791T/36 divided by T:B ratio for Ig2b) was 2.16 on Day 1 and 6.48 on Day 7. (————) Tumor; (- - - - -) blood.

Initial studies, in which different amounts of 791T/36 antibody were injected in different experiments, suggested that there was good correlation between tumor size and the proportion of injected radioactivity localizing within the tumor (Pimm et al., 1982a). This correlation was confirmed in controlled experiments in which mice received a standard 30-μg dose of radiolabeled 791T/36 and the tissue distribution was determined 3 days later. The mice bore tumors of different sizes (weights varying from 55 to 800 mg), and it was found that the resultant relationship between tumor size and uptake of radioactivity was linear (Fig. 5). In the experiment shown, the 55-mg tumor contained 90 ng of antibody, and the 800-mg tumor contained 250 ng.

B. Localization in Cancer Patients

Clinical studies have been undertaken to determine the localization of 791T/36 in human cancer patients, on the basis of the information gained with xenografts. In view of the rarity of osteogenic sarcoma, it was decided to exploit the cross-reactive properties of the antibody by initiating a phase I-II clinical trial on patients with colorectal carcinoma (Farrands et al., 1982). As indicated in Table I, the 791T/36 antibody bound to three of five colon carcinoma cell lines, and subsequent studies indicated that it was able to localize in a proportion of a series of xenografts established from primary colon carcinoma

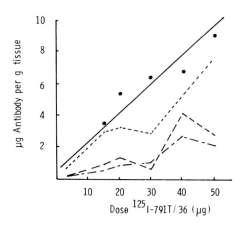

Fig. 4.   Correlation between dose of ^{125}I-labeled 791T/36 and localization in tumor and other organs.   791T-Xenografted mice were given ^{125}I-labeled 791T/36 by ip injection and radioactivity measured 3 days later.   (———) Tumor; (-----) blood; (————) spleen; (—·—·—) liver.

fragments (P. Farrands, personal communication).   In the clinical trial, patients received 200 µg 791T/36 antibody labeled with 1.5 mC of ^{131}I.   Samples of blood plasma taken 1-2 days after injection showed that circulating radioactivity was associated with a 7S region after Sephacryl S-300 chromatography and that it bound specifically to 791T target cells *in vitro*.   It was thus clearly associated with active antibody.   External ^{131}I images of the patients were obtained with a gamma camera 1, 2, or 3 days after intravenous antibody infusion, and blood pool images were obtained following injection of [^{99m}Tc]pertechnetate or [^{113}In]indium chloride for purposes of computerized enhancement.

Of 11 patients with primary or metastatic tumors who were studied, in 9 of them accurate tumor localization was seen (Table II).   In one patient localization was masked because of the disposition of the tumor behind the urinary bladder, which itself gave an image due to excreted ^{131}I.   Resected specimens from five patients with primary tumors were separately measured; and these showed increased ^{131}I uptake in the tumor compared with surrounding material in four cases (Farrands *et al*., 1982).   Perhaps the most exciting aspect of this series of patients, however, was the fact that metastatic deposits gave positive images as well as primary tumors.

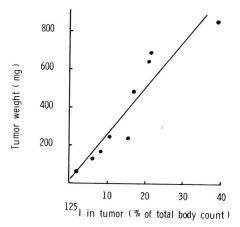

Fig. 5. Correlation between weight of 791T xenograft and tumor uptake of ^{125}I-labeled 791T/36 antibody. Tumor-bearing mice were killed 2 days after ip injection of ^{125}I-labeled 791T/36, and the radioactivity in the tumor was expressed as a percentage of the total body radioactivity.

IV. DRUG-TARGETING STUDIES

A. Cytotoxic Drugs

1. *In Vitro Studies*

Current emphasis is on the use of tumor-seeking antibodies to target directly acting agents such as toxins or cytotoxic drugs. Plant toxins and their A chains are an attractive proposition in this regard because of their potency (Thorpe and Ross, 1982). Indeed it has been estimated that entry of a single molecule of some toxins (e.g., ricin, diphtheria toxin) can result in death of a cell (Yamaizumi *et al.*, 1978; Eiklid *et al.*, 1980). However, because of their efficiency it is important that antibodies used to target toxins are specific only for the target tumor cells. In practice the necessary degree of specificity may not be possible to achieve. Although it may be possible to employ toxin-antibody conjugates safely by careful dose schedules, another alternative is to use antibodies to target drugs that are already used clinically and whose side effects are considered tolerable.

In our laboratory we have been evaluating the effects on cultured tumor cells of conjugates prepared between the 791T/36 monoclonal antibody and drugs such as vindesine and methotrexate. Vindesine-791T/36 conjugates were prepared by external collaborators and tested in our laboratory for cytotoxicity against various tumor cell lines in comparison with free vindesine (VDS), after confirming by competitive binding experiments that the conjugates

TABLE II. External Imaging of Colorectal Carcinomas with ^{131}I-Labeled 791T/36 Monoclonal Antibody

Patient number	Macroscopic tumor	Site of image	Tumor:nontumor ratio[a]
1	Primary carcinoma	Primary in pelvis	8.0:1
2	Primary carcinoma	Primary in pelvis	2.1:1
3	Primary carcinoma	Negative (behind bladder)	
4	2 Primary carcinomas	Both primaries	2.1:1
5	Primary carcinoma	Primary in pelvis	1.5:1
6	Disseminated carcinoma, omental metastasis	Primary pelvis mass and secondary	--
7	Disseminated carcinoma, liver metastasis	Liver metastasis	5.1:1
8	Disseminated carcinoma, liver metastasis	Liver metastasis	4.4:1
9	Inoperable carcinoma, treated by radio-therapy (30 Gy)	Negative	--
10	Disseminated carcinoma, liver and brain metastases	Liver and brain metastases	4.0:1
11	Disseminated carcinoma, pelvic recurrence	Recurrent tumor	4.3:1

[a]Tumor:nontumor ratio is the ratio of radioactivity concentreated over the area of the macroscopic tumor, divided by the mean radioactivity in adjacent areas.

retained antibody activity (Embleton *et al.*, 1983). The conjugate and the parent drug were assayed for their ability to inhibit the uptake of [^{75}Se]selenomethionine by the target cells, it having been established that ^{75}Se uptake correlated extremely well with the numbers of cells surviving toxicity. Representative results with this assay are illustrated in Fig. 6, depicting the relative effects of VDS-791T/36 and VDS on osteogenic sarcoma 791T, melanoma Mel-57, and ovarian carcinoma PA-1. Treatment with the conjugate markedly inhibited protein synthesis (^{75}Se uptake) by 791T cells in a dose-related manner but had no effect on Mel-57 or Pa-1, which are both antigen-negative with respect to the 791T/36 antibody (see Table I). That this was not a result of inherent resistance to VDS on the part of Mel-57 and PA-1 is indicated by the fact that all three cell lines showed comparable susceptibility to VDS alone. It is thus apparent that the coupling of VDS to monoclonal antibody confers specificity for cells to which the antibody can bind. The

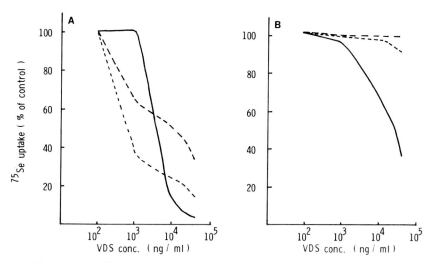

Fig. 6. Effect of (A) vindesine (VDS) and (B) VDS-791T/36 conjugate monoclonal antibody on survival of tumor cells in culture. Cells were treated with the agent for 15 min, then washed and cultured for 24 h. They were then labeled for 16 h with ^{75}Se selenomethionine and washed three times. Uptake of ^{75}Se by treated cells is expressed as a percentage of that in controls (treated with PBS). 791T (————) was an osteogenic sarcoma line, and Mel-57 (- - - -) and PA-1 (— — —) were a noncross-reactive melanoma and ovarian carcinoma, respectively.

overall toxicity of the drug VDS is greatly reduced by antibody coupling (Embleton *et al.*, 1983), and it is probable that targeting by the antibody compensates for this reduction in the case of 791T cells. Further tests confirmed that conjugates were active against other cells that react with 791T/36 (osteogenic sarcomas 788T, 2 OS, and T278) but not against nonreactors (bladder carcinoma T24 and melanoma RPMI 5966) (Embleton *et al.*, 1983). In these studies application of 791T/36 antibody alone had no cytotoxic effect.

Similar experiments were performed using conjugates of methotrexate (MTX) and 791T-36 in which both drug and antibody were linked to human serum albumin as a carrier (Garnett *et al.*, 1983). An example of one such experiment shows that MTX-791T/36 conjugate was as cytotoxic for 788T osteogenic sarcoma cells as unconjugated MTX (Fig. 7A), whereas MTX linked to human serum albumin (MTX-HSA) was approximately 500 times less toxic than either MTX or MTX-791T/36, based on their LD_{50} values. With bladder carcinoma T24 (Fig. 7B), the MTX-791T/36 conjugate was much less active than MTX, being more closely comparable with MTX-HSA. These results support those obtained with VDS-791T/36 conjugate, in that conjugation of the drug to a protein tends to reduce markedly the inherent toxicity of the drug, except in combinations in which the conjugate is targeted to a particular cell line by the monoclonal antibody.

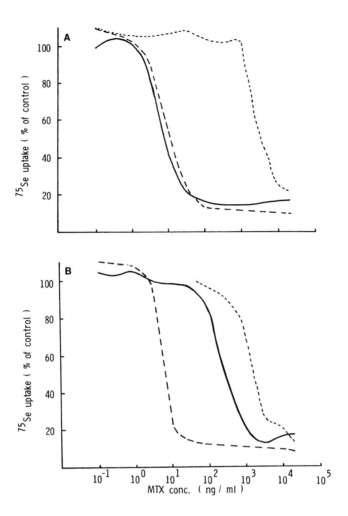

Fig. 7. Effect of (————) methotrexate (MTX), (———)
MTX-791T/36 monoclonal antibody conjugate, and (-----) MTX-human
serum albumin conjugate (MTX-HSA) on tumor cell survival. The
MTX-791T/36 conjugate was formed using HSA as a bridge. Target
cells were continuously exposed to the agents for 24 h in culture
before labeling for 16 h with [^{75}Se]selenomethionine. (A) Osteogenic sarcoma 788T cells; (B) bladder carcinoma T24 cells.

2. *Drug-Antibody Conjugates in Vivo*

Following the demonstration of selective *in vitro* cytotoxicity
against relevant target cells, it is necessary to determine the
effectiveness of drug-antibody conjugates *in vivo*. This raises
many questions including the choice of model, route of administration, dose of conjugate, and number of individual treatments.
Although informed guesses can be made by extrapolating data from

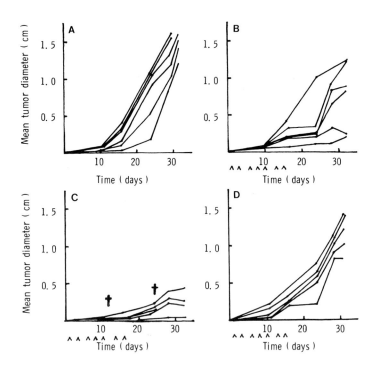

Fig. 8. Effect of vindesine (VDS), VDS-791T/36 conjugate, and 791T/36 alone on xenografts of 791T in athymic mide. Each agent was given in seven equal treatments at the time intervals indicated (^). The total doses received by each mouse were equivalent to 19.2 mg/kg body weight VDS and 500 mg/kg 791T/36 antibody. (A) Untreated controls; (B) VDS-791T/36 conjugate, each treatment 55 μg VDS and 1.5 mg Ab; (C) VDS alone, each treatment 55 μg; (D) 791T/36 alone, each treatment 1.5 mg.

antibody localization and *in vitro* cytotoxicity studies, answers to these questions can only be obtained with certainty by empirical means and will involve painstaking development work.

In our initial studies with a VDS-791T/36 conjugate we have used xenografts of osteogenic sarcoma 791T in immune-deprived mice as a tumor model. Tumor cells (10^6) were inoculated sc into the flank of several groups of mice and different groups were treated with conjugate, VDS, or 791T/36 antibody alone by ip injection. In the experiment illustrated in Fig. 8, these agents were administered in seven equal doses on Days 1, 3, 6, 8, 10, 13, and 15 after injection of the tumor cells, the total doses being equivalent to 19.2 mg VDS and 500 mg antibody per kilogram of body weight. There was considerable variation of tumor growth between individuals in any one group, but the overall trend was a reduced rate in mice treated with VDS or VDS-791T/36 conjugate, whereas animals given antibody alone were similar to the untreated controls. The free drug produced greater inhibition of tumor growth than the conjugate but was toxic to the mice at the dose

administered, resulting in two deaths (see crosses, Fig. 8C) in
the VDS group of six mice. The conjugate, however (Fig. 8B), was
completely nontoxic systemically. Toxicity studies performed
elsewhere (G. Rowlands, personal communication) confirm that VDS-
antibody conjugates are generally at least 50 times less toxic
than VDS alone.

The conclusion to be drawn from such results is that although
drug-antibody conjugates may be no more active than free drug at
equivalent drug doses at their present stage of development, they
are far safer to use and cause fewer untoward side effects. This
may allow higher doses to be administered, and combined with more
efficient conjugation procedures, this offers the hope of increased
therapeutic effectiveness in the future.

B. Biological Response Modifiers (BRM)

Our initial choice of BRM for antibody-targeting studies was
human lymphoblastoid interferon (IFN), since IFNs have been shown
to have two modes of action on tumor cells. They activate cytolytic cells such as natural killer (NK) cells (Berthold *et al.*,
1981) and may exert direct cytostatic effects on tumor cells,
particularly osteogenic sarcoma (Strander and Einhorn, 1977).
However, direct cytostasis was ruled out in the case of osteogenic
sarcoma 791T following assays in which the tumor cells were cultivated with IFN for periods of between 1 and 6 days without significantly affecting rates of cell division. Also, xenografts of
791T in nude mice were not suppressed by administration of IFN.

Since 791T cells were not susceptible to cytostasis, the effect of IFN on cytolysis mediated by NK cells was explored.
Peripheral blood lymphocytes from normal human donors were
cultured with ^{51}Cr-labeled 791T or erythroleukemia K562 target
cells for 6 h, using effector: target cell (E:T) ratios of
12.5:1, 6.25:1, and 3.125:1. Percentage cytotoxicity was plotted
against E:T ratios to obtain regression lines that passed through
the origin, the slope of these plots being directly proportional
to the frequency of NK cells in the lymphocyte population (Brooks
and Flannery, 1980). Using this assay system the effect of IFN
was assayed by incubating the lymphocytes with IFN (200 units/ml)
for 1 h at 37°C followed by three washes, before adding them to the
target cells. Conjugates of IFN-791T/36 were prepared by linking
affinity-purified antibody and IFN with *N*-succinimidyl-3-(2-pyridyl-
dithio)-proprionate (SPDP).

The NK-activating properties of both IFN and IFN-791T/36 were
assessed against 791T and K562 targets, and it was ascertained that
the conjugate retained most of the activation potential of the unconjugated IFN (Table III). In the case of 791T targets this was
sufficient to augment NK cell cytotoxicity by 315%. A more
exacting experiment was then performed that was intended to mimic
the targeting of IFN to tumor cells and the resultant activation

TABLE III. Augmentation of Cytolysis by Natural Killer Cells:
Effect of Interferon-791T/36 Monoclonal Antibody Conjugate[a]

Target cells	Effector cell treatment[b]	Cytotoxicity (slope ± SD)	Increase in cytolysis (%)
K562	None	8.2 ± 0.2	
K562	IFN	19.3 ± 0.3	235 ($p < .001$)
K562	IFN-791T/36 conjugate	11.5 ± 0.2	140 ($p < .001$)
791T	None	2.1 ± 0.3	--
791T	IFN	8.9 ± 1.1	415 ($p < .001$)
791T	IFN-791T/36 conjugate	6.8 ± 0.2	315 ($p < .001$)

[a]These data were compiled from Flannery et al. (1982).

[b]Effector cells were peripheral blood lymphocytes. Cells were pretreated with IFN or conjugate at 200 IFN units/ml for 60 min at 37°C before being added to ^{51}Cr-labeled cells.

of NK cells in the local environment. 791T target cells were pre-incubated with IFN-791T/36 and washed, then added to a mixed culture of normal lymphocytes and ^{51}Cr-labeled K562 third-party cells (Table IV). This resulted in augmentation of NK activity against the K562 cells. Pretreatment with a mixture of IFN and 791T/36 rather than conjugate did not result in augmentation, however. Also, T24 bladder carcinoma cells pretreated with the conjugate failed to augment cytotoxicity. These experiments were interpreted as suggesting that IFN specifically targeted and bound to tumor cells by monoclonal antibody might locally recruit cytotoxic effector cells, which could react against surrounding tumor cells in addition to those bearing the bound conjugate. The species specificity of human IFNs unfortunately limits the possibilities of testing this hypothesis in vivo using xenografted tumors in immune-deprived murine hosts, but the same basic approach should be applicable to virtually any BRM with less species-restricted activity.

V. CONCLUSIONS

The use of monoclonal antibodies for localizing tumors will clearly have considerable potential for the detection and treatment of metastases. Detection of metastases by external gamma scintigraphy, and the targeting of antitumor agents by antibodies

TABLE IV. Augmentation of Cytolysis by Natural Killer Cells: Lysis of Third-Party Cells (K562) Mediated by Cell-Bound Interferon-791T/36 Monoclonal Antibody Conjugate[a]

Tumor cell pretreatment[b]	Treated cells	Cytotoxicity (slope ± SD)	Increase in cytolysis (%)
Medium	791T	6.7 ± 0.4	--
IFN + 791T/36 (mixture)	791T	7.5 ± 0.6	112 (n.s.)
IFN-791T/36 conjugate	791T	14.4 ± 2.0	215 (p < .01)
Medium	T24	8.2 ± 2.0	--
IFN + 791T/36 (mixture)	T24	7.8 ± 0.2	95 (n.s.)
IFN-791T/36 conjugate	T24	8.7 ± 0.3	106 (n.s.)

[a]These data were compiled from Flannery *et al.* (1982).

[b]Tumor cells were incubated for 1 hr at 37 C with IFN-791T/36 conjugate or a nonconjugated mixture of IFN and 791T/36, and then washed. They were then added to a mixed culture of peripheral blood lymphocytes and ^{51}Cr-labeled third-party cells (K562).

[c]n.s., Not significant.

must result in improved therapy. However, these approaches are still experimental, and there are many problems yet to be resolved. The most basic requirement is a monoclonal antibody that reacts specifically with tumor-associated antigens and can be obtained in high yields. In real terms most antitumor monoclonal antibodies so far produced have reacted preferentially rather than solely with tumor cells, but so long as binding to normal cells does not produce an adverse reaction, this is an acceptable level of specificity. With the increasing repertoire of monoclonal antibodies against human tumors that is becoming available, it may be that some will show even greater specificity for neoplastic cells.

It is clear from our studies on *in vivo* localization of 791T/36 in human osteogenic sarcoma xenografts that the fate of parenterally inoculated antibody is influenced by a complex set of events. Some factors, such as rate of catabolism, will depend largely on the quality of the preparation. This can be affected by labeling procedures, since it is known that relatively minor degrees of substitution of amino acid residues can severely impair the functions of immunoglobulins. It is for this reason that it may be necessary to insert spacer molecules in the construction of antibody-drug conjugates, as we have done in the case of methotrexate-791T/36 conjugates, where human serum albumin was used as a bridge. However, the fate of these large complexes *in vivo* may prove to be quite different from that of free radio-labeled antibody.

   In addition to tracing the localization of antibody to tumors, it is important to determine the degree of penetration. Our studies with 791T/36 indicate that the antibody becomes associated primarily with the periphery of the tumor with fairly limited intratumor penetration (Pimm *et al.*, 1982a). This is a finding encountered by other groups investigating monoclonal antibody localization in human tumor xenografts (Moshakis *et al.*, 1981; Epenetos *et al.*, 1982b), and presumably will depend on multiple factors such as blood flow through tumors, antibody levels in blood, and probably circulating sequestered antigen levels. From these comments it is obvious that greater attention must be paid to the penetration of tumor masses when considering drug targeting by monoclonal antibodies.

   Another potential problem is the heterogeneity of expression of cell surface antigens by cell populations within tumors. It has been shown that cell lines established from different meta-stases of a primary human melanoma had markedly different surface antigen phenotypes when typed by a series of sera and monoclonal antibodies (Albino *et al.*, 1981), and this suggests that a single antibody may not be sufficient to detect all metastases, although it is clear from our studies with 791T/36 that an antibody that recognizes a fairly widespread antigen has definite potential in this regard. Problems of antigenic heterogeneity could, in any case, be overcome by the use of an appropriate battery of monoclo-nal antibodies recognizing a range of antigens.

   Not the least of the variables affecting the performance of monoclonal antibodies for tumor detection or drug targeting is the rate of removal from the circulation of the host. If removal is rapid, one might expect improved tumor localization due to a lower blood pool background, but this has not proved to be the case where $F(ab)_2$ or Fab fragments have been used. These tend to be catabolized more readily than intact Ig, but in at least one study they were less effective than intact anti-CEA antibody for localizing tumors (Gaffar *et al.*, 1982). Since most of the mono-clonal antibodies to human tumors so far produced are murine anti-bodies, one of the factors leading to their possible deactivation and removal in patients is their antigenicity in the human host. The production of antibodies to mouse Ig has been documented in a phase I clinical trial in the treatment of gastrointestinal tumors with monoclonal antibody (Sears *et al.*, 1982). However, one impor-tant point is that this was not accomplished by adverse reactions on the part of the patient.

   It can be seen from the considerations just outlined that there are still many problems to be analyzed and solved before monoclonal antibodies can be applied routinely to the management of human can-cer, and obviously it is too soon to predict with certainty whether antibody-targeted antitumor agents will be a universally practicable form of therapy. However, there is enormous scope for improving the current techniques of radioimaging and chemical coupling of agents to antibodies, and on the basis of achievements at the present early stage of development, the future appears to hold great promise.

ACKNOWLEDGMENTS

    This work was supported by a grant from the Cancer Research Campaign, London, England. The authors wish to acknowledge the collaboration of Professor J. D. Hardcastle, Messrs. A. C. Perkins and P. A. Farrands, and Drs. M. Garnett, G. F. Rowland, R. G. Simmonds, G. R. Flannery and J. D. Gray, and Miss J. Pelham. Human lymphoblastoid interferon was kindly provided by Dr. K. Fantes, Burroughs Wellcome Ltd., United Kingdom.

REFERENCES

Albino, A. P., Lloyd, K. O., Houghton, A. N., Oettgen, H. F., and Old, L. J. (1981). *J. Exp. Med. 154*, 1764-1778.
Arnon, R. (1979). *In* "Tumor-Associated Antigens and Their Specific Immune Responses" (F. Spreafico and R. Arnon, eds.), pp. 287-304. Academic Press, London.
Baldwin, R. W., Embleton, M. J., and Price, M. R. (1981). *Mol. Aspects Med. 4*, 329-368.
Berthold, W., Masucci, M. G., Klein, E., and Strander, H. (1981). *Hum. Lymphocyte Differ. 1*, 1.
Bloom, E. T., Fahey, J. L., Peterson, I. A., Geering, G., Bernhard, M., and Trempe, G. (1973). *Int. J. Cancer 12*, 21-31.
Brooks, C. G., and Flannery, G. R. (1980). *Immunology 39*, 187-194.
Deng, C., Terasaki, P. I., El-Awar, N., Billing, R., Cicciciarelli, J., and Lagrasse, L. (1981). *Lancet 8217*, 403-405.
Eiklid, K., Olsnes, S., and Pihl, A. (1980). *Exp. Cell Res. 126*, 321-326.
Embleton, M. J., Gunn, B., Byers, V. S., and Baldwin, R. W. (1981a). *Br. J. Cancer 43*, 582-587.
Embleton, M. J., Gunn, B., Byers, V. S., and Baldwin, R. W. (1981b). *Transplant. Proc. 12*, 1966-1969.
Embleton, M. J., Rowland, G. F., Simmonds, R. G., Jacobs, E., Marsden, C. H., and Baldwin, R. W. (1983). *Br. J. Cancer*, in press.
Epenetos, A. A., Britton, K. E., Mather, S., Shepherd, J., Granowska, M., Taylor-Papadimitriou, J., Nimmon, C. C., Durbin, H.,

Hawkins, L. R., Malpas, J. S., and Bodmer, W. F. (1982a). *Lancet*
11, 999-1004.
Epenetos, A. A., Nimmon, C. C., Arklie, J., Elliot, A. T.,
Hawkins, L. A., Knowles, R. W., Britton, K. E., and Bodmer, W. F.
(1982b). *Br. J. Cancer 46*, 1-8.
Farrands, P. A., Perkins, A. C., Pimm, M. V., Hardy, J. D.,
Embleton, M. J., Baldwin, R. W., and Hardcastle, J. D. (1982).
Lancet 11, 397-400.
Flannery, G. R., Pelham, J. M., Gray, J. D., and Baldwin, R. W.
(1982). *J. Cell. Biochem. 6* (Suppl.), 101.
Gaffar, S. A., Bennet, S. J., Deland, F. H., Primus, F. J., and
Goldenberg, D. M. (1982). *Proc. Am. Assoc. Cancer Res. 23*, 249.
Garnett, M. C., Embleton, M. J., Jacobs, E., and Baldwin, R. W.
(1983). *Int. J. Cancer 31*, 661-670.
Gilliland, D. G., Steplewski, Z., Collier, R. J., Mitchell, K. F.,
Chang, T. H., and Koprowski, H. (1980). *Proc. Natl. Acad. Sci.*
(USA) 77, 4539-4543.
Goldenberg, D. M., Kim, E. E., Deland, F. H., Bennet, S., and
Primus, F. J. (1980). *Cancer Res. 40*, 2984-2992.
Greaves, M. F., Verbi, W., Kemshead, J., and Kennet, R. (1980).
Blood 56, 1141-1144.
Hosoi, S., Nakamura, T., Higashi, S., Yamamuro, T., Toyama, S.,
Shinomiya, K., and Mikawa, H. (1982). *Cancer Res. 42*, 654-659.
Irie, R. F., and Morton, D. L. (1974). *J. Natl. Cancer Inst.*
(US) 52, 1051-1057.
Köhler, G., and Milstein, C. (1975). *Eur. J. Immunol. 6*, 511-519.
Lederer, E. (1980). *In* "Immunology 80: Progress in Immunology IV"
(M. Fougereau and J. Dausset, eds.), pp. 1194-1211. Academic
Press, London.
Mach, J. P., Buchegger, F., Forni, M., Richard, J., Berche, C.,
Lambroso, J. D., Schreyer, M., Giradet, C., Accola, R., and
Carrel, S. (1981). *Immunol. Today 2*, 239-249.
Moore, M., and Hughes, L. A. (1973). *Br. J. Cancer 28* (Suppl. 1),
175-184.
Morton, D. L., and Malmgren, R. A. (1968). *Science (Washington,*
D.C.) 162, 1279-1281.
Moshakis, V., McIllhinney, R. A. J., and Neville, A. M. (1981).
Br. J. Cancer 44, 663-669.
Old, L. J. (1981). *Cancer Res. 41*, 361-375.
Pimm, M. V., Hopper, D. G., and Baldwin, R. W. (1976). *Br. J.*
Cancer 34, 368-373.
Pimm, M. V., Embleton, M. J., Perkins, A. C., Price, M. R.,
Robins, R. A., Robinson, G. R., and Baldwin, R. W. (1982a).
Int. J. Cancer 30, 75-85.
Pimm, M. V., Jones, J. A., Price, M. R., Middle, J. G.,
Embleton, M. J., and Baldwin, R. W. (1982b). *Cancer Immunol.*
Immunother. 12, 125-134.
Price, M. R., Pimm, M. V., Dawood, F. A., Embleton, M. J., and
Baldwin, R. W. (1982). *In* "Tumor Progression and Markers"
(K. Lapis and A. Jeney, eds.), pp. 427-437. Kugler, Amsterdam.

Sears, H. F., Atkinson, B., Mattis, J., Ernst, C., Herlyn, D.,
Steplewski, Z., Hayry, P., and Koprowski, H. (1982). *Lancet i*,
762-765.
Sone, S., and Fidler, I. J. (1982). *Cancer Immunol. Immunother.*
12, 203-209.
Strander, H., and Einhorn, S. (1977). *Int. J. Cancer 19*, 468-473.
Thorpe, P. E., and Ross, W. C. J. (1982). *Immunol. Rev. 62*, 119-
158.
Thorpe, W. P., Parker, G. A., and Rosenberg, S. A. (1977).
J. Immunol. 119, 818-823.
Trowbridge, J. S., and Domingo, D. J. (1981). *Nature (London) 294*,
171-173.
Yamaizumi, M., Mekada, E., Uchida, T., and Okada, Y. (1978).
Cell 15, 245-250.

DISCUSSION

COHEN: I see some theoretical problems with the interferon-conjugated antibody. First, in most solid tumors, lymphocytes are in regions outside of islands of tumor, not sprinkled within. Therefore, it's hard to envision the coupling you postulate in an *in vivo* system. Second, there is no experimental evidence that would suggest that local activation of killer cell activity would be more effective than systemic activation; it could actually be less!

EMBLETON: The interferon (IFN)-monoclonal antibody studies were performed only *in vitro* because the human lymphoblastoid INF we used could not activate mouse NK cells and was not testable against xenografts *in vivo*. The regional distribution of natural killer cells within tumors may indeed be a problem, which we have not been able to investigate. It is possible that distribution may be modified by IFN-mediated recruitment. I agree that we do not yet know whether local activation of natural killer cells would be more beneficial than systemic activation.

GOLUB: The antibody-IFN conjugate is a very creative approach, but I don't understand why it works. One would expect the antibody to mediate ADCC with or without IFN.

EMBLETON: The 791T/36 antibody does not mediate ADCC against 791T osteogenic sarcoma or other target cells. These experiments were controlled positively by showing simultaneously than anti-Chang serum mediates ADCC against all targets tested.

COCHRAN: We find that it is necessary to undertake histological
            localization of antibody for accumulated assessment of
            specificity--*in vitro* techniques give only a partial
            view. Are you currently employing a histological ap-
            proach?

EMBLETON: We have begun to investigate the reactivity of our
            monoclonal antibody 791T/36 by immunohistology on fro-
            zen sections of normal human tissues, and find areas
            of reaction in the stroma of some tissues that would
            not be detected in cell-binding assays.

KOBAYASHI: Can the antibody penetrate the tumor cells located in
            the central area of the tumor tissue where the growth
            fraction is probably low?

EMBLETON: Autoradiographs of tumor indicate that the antibody
            is concentrated at the periphery of the tumor, with
            only slight penetration to the interior.

LIOTTA: What is the smallest sized tumor detectable by this
            method? From the point of view of the circulating
            monoclonal antibody, it can't "see" the tumor cell
            out in the tissue. Therefore, the monoclonals have to
            leak out nonspecifically in all tissues. What mecha-
            nism washes out unbound antibodies?

EMBLETON: The smallest tumor we have detected in xenografts was
            50 mg; this would presumably not be detectable in a
            human patient. The level of antibody in normal tissues
            equilibrates with that in the blood, and the half-life
            of radiolabeled antibody in the circulation is about
            24 hr. By 7 days the levels in blood and normal tissues
            are low, while the level of antibody within the tumor
            becomes higher than in blood at 24 hr and remains fairly
            stable for at least 7 days. Unbound antibodies in nor-
            mal tissues presumably enter the blood by diffusion and
            are inactivated by the liver and secreted via the kid-
            neys.

POSTE: Comment: I would like to add to the list of problems
            that you stated at the end concerning the use of drug-
            antibody conjugates in therapy. My laboratory has
            recently completed studies using drug-antitumor antibody
            complexes, and also liposomes containing cytotoxic drugs
            and bearing antitumor monoclonal antibodies on their
            surface. Even though these modalities may interact with
            tumor cells, significant uptake of drug-antibody/drug-
            liposome antibody complexes also occurs into mononuclear
            phagocytes of the RES and in the circulation, presumably
            as a result of binding of antibodies to FC receptors on

these cells. This event results in toxic destruction
of these cells. If studies are done with metastatic
tumor models, rather than the nonmetastizing tumors
typically used in your studies to date, one finds that
both drug-antibody and drug-liposome-antibody complexes
produce a marked enhancement of metastasis. I, thus,
consider that the altered *pharmacodistribution* of drug-
antibody conjugates may pose serious risks in the
important host defense functions performed by mononuclear phagocytes.

EMBLETON: In our studies we see no preferential uptake of
labeled antibody or labeled antibody-vindesine conjugate into the liver on the basis of tissue:blood
ratios (radioactivity per gram of tissue divided by
radioactivity per gram of blood). Liver levels are at
the same background level as other normal tissues and
much less than in the tumor. If antibody-vindesine
conjugate is taken up into reticuloendothelial cells,
it may cause less damage than many other drugs or plant
toxins owing to its specificity for the mitotic phase
of the cell cycle.

PART VB

Chairpersons

M. J. Embleton
Kikuo Nomoto

CHAPTER 28

EXPERIMENTAL IMMUNOTHERAPY OF HUMAN MELANOMA WITH HUMAN MONOCLONAL
ANTIBODY TO A TUMOR ANTIGEN (OFA-I-2) USING ATHYMIC NUDE MICE

Mitsuo Katano
Reiko F. Irie

Division of Surgical Oncology
University of California at Los Angeles School of Medicine
Los Angeles, California

I. INTRODUCTION

Georges Köhler and Cesar Milstein (1975) introduced the hybridoma technology. Thereafter, many monoclonal antibodies
against human tumor cells have been reported (Koprowski *et al.*,
1979; Dippold *et al.*, 1980). Monoclonal antibodies are now

thought to be one of the most hopeful weapons against cancer. All
of these monoclonal antibodies, however, originated from murine
cells but not from human cells. While some investigators (Miller
et al., 1982) suggest that mouse monoclonal antibodies could be
therapeutically useful for human cancer, others (Stevenson and
Stevenson, 1980) emphasize the potential disadvantages of those
foreign substances in clinical application. Some, but by no means
all, of the problems may be overcome by using human monoclonal
antibody.

We have established two Epstein-Barr virus-transformed human
B-lymphoblastoid cell lines, L55 and L72, that produce human antibody against a human tumor-associated membrane antigen (OFA-I)
(Irie *et al.*, 1976, 1981, 1982). L55 produced IgM antibody
(anti-OFA-I-1) directed against a membrane antigen (OFA-I-1) of
various histological types of human malignant cells (Irie *et al.*,
1982). L72 secrete IgM antibody (anti-OFA-I-2) directed against a
membrane antigen (OFA-I-2) of tumors only of neuroectodermal
origin (Irie *et al.*, 1982). L55 ceased secreting antibody
6 months after the culture. In contrast, the anti-OFA-I-2-
producing cell line, L72, has continuously produced antibody for
more than 1 year. Therefore, anti-OFA-I-2 can be collected in
large amounts from L72 spent medium.

We previously reported that OFA-I was immunogenic in adult
humans and could induce IgM-class antibody in serum of melanoma
patients (Irie *et al.*, 1976, 1979), and that serum anti-OFA-I
titer showed a positive correlation with clinical prognosis of
melanoma patients (Jones *et al.*, 1981). This fact, coupled with
the finding that serum anti-OFA-I is cytotoxic in the presence of
either rabbit or human complement to OFA-I-positive tumor cells
(Sidell *et al.*, 1979), suggests that IgM anti-OFA-I could confer
some protection against tumor growth *in vivo*. These findings indicated to us a strong potential for clinical application of this
L72 lymphoblastoid cell secreting anti-OFA-I-2.

Several reports have shown that human tumors transplanted
into athymic nude mice not only preserved the biological and
biochemical characteristics of the tumor origin, but also sometimes had a similar sensitivity to chemotherapy to that of the
human tumor. These findings have stressed the potential value of
the nude mouse system in testing the *in vivo* effect of L72
producing anti-OFA-I-2 on transplantable human melanomas.

This chapter describes the purification procedure of the human
IgM anti-OFA-I-2 antibody from spent medium, the monoclonal character of this antibody determined by agarose isoelectric focusing
(IEF) technique, and finally the experimental passive immunization
by human monoclonal antibody (anti-OFA-I-2) using a nude mouse
system to assess human application of this antibody.

II. CHARACTERIZATION OF ANTI-OFA-I-2

A. Purification of Anti-OFA-I-2

IgM anti-OFA-I-2-producing lymphoblastoid cells (L72) were
cultured in 1-5% fetal calf serum (FCS) containing RPMI 1640
medium (Irie *et al.*, 1982). Antibody titer was tested every 3-4
days after culture by immune adherence (IA) assay using a OFA-I-2-
positive human melanoma cell line (M14) as the target (Irie *et al.*,
1974). Antibody-positive spent medium was collected from
cultures, and concentrated by ultrafiltration. Albumin derived
from FCS and some other proteins were removed in the supernatant
by 50% ammonium sulfate precipitation. An IgM-rich fraction was
further purified by dialyzing the above precipitate against distilled water. After dissolving the precipitate in phosphate-
buffered saline (PBS), it was centrifuged at 100,000 g for 90 min
to remove cell membrane-derived large molecules and protein aggregates. Clear supernatants were collected and stored at -190°C
until used (partially purified anti-OFA-I-2). At this stage, more
than 80% of the protein was human IgM. Antibody titer recovery
was over 100%, which may reflect removal of factor(s) inhibiting
antibody binding to tumor target cells by the IA assay. Protein
and IgM contents were measured by Coomassie brilliant blue binding
assay (Bradford, 1976) and radioimmunoassay (Pierce and Klinman,
1975), respectively.

Partially purified anti-OFA-I-2 fractions were applied to a
Sephacryl S-300 superfine column and eluted with PBS. Fractions
of 5 ml were collected and assayed for total protein, IgM content,
and antibody titer. The three fractions after the first excluded
peak showed an equal concentration of protein and human IgM.
These three fractions were combined together and used as a final
purified anti-OFA-I-2. Antibody titer was detected only in human
IgM-positive fractions.

The purity of human IgM anti-OFA-I-2 isolated by gel filtration was assessed by SDS-polyacrylamide gel electrophoresis. As
shown in Fig. 1, when a sample was prepared under reducing conditions using 0.1 *M* DTT before the run, only two bands representing
IgM heavy and light chains were detected.

The yield of IgM, antibody titer, and purity are summarized in
Table I.

B. Determination of Monoclonal Character of Anti-OFA-I-2

Awden *et al.* (1968) reported the method of isoelectric focusing (IEF) in thin-layer polyacrylamide gel to analyze IgG heterogeneity; this method was not useful in our studies, probably
because of severe restrictions of mobility of large proteins like
IgM immunoglobulins in the polyacrylamide gel. Thus, native IgM

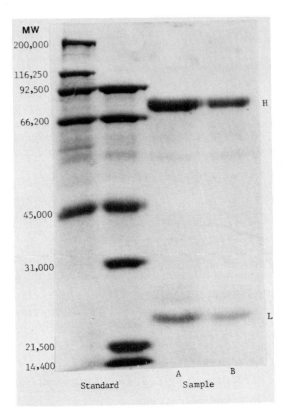

Fig. 1. SDS-polyacrylamide gel electrophoresis of a purified anti-OFA-I-2 fraction. The sample was prepared in the presence of 0.1 M DTT. H, Heavy chain; L, light chain. The following standards (indicated by their molecular weights) were used: myosin (200,000), β-galactosidase (116,250), phosphorylase B (92,500), bovine serum albumin (66,200), ovalbumin (45,000), carbonic anhydrase (31,000), soybean trypsin inhibitor (21,500), and lysozyme (14,400).

must be altered to its monomers using reducing agents and heat treatment prior to application to polyacrylamide gel IEF. Unfortunately, these treatments often may give rise to artifactual heterogeneity of immunoglobulin isoelectric pattern. Rosen et al. (1979) reported that agarose IEF could be used to determine the monoclonality of native IgM. They showed that the resolving power is comparable to that obtained in thin-layer IEF in polyacrylamide gel. Therefore, to determine the monoclonality of L72 producing IgM antibody, we used the agarose IEF technique. Purified IgM fraction was electrophoresed on agarose, and focused proteins were stained with Coomassie brilliant blue R-250. Isoelectric focusing was performed in 10% D-sorbitol, 0.8% agarose in the presence of 2% Ampholine, pH 3.5-9.5. Aliquots of 10 µl

TABLE I. Purification of Anti-OFA-I-2 from L72 Spent Medium

Fraction of L72 spent medium	Protein (mg)	IgM (mg)	Purity (%)	Recovery in IA activity
L72 spent medium[a]	560	4.6	0.8	1
Ammonium sulfate ppt	230	4.3	1.9	0.9
Water ppt	5.5	4.0	72.7	1
Sephacryl S-300 column purified fraction[b]	2.9	2.9	100.0	0.8

[a]One liter of spent medium of L72 cells grown in 1% FCS containing RPMI 1640 was used as a starting material.

[b]The fractions showing an equal concentration of protein and IgM obtained from Sephacryl S-300 superfine column were combined together.

of the samples, soaked in Paratex filter pads, were applied to the gel surface. The following electrofocusing conditions were used for IgM separation: 20 min at 100 V (max. 5 mA); 30 min at 200 V; the sample filter pads were then removed, and focusing was continued at 6.2 W constant power (max. 1000 V) for 60 min. As shown in Fig. 2, the IgM fraction was focused only on one isoelectric point, pH 8.0. When 10-20 L72 cells were planted in Costar 96-well microplates using irradiated human peripheral blood lymphocytes as a feeder layer, the spent medium from all of the wells became anti-OFA-I-2 antibody-positive within 3 weeks. When antibodies from two randomly selected subclones, L72-2X and L72-63, were analyzed by IEF together with the original L72 antibody, IgM fractions from all three focused in an identical region at pH 8.0 (Fig. 2). The same IgM fractions from L72, L72-2X, and L72-63 were electrophoresed after absorption by OFA-I-2-positive human melanomas. As shown on the right side of each IgM IEF, the pH 8.0 band completely disappeared, indicating that all of the IgM had specificity for OFA-I-2 antigen.

To identify the focused protein as human IgM, immunofixation was performed. In this test, concentrated L72 spent medium was used rather than purified IgM. After focusing, the agarose plate was overlaid with rabbit anti-human γ-, μ-, κ-, and λ-chain specific antibodies. As shown in Fig. 3, anti-μ and -κ antibodies were reactive with the protein. However, antibodies to γ and λ were devoid of reactivity.

These findings indicated that the human IgM secreted by the L72 cell line was of monoclonal origin with specificity for OFA-I-2.

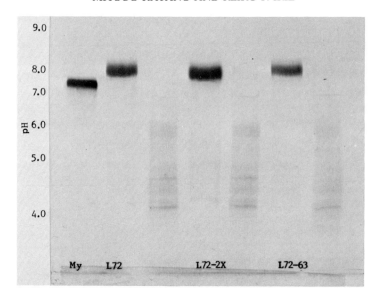

Fig. 2. Agarose IEF of purified IgM anti-OFA-I-2 fraction
from spent medium of L72 and L72 subclones (L72-2X and L72-63).
Samples of 10 µl (4 mg/ml) were applied to the gel surface.
L72 and L72 subclones purified IgM anti-OFA-I-2 fractions preab-
sorbed by OFA-I-2-positive Ml4 melanoma cells (right-hand lane of
each IgM fraction). IgM from serum of a patient with
Waldenström's macroglobulinemia (My).

C. Complement-Dependent Cytotoxicity of OFA-I-2-Positive Tumor
   Cells by Purified Anti-OFA-I-2

To examine if purified anti-OFA-I-2 retained its cytotoxic activity, the complement-dependent cytotoxicity assay was performed
using OFA-I-2-positive human melanoma cell line Ml4 as target
cell. Fifty microliters of Ml4 cell suspension adjusted to
5×10^5 cells/ml, 50 µl of anti-OFA-I-2 in serial dilution, and
50 µl of fourfold-diluted fresh rabbit or human serum used as complement sources, were mixed and incubated at 37°C for 90 min.
Fresh human AB serum used as a second complement source was absorbed prior to use by Ml4 cells at 0°C to remove natural antibody.
Dead cells were determined after the addition of 150 µl of 0.5%
trypan blue dye solution. As shown in Fig. 4, when OFA-I-2-posi-
tive Ml4 cells were exposed to antibody and rabbit complement,
various degrees of cytotoxicity were obtained depending on the antibody concentration. Complement alone or antibody alone had no
cytotoxic effect. Although the percentage cytotoxicity was lower,
human complement was also effective.

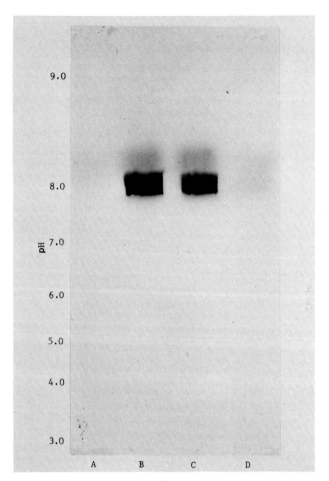

Fig. 3. Agarose IEF of L72 spent medium followed by immunofixation with rabbit anti-human immunoglobulins.   L72 spent medium
was concentrated 100-fold by ultrafiltration.   Concentrated L72
spent medium was applied to the gel surface.   After focusing, the
focused proteins were overlaid with rabbit anti-human (A) γ-,
(B) μ-, (C) κ-, and (D) λ-chain specific antibodies and incubated
at 37°C for 1 hr in a humidity chamber.

III.   EXPERIMENTAL IMMUNOTHERAPY USING NUDE MICE INOCULATED
        WITH HUMAN MELANOMAS

A.   Simultaneous Inoculation of Melanoma Cells and Anti-OFA-I-2

The *in vivo* cytotoxic effect of antibody was assessed using
homozygous athymic male CD-1 nude mice inoculated with human melanoma.   Various human melanoma cell lines were tested for the
growth rate and tumor-free interval by subcutaneous tumor inocula-

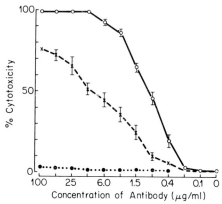

Fig. 4. Complement-dependent cytotoxicity of purified anti-
OFA-I-2 against M14 cells using rabbit (o——o) or human (x----x)
complement. Complement alone (●) or antibody alone (•••••) had
no cytotoxic effect. Vertical bars, ±SE. Cytotoxicity assay was
performed as described in text (Section II,C).

tion. M14 and M24 were chosen as OFA-I-2-positive and -negative
melanomas, respectively, because both cells showed a similar
growth pattern in the CD-1 nude mice. A protocol for experimental
passive immunotherapy using anti-OFA-I-2 was developed. Human
melanoma cells in the concentration of 2 × 10^6 cells/ml were mixed
with an equal volume of 500 µg/ml of 10 µg/ml of anti-OFA-I-2 *in
vitro*, and 0.2 ml of the mixture was inoculated subcutaneously in
the anterior thoracic region of CD-1 nude mice. The duration from
tumor inoculation to the appearance of a visible tumor mass was
recorded as the tumor-free interval. Table II shows the mean
tumor-free interval after inoculation of the mixture of M14 or M24
and 50 µg of anti-OFA-I-2. The mean tumor-free interval in the
control group was 12 days, and in the antibody-sensitized M14-
inoculated group the interval was 30 days. The difference in
tumor-free interval between the two groups was statistically significant (*p* = .01). However, there was no significant difference
in tumor-free interval between the control and the antibody-treated
M24-inoculated group. Nonrelevant human IgM from a myeloma patient's serum did not affect the tumor-free interval in M14-
inoculated mice either.
    The dose dependence for the antitumor effect of the antibody
was tested. CD-1 mice were inoculated subcutaneously with 2 × 10^5
cells/ml M14 together with different concentrations of anti-OFA-I-2.
The antitumor effect of the antibody was totally dependent on the
concentration of antibody used (100 µg to 1 µg) (data not shown).
However, none of these doses resulted in a complete rejection of
the tumor, which probably means that anti-OFA-I-2 did not generate
complete rejection due to complement activities in CD-1 nude mice.
As shown in Table III, their complement titers in complement-
dependent cytotoxicity were extremely low, when compared with that

TABLE II. Tumor-Free Interval of CD-1 Nude Mice Inoculated Subcutaneously with OFA-I-2-Positive (M14) or -Negative (M24) Human Melanoma and Anti-OFA-I-2

Tumor (2×10^5 cells/mouse)	Tumor admixed with	(IgM) (μg)	No. of tumor takes/no. of mice tested	Tumor-free interval (mean days)
M14	Anti-OFA-I-2	50	11/11	30
		1	3/3	12
	Anti-OFA-I-2-negative fraction[a]	1	11/11	12
	Serum from patient with IgM myeloma	50	4/4	13
M24	Anti-OFA-I-2	50	4/4	9
	Anti-OFA-I-2-negative fraction	1	4/4	9

[a] L72 often changes to anti-OFA-I-2-nonproducing cells several months after the continuous culture. Anti-OFA-I-2-negative fraction was prepared from non-antibody-producing L72 culture using the same method and conditions as that of anti-OFA-I-2 preparation from antibody-producing L72 spent medium.

TABLE III. Complement-Dependent Cytotoxicity of Anti-OFA-I-2 against M14 Cells

Antibody (µg/ml)	Complement sources[a]	Percentage cytotoxicity (mean ± SD)[b]
0	None	8.0 ± 4.7
100	None	8.7 ± 4.7
0	Rabbit	7.3 ± 7.3
100	Rabbit	89.0 ± 6.7
0	Human	8.0 ± 3.7
100	Human	62.0 ± 7.3
0	CD-1 Nude mouse	2.4 ± 2.3
100	CD-1 Nude mouse	23.5 ± 8.1

[a]Fourfold-diluted fresh rabbit or human serum and threefold-diluted CD-1 male nude mouse serum were used as complement sources.
[b]Complement-dependent cytotoxicity was assayed as described in the text (Section II,C).

of rabbit or human serum. In fact, when M14 cells were mixed with antibody and rabbit complement *in vitro* at 4°C, and then inoculated subcutaneously at CD-1 mice, approximately half of the mice did not have visible tumor nodules by 3 months observation.

B. Intratumor Injection of Anti-OFA-I-2

We first examined whether the cells in the tumor nodules growing in nude mice express OFA-I-2 antigenicity. One million M14 or M24 cells were inoculated subcutaneously in the anterior thoracic region of CD-1 nude mice. By 4 to 5 days after the tumor inoculation, all the mice showed a visible tumor nodule at the inoculated site. At 2 and 4 weeks after the subcutaneous inoculation of M14 or M24, tumor nodules were excised and minced, and the IA assay was performed on these cells using purified anti-OFA-I-2. As shown in Table IV, OFA-I-2 antigenicity was maintained in M14 cells grown in nude mice. In contrast, the OFA-I-2-negative M24 cells in culture were transformed to become slightly positive in the nude mice. But the antigenicity was minimal as compared to that of M14.

Subsequently, 1×10^6 M14 cells were inoculated subcutaneously in CD-1 nude mice. Ten days after the inoculation, mice bearing the same-sized tumors were selected and randomly divided into four groups as shown in Fig. 5. Tumors receiving antibody alone were slightly suppressed. Tumors receiving antibody and rabbit complement were significantly suppressed. No tumor suppression effects were observed in M24 nodules by the antibody and complement (data not shown).

TABLE IV. OFA-I-2 Antigenicity on M14 and M24 Cells Grown in CD-1 Nude Mice

Tumor	Tumor grown in	Number of specimens tested	IA_{50} with anti-OFA-I-2
M14	Nude mice		
	2 weeks	3	800-3200
	4 weeks	4	1600-3200
	Tissue culture	6	800-3200
M24	Nude mice		
	2 weeks	2	10, 100
	4 weeks	2	10, 40
	Tissue culture	2	1, 1

IV. SUMMARY

The results from experimental immunotherapy indicate that human monoclonal anti-OFA-I-2 may be useful for the suppression of OFA-I-2-positive tumors if tumors can be directly exposed to the antibody.

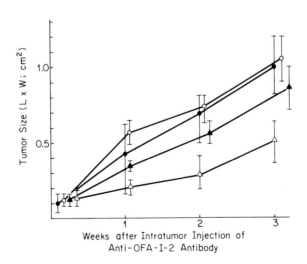

Fig. 5. Suppression of tumor growth by intratumor injection of anti-OFA-I-2 in subcutaneous nodules of human melanoma (M14). Anti-OFA-I-2-negative fraction alone (●——●), n = 5). Rabbit complement alone (o——o, n = 4). Anti-OFA-I-2 alone (▲——▲, n = 4). Anti-OFA-I-2 and rabbit complement (Δ——Δ, n = 4). Vertical bars, ±SE.

For example, the circulating tumor cells that cause metastases might be killed by this antibody.

Systemic administration of antibody may play an important role in elimination of subclinical tumor deposits or circulating tumors in patients either during or after operation. A direct administration of antibody to tumor sites, including primary and metastatic tumors, may be therapeutically effective.

Another therapeutic approach using anti-OFA-I-2 will be construction of toxic conjugates with anti-OFA-I-2. This takes advantage of the specificity of the monoclonal antibody for delivery of a killing agent to OFA-I-2-positive tumors. Linking anti-OFA-I-2 to radioisotopes may be also possible for localized radiotherapy.

We are now studying the possibility of early diagnosis by detection of circulating OFA-I-2 antigen using anti-OFA-I-2 antibody.

REFERENCES

Awden, Z. L., Williamson, A. R., and Askonas, B. A. (1968). *Nature (London) 219*, 66.
Bradford, M. M. (1976). *Anal. Biochem. 72*, 248.
Dippold, W. G., Lloyd, K. O., Li, L. T. C., Ikeda, H., Oettgen, H. F., and Old, L. J. (1980). *Proc. Natl. Acad. Sci. (USA) 77*, 6114.
Irie, R. F., Irie, K., and Morton, D. L. (1974). *J. Natl. Cancer Inst. (US) 52*, 1051.
Irie, R. F., Irie, K., and Morton, D. L. (1976). *Cancer Res. 36*, 3510.
Irie, R. F., Jones, P. C., Morton, D. L., and Sidell, N. (1981). *Br. J. Cancer 44*, 262.
Irie, R. F., Sze, L. L., and Saxton, R. E. (1982). *Proc. Natl. Acad. Sci. (USA) 79*, 5666.
Jones, P. C., Sze, L. L., Liu, P. Y., Morton, D. L., and Irie, R. F. (1981). *J. Natl. Cancer Inst. (US) 66*, 249.
Köhler, G., and Milstein, C. (1975). *Nature (London) 256*, 495.
Koprowski, H., Steplewski, Z., Herlyn, D., and Herlyn, M. (1979). *Proc. Natl. Acad. Sci. (USA) 75*, 3405.
Miller, R. A., Maloney, D. G., Warnke, R., and Levy, R. (1982). *New Engl. J. Med. 306*, 517.
Pierce, S. K., and Klinman, N. R. (1975). *J. Exp. Med. 142*, 1165.
Rosen, A., Ek, K., and Aman, P. (1979). *J. Immunol. Methods 28*, 1.
Sidell, N., Irie, R. F., and Morton, D. L. (1979). *Cancer Immunol. Immunother. 7*, 151.
Stevenson, F. K., and Stevenson, G. T. (1980). *Br. J. Cancer 42*, 495.

CHAPTER 29

POSTOPERATIVE LONG-TERM IMMUNOSTIMULATORY
PROTEIN-BOUND POLYSACCHARIDE KUREHA (PSK) THERAPY
FOR ADVANCED GASTRIC CANCER

Ryunosuke Kumashiro
Youichiro Hiramoto
Takeshi Okamura
Tadashi Kano
Chiaki Sano
Kiyoshi Inokuchi

Second Department of Surgery
Kyushu University School of Medicine
Fukuoka, Japan

BASIC MECHANISMS AND CLINICAL TREATMENT
OF TUMOR METASTASIS

I. INTRODUCTION

Postoperative adjuvant chemotherapy has been given much attention in the last two decades, but few adjuvant chemotherapy
regimens have been clinically effective for the treatment of
gastrointestinal cancer (Longmire *et al.*, 1968; Higgins *et al.*,
1971; Laurence *et al.*, 1975).
Improvement in the survival rate in patients treated with
curative surgery and adjuvant chemotherapy has been reported in
Japan (Hattori *et al.*, 1972; Imanaga and Nakazato, 1977).
Postoperative long-term cancer chemotherapy (PLCC) was found
by our group to be effective for patients with gastric cancer
(Kaibara *et al.*, 1976). In this PLCC regimen, we prescribed
protein-bound polysaccharide Kureha (PSK), an immunostimulator,
plus mitomycin C (MMC), and Tegafur in an attempt to improve the
immunological response in these patients.
This report is concerned with the enhancement of effects of
MMC and Tegafur by the immunostimulator PSK (Akiyama *et al.*,
1977).

II. MATERIALS AND METHODS

A. Patients

We separated 325 Japanese patients with stages III and IV
gastric cancer treated in the Second Department of Surgery at
Kyushu University Hospital (Fukuoka, Japan) into three groups and
two subgroups.
From 1964 to 1970, 131 gastrectomized patients with stages III
and IV gastric cancer were given no chemotherapy (no chemo group).
From 1964 to 1970, 103 gastrectomized patients with stages III and
IV gastric cancer were intraoperatively treated only with 20 mg
mitomycin C (MMC group). From 1964 to 1979, 91 patients with
stage III and IV gastric cancer and who underwent gastrectomy,
were treated by postoperative long-term cancer chemotherapy (PLCC
group).
The regimen of the PLCC group was as follows: 20 mg of MMC
intravenously (iv) administered intraoperatively, and 10 mg of MMC
iv 4 weeks after surgery. Thereafter, patients received 10 mg of
MMC iv every 3 months for as long as 2 years. Oral administration of Tegafur (600 mg/day) was prescribed from Day 7 until
2 years postoperatively, and was or was not followed by the administration of PSK (3 g/day) from Day 7 until 2 years postoperatively.
Among 91 patients treated with PLCC, 25 with stage III and
9 patients with stage IV received PSK, while 45 in stage III and

12 in stage IV did not receive PSK. These 70 were divided into
two subgroups: PLCC with PSK and PLCC without PSK. The efficacy
of PSK was examined by comparing the results obtained with these
two subgroups.

Anticancer agents were prescribed according to the following
criteria: (1) age not over 70, (2) weight over 40 kg, (3) 30-
min value of BSP not less than 15%, (4) 15-min value of PSP not
less than 20%, and (5) no abnormal ECG findings.

B. Immunosuppressive Acidic Protein (IAP) Levels in Patients
   after gastrectomy

The levels of IAP in serially obtained sera before and after
the operations on patients with gastric cancer were examined
using the single radial immunodiffusion method (Tamura *et al.*,
1978).

C. Staging

Staging for each case followed the general rules for gastric
cancer study in surgery and pathology in Japan (Japanese Research
Society for Gastric Cancer, 1973). Extent of lymph node metastasis and serosal invasion were designated as (n) and (s),
respectively, according to the respective rules. This study
involved patients with stages III and IV gastric cancer.

D. Statistical Analysis

Survival rate was calculated by the actuarial survival rate;
for statistical analysis, the χ^2 test was used.

III. RESULTS

A. Prognostic Factors

As shown in Table I, the number of patients with stage III
gastric cancer and prognostic factors such as serosal invasion
and lymph node metastasis did not significantly differ among the
three groups, including the two subgroups (i.e., PLCC with PSK
and PLCC without PSK).

Prognostic factors of patients with stage IV gastric cancer
are shown in Table II. There were no significant differences
among the three groups and the two subgroups.

TABLE I

Distribution of Prognostic Factors and Doses of Drugs in Stage III gastric Cancer Patients

	No chemotherapy group	MMC group	PLCC group	PLCC with PSK subgroup	PLCC without PSK subgroup
Number of cases	112	69	70	25	45
Serosal invasion (s_2)	63/112 (56.3%)	34/69 (49.3%)	35/70 (50.0%)	16/25 (64.0%)	18/45 (40.0%)
Lymph node metastasis (n_2)	18/112 (16.1%)	7/69 (10.1%)	8/70 (11.4%)	1/25 (4.0%)	8/45 (20.0%)
Serosal invasion + lymph node ($s_2 + n_2$)	31/112 (27.7%)	28/69 (40.6%)	27/70 (38.6%)	8/25 (32.0%)	18/45 (40.0%)
Mean doses of MMC (mg)	0	20.8 ± 7.2	54.7 ± 33.7	38.5 ± 27.5	59.4 ± 34.3
Mean duration of Tegafur (months)	0	0	8.1 ± 5.2	9.5 ± 5.6	6.6 ± 3.3
Mean duration of PSK (months)	0	0	3.3 ± 4.5	9.6 ± 11.4	0

TABLE II

Distribution of Prognostic Factors and Doses of Drugs in Stage IV Gastric Cancer Patients

	No chemotherapy group	MMC group	PLCC group	PLCC with PSK subgroup	PLCC without PSK subgroup
Number of cases	19	34	21	9	12
Serosal invasion (s_3)	12/19 (63.1%)	18/34 (52.9%)	12/21 (57.1%)	6/9 (66.7)	8/12 (66.7%)
Lymph node metastasis (n_3)	6/19 (31.6%)	13/34 (38.2%)	9/21 (42.9%)	3/9 (33.3%)	4/12 (33.3%)
Serosal invasion + lymph node ($n_3 + s_3$)	1/19 (5.3%)	3/34 (8.8%)	0/21 (0%)	0/9 (0%)	0/12 (0%)
Mean doses of MMC (mg)	0	22.0 ± 9.4	59.3 ± 34.0	60.0 ± 31.6	58.8 ± 32.6
Mean duration of Tegafur (months)	0	0	9.8 ± 8.8	13.3 ± 9.9	4.2 ± 1.3
Mean duration of PSK (months)	0	0	5.4 ± 9.5	15.9 ± 10.4	0

B. Drugs

   The mean doses of drugs administered to each group of stage
III gastric cancer patients are listed in Table I.
   Mean doses of MMC were 54.7 ± 33.7 mg in the PLCC group,
20.8 ± 7.2 mg in the MMC group, 38.5 ± 27.5 mg in the PLCC with
PSK subgroup, and 59.4 ± 34.3 mg in the PLCC without PSK subgroup. Tegafur was administered for 6 to 10 months, and PSK was
given for 3 to 10 months.
   Doses of MMC, Tegafur, and PSK in stage IV gastric cancer
patients after curative operation are shown in Table II.
   Mean doses of MMC were 59.3 ± 34.0 mg in the PLCC group,
22.0 ± 9.4 mg in the MMC group, 60.0 ± 31.6 mg in the PLCC with
PSK subgroup, and 58.8 ± 32.6 mg in the PLCC without PSK subgroup.
   Duration of Tegafur ingestion was 9.8 ±8.8 months in the PLCC
group, 13.3 ± 9.9 months in the PLCC with PSK subgroup, and
4.2 ± 1.3 months in the PLCC without PSK subgroup.
   PSK was given for 5.4 ± 9.5 months in the PLCC group and
15.9 ± 10.4 months in the PLCC with PSK subgroup.

C. Survival Rate

1. *PLCC Group, MMC Group, and No Chemotherapy Group*

   In the curative patients with stage III gastric cancer, the
5-year survival rates were 61.4% in the PLCC group, 44.9% in the
MMC group, and 44.1% in the no chemo group, as shown in Fig. 1.
There was a significant difference between the rates in the PLCC
and no chemo groups (p = .0230), and also a somewhat significant
difference between the PLCC group and the MMC group (p = .0637).
   Survival rates for stage IV gastric cancer patients after
curable operation were 52.4% in the PLCC group, 20.6% in the MMC
group, and 21.1% in the no chemo group, as shown in Fig. 2.
There was a significant difference between the PLCC and MMC
groups (p = .0317), and also a somewhat significant difference
between the PLCC and no chemo groups (p = .0849).

2. *Survival Rate in Patients Treated with PLCC and with or
    without PSK*

   Survival rates in patients treated with PLCC with PSK administration were 68.0% in stage III, and 66.7% in stage IV, while
those of patients treated with PLCC without PSK administration
were 57.8% in stage III and 41.7% in stage IV. The survival rates
of PLCC-treated patients in the PSK subgroup were better than
those of the PLCC without PSK subgroup, but there were no significant differences.

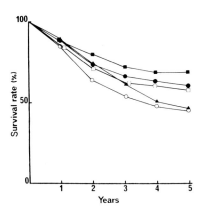

Fig. 1. Actuarial survival curves in stage III gastric cancer patients after curative surgery. ●——● PLCC (61.4%); ■——■ PLCC with PSK (68.0); □——□ PLCC without PSK (57.8%); ▲——▲ MMC (44.9%); ○——○ no chemotherapy (44.1%).

However, survival rates of the PLCC with PSK subgroup in stage III were higher than those of the MMC group ($p = .079$), and better than those of the no chemo group ($p = .050$).

Survival rates of the PLCC with PSK subgroup in stage IV were also higher than those of the MMC group ($p = .0216$), and higher than those in the no chemo group ($p = .0534$).

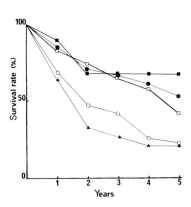

Fig. 2. Actuarial survival curves in stage IV gastric cancer patients after curative surgery. ●——● PLCC (52.4%); ■——■ PLCC with PSK (66.7%); □——□ PLCC without PSK (41.7%); ▲——▲ MMC (20.6%); ○——○ no chemotherapy (21.1%).

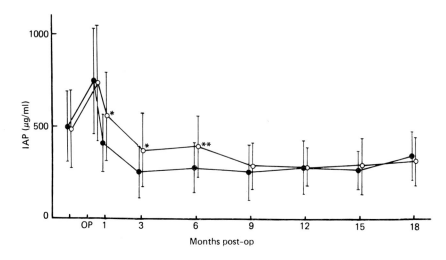

Fig. 3. Serum IAP levels in patients with stage III gastric cancer. ●——● PLCC with PSK ($n = 25$); ○——○ PLCC without PSK ($n = 18$). * $p < .1$; ** $p < .05$.

D. IAP Level

The levels of IAP in patients with stage III gastric cancer who were given or not given PSK are shown in Fig. 3.

The levels of IAP at 1, 3, and 6 months after the surgery were significantly lower in the PLCC with PSK subgroup in stage III gastric cancer ($p < .05$).

As shown in Fig. 4, the levels of IAP in patients with stage IV gastric cancer at 3 months after surgery were significantly lower in the PLCC with PSK subgroup ($p < .1$).

IV. DISCUSSION

Postoperative long-term cancer chemotherapy, (PLCC) is mainly prescribed on an outpatient basis and long-term oral administration of Tegafur and PSK was prescribed in addition to the intermittent iv injection of MMC. Oral Tegafur is one of the most effective drugs for PLCC, has fewer side effects, and seems to be particularly effective for gastric cancer.

Our former results (Kaibara et al., 1976) in cases of stage IV gastric cancer patients treated with PLCC were confirmed in the present study, from the viewpoint of the 5-year survival rate. Our PLCC regimen was also effective for improving the 5-year survival rate in stage III gastric cancer patients. Moreover, the 5-year survival rates were significantly improved with PLCC especially when PSK was included.

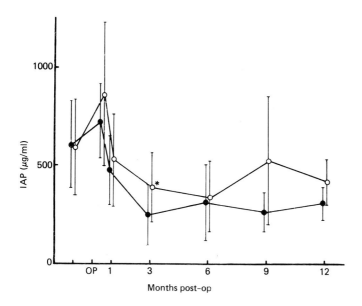

Fig. 4. Serum IAP levels in patients with stage IV gastric cancer. ●————● PLCC with PSK (n = 23); O————O PLCC without PSK (n = 6). * p < .1.

Hattori et al. (1979) suggested that the combined use of PSK with other anticancer drugs having cytocidal action accounted for the good results in clinical trials. Furthermore, PSK seems to be one of the most suitable and available immunostimulators for the treatment of gastric cancer.

The immune response deteriorates in cancer patients (Garrioch et al., 1973; Kumashiro, 1976), and certain anticancer drugs (Santos, 1974) lead to disturbances in immunological functions. The enhancement by PSK of the effects of MMC and Tegafur on survival seems to be due to an improvement in the diminished immunological resistance against cancer.

The acronym PSK describes a protein-bound polysaccharide derived from Basidiomycetes. Nomoto et al. (1975) reported that the administration of PSK improved antibody-forming capacities and that the depression of immunity in tumor-bearing mice returned to normal levels with ingestion of PSK. Matsunaga et al. (1980) reported that PSK is most effective for removing the immunosuppressive serum factor from the tumor-bearing animals.

Tamura et al. (1981) noted abnormal levels of immunosuppressive acidic protein (IAP) in cancer patients. This protein was found to suppress both phytohemagglutinin-induced lymphocyte blast formation and mixed lymphocyte reaction in vitro, and it was suggested that this protein impaired the immunological surveillance mechanism in cancer patients.

We reported that the levels of immunosuppressive acidic protein were increased in gastric cancer patients (Hiramoto et al., 1983).

In this study, however, the serial levels of IAP returned to normal in the PSK-treated patients. Such early normalization of IAP in cases of advanced gastric cancer may play a role in the improvement of immunological resistance in these patients.

The study described here is a retrospective analysis of the effects of PSK in postoperative treatment of patients with gastric cancer. Randomized prospective studies on PSK for the postoperative long-term treatment of cancer patients are under way.

V. SUMMARY

Five-year survival rates in stages III and IV gastric cancer patients were improved when PSK, an immunostimulator derived from Basidiomycetes, was prescribed in addition to mitomycin C and Tegafur.

REFERENCES

Akiyama, J., Kawamura, T., Gotohda, E., Yamada, Y., Hoshokawa, M., Kodama, T., and Kobayashi, H. (1977). *Cancer Res. 37*, 3042-3045.
Garrioch, D. B., Good, R. A., and Gatti, R. A. (1973). *Lancet 1*, 618-619.
Hattori, T., Mori, A., Hirata, K., and Ito, I. (1972). *Gann 63*, 517-522.
Hattori, T., Niimoto, M., Nakano, A., Oride, K., Takiyama, W., and Nishimawari, K. (1979). *Jpn. J. Surg. 9*, 110-117.
Higgins, G. A., Dwight, R. A., Smith, J. V., and Kenhn, R. J. (1971). *Arch. Surg. 102*, 339-343.
Hiramoto, Y., Nozuka, T., Sano, C., Abe, Y., Masuda, H., Kumashiro, R., Tamada, R., Kano, T., and Inokuchi, K. (1983). *Clin. Immunol. 15 (Suppl. 7)*, 100-105.
Imanaga, H., and Nakazato, H. (1977). *World J. Surg. 1*, 213-221.
Japanese Research Society for Gastric Cancer (1973). *Jpn. J. Surg. 3*, 61-71.
Kaibara, N., Soejima, K., Nakamura, T., and Inokuchi, K. (1976). *Jpn. J. Surg. 6*, 54-59.
Kumashiro, R. (1976). *Fukuoka Acta Med. 67*, 339-349.
Laurence, W., Terz, J. J., Horsley, S., Donaldson, M., Lovett, W. L., Brown, P. W., Ruffner, B. W., and Regelson, W. (1975). *Ann. Surg. 181*, 616-623.
Longmire, J. R. W. P., Kuzma, J. W., and Dixon, W. J. (1968). *Ann. Surg. 167*, 293-312.

Matsunaga, K., Tsuru, S., Morita, I., Oguchi, Y., Fujii, T.,
  Yoshikumi, C., Hatta, T., and Nomoto, K. (1980). *Gan to
  Kagakuryoho* 7, 496-503.
Nomoto, K., Yoshikumi, C., Matsunaga, K., Fujita, T., and
  Takeya, K. (1975). *Gann 66*, 365-374.
Tamura, K., Shibata, Y., Matsuda, Y., and Ishida, N. (1978).
  Igakunoayumi 105, 668-670.
Tamura, K., Shibata, Y., Matsuda, Y., and Ishida, N. (1981).
  Cancer Res. 41, 3244-3252.

CHAPTER 30

THE ANTITUMOR AND TUMOR METASTASIS-INHIBITORY ACTIVITIES
OF LENTINAN IN PRECLINICAL ANIMAL MODELS
AND ITS POSSIBLE IMMUNE MECHANISM

Goro Chihara

National Cancer Center Research Institute
Tokyo, Japan

I. INTRODUCTION

In Oriental medicine practice in Asian countries, some kinds
of fungus of the class Basidiomycetes have been known for centuries as a folk remedy to be effective for cancer patients. On
the basis of this viewpoint, we reexamined the antitumor activity
of numerous folk remedies and isolated a polysaccharide with

BASIC MECHANISMS AND CLINICAL TREATMENT
OF TUMOR METASTASIS

marked antitumor activity from hot-water extract of the fruit
body of *Lentinus edodes* (Berk.) Sing., the most popular edible
mushroom in Japan, and named it lentinan (Chihara *et al.*, 1969,
1970).

Lentinan is a fully purified neutral polysaccharide, and its
physicochemical properties are strictly characterized. The
chemical structure of lentinan is a β-(1→3)-D-glucan, having two
β-(1→6)-D-glucopyranoside branches for every five β-(1→3)-D-gluco-
pyranoside linear linkages (Sasaki and Takasuka, 1976), with
right-handed triple-helical structure (Bluhm and Sarko, 1977).
The molecular weight is about 4×10^5 to 8×10^5. Lentinan is
composed of only glucose with no other sugar component.
Elementary analysis verified the molecular formula as $(C_6H_{10}O_5)_n$,
consistent with structural elucidation, and nitrogen, phosphorus,
and sulfur cannot be detected. Therefore, the biological activities of lentinan are completely reproducible from lot to lot.
This is one of the most important characteristics of lentinan for
its basic immunopharmacological consideration and for its possible
clinical use.

It has been confirmed that lentinan has strong antitumor and
metastasis-inhibitory activities in syngeneic hosts as well as
allogeneic hosts, and that it prevents chemical and viral oncogenesis. This chapter concerns the preclinical evaluation of
lentinan for cancer patients in animal models and its unique
mechanism in host defense against cancer.

II.   ANTITUMOR AND METASTASIS-INHIBITORY ACTIVITIES OF LENTINAN
      IN ANIMAL MODELS

A. Allogeneic Tumors

In 1969 we reported that lentinan brought about complete regression in solid types of sarcoma 180 transplanted subcutaneously
in SWM/Ms or ICR mice when administered at a dose of 1 mg/kg for
10 days intraperitoneally (Chihara *et al.*, 1969, 1970). Lentinan
also has a prominent antitumor effect against Ehrlich carcinoma
and CCM adenocarcinoma in mice (Maeda *et al.*, 1973), and against
Walker carcinoma 256 (T. Shiio, personal communication), AH-130,
AH-41C, AH-44, and AH-66 hepatoma in rats (Sato, 1980).

Several interesting characteristics were observed in the antitumor action of lentinan.

1. Lentinan does not show any direct cytotoxicity against
tumor cells, and its action is host mediated (Maeda and Chihara,
1973a).

2. The antitumor action of lentinan is systemic. Although
lentinan is effective by intravenous, intraperitoneal, or intramuscular injection, there is no evidence of the effectiveness of

lentinan by intratumoral or lesional injection different from
BCG-CWS in guinea pigs.

3. There are interesting phenomena of optimal dose and timing
in the administration of lentinan. A higher injected dose of
lentinan does not show any antitumor effect, and this phenomenon
of optimal dose is also observed in various immunological
responses by lentinan.

4. There are marked differences in the antitumor effect
against sarcoma 180 among various strains of mouse. A/J, DBA/2,
SWM/Ms, and CD-1 mice are high responders, and C57BL/6 and
C3H/HeN mice are low responders with regard to the antitumor effect of lentinan, and CBA and BALB/c mice are medium responders.
These responses to lentinan action in their Fl hybrids and back-
cross mice are regulated by their parent mice (Zákány et al.,
1980a; Suga et al., 1984).

B. Syngeneic Tumors

Using high-responder mice such as A/J, DBA/2, or SWM/Ms with
a suitable dose and with a strictly planned timing of lentinan
administration, lentinan was very effective against various kinds
of tumors in syngeneic and even autochthonous hosts as well as in
allogeneic hosts.

A/Ph(A/J) mice are one of the highest responders to lentinan
action, and a 3-methylcholanthrene-induced A/Ph.MC.Sl-fibrosarcoma
transplanted subcutaneously in syngeneic A/Ph mice regressed
completely with a lentinan dose of 1 mg/kg for 10 days by intraperitoneal injection (Zákány et al., 1980a). Lentinan, however,
did not show any antitumor effect against Meth-A fibrosarcoma
transplanted in low-responder BALB/c mice.

Lentinan inhibits considerably the growth of mastocytoma
P815, L5178Y lymphoma, or MM46 carcinoma transplanted in syngeneic
mice without any combination therapy of cancer chemotherapeutic
agent (Akiyama et al., 1981). In these cases, the timing of
lentinan administration is very important for its antitumor effects. Optimal timing for administration of lentinan appears to
be 2 or 3 weeks after P815 transplantation in DBA/2 mice. The
results showing the same tendency regarding the timing of administration were also obtained in L5178Y-DBA/2 and MM46-C3H/He
syngeneic systems. Complete regression (100%) of syngeneic MM46
carcinoma was observed when 5 mg/kg lentinan were administered
twice at 13 and 15 days after tumor inoculation. This is the
best timing for this type of cancer.

C. Autologous Tumors

Lentinan was effective against methylcholanthrene (MC) -induced
primary tumor in combination therapy with cyclophosphamide (CY)
(Shiio and Yugari, 1981). When the tumor induced by MC attained a
diameter of about 8 mm, 100 mg/kg of CY were administered, and
1 mg/kg of lentinan was injected intraperitoneally once a day for
20 days, from 3 weeks after CY injection. This resulted in a prolongation of survival time of greater than 200% compared with
control mice. Such a prolongation of survival was not observed
when lentinan was given before CY, nor when the two were given at
the same time.

D. Effect on Tumor Metastasis

The most promising target for lentinan application in humans
may be its preventive effect against micrometastasis and/or
recurrence after surgical operation. As shown in Fig. 1, lentinan
prevented completely the reappearance of tumor after resection of
MH134 carcinoma transplanted in the footpad of C3H/He mice when
1 mg/kg of lentinan was administered ip once a day for 10 days
from day 1 after the surgical operation, whereas about 70% of
control mice receiving only surgical treatment died at 8 weeks
after tumor inoculation. Pretreatment with lentinan before surgical operation was not so effective.
The similar protective effects of lentinan were observed in
P388 and Ll210 lymphoma metastasis (Shiio and Yugari, 1981).
Lentinan also suppressed markedly the metastasis of Lewis lung
cancer after the amputation of the footpad with tumor.

E. Prevention of Carcinogenesis

Lentinan prevents chemical and viral carcinogenesis. When
1 mg/kg of lentinan was injected ip once a day for 10 days from
3 weeks after methylcholanthrene inoculation in SWM/Ms mice, the
incidence of tumors was only about 30% at Week 30 after methylcholanthrene inoculation, while it was 83% in control mice without
lentinan treatment. Similar results were obtained when DBA/2 mice
were used, but not when BALB/c mice were used (Suga et al.,
1984).
Lentinan also prevents adenovirus oncogenesis (Hamada, 1981).
Human adenovirus type 12 (Ad-12) is highly oncogenic in mice,
when the virus is inoculated to newborn animals. The incidence of
tumor in C3H/He mice infected with 1×10^7 $TCID_{50}$ of Ad-12 at
birth was 78.6% (11 of 14) at 80 days after infection. However,
a most efficient inhibition of tumor growth was observed when the
infected C3H/He mice received three injections of lentinan

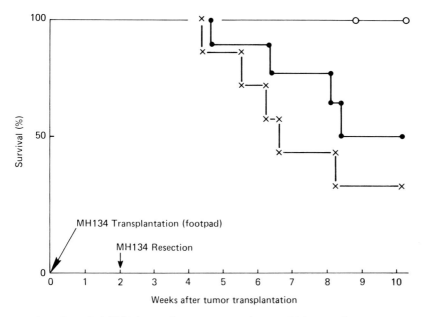

Fig. 1. Inhibition of postoperative MH134 carcinoma metastasis by ip lentinan administration. (O) Surgery + lentinan
1 mg/kg × 10 days (Days 15-28); (●) surgery + lentinan 1 mg/kg
× 10 days (Days 1-14); (X) surgery only (control). (From Shiio
and Yugari, 1981.)

(10 mg/kg on each of Days 14, 16, and 18) after Ad-12 infection,
resulting in a reduction of tumor incidence to 40% (6 of 15,
$p < .05$). Treatment of mice at other times, earlier or later than
the above timing, was less effective.

Lentinan is effective in various viral infections. Of mice
infected with VSV encephalitis virus, about 100% of mice survive
after treatment with lentinan, whereas 80% of the control mice
inoculated with this virus die after 2 weeks. Lentinan is also
effective against infection with Abelson virus in terms of its
marked effect in prolonging the survival of infected animals
(Chang, 1981).

III. POSSIBLE IMMUNE MECHANISMS

Among the well-known immunopotentiators such as BCG,
Conynebacterium parvum, liposaccharide (LPS), or zymosan, lentinan
appears to represent a unique class of immunological adjuvant. We
postulate the existence of three major pathways in the action
mechanism of lentinan for target cell destruction: (1) helper
T-cell-oriented specific immunopotentiation, which is the most important property of lentinan different from many other immuno-

TABLE I

Various Immunological and Physiological Activities of Lentinan

Activity	Effect	References
T-Cell participation		
Neonatal thymectomy	No antitumor effect	Maeda and Chihara (1971)
Antilymphocyte serum	Decreased antitumor effect	Maeda et al. (1971)
Cytotoxic T cell (in vitro and in vivo)	Augmentation	Hamuro et al. (1978a,b)
Helper T cell	Activation	Haba et al. (1976)
Suppressor T cell	No induction	J. Hamuro (Personal communication)
Delayed Hypersensitivity	Potentiation	Zákány et al. (1980b)
Natural killer cell (in vivo only)	Activation	Akiyama et al. (1981)
T-Derived CSF	Augmented production	Hamuro et al. (1982)
Macrophage participation		
Phagocytic macrophage (in vitro and in vivo)	No activation	Maeda and Chihara (1973a)
Cytotoxic macrophage; (in vitro)	No activation	Hamuro et al. (1980)
Cytotoxic macrophage (in vivo)	Activation	Hamuro et al. (1980)
Suppressor macrophage	No induction; Suppressed PGs release	Hamuro et al. (1979)
Local cellular reaction	Infiltration around tumor	Tokuzen (1971)
Interleukin-1 production	Augmentation	Yoshimoto et al. (1982)
Serum factor		
Complement system alternative, classical	Activation	Okuda et al. (1972) K. Nishioka (Personal communication)
C3	Increase	A. J. S. Davies (Personal communication)
Serum amyloid P	Increase	
Haptoglobin	Increase	Manabe et al. (1983)
Ceruloplasmin	Increase	Ito et al. (1980)
Hemopexin	Increase	Torikai et al. (1981)
Lysozyme activity	Activation	G. Chihara (unpublished observation)

stimulants, (2) complement-macrophage-mediated nonspecific immunopotentiation, and (3) nonimmunological stimulation of host
defense mechanisms through acute-phase proteins, complement
components, colony-stimulating factor, and serum bioactive factors. Various immunological and physiological properties of
lentinan are summarized in Table 1.

A. Helper T-Cell-Oriented Specific Immunopotentiation

One of the distinguishing characteristics of lentinan is its
capacity to act as T-cell immune adjuvant. The antitumor activity
of lentinan against sarcoma 180 does not appear in neonatally
thymectomized mice (Maeda and Chihara, 1971, 1973a) and is considerably suppressed by the administration of antilymphocyte serum
(Maeda et al., 1971) and by whole-body irradiation (400 rad)
within 3 days of tumor transplantation (Maeda and Chihara, 1973b).
The growth-inhibitory effect of lentinan against methylcholanthrene-induced syngeneic KKN1 fibrosarcoma is also abolished in
nude mice (Yamada et al., 1981). In another experimental system,
lentinan markedly enhances the antibody production against SRBC
in CBA mice only in the presence of T lymphocytes (Dresser and
Phillips, 1974). These experimental results support the concept
that the antitumor activity of lentinan requires intact immunocompetent T-cell compartments, and the activity is mediated
through a thymus-dependent immune mechanism.
First, lentinan triggers the increased production of lymphocyte-activating factor, interleukin-1 (IL-1), by direct impact of
macrophages. The augmented production of IL-1 was observed when
peritoneal macrophages were cocultivated for 48 hr with 5 to
25 µg/ml of lentinan in vitro as shown in Fig. 2. Furthermore,
the augmented production of IL-1 from macrophages was also confirmed by cocultivation of macrophage cell line P388D$_1$ with lentinan (Akiyama et al., 1981; Yoshimoto et al., 1982; Hamuro and
Chihara, 1984).
As is well known, IL-1 is capable of differentiating thymic
premature T cells into immunocompetent mature T cells. Thus, increased production of IL-1 results in augmented maturation of
activated helper T lymphocytes capable of inducing some kinds of
lymphokines such as interleukin-2 (IL-2). This results in the
augmented generation of effector killer T cells, and humoral
antibodies. Lentinan augments generation of antigen-specific
cytotoxic T lymphocytes (CTL) against alloantigen and haptenated
syngeneic cells in vitro (Hamuro et al., 1978a) and in vivo
(Hamuro et al., 1978b).
To evaluate the validity of the reaction scheme presented,
generation of allokiller cells from thymocytes was tested.
Thymocytes, harvested from responder DBA/2 mice treated with
lentinan, induce augmented generation of allokiller cells in the
presence of IL-2. This demonstrates that thymocytes of lentinan-

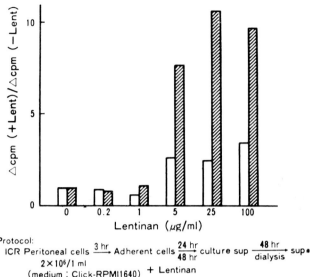

Fig. 2. *In vitro* augmented generation of lymphocyte-activating factor (IL-1) from peritoneal macrophages by lentinan. White bars, 24-hr culture; crosshatched bars, 48-hr culture. (From Yoshimoto *et al.*, 1982.)

injected mice are more reactive to IL-2. In syngeneic tumor-bearing systems such as P815-DBA/2, generation from thymocytes of allokiller cells is considerably suppressed even in the presence of IL-2. This generation, however, was restored to the level of non-tumor-bearing mice by the injection of lentinan. The generation of allokiller cells from splenocytes was also restored from null to around 40% in the absence of IL-2. These results are possible to explain by the augmented induction of mature T cells reactive to IL-2 as a second signal. Furthermore, most interestingly, spleen cells harvested from syngeneic mastocytoma P815-bearing DBA/2 mice that received triple ip injection of lentinan 2 weeks after P815 transplantation were able to generate significant levels of antisyngeneic P815 killer cells in the presence of IL-2, as shown in Fig. 3 (Akiyama *et al.*, 1981).

Lentinan is a good restorer or potentiator of humoral immune responses. The mice pretreated with cell-free Ehrlich ascites fluid are selectively depressed in their helper T-cell activity, when using DNP-bacterial α-amylase as hapten carrier. Lentinan is able to restore such suppressed immune response to an almost normal state (Haba *et al.*, 1976). A similar result was obtained in the delayed hypersensitivity reaction.

As far as other important effector NK cells are concerned, lentinan does augment NK activity in spleen cells or peritoneal exudate cells when administered into NK high-responder C3H/He mice, but does not when administered into BALB/c mice. Lentinan, however, does not activate NK cells when incubated *in vitro* as poly I:C or *C. parvum* does, but it augments *in vitro*

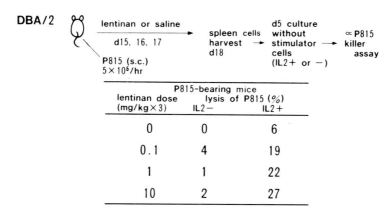

lentinan dose (mg/kg × 3)	P815-bearing mice lysis of P815 (%)	
	IL2−	IL2+
0	0	6
0.1	4	19
1	1	22
10	2	27

Fig. 3. Augmented killer T induction against syngeneic tumor in DBA/2 mice by the administration of lentinan. IL2, interleukin 2; E:T (effector:target cell ratio) = 50 (culture base); killer assay, 3-hr ^{51}Cr-release assay. (From Akiyama et al., 1981.)

generation of NK cells cultured with poly I:C or IL-2 when spleen cells harvested from lentinan-treated mice are used. Lentinan might stimulate NK cells via a T-cell-dependent pathway but not via macrophages or interferon (Hamuro and Chihara, 1984).

B.   Complement-Macrophage-Mediated Nonspecific Immunopotentiation

There is another pathway of complement-macrophage-induced non-specific immunopotentiation by lentinan. The antitumor effect of lentinan against sarcoma 180 is blocked by antimacrophage agents such as carrageenan or silica (G. Chihara and T. Shiio, unpublished). Lentinan, however, does not enhance the in vivo phagocytic activity of macrophages according to the conventional carbon clearance method (Maeda and Chihara, 1973a), and also does not enhance such activity in in vitro experiments, in contrast with C. parvum, BCG, or zymosan. Lentinan should not be called an RES stimulant in this sense.
Lentinan enhances the cytotoxic and cytostatic activities of peritoneal exudate cells against various tumor cells in vivo (Maeda and Chihara, 1973b). For example, the peritoneal macrophages harvested from CBA mice 10 days after triple injections of 10 mg/kg of lentinan display 76% lysis against P815 mastocytoma labeled with Cr^{51}, while the lysis in the control mice is only 2.5% (Hamuro et al., 1980). This activity is nonspecific and appears with many other tumors. Lentinan, however, does not enhance the cytotoxic activity of macrophages in in vitro experiments.
The activation of cytotoxicity of macrophages is considered to be a result of complement C3-splitting activity of lentinan. Lentinan has the ability to split C3 into C3a and C3b, which is able to be expressed as 96% reduction of hemolytic activity in

vitro (Okuda *et al.*, 1972). Lentinan activates considerably the
alternative pathway of the complement system. Complement C3
splitting is also one of the first reactions to lentinan in the
host, which undergoes nonspecific activation of macrophages
(Hamuro *et al.*, 1980).

C. Nonimmunological Potentiation of Host Defense Mechanisms

    Besides specific or nonspecific immunopotentiation, lentinan
displays an interesting role of nonimmunological potentiation of
defense mechanisms of hosts.
    Lentinan increases histamine or serotonin sensitivity in mice,
and by contrast, is able to protect *pertusis*-treated mice from
histamine shock (Homma and Kuratsuka, 1973). It seems relevant
to examine the effect of lentinan in preventing toxic death due
to the administration of vincristine or cyclocytidine. Toxic
death from the administration of 500 mg/kg of cyclocytidine alone
for 20 days occurred in 7 of 17 mice, but this toxic effect was
apparently suppressed when lentinan was used in combination with
cyclocytidine therapy for a comparable period, in that there was
no death (Tokuzen *et al.*, 1976). The effect on vascular permeability of bioactive amines might play some part in the
mechanism of action of lentinan.
    Next, we found a transitory and marked increase in several
kinds of serum protein components and serum biological active
factors with a peak at 4 to 7 days after the administration of
lentinan (Maeda *et al.*, 1974). These protein components have been
identified as acute-phase proteins such as haptoglobin, hemopexin,
ceruloplasmin, haptoglobin-hemoglobin complex (Manabe *et al.*,
1983; Ito *et al.*, 1980; Torikai *et al.*, 1981), and serum amyloid
P (A. J. S. Davies, personal communication). Lentinan may have
relevance in maintaining biochemical homeostasis of the host in
addition to immunological homeostasis. Ceruloplasmin possesses a
protective effect against the lowering of liver catalase activity
triggered by toxohormone, and it can be used as a therapeutic
agent for human aplastic anemia and cachexia. In addition, a considerable increase in the absolute value of C3 and total complement
components are also observed (A. J. S. Davies and K. Nishioka,
personal communication).
    Lentinan also increases various kinds of biological activities
in the serum of mice, besides the increase of serum protein components detected by electrophoresis. One of the most important bioactive factors detected in serum from lentinan-treated mice has
been functionally assigned the name, colony-stimulating factor
(CSF). The augmented production of CSF in the serum showed two
peaks 3 hr and 3 days after lentinan application. The CSF observed in the early phase was confirmed to have been generated
from alveolar macrophages, and that in the later phase from mature
T cells (Hamuro *et al.*, 1982). Lentinan seems to activate a fun-

damental host defense mechanism according to prolifaration of
leukocytes, bone marrow cells, or various other kinds of immunocompetent cells. This is a general potentiation of host resistance
against cancer and infections.

IV. TOXICOLOGY

    The acute and subacute toxicities of lentinan have been ex-
amined mostly by intravenous injection into mice, rats, dogs, and
monkeys. In any species tested, the LD_{50} of lentinan was more
than 100 mg/kg. In anaphylaxis tests, none of the guinea pigs
preinjected with lentinan were hypersensitized by intravenous or
intracutaneous injection with lentinan. Potential for chronic
toxicity to lentinan was examined by daily iv injection of lentinan
into rhesus monkeys for 26 weeks; the control and lentinan-treated
groups showed neither side effects nor histological changes.
Accordingly, the regular dose of lentinan in clinical trials
(1 mg by intravenous injection for humans) is quite safe (Sortwell
et al., 1981; Chesterman et al., 1981).

V. CONCLUSION

    Lentinan is now universally recognized as being the most potent
presently known immunopotentiator, and its biological and immunopharmacological characteristics are distinguished from those of
other immunostimulants such as BCG and related substances,
C. parvum, levamisole, LPS, poly I:C, or interferon. Low toxicity
is also an important characteristic of lentinan when compared with
other chemotherapeutic agents possessing detrimental toxic side
effects. The characteristics of lentinan described in this chapter
are very hopeful for cancer patients.
    Nevertheless, cancer immunotherapy is extremely difficult.
Lentinan can be effective against human cancer only when used in
conjunction with other therapy under strictly planned timing and
schedules, and only when the host-tumor relationship is in good
agreement with such treatment. We consider that lentinan would
be most effective against cancer micrometastasis after surgery or
radiotherapy, because lentinan causes complete regression of small
numbers of cancer cells in the animal models, for example, 3 weeks
after methylcholanthrene inoculation or soon after amputation of
foodpad with tumor. To utilize as effectively as possible the
characteristics of lentinan, the most important and urgent task
for clinical immunologists might be to determine the parameters of
the host-tumor relationship that is most beneficial for the

application of lentinan as an immunomodulating agent for therapeutic and prophylactic treatment against cancer.

ACKNOWLEDGMENT

I would like to express my sincerest thanks to a number of
excellent colleagues who have been very helpful throughout the
course of this work. These individuals include Drs. Yukiko,
Y. Maeda, Junji Hamuro, Tsuyoshi Shiio, Katsumi Suzuki,
Takuma Sasaki, and Mrs. Kazuko Ishimura-Yamaoka.

REFERENCES

Akiyama, Y., Kashima, S., Hayami, T., Izawa, M., Mitsugi, K., and
    Hamuro, J. (1981). *In* "Manipulation of Host Defense Mechanisms"
    (T. Aoki, I. Urushizaki, and E. Tsubura, eds.), pp. 227-238.
    Excerpta Medica, Amsterdam.
Bluhm, T. H., and Sarko, A. (1977). *Can. J. Chem.* 55, 293.
Chang, K. S. S. (1981). *In* "Manipulation of Host Defense
    Mechanisms" (T. Aoki, I. Urushizaki, and E. Tsubura, eds.),
    pp. 88-100. Excerpta Medica, Amsterdam.
Chesterman, H., Heywood, R., Allen, T. R., Street, A. E.,
    Edmondson, N. A., and Prentice, D. E. (1981). *Toxicol. Lett. 9*,
    87.
Chihara, G., Maeda, Y. Y., Hamuro, J., Sasaki, T., and Fukuoka, F.
    (1969). *Nature (London) 222*, 687.
Chihara, G., Hamuro, J., Maeda, Y. Y., Arai, Y., and Fukuoka, F.
    (1970). *Cancer Res. 30*, 2776.
Dresser, D. W., and Phillips, J. M. (1974). *Immunology 27*, 895.
Haba, S., Hamaoka, T., Takatsu, K., and Kitagawa, M. (1976). *Int.
    J. Cancer 18*, 93.
Hamada, C. (1981). *In* "Manipulation of Host Defense Mechanisms"
    (T. Aoki, I. Urushizaki, and E. Tsubura, eds.), pp. 76-84.
    Excerpta Medica, Amsterdam.
Hamuro, J., and Chihara, G. (1984). *In* "Immunomodulating Agents:
    Properties and Mechanisms" (R. L. Fenichel and M. A. Chirigos,
    eds.), pp. 409-436. Dekker, New York.
Hamuro, J., Wagner, H., and Röllinghoff, M. (1978a). *Cell. Immunol*
    38, 328.
Hamuro, J., Röllinghoff, M., and Wagner, H. (1978b). *Cancer Res.*
    38, 3080.
Hamuro, J., Röllinghoff, M., Wagner, H., Seitz, M., Grimm, W., and
    Gemsa, D. (1979). *Z. Immune-Forsch. 155*, 248.
Hamuro, J., Röllinghoff, M., and Wagner, H. (1980). *Immunology*
    39, 551.

Hamuro, J., Akiyama, Y., Iguchi, Y., Izawa, M., and Matsuo, T. (1982). *Int. J. Immunopharmacol.* 4, 268.

Homma, R., and Kuratsuka, K. (1973). *Experientia 39*, 551.

Ito, O., Torikai, T., Satoh, M., and Osawa, T. (1980). *Gann 71*, 644.

Maeda, Y. Y., and Chihara, G. (1971). *Nature (London) 229*, 634.

Maeda, Y. Y., and Chihara, G. (1973a). *Int. J. Cancer 11*, 153.

Maeda, Y. Y., and Chihara, G. (1973b). *Gann 64*, 351.

Maeda, Y. Y., Hamuro, J., and Chihara, G. (1971). *Int. J. Cancer 8*, 41.

Maeda, Y. Y., Hamuro, J., Yamada, Y. O., Ishimura, K., and Chihara, G. (1973). *Ciba Found. Symp. New Ser. 18*, 259-286.

Maeda, Y. Y., Chihara, G., and Ishimura, K. (1974). *Nature (London) 252*, 250.

Manabe, T., Takahashi, Y., Okuyama, T., Maeda, Y. Y., and Chihara, G. (1983). *Electrophoresis 4*, 242.

Okuda, T., Yoshioka, Y., Ikekawa, T., Chihara, G., and Nishioka, K. (1972). *Nature New Biol. 238*, 59.

Sasaki, T., and Takasuka, N. (1976). *Carbohyd. Res. 47*, 99.

Sato, H. (1980). *Gan to Kagakuryoho 7*, 1694.

Shiio, T., and Yugari, Y. (1981). *In* "Manipulation of Host Defense Mechanisms" (T. Aoki, I. Urishizaki, and T. Tsubara, eds.), pp. 29-42. Excerpta Medica, Amsterdam.

Sortwell, R. J., Dawe, S., Allen, D. G., Street, A. E., Heywood, R., Edmondson, N. A., and Copinath, C. (1981). *Toxicol. Lett. 9*, 81.

Suga, T., Shiio, T., Maeda, Y. Y., and Chihara, G. (1984). *Cancer Res. 44*, 5132.

Tokuzen, R. (1971). *Cancer Res. 31*, 1590.

Tokuzen, R., Okabe, M., and Nakahara, W. (1976). *Gann 67*, 327.

Torikai, T., Itoh, O., Sato, M., Okumara, O., and Osawa, T. (1981). *Gann 72*, 92.

Yamada, Y., Kubota, T., Hanatani, Y., Matsumoto, S., Kumai, K., Ishibiki, K., and Abe, O. (1981). *In* "Manipulation of Host Defense Mechanisms" (T. Aoki, I. Urishizaki, and E. Tsubura, eds.), pp. 219-225. Excerpta Medica, Amsterdam.

Yoshimoto, R., Akiyama, Y., Hayami, T., Iguchi, Y., Izawa, M., and Hamuro, J. (1982). *Int. J. Immunopharmacol. 4*, 267.

Zákány, J., Chihara, G., and Fachet, J. (1980a). *Int. J. Cancer 25*, 371.

Zákány, J., Chihara, G., and Fachet, J. (1980b). *Int. J. Cancer 26*, 783.

CHAPTER 31

LENTINAN: BIOLOGICAL ACTIVITY AND CLINICAL TRIAL

Tetsuo Taguchi

Department of Oncologic Surgery
The Research Institute for Microbial Diseases
Osaka University
Osaka, Japan

I. CHARACTERISTICS OF LENTINAN IN ANIMAL EXPERIMENTS

Lentinan, a purified polysaccharide extracted from *Lentinus edodes* (edible Japanese mushroom), has been studied by Chihara and colleagues (Chihara *et al.*, 1969). Lentinan is composed of a β-(1$\to$3)-D-glucan as a main chain with some β-(1$\to$6)-glucopyranoside branchings. Its biological and immunological characteristics have been precisely investigated in animal experiments, with the finding that it has antitumor effects on allogeneic and syngeneic transplanted tumors, and on autochthonous tumors in combination treatment with chemotherapeutic agents, surgery, or irradiation, or by single administration alone (Table I). Furthermore, it has been found that lentinan stimulates host defense mechanisms against bacterial, viral, and parasitic infections (Chihara and Taguchi, 1982).

549

TABLE I

The Antitumor Activity of Lentinan

Tumors[a]	Hosts	Dose (mg/kg × days)	Tumor inhibition ratio (%)[b]
Allogeneic			
Sarcoma 180	CD-1/ICR	1 × 10	100
	A/J	4 × 5	96.5
	DBA/2	4 × 5	100
Ehrlich carcinoma	CD-1/ICR	1 × 10	54.7
CCM Adenocarcinoma	SWM/Ms	0.5 × 10	65.3
Syngeneic			
A/Ph. MC. Sl-Fibrosarcoma	A/Ph(A/J)	1 × 10	100
MM46 Carcinoma	C3H/HeN	5 × 2	100
L5178Y Lymphoma	DBA/2	10 × 3	89
P815 Mastocytoma	DBA/2	5 × 4	82
EL4 Lymphoma	C57BL/6	10 × 1	72
MM102 carcinoma	C3H/HeN	10 × 1	60
Lewis lung cancer	C57/BL/6	1 × 6	59.3
B16 Melanoma	BDF$_1$	1 × 5	50.7
SR-C3H/He Sarcoma	C3H/He	1 × 10	47.5
Autologous			
MC-Induced primary tumor	C3H/HeN	1 × 20 (CY: 100 × 1)[c]	Over 200% survival
Prevention of carcinogenesis			
Methylcholanthrene-induced	SWM/Ms	1 × 10	83 → 33%[d]
Adenovirus type 12-induced	C3H/He	1 × 10	Marked

[a]All tumors are solid form implanted sc.

[b]Tumor inhibition ratio = (C-T)/T × 100 (C, average tumor weight of control mice; T, that of lentinan-treated mice).

[c]Tumor diameter was 8 mm on Day 0, when 100 mg/kg cyclophosphamide were injected ip.

[d]Determination at 30 weeks after methylcholanthrene treatment.

Immunological and physiological studies of lentinan have shown that it has affected T-helper cells and Ia[+] macrophages to produce cytotoxic T cells, and it has augmented macrophages and/or natural cytotoxicities against tumor cells (Table II) (Chihara and Taguchi, 1982).

Based on these experimental results, Chihara and colleagues have presented the possible mode of action of lentinan for target cells (Fig. 1) (Chihara and Taguchi, 1982).

TABLE II

Various Immunological and Physiological Activities of Lentinan

Activity	Effect
T-Cell participation	
Neonatal thymectomy	Abolish antitumor effect
Antilymphocyte serum	Decrease antitumor effect
Nude mice	Decrease antitumor effect
Helper T cell, *in vitro*	Not observed
Helper T cell, *in vivo*	Restoration or potentiation
Cytotoxic T cell, *in vitro*	Augmentation
Cytotoxic T cell, *in vivo*	Augmentation
Suppressor T cell	Not observed
NK Cell participation	
NK Cell activity, *in vitro*	Not observed
NK Cell activity, *in vivo*	Potentiation
Macrophage participation	
Carrageenan or silica	Abolish antitumor effect
Macrophage phagocytic, *in vitro*	Not observed
Macrophage phagocytic, *in vivo*	Weak effect
Macrophage cytotoxic, *in vitro*	Not observed
Macrophage cytotoxic, *in vivo*	Activation
Macrophage suppressive	Decrease prostaglandin release
Antibody formation	
Antibody for SRBC	Increase with T cells
Antibody for BSA, SRBC	Increase
ADCC	Activation
Cellular reactions	
Delayed hypersensitivity, *in vivo*	Restoration or stimulation
Local cellular reaction	Stimulation around tumor
Granuloma formation	Increase around Shistosoma
Complement participation	
Alternative pathway	Activation
C3-Splitting activity	Activation
Factor B	Increase
C3 absolute value	Increase
Total complement value	Increase
Classical pathway	Activation
Serum proteins or factors	
Lentinan-induced serum proteins (LA, LB, LC)	Increase (temporarily)
Ceruloplasmin	Increase
Hemopexin	Increase
Serum amyloid P factor	Increase
Serum lysozyme activity	Activation
Colony-stimulating factor	Increase
Interferon *in vitro*	Not observed
Interferon *in vivo*	Increase poly I:C activity
Tumor necrosis factor (TNF)	Not observed

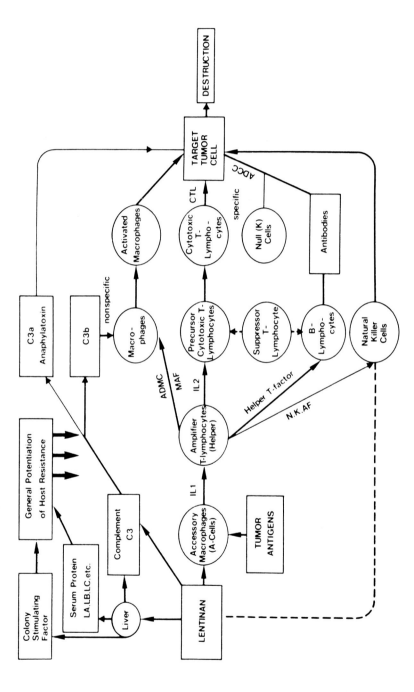

Fig. 1. Possible mode of action of lentinan for target cell destruction. ADMC, Antibody-Dependent Macrophage Cytotoxicity; MAF, Macrophage Activating Factor; N.K.AF, Natural Killer Activating Factor.

II. CLINICAL STUDIES OF LENTINAN ON NEOPLASTIC DISEASES
     IN HUMANS

A. Phase I Study

   These distinct characteristics of lentinan as revealed in animal models have indicated that there should be an effect to human
malignant tumors that is somewhat different from the known antitumor agents. Therefore, after the completion of acute, subacute,
and chronic toxicological studies, a phase I study has been conducted on 50 patients with malignant diseases, such as gastric,
colorectal, breast, and other types of cancer, in order to determine the administration dosage (Taguchi et al., 1979, 1981).
Three dose levels (0.5, 5.0, and 50 mg/person) have been tested
with consecutive or intermittent intravenous injection.
   Three kinds of side effects have been observed among the
50 patients (i.e., liver dysfunction detected with GOT, GPT, a
feeling of heaviness in the chest, and petechiae on the legs,
each in one case). All symptoms have been transitional and not
serious. Considering the fact that petechiae have been observed
at doses of 50 mg/person/day with consecutive administration for
1 week, recommended dosage has been determined as 0.5 to 5.0
mg/person/day.

B. Phase II Study

   On the basis of the results of the phase I study, a phase II
trial has been carried out on 126 patients with various types of
advanced cancer, to investigate the optimal method of administration of lentinan (Taguchi et al., 1981a,b). The 126 patients
included 60 cases of gastric or colorectal cancer, 15 of breast
cancer, 10 of liver cancer, and 41 cases of other types of cancer.
Lentinan was administered intravenously in doses of 0.5, 1.0, or
5.0 mg/person consecutively or intermittently in combination
treatment with chemotherapeutic agents such as 5-FU, mitomycin C,
and/or Tegafur, or with single administration of lentinan alone.
   Antitumor effectiveness and improvement of host immune
responses have been measured by employing the PPD skin test or
peripheral blood lymphocyte (PBL) counts to determine the optimum
administration conditions of lentinan. The 126 eligible patients
have been stratified with lentinan administration intervals of
once or twice a week, or three to seven times a week, and stratified with administration of lentinan only or in combination with
various chemotherapeutic agents. The results of analyses of
antitumor effects and improvement in host immune responses have
suggested that lentinan should be administered once or twice a
week at doses of 0.5 or 1.0 mg/person/day in combination with
chemotherapeutic agents.

C. Phase III Study

     To clarify the clinical efficacy of lentinan for patients
with cancer, a phase III study of randomized controlled trials
has been conducted on patients with advanced or recurrent gastric
or colorectal cancer (Furue et al., 1981). Lentinan has been
administered intravenously at doses of 1 mg/person/day twice a
week or 2 mg/person/day once a week in combination with chemotherapeutic agents such as 5-FU + mitomycin C (MF) or Tegafur
(FT). Control treatments consisted of administering chemotherapeutic agents alone. In MF treatment, mitomycin C was
administered intravenously at doses of 4 mg/person/day twice a
week for the first 2 weeks, followed by the same dose once a week.
In FT treatment, Tegafur was administered in doses of 400 to
1200 mg/person/day by mouth, intravenous injection, or suppository.
Lentinan has been prepared as a lyophilized vial composed of 1 mg
of lentinan, 40 mg of mannitol, and 4 mg of dextran-40 as exci-
pients. In gastric cancer patients, 60 cases were eligible for
MF, 76 cases for MF + lentinan, 72 cases for FT, and 77 cases for
FT + lentinan. In patients with colorectal cancer, 17 cases
were eligible for FT and 23 cases for FT + lentinan.
     Clinical efficacies were evaluated with regard to life span
prolongation effects, antitumor effects, and side effects. Life
span prolongation effects were evaluated by Kaplan-Meier's survival
curve with statistical examination using a generalized Wilcoxon's
test. Antitumor effects were examined statistically with Fisher's
test. Figures 2 and 3 indicate that there were distinct life span
prolongation effects in the lentinan-treated group with statistical significance ($p < .01$ or $p < .05$). Antitumor effects are shown
in Table III, which indicates that better results were achieved in
the lentinan-treated group. Concerning suspected side effects of
lentinan administration, the following symptoms were observed in
13 patients: a feeling of heaviness in the chest (four cases),
and nausea and vomiting in three cases. All of these results are
similar to those of the phase I and II studies, and every side
effect has been transitional and not serious.
     Because lentinan has been shown in animal experimental models
to be a nonspecific immunoaugmenting agent, the effects of lentinan
on the host immune system in humans were studied through the
phase III study. Improvement in host immune response was
evaluated by PPD skin tests and peripheral lymphocyte counts, both
as immunoparameters. Incidence rates on positive increase in each
parameter have been higher in the lentinan-treated group than in
the control group (Table IV).

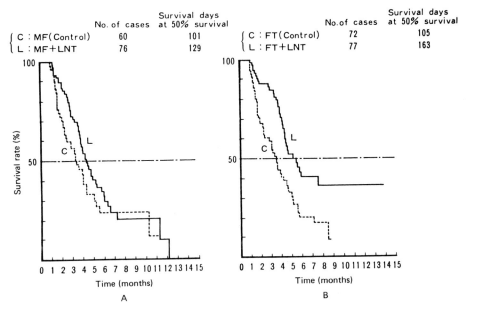

	No. of cases	Survival days at 50% survival		No. of cases	Survival days at 50% survival
C : MF(Control)	60	101	C : FT(Control)	72	105
L : MF+LNT	76	129	L : FT+LNT	77	163

Fig. 2.   Effect of lentinan (LNT) on survival curve in patients with advanced or recurrent gastric cancer.   (A) MF ($p < .05$), $z = -2.1985$; (B) FT ($p < .01$, $z = -3.7771$).

	No. of cases	Survival days at 50% survival
C : FT(Control)	17	94
L : FT+LNT	23	200

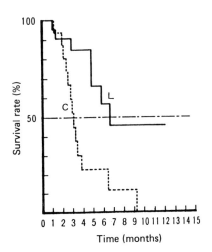

Fig. 3.   Effect of lentinan (LNT) on survival curve in patients with advanced or recurrent colorectal cancer ($p < .05$, $z = -2.4814$).

TABLE III

Effect of Lentinan (LNT) on Regression of Solid Tumor
in Patients with Measurable or Evaluable Lesions

Therapies	Number of cases (A)	Number of PR or CR cases[a] (B)	Rate of positive response (B/A) × 100 (%)	Statistical examination (Fisher test)
Gastric cancer				
MF	39	2	5.1	p = .4585
MF + LNT	52	6	11.7	
FT	55	1	1.8	p = .0114
FT + LNT	48	8	16.3	
Colorectal cancer				
FT	11	0	0	p = .4923
FT + LNT	15	2	13.3	

[a]PR, partial regression; CR, complete regression.
[b]Significant.

III. CONCLUSION OF PHASE III STUDY ON PATIENTS WITH GASTRO-
      INTESTINAL CANCER

These results show that lentinan should be effective for patients with advanced or recurrent gastric or colorectal cancer in
combination with chemotherapeutic agents such as MF or FT.

TABLE IV

Effect of Lentinan (LNT) on Host Immune Response,
Measured by PPD Skin Test (PPD) and Peripheral Blood Lymphocyte Counts (PBLC)

Criteria	Treatments	Number of cases tested (A)	Number of positive cases[a]	Rate of positive cases (%)	Statistical examination (Fisher test)
PPD	MF or FT	68	6	9	$\chi^2 = 1.9427$, $p = .1634$
	MF or FT + LNT	102	18	18	
PBLC	MF or FT	101	32	32	$\chi^2 = 4.5317$, $p = .0333$
	MF or FT + LNT	120	56	47	

Positive case in PPD: Diameter (ϕ) of reaction area changed from $\phi < 10$ to $\phi \geq 10$ mm. Positive case in PBLC: $(N-Nc)/Nc \times 100 = A \geq 20$ (%). N, Maximum PBLC observed during trial; Nc, PBLC at commencement of trial.

REFERENCES

Chihara, G., Maeda, Y., Hamuro, J., Sasaki, T., and Fukuoka, F.
  (1969). *Nature 222*, 687-688.
Chihara, G., and Taguchi, T. (1982). *Sigmatau 2*, 93-104.
Furue, H., Itoh, I., Kimura, T., Kondo, T., Hattori, T., Ogawa,
  N., and Taguchi, T. (1981). *Gan-to-Kagakuryoho 8*, 944-966.
Taguchi, T., Nakano, Y., Urushizaki, I., Kure, T., Ishitani, K.,
  Saito, T., Wakui, A., Takahashi, K., Koyama, Y., Kimura, T.,
  Furue, H., Kusama, S., Tomiyama, J., Itoh, I., Tominaga, T.,
  Majima, H., Kondo, T., Kamei, H., Terabe, K., Kamisaki, G.,
  Mori, T., Yayoi, K., Masaoka, T., Kimura, I., Onoshi, T.,
  Inokuchi, K., and Kumashiro, R. (1979). *Gan-to-Kagakuryoho 6*,
  619-626.
Taguchi, T., Furue, H., and Majima, H. (1981). *Gan-to-Kagakuryoho
  8*, 422-440.
Taguchi, T., Aoki, T., Furue, H., and Majima, H. (1981). *In*
  "Manipulation of Host Defense Mechanisms", ICS 576, (T. Aoki,
  I. Urushizaki, and E. Tsubura, eds.), pp. 259-266. Excerpta
  Medica, Amsterdam.
Taguchi, T. (1979). *In* "Recent Results in Cancer Research"
  (G. Bonnadonna, G. Mathe, and S. E. Salmon, eds.), Vol. 68, pp.
  236-240.
Torisu, M., Fukawa, M., Nishimura, M., Harasaki, H., Kai, S., and
  Tanaka, J. (1975). *In* "International Conference on Immunotherapy
  of Cancer" (C. H. Southman and H. Friedman, eds.) Vol. 277, pp.
  160-186. *Ann. N.Y. Acad. Sci.*, New York.
Torisu, M., Miyahara, T., Fujiwara, H., Ohsato, K., Okano, H.,
  Fukawa, M., and Harada, M. (1977). *In* "Immunotherapy of Malignant
  Disease" (H. Reiner, ed.), pp. 137-142. F. K. Schattauer Verlag,
  Stuttgart.
Torisu, M., Miyahara, T., Yamamoto, T., Harada, M., Fujiwara, H.,
  Kitamura, Y., Jimi, M., Ohsato, K., Tanaka, J., and Fukawa, M.
  (1978). *Gann Monogr. 21*, 173-179.
Tsukagoshi, S., and Ohashi, F. (1974). *GANN 65*, 557-558.
Tsukahara, Y., Siozawa, I., Noguchi, H., Iwai, S., and Fukuta, T.
  (1979). *Acta Obst. Gynec. Jpn. 31*, 889-893.
Usui, S., Urano, M., Koike, S., and Kobayashi, Y. (1976). *J.
  Natl. Cancer Inst. 56*, 185-187.
Yokoe, N., Kato, H., Takemura, S., Yoshikawa, T., Kondo, M.,
  Hosokawa, K., and Kodama, M. (1979). *Jap. J. Clin. Oncol. 9*,
  209-214.
Yoshikumi, C., Fujii, T., Matsunaga, K., Morita, I., Yagihashi, Y.,
  Arakawa, Y., Toyoda, Y., Furusho, T., Hotta, T., Nomoto, K., and
  Takeya, K. (1975). *GANN 66*, 649-654.

PART VC

Chairpersons

Donald L. Morton
Motomichi Torisu

CHAPTER 32

NEW HORIZONS IN SURGICAL ONCOLOGY: MALIGNANT MELANOMA[1]

Donald L. Morton
Rishab K. Gupta
James F. Huth

Division of Surgical Oncology
John Wayne Clinic and Armand Hammer Laboratories
Jonsson Comprehensive Cancer Center
University of California at Los Angeles School of Medicine
Los Angeles, California
and
Surgical Services
Veterans Administration Medical Center
Sepulveda, California

[1]Supported by Grants CA12582, CA29605, CA09010, and CA30019,
awarded by the National Cancer Institute, DHHS; and by Medical
Research Services of the Veterans Administration.

I.   INTRODUCTION

Our early studies demonstrating that patients with malignant
melanoma formed antibodies reactive with cell surface and intra-
cytoplasmic antigens detectable by immunofluorescent techniques
provided the justification for clinical trials of immunotherapy
(Morton et al., 1968). In 1970, we observed remarkable regres-
sions of intradermal metastases in patients with disseminated
melanoma after tumor deposits were injected with viable BCG
organisms. The incidence of tumor regression was correlated with
the presence of delayed hypersensitivity reactivity on skin testing (Morton et al., 1970). We observed regression of up to 90%
of the injected lesions in immunocompetent patients. In addition,
15-20% of uninjected lesions also regressed, suggesting that the
BCG immunotherapy had a systemic effect. However, patients who
were anergic to skin testing materials and those with large tumor
burden metastatic to liver, lung, and brain or bulky subcutaneous
disease had little or no response to immunotherapy.
Evidence that BCG induced a systemic antitumor effect led to
the study of BCG immunotherapy as an adjuvant during the postoperative period for patients with melanoma metastatic to regional
lymph nodes who were clinically free of disease following surgical
lymphadenectomy. This study was simultaneously controlled but
nonrandomized, and consisted of patients who were treated in our
institution by surgery alone or who had surgery and postoperative
immunotherapy. The initial results of this study, reported in
1974 (Morton et al., 1974) and 1976 (Eilber et al., 1976), suggested that BCG adjuvant immunotherapy was of benefit to patients
with melanoma metastatic to regional lymph nodes in that BCG
appeared to reduce the early postoperative recurrence rate and
prolong survival. These encouraging results led us to undertake
a prospective randomized trial to evaluate postoperative adjuvant
immunotherapy in patients with melanoma metastatic to regional
nodes.

II. PROSPECTIVE RANDOMIZED CLINICAL TRIAL OF BCG ADJUVANT
     IMMUNOTHERAPY

A.   Patients and Methods

This clinical trial, completed in 1978, consisted of patients
who were randomized into one of three treatment categories:
Surgery only (48), surgery and BCG (49), and surgery, BCG, and
tumor cell vaccine (TCV) (52). Ten patients were excluded from
the analysis for protocol violations. Analysis was performed on
139 patients at a median follow-up of 62 months. Patients who

TABLE I

Clinical Characteristics of Treatment Groups in
Stage II Melanoma: Clinical Trial

Randomization factors	Control (surgery only)	BCG + surgery	BCG + TCV + surgery
Number of patients	46	45	48
Age (mean years)	42	44	42
Sex			
Male	34	33	34
Female	12	12	14
Lymph node status			
Clinically Positive	33	34	34
Clinically Negative	13	11	14

TABLE II

Recurrence and Survival Rates
in 139 Stage II Melanoma Patients: Clinical Trial

	Control (surgery only)	BCG + surgery	BCG + TCV + surgery
Number of patients	46	45	48
Number of recurrences	27	28	24
Number of deaths	24	21	23
Recurrence rate at 2 years (%)	48	49	52
Survival rate at 2 years (%)	61	80	63
Survival rate at 4 years (%)	47	53	54
Percentage of patients surviving at least 1 year after recurrence	26	56	21

developed disease recurrence continued to receive adjuvant therapy
if assigned to an adjuvant group but also received chemotherapy
consisting of DTIC in combination with BCNU or CCNU or high-dose

methotrexate. Patients in the control group who had disease
recurrence received the same chemotherapy.

B. Results

    Tables I and II show the clinical characteristics of these
patients and their recurrence and survival rates. Unfortunately,
the results of this randomized trial were not nearly as
impressive as the earlier trial, and, as shown here, although it
appeared that the group receiving BCG was surviving longer than
the controls, with increasing time the arms came together and
these differences were not statistically significant for survival.
However, if we look at the time from recurrence to death, we
again see that there was a therapeutic effect from BCG that was
highly significant statistically (p = .01). The only other apparent effect of BCG was the fact that these patients were more
likely to have local regional recurrences and less likely to have
visceral or brain recurrences as their first site of recurrence
(Morton *et al.*, 1981).

II. INVESTIGATION OF REASONS FOR DIFFERENCES IN TRIAL RESULTS

    Obviously, we were concerned about the differences between
these two trials, and we compared the two in terms of controls
versus the adjuvant treatment groups. We found that patients
treated with BCG had almost identical survival rates at 2 and
3 years. However, the most striking differences were found in
the two control groups--60% survival at 2 years in the second
trial and only 38% in the first trial. Three-year survival was
50% in the second trial versus 28% in the first trial. The difference between the two studies were in the control groups--in
the second study the surgery-only group did so well that we could
not demonstrate a significant effect for adjuvant therapy.

A. Natural Course of Melanoma

    This finding led us to a study of the natural history of
melanoma (Morton *et al.*, 1981). We assessed the effect on survival of histological and clinical features in 150 stage II melanoma
patients seen at UCLA between January 1954 and June 1976. These
patients had been treated by lymphadenectomy but had received
neither chemotherapy nor immunotherapy, and were representative
of the types of patients who would constitute a stage II adjuvant
therapy protocol. Their clinical course until the point of

development of postlymphadenectomy metastases represented the "natural history" of patients treated by surgery alone.

B. Study Parameters

Putative prognostic factors included age, sex, parity, site of primary tumor, presence of satellitosis, clinical status of nodes, histological characteristics of the primary lesion (Clark's level, thickness of tumor, presence and width of ulceration, and number of mitoses/high power field), time from biopsy of primary tumor to lymphadenectomy, and number of positive nodes. Survival for the entire group at 1, 2, 5, and 10 years was estimated to be 73, 55, 37, and 33% by Kaplan-Meier estimate. Univariate analyses showed that thickness of the primary lesion ($p < .001$), width of ulceration ($p = .003$), absence of ulceration ($p = .024$), and number of positive nodes ($p = .033$) were prognostic for survival. In multivariate analysis by the Cox procedure, thickness of the primary ($p = .001$) and number of melanoma-containing nodes ($p = .043$) were prognostic for survival. Location of the primary tumor became marginally significant ($p = .12$) in the multivariate model. These findings demonstrated the prognostic importance of characteristics of both the primary lesion and the extent of regional dissemination.

C. Implications of Results

The results of these studies showed that stage II melanoma patients are not a homogeneous group at all. To underline this fact, we plotted a histogram of survival time for the patients in this surgery-only group, and found three different subpopulations. There was a large group of patients who died within the first 14 months of lymphadenectomy, a second group who died more slowly over a 48-month period, and a third that only had sporadic deaths. We hypothesized that the first group represented those patients who had large tumor burden with a high incidence of subclinical metastases or who had a weakened immune response. The second group seemed to have a lesser tumor burden and a stronger immune response, and the third was representative of those patients who remain free of disease for years with only an occasional death between the fifth and fifteenth years. It seemed to us that these observations would have extraordinary implications for cancer therapy in general and for further clinical adjuvant trials in particular. The patients in group 1 were unlikely to benefit from immunotherapy as an adjunct to their surgeries because of their high residual disease. In contrast, the patients in group 3 were going to be cured by their surgeries, and they, too, could derive no benefit from any additional treatment. Theoretically, then, we had group 2, a relatively small number of patients whose disease might be influenced by adjuvant therapy.

This natural history study analyzed 13 factors in an attempt to identify that small middle group of patients who could benefit from adjuvant therapy. The heterogeneity of the entire stage II group of patients very nearly defeated our purpose. After all, we could only measure the tumor we removed from the patient, whereas survival depended on the amount of tumor that remained after the surgical procedure. We began looking at various assays that might allow us to separate these three groups of patients.

IV. IDENTIFICATION OF PATIENTS WHO CAN BENEFIT FROM ADJUVANT
     THERAPY

A. Role of Circulating Immune Complexes

The phenomenon of *in vitro* antigen modulation, capping, and shedding after exposing melanoma cells to antibody had been described, and cultured melanoma cells were shown to shed antigen spontaneously into culture medium. We hypothesized that part or all of the antigens shed into the circulation could complex with humoral antibodies to form circulating immune complexes (CIC). Analyses of sequential serum samples from melanoma patients for antitumor antibody by the complement fixation assay had shown significant levels of anticomplementary activity just before or at the time of clinically detectable tumor recurrence (Gupta and Morton, 1978; Gupta *et al.*, 1979). Many of these samples were also capable of inhibiting mitogen-induced lymphocyte blastogenesis (Rangel *et al.*, 1977). We reasoned that an assessment of CIC might be useful for following the clinical course of melanoma patients.

Serum samples from 341 melanoma patients were randomly selected for study (Gupta and Morton, 1981). None of the patients had received immunotherapy, chemotherapy, or radiation therapy at the time of serum sampling. Patients ranged in age from 10 to 80 years, and the population was distributed evenly between male and female. Control sera were procured from the various clinics and included samples from patients who had immune complex diseases (hepatitis, acute viral infections, glomerulonephritis, rheumatoid arthritis, systemic lupus erythematosus) and samples from apparently healthy normal donors. The microcomplement consumption technique was used to assess anticomplementary activity of each test serum.

1. Evaluation Methods

Body burden of tumor at the time of serum sampling was roughly approximated in terms of weight. Size and number of palpable tumor masses and tumor nodules seen on radiological films, scans, and tomograms were determined. It was arbitrarily assumed that a 1.0-cm^3 nodule weighed about 1.0 g. Based on these estimations, melanoma patients were grouped into categories: no evidence of disease to <1 g tumor (NED), 1 to <100 g tumor (medium tumor burden), and $\geq$100 g tumor (high tumor burden). Patients in the NED group had no detectable disease by physical and radiological examinations. Patients in the medium tumor burden group had from small to fairly large pulmonary or subcutaneous metastases. Patients in the high tumor burden group had grossly large tumor masses. The incidence of positive anticomplementary activity was highest (71%) for the medium tumor burden group, and it was significantly lower in the NED and high tumor burden groups (35 and 31%, respectively).

2. Results

In some patients whose serum samples were studied for over a year, the anticomplementary activity decreased below detectable levels as tumor burden increased or persisted over a period of several months. In some patients, serum samples began to consume complement 2-4 weeks before their recurring tumors were clinically detectable. Antibody levels against autologous and allogeneic melanoma cells also increased. However, the antibodies declined to undetectable levels in serum samples taken shortly before death. Anticomplementary activity also decreased at this time.

We found that 43% (147 of 341) of melanoma sera were positive for anticomplementary activity compared to 13% (31 of 245) of sera from healthy normal donors (p <0.05). The non-cancer patients with suspected immune complex diseases had a 68% incidence of anticomplementary activity. Positive anticomplementary activity was lower in melanoma patients with no evidence of disease or with high tumor burden than in patients with medium tumor burden. Assuming that anticomplementary activity was due to immune complexes, then this lower incidence could be the result of antibody excess in sera from patients with low tumor burden (<1 g) and of antigen excess in sera from patients with high tumor burden (>100 g). Therefore, the quantity or composition of the immune complexes in these extreme groups would be such that neither could consume complement.

Analysis of anticomplementary activity in sequential serum samples from several melanoma patients revealed that some samples consumed significant amounts of complement in the absence of clinically detectable tumor, whereas some had no anticomplementary activity despite evidence of disease. Some patients who were disease free had serum samples that were anticomplementary during the disease-free interval. These patients generally had disease recurrence within 6 months. In some patients, serum anticomplementary activity decreased as tumor burden increased. Analyses of serial serum samples from these patients for complement-fixing antibody levels revealed that the disappearance of antibody was concomitant with or just before a decrease in anticomplementary activity. These findings suggested that the antigens were complexing with virtually all of the circulating antibody to produce antigen excess in the circulation. These complexes together with the excess free antigen could directly or indirectly produce the immunosuppressive serum factors that would block further production of antibody.

Melanoma sera with anticomplementary activity and free antigen were more inhibitory to .PHA-induced blastogenesis than sera with anticomplementary activity alone. The inhibition appeared to be abrogated by antibody excess, that is, sera that were anticomplementary and that contained detectable levels of antibody.

B. Radioimmunoassay Studies

With the development of a radioimmunoassay (Gupta and Morton, 1982), we could look at a series of patients by relating antibody titer, antigen titer, and immune complexes to body burden of tumor, and we found that the antibody titer was highest in those who were free of disease or who had small tumor burdens that we could see clinically. The titer fell relatively abruptly in those who had an intermediate tumor burden, and fell progressively in those with advanced disease of an estimated 100-g tumor burden. The antigen titer was lowest in those who were clinically free of disease and then rose abruptly in those with intermediate tumor burden. However, the antigen titer was highest in the patients with advanced disease. The immune complexes were lowest in the tumor-free group, reached a peak in the intermediate tumor burden group, and fell to undetectable levels in the group with advanced disease. These findings led us to hypothesize that there might be a relationship between body burden of tumor following surgery and these three components of the immune response.

C. Competitive Inhibition Enzyme Immunoassay Studies

Another assay, the competitive inhibition enzyme immunoassay (EIA), was used to monitor antigen levels in the 24-hr urine samples of 153 stage II and III melanoma patients. Of 89 patients who had clinical evidence of persistent disease, 74 (83%) were positive for urinary antigen. The remaining 15 patients were negative for antigen in the urine, although 10 of these patients had far advanced disease, a condition known to cause decreased antigen titer. Five patients had moderate tumor burden and no

TABLE III

Urine Antigen Assay Results: Stage II Postlymphadenectomy

Antigen assay	Recurrence	No recurrence	Total
Positive	17	8	25
Negative	0	32	32
Total	17	40	57

antigen detectable in the urine. Seven stage II patients had urine samples collected before and after lymphadenectomy; six (86%) were positive for antigen before the procedure. One patient who was antigen negative had microscopic tumor in one axillary lymph node. Fifty-seven stage II patients were followed at regular intervals after lymphadenectomy with urine collections and physical examinations that included chest roentgenographs. Of the 25 patients who developed positive antigen titers, 17 (68%) developed disease recurrence. The 32 patients whose urine remained negative for urinary antigens are free of disease (Table III) (Huth *et al.*, 1981).

There was a high degree of correlation between observable disease and positive antigen titers in the 89 patients with evaluable disease. Excretion of tumor-associated antigens appeared to be dependent on the deposition of circulating immune complexes within the glomerular basement membrane of the kidney. We could demonstrate a correlation between the presence of circulating immune complexes and urinary antigen excretion.

V. CONCLUSIONS

Now if we combine all this information, we find that if we look at disease recurrence in melanoma patients versus the presence of serum antigen and complexes, those patients who are antigen negative and complex negative have a relatively high long-term survival rate, whereas patients who are antigen positive, whether or not they have enough antibody to make complexes, have very rapid disease recurrence. Patients who are antigen negative but complex positive have an intermediate disease recurrence rate. Then, if we look at the presence of antibody, we find that those patients who are antibody positive and complex negative will probably be long-term disease-free survivors. Those who are antibody negative and complex negative or positive will have early disease recurrences, and those who are antibody positive and complex positive will be in the intermediate group.

When the urinary antigen assay was combined with the antigen-antibody-immune complex information, we found that patients who were positive for urinary antigen had immune complexes in their serum, and that those patients who were urinary antigen negative were also free of immune complexes. There appeared to be a close relationship between the presence of antigen in the urine and disease status. For example, there was a dramatic increase in urinary antigen with tumor necrosis caused by chemotherapy, hyperthermia, or radiation, yet there was a decrease to nondetectable levels when tumor was removed. Its presence appears to portend subclinical disease in the postoperative patient. Urinary antigen titers will also drop dramatically as disease advances.

To summarize our findings, we found that our clinical trials were based on some factors that had little relationship to the true problem of the postoperative stage II melanoma patient. There were at least 20 stratification factors involving the relationships of serum antigen to antibody and immune complexes that influenced survival in the patients involved in these trials. We found that adjuvant therapy would only benefit the true stage II patient and would have no effect on those whose disease had progressed subclinically to stage III or whose disease could be cured by the surgical procedure itself. These findings should permit us to design clinical trials based on what is truly happening in this most heterogeneous group, rather than assuming that all stage II melanoma patients will respond to therapeutic manipulations.

REFERENCES

Eilber, F. R., Morton, D. L., Holmes, E. C., Sparks, F. C., and Ramming, K. P. (1976). *N. Engl. J. Med.* *294*, 237.

Gupta, R. K., and Morton, D. L. (1978). *Fed. Proc. Fed. Am. Soc. Exp. Biol.* *37*, 1595.

Gupta, R. K., and Morton, D. L. (1981). *In* "Fundamental Mechanisms in Human Cancer Immunology" (J. Saunders, J. Daniels, B. Serrou, D. Rosenfeld, and C. Denney, eds.), pp. 305-320. Elsevier/North Holland, New York.

Gupta, R. K., and Morton, D. L. (1982). *In* "Melanoma Antigens and Antibodies" (R. Reisfeld and S. Ferrone, eds.), p. 139. Plenum, New York.

Gupta, R. K., Theofilopoulos, A. N., Dixon, F. J., and Morton, D. L. (1979). *Cancer Immunol. Immunother.* *6*, 211.

Huth, J. F., Gupta, R. K., and Morton, D. L. (1981). *Surg. Forum* *32*, 417.

Morton, D. L., Malmgren, R. A., Holmes, E. C., and Ketcham, A. S. (1968). *Surgery* *64*, 233.

Morton, D. L., Eilber, F. R., Malmgren, R. A., and Wood, W. C. (1970). *Surgery 68*, 158.

Morton, D. L., Eilber, F. R., Holmes, E. C., Hunt, J. S., Ketcham, A. S., Silverstein, M. J., and Sparks, F. C. (1974). *Ann. Surg. 180*, 635.

Morton, D. L., Eilber, F. R., Weisenburger, T. H., and Liu, P.-Y. (1981). *Adjuvant Ther. Cancer 3*, 241.

Rangel, D. M., Gupta, R. K., Golub, S. H., and Morton, D. L. (1977). *Proc. Am. Assoc. Cancer Res. 18*, 184.

CHAPTER 33

IN VIVO AND IN VITRO EXPERIMENTS USING OK-432
AS AN IMMUNOBIOLOGICAL RESPONSE MODIFIER

Takashi Hoshino

Department of Immunology
Fukui Medical School
Fukui, Japan

Atsushi Uchida

Institute for Applied and Experimental Oncology
University of Vienna
Vienna, Austria

BASIC MECHANISMS AND CLINICAL TREATMENT
OF TUMOR METASTASIS

I. INTRODUCTION

It has been known for many years that accidental complication
with erysipelas (*Streptococcus hemolyticus* infection) often brings
about temporal benefits in patients with malignant diseases, suggesting that this particular bacillus has a potential activity
against cancer through modification of the host defense mechanism.
Okamoto and associates (1967), who were studying anticancerous
microorganisms, discovered a useful preparation of this group of
the bacilli and designated it as OK-432.

OK-432 is produced by incubating the culture of the low-
virulent SU strain of type III, group A *Streptococcus pyogenes* of
human origin, treating with penicillin G potassium, and then
lyophilizing the incubation mixture. A unit of KE (Klinische
Einheit) is used to express the strength of the preparation, with
1 KE corresponding to 0.1 mg dried bacilli. It is parenterally
given through any route suspended in saline or any other suitable
medium. A lack of growing capacity of the bacilli has been confirmed by animal inoculation study as well as by cultivation in
various media following treatment with penicillinase to decompose
penicillin. Since 1975, when the preparation was given approval
by the Japanese Ministry of Health and Welfare for marketing on
the basis of the results of preliminary experimental and clinical
use showing its adequate antitumor activity with confirmed safety,
OK-432 has been widely prescribed to treat cancer patients in
Japan and in South Korea. Despite the favorable results it has
achieved in prolonging survival and lessening clinical symptoms
of treated patients, its mechanisms of action and the best route
of administration have not yet been fully defined. This chapter
gives an overview of the clinical effectiveness and the immunopharmacological functions of OK-432 as a biological response
modifier, on the basis of the results of our own *in vivo* and *in
vitro* studies supplemented with published articles and orally presented papers by the many outstanding investigators who have
conducted excellent studies on this interesting treatment modality.

II. CLINICAL STUDIES OF OK-432 TREATMENT

In 1980, we first reported the results of a randomized comparative study on OK-432 immunotherapy (Uchida and Hoshino, 1980a).
A series of 44 patients with adenocarcinoma of the stomach and
36 patients with adenocarcinoma of the lung, all of whom were very
advanced (i.e., in clinical stages III or IV), were divided into
two groups. The patients in the study group received OK-432,
5-10 KE/day in combination with 5-FU, while the control group received 5-FU only. Although most of the patients had rather a

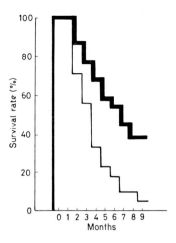

Fig. 1. Comparison of survival time between group treated
with (heavy line) and without (light line) OK-432 in patients
with cancer of the stomach and lung.

downhill disease course because of extensive metastasis of the
original tumor, survival times after the initiation of the therapy
were much longer in patients who received chemoimmunotherapy with
5-FU and OK-432 than in those given chemotherapy with 5-FU alone
(Fig. 1). The most conspicuous effect of OK-432 therapy was observed in the 12-months survival rates, which exceeded 23% in the
study groups, while all patients treated with 5-FU alone died
within 10 months. The results clearly indicated that OK-432 immunotherapy was effective at least in life prolongation, even in
advanced cancer of the stomach and the lung. The immunological
studies performed on those patients given OK-432 showed quantitative and qualitative effectiveness on impaired cell-mediated
immunity after the therapy. When the *in vitro* lymphocyte parameters were compared before and 4 weeks after daily intradermal
OK-432 injections, there were increased absolute lymphocyte counts
above 1500 per cubic millimeter and normalizing T-cell rate in
almost all cases, and increased PHA or Con-A blastogenesis up to
the normal ranges in about half the cases, respectively.
      Until our report there were few articles concerning small com-
parative studies on the effect of OK-432 in malignant diseases.
Nakazato and colleague (1976) of the Tokai Cooperative Study
Group of adjuvant immunochemotherapy of stomach cancer demonstrated a statistically significant prolongation of survival time
in 26 patients who underwent noncurative surgical resection and
were treated with so-called MFC chemotherapy (i.e., mitomycin C,
5-FU, and cytosine arabinoside) plus OK-432 immunotherapy, compared to that in 19 patients whose surgical treatment was similar
but who received MFC only. Kimura and associates (1976) demonstrated a significant prolongation of survival time in 22 patients
with stage III and IV lung cancer treated with induction chemo-

therapy in combination with a maintenance dosage of OK-432 compared to that in 26 historical control patients who received
induction chemotherapy alone. The median survivals of the study
group and the control were 6 and 4 months, respectively.

Following those two studies and our own reports, many clinical
experiments were designed and carried out in Japan to confirm the
clinical effectiveness and to analyze the immunological efficacy
of OK-432 (Suga *et al.*, 1977; Yasue *et al.*, 1981). In September
1982, the results of larger and well-organized comparative clinical studies on OK-432 immunotherapy were presented at the
International Cancer Congress held in Seattle, Washington. Some
of these results will be discussed here.

For lung cancer, an excellent randomized comparative study was
performed by Watanabe and Iwa (1982). A total of 211 patients
with lung cancer of various cell types and clinical stages was
randomized into two groups. Combination chemotherapy with cyclophosphamide, Adriamycin (doxorubicin), and 5-FU for adenocarcinoma,
and carboquinone, Adriamycin, and 5-FU for epidermoid carcinoma
were given with or without immunotherapy with OK-432. With a con-
firmation that the background profile of patients is not
different between the two groups, a comparative analysis was
performed on the effectiveness of the therapy. It was found
generally that the survival rate in a total of 108 patients given
immunochemotherapy was significantly higher than that of 103
patients given chemotherapy alone. When the patients were divided
by clinical stages, the 3-year survival rates in the immunochemotherapy and the simple chemotherapy group were 71.1 and 48.1%,
respectively, in the cases of stages I and II, and 23.8 and 8.6%,
respectively, in the cases of stage III. These differences
between groups were highly significant. Of much interest is a
striking prolongation of survival time in patients showing positive
skin test against SU antigen, one of the polysaccharide antigenic
substances in OK-432, at 3 months after the initiation of the
therapy, compared to survival time in patients with negative skin
test. The data indicate that patients who were immunologically
capable of responding to OK-432 administration could live much
longer than patients who were unable to respond to SU even after
repeated immunization.

A randomized comparative study done by the Brain Tumor Adjuvant
Immunotherapy Study Group, conducted by Takakura (1982), disclosed
an advantage of OK-432 immunotherapy in patients undergoing surgical removal of malignant glioma. A significantly higher survival
rate was observed in 30 patients given radiotherapy plus ACNU in
combination with OK-432, compared to that in 28 patients given
radiotherapy plus ACNU alone.

Shirakawa (1982) reported more favorable remission-prolonging
effects of separate treatment with OK-432 than of maintenance
chemotherapy in patients with malignant lymphoma. After induction
of complete remission by a fixed schedule of combination chemotherapy, a total of 55 patients, 25 with Hodgkin's disease and

30 with non-Hodgkin's lymphoma, were randomly divided into two
groups, one receiving OK-432 alone and the other maintenance
combined chemotherapy. In both groups of Hodgkin's and non-
Hodgkin's disease patients, significantly better prognoses of
lower relapse rate and longer duration of remission were observed
in the patients given OK-432 alone than in those who were treated
with chemotherapy during the remission. The results of a randomized comparative study performed by the Japan Cooperative Study
Group for Malignant Melanomas headed by Hayasaka *et al.* and
presented at the Sixteenth International Congress of Dermatology
held in Tokyo in May 1982, also showed a statistically significant
increase in 3-year survival rate of 46% in 83 patients treated
with chemotherapeutic agents and OK-432, as compared to 20% in 84
patients treated with chemotherapeutic agents alone.
    Summarizing these clinical studies, it was certainly recog-
nized that OK-432 administration, either alone or in combination
with other chemotherapeutic agents, to patients with various
types of malignant tumors successfully prolonged the survival time
even in advanced cases. Use of OK-432 has proved to be effective
not only in producing a remission together with chemotherapy or
radiotherapy but also in extending the duration of disease-free
periods. Patients successfully treated with OK-432 demonstrated
recovery of immune response to recall antigens *in vivo* and increase
of mitogenic blastogenesis of lymphocytes *in vitro*. These data
suggest that the mechanisms of action of OK-432 are not directly
tumoricidal but seem to operate through activation of the host
defense mechanisms. Thus, it would be of special interest to know
the effective mechanisms of this preparation, particularly its
immunological functions.

III. IMMUNOLOGICAL STUDIES ON OK-432

    So far a number of *in vivo* and *in vitro* studies concerning the
immunological function of OK-432 have been carried out, and the
results have been reported in both domestic and foreign medical
journals (Micksche *et al.*, 1982; Moriyasu *et al.*, 1982). This
chapter, however, will concentrate on certain restricted but important effects of OK-432, mainly on T cells, macrophages, and NK
cells.

A. Activation of T Cells and Macrophages

    OK-432 has been found to activate T cells and macrophages *in
vivo* and *in vitro*. The results of our study (Uchida and Hoshino,
1980b) on patients with cancer of the stomach and lung disclosed
that certain subclasses of suppressor T cells are responsible for

the impaired mitogenic blastogenic response of lymphocytes. OK-432 therapy for 4 weeks produced disappearance of such suppressor cells resulting in recovery of blastogenesis (Uchida and Hoshino, 1980c). Hojo and Hashimoto (1981) demonstrated in rats bearing bladder carcinoma that intraperitoneal injection of OK-432 produced selective cytolytic T cells, nonselective cytolytic non-T cells, and cytostatic macrophages. According to Kai and associates (1979), OK-432 was found to enhance the cellular and humoral immune responses that require the contributions of T cells. They demonstrated increases in direct cytotoxicity of spleen cells and delayed footpad reaction after immunization with chicken red blood cells and augmentation of anti-hapten antibody production by enhancement of helper T-cell activity in mice given OK-432.

In vivo and *in vitro* macrophage-activating functions of OK-432 have been known since the preparation was first used as an immunostimulant. The mechanisms of such macrophage activation have been studied from different aspects of interest. Among them, the most important activating function of macrophages must be related to cytotoxic activity by self-phagocytosis, followed by cytolysis and mediation of immunocytocidal functions of other immunocytes.

A study on cytostatic activity made by Matsunaga and associates (1980) showed that human circulating monocytes cultured in the presence of an immunostimulant such as OK-432 exhibited increased phagocytic activity. For the binding macrophage and target cell, Torikai and his group (1980) disclosed an enhancement of macrophage-mediated cytotoxicity in mice treated with OK-432 by increasing serum level of antitumor protein LB, which was later identified to be hemopexin (Torikai *et al*., 1981) and was proved to potentiate the intimate binding between target tumor cell and OK-432-elicited macrophage.

For the actual cytolytic mechanisms of OK-432-activated macrophage, two important reports will be discussed. Saito and Tomioka (1979) demonstrated that OK-432-stimulated macrophages were highly responsive to wheat germ lectin, which is known to be a potent triggering agent for hydrogen peroxide release. Murayama (1982) discovered that triggering mechanisms of OK-432 for cytotoxic activity of macrophages were mediated by formation of complexes of OK-432 and the third component of complement (C3) and thus obtained C3-OK-432 complex bound to the resident macrophages, followed by their augmentation of cytotoxic activity against tumor cells.

These reports suggest to us that the mechanisms of OK-432 activation of macrophages are not simple but might be involved in multiple functions of these complicated cells. In any case, a study made by Mashiba and associates (1979) is important from the clinical point of view. They proved that the macrophage-activating function of OK-432 was well displayed even when it was given to mice in combination with chemotherapeutic agents. Acid phosphatase activity and mobility of the peritoneal macrophages were enhanced and followed by strengthened cytostatic activity after injection of mitomycin, cyclophosphamide, and 5-FU together with OK-432.

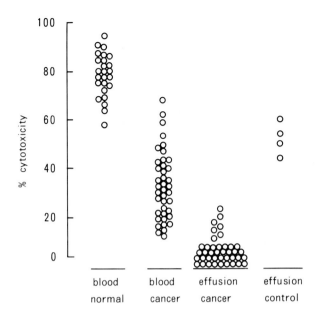

Fig. 2. Natural killer activity of mononuclear cells from blood and cancerous pleural effusion against K562. Control effusion was obtained from patients with inflammatory pleurisy. Incubation was for 4 hr at 37°C (E:T = 40:1).

B. Augmentation of NK-Cell Activity

It is widely accepted that NK cells may play an important role in tumor resistance, especially in protecting tumor metastases, although the actual biological significance is not clearly understood. Our studies demonstrated an augmentation of NK activity of mononuclear cells (MC) after *in vivo* injection or *in vitro* incubation (Uchida and Micksche, 1981, 1982a; Uchida *et al.*, 1982a) with OK-432 in patients with cancer. The results will be briefly discussed.

1. NK Activity of Mononuclear Cells in Circulating Blood (PB-MC) and Carcinomatous Pleural Effusion (PE-MC)

Sixty patients with malignant solid tumors who were not receiving anticancerous drugs and 44 roughly age-matched healthy men were subjected to study as experimental and control groups. Circulating blood MC (PB-MC) and PE-MC from patients with breast and lung cancer showed moderate impairment and marked reduction or even complete absence of NK activity, respectively, compared to NK activity of PB-MC from normal subjects (Fig. 2).
A single injection of 5 KE OK-432 to the study patients resulted in an increase in NK activity of PB-MC of up to 180% of the

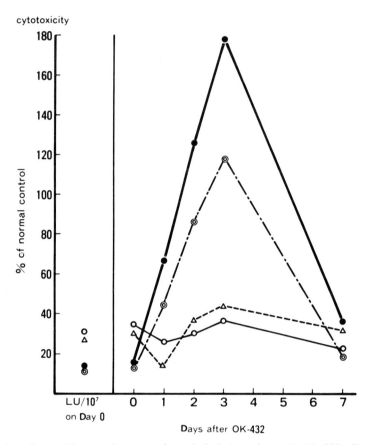

Fig. 3. Effect of systemic administration of OK-432 (1 KE on Day 0) on NK activity. Effect on NK activity varied with route of administration: ●, iv; ◎, id; △, im; ○, none.

pretreatment level, with a peak in 3 days and a subsequent rapid decrease to the original low levels in 7 days (Fig. 3). The extent of NK augmentation by OK-432 was dependent on the route of administration. The highest NK augmentation was achieved through intravenous injection, followed by the intradermal route. Since human NK activity is exerted by large granular lymphocytes (LGL), time course change in LGL count and rate of LGL-target conjugates were examined, but those values were fairly stationary even after OK-432 administration. Thus, the NK-augmentative effect of OK-432 might be derived from an enhancement of the lytic function of NK cells.

Similar *in vivo* effects of OK-432 on NK activity have been demonstrated by a few other investigators. Oshimi and co-workers (1980a) showed a significant increase in NK activity after daily intramuscular injections of OK-432 in patients with cancer, with the maximum level on Day 3 and a subsequent decline despite continued daily injections until Day 6 when NK activity dropped to the pretreatment level.

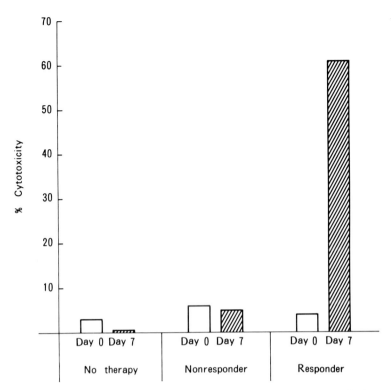

Fig. 4.   Enhancement of pleural effusion NK-cell activity by intrapleural injection of 10 KE OK-432 on Day 0 (E:T = 40:1).

To clarify the effect of OK-432 therapy at the site of malignant cell proliferation, NK activity of PE-MC was traced after intrapleural injection of 5 to 10 KE OK-432 in 12 patients with malignant pleural effusion as the most appropriate model for a study of local immunity against cancer (Fig. 4).   A marked increasing recovery of NK activity of PE-MC was observed 7 days after the injection in 10 patients who clinically responded to OK-432 by conspicuous reductions in the amount of effusion or number of tumor cells.   However, NK activity remained low or absent in two patients who did not respond to the OK-432 therapy.   Thus, it is clearly shown that the effectiveness of OK-432 in reducing carcinomatous effusion is manifested through increasing NK activity (Uchida and Micksche, 1983).

2.   Role of Macrophage in NK-Cell Activity

In searching for the cause of the marked decrease in or even absence of NK activity of PE-MC fractionation of the cells, an attempt was made to isolate the responsible components (Uchida and Micksche, 1982b).   The frequency of LGL in effusion cells was comparable to that in blood lymphocytes, suggesting that the cause of absent NK activity is not a reduction of LGL.   Natural killer

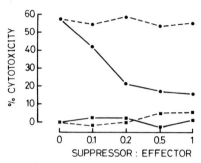

Fig. 5. Suppression of NK activity of indicator lymphocytes
(PBL) from a normal man by macrophages obtained from patients with
cancer. ●——●, Cancer PE-MC; ●---● cancer PB-MC; ■——■ normal
PBL + cancer PE-MC; ■·■, normal PBL + cancer PB-MC. K562 target
cells (E:T = 20:1).

activity of PB-MC from normal humans deteriorated when they were
mixed with PE-MC from cancer patients, suggesting the presence of
strong NK-suppressing components in PE-MC. Sephadex G-10 column
passage of PE-MC abrogated the NK-suppressing capacity, and the
G-10-passed cells not only responded to OK-432 with increased NK
activity but also displayed adequate NK activity after a 24-hr
incubation (Fig. 5). Sephadex G-10-adherent cells, in contrast,
possessed marked NK-suppressing ability to normal allogeneic as
well as autologous circulating lymphocytes with a dose-response
relationship.

This study confirmed that carcinomatous pleural effusion contains macrophages that suppress the development and maintenance
of NK activity of lymphocytes. Intrapleural injection of OK-432
abrogated the suppressing activity of macrophages, resulting in
a recovery of NK activity of PE-MC followed by a reduction of effusion (Fig. 6).

Similar NK-suppressing macrophages or monocytes were discovered by us (Uchida et al., 1982b) in the circulating blood of
postoperative cancer patients, and this may cause development of
the metastasis often observed after major surgery for removal of
the cancer focus. Monocytes separated from heparinized venous
blood (PBMO) from patients and controls by adherence to a plastic
surface were incubated with lymphocytes from blood (PBL) of a normal subject for 12 hr, then the monocytes were removed by passage
through Sephadex G-10 column to collect the indicator lymphocytes,
of which NK activity was determined. It was found that the monocytes obtained from patients within 24 hr after operation were
capable of suppressing NK activity in a dose-response manner. The
suppressor monocytes were recognized in 12 of 16 cases of cancer
of the breast, whereas 1 of 10 preoperative period of these
patients and none of control subjects with major noncancerous
operation possessed such NK-suppressive monocytes (Figs. 7 and 8).

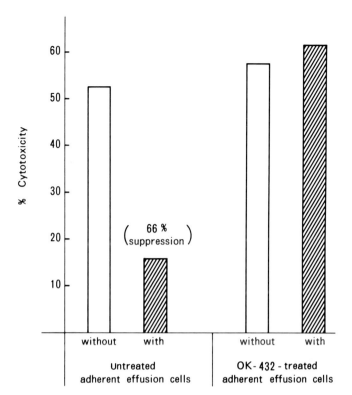

Fig. 6. Reduction of NK-suppressor cells by intrapleural injection of OK-432. Blood lymphocytes were cultured for 24 hr with
or without adherent effusion cells before and 7 days after the
first intrapleural injection of OK-432 (E:T = 40:1).

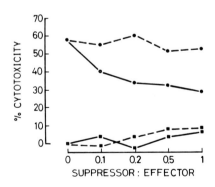

Fig. 7. Suppression of NK activity of indicator lymphocytes
(PBL) from a normal man by monocytes (PBMO) obtained from patients
with cancer of the breast before and after surgical removal of the
tumor. ■---■, Pre-op PBMO; ■——■, post-op PBMO; ●---●, normal PBL
+ pre-op PBMO; ●——●, normal PBL + post-op PBMO. K562 target
cells (E:T = 20:1).

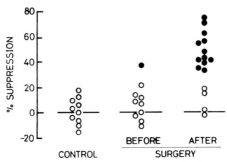

Fig. 8. NK suppression by monocytes before and after surgical removal of breast cancer. Suppressor: effector ratio = 0.2:1. ●, $p < .05$.

Of interest was that the postoperative NK-suppressive mono-cytes were abrogated if the patients were given OK-432 3 days prior to the operation. This treatment were considered to prevent a collapse of the postoperative NK activity, since the maximum rise in NK activity is achieved in 3 days following OK-432 admini-stration (Fig. 9). Although the mechanism of the appearance of postoperative suppressive monocytes is not clarified yet, it is expected that such prophylactic immunotherapy with OK-432 to pa-tients undergoing a major surgical procedure to remove cancer tissue might effectively prevent the postoperative metastasis due to hematogenous dissemination of tumor cells.

3. In Vitro Augmentation of NK Activity by OK-432

In vitro incubation of mononuclear cells with OK-432 resulted in a dose-dependent and time of incubation-dependent augmentation of NK activity in both normals and patients with cancer (Uchida and Micksche, 1981). The enhancement of NK activity by OK-432 was observed as early as 4 hr preincubation, with the peak effect as around 20 hr incubation (Fig. 10). The mode of intensity of cyto-toxic activation of OK-432 was dose dependent, with the maximum effect at the concentration of 0.5 KE/ml (Fig. 11). The manifes-tation of OK-432-induced NK augmentation required active cell metabolism, RNA and protein synthesis, but no DNA synthesis of lymphocytes. Percoll fractionation study disclosed that the ac-tual augmentation of NK activity is merely performed by the LGL fraction. Incubation with OK-432 altered neither the rate of LGL and target cell conjugation nor participation of monocytes or macrophages.

Addition of anti-α-interferon antibody to OK-432 incubation mixture did not completely inhibit the boosting activity of OK-432 (Fig. 12). These results suggest that OK-432 augments the cytotoxic activity of LGL having the ability to recognize target cells not simply depending on α-interferon production. However,

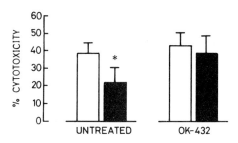

Fig. 9.   Postoperative reduction of NK activity and its prevention by prophylactic immunotherapy with OK-432.   Before surgery
(white bars); after surgery (black bars).   K562 target cells
(E:T = 20:1).   Vertical bars, SEM.   *, p < .05.

Wakasugi (Wakasugi *et al*., 1981; Wakasugi, 1982) demonstrated
NK-activating ability in the supernatant fraction after incubation of lymphocytes with OK-432, which was identified as interferon (IFN) and interleukin-2 (IL-2).   They also showed that
neither monocytes nor macrophages are involved in the NK-augmen-
tation process by OK-432.   Oshimi and his group (1980b) demonstrated
in mice that the cells involved in OK-432 augmentation for NK activity are sensitive to anti-asialo Gm_1 antibody complement.   These
experimental results suggest that OK-432-induced augmentation takes
place via LGL in humans and asialo Gm_1-positive cells in mice
through mediation of at least immune IFN and IL-2.   Actually, Saito
and associates (1982) demonstrated production of γ-IFN from mouse
spleen cells stimulated with OK-432.   Interferon was detected as

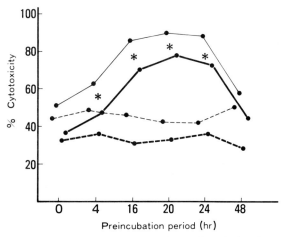

Preincubation period (hr)

Fig. 10.   Kinetics of augmentation of cytotoxic activity against
K562 cells (Ly) by OK-432) (0.5 KE/ml); effect of preincubation
period. ●----●, Normal Lys; ●---●, cancer Ly; ●——●, normal Ly
+ OK-432; ●——●, cancer Ly + OK-432 (E:T = 20:1).   *, p < .05.

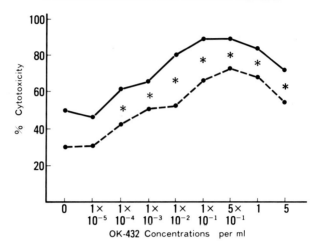

Fig. 11. Augmentation of cytotoxic activity against K562
cells by doses of OK-432. Incubation time, 20 hr (E:T = 20:1).
●——●, Normal Ly; ●---●, cancer Ly. *, *p* < .05.

early as 4 hr incubation and reached the maximum level in
24 hr.

This kinetics pattern of IFN production is comparable to
that seen in NK augmentation of human lymphocytes by OK-432.
Ishida and colleague (1982) have extensively studied lymphokine
production by OK-432-primed lymphocytes in mice. They proved

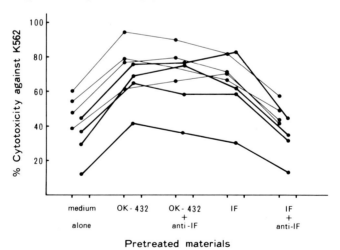

Fig. 12. Effects of anti-interferon antibodies (1 × 10^4
units/ml) of cytotoxic activity of lymphocytes by OK-432 and
α-interferon (500 units/ml). ●——●, Normal donor; ●——●, cancer
patient. Preincubation time, 20 hr (E:T = 20:1).

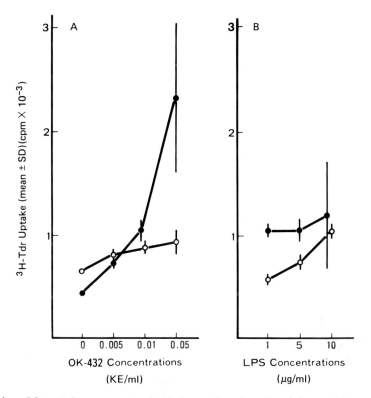

Fig. 13. Enhancement of IL-1 production by (A) OK-432 and (B) Lipopolysaccharides (LPS) (dose dependency). ○ , Control; ● , Day 4 PEC.

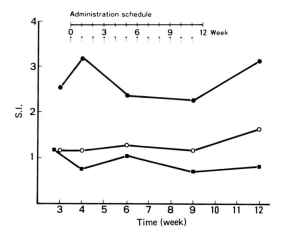

Fig. 14. Effect of OK-432 (0.05 KE/ml) on production of IL-2 (long-term administration). ○ , None added; ● , OK-432; ■ , Con A 5 μg/ml. Administration: (↑) OK-432 1 KE/mouse ip, 1 KE/week.

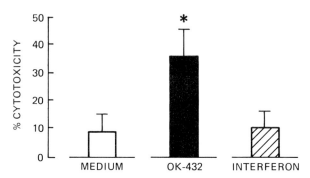

Fig. 15.   OK-432-induced autologous lymphocyte cytotoxicity.
Fresh tumor cells labeled with ^{51}Cr were incubated with self
peripheral blood lymphocytes previously activated by OK-432 or
α-interferon, and 5-hr release was determined.   Vertical bars,
SEM.   E:T = 40:1, * p < .05, n = 8.

that a large amount of IFN, consisting mainly of γ-IFN but also
some α- and β-IFN, is produced by OK-432-presensitized spleen
cells but not by BCG-primed lymphocytes.   A preliminary report by
Ichimura (unpublished) showed that IL-1 as well as IL-2 is also
produced by OK-432 stimulation (Figs. 13 and 14).   Thus, the augmentation of NK activity by OK-432 must be the result of production
of multiple lymphokines and probably monokines.

C.   Augmentation of Autologous Cytotoxicity by OK-432

    Because augmented NK activity of lymphocytes induced by stimu-
lation with OK-432 must work to kill self tumor cells in or
around the original and metastatic sites, autologous cytotoxicity
was examined on the tumor cell separated from pleural effusion.
Circulating blood MC incubated with OK-432 definitely showed a
higher rate of lymphocyte cytotoxicity against ^{51}Cr-labeled self
tumor cells than that of unstimulated PB-MC or PB-MC stimulated
with α-IFN (Uchida and Micksche, 1983) (Fig. 15).   A similar
autologous cytotoxicity was attempted in malignant lymphoma.
Naturally, the autologous cytotoxicity by unstimulated PB-MC was
absent in all cases, but preincubation of PB-MC with OK-432 for
16 hr resulted in development of cytotoxic ability against autologous tumor cells.   Preincubation of PB-MC with α-IFN or IL-2, however, failed to produce autologous cytotoxicity (Yagita and
Hoshino, 1983) (Fig. 16).

Case #	Histological Diagnosis	% Cytotoxicity of PB-MN from patient				% Cytotoxicity of PB-MN from normal subject			
		(−)	OK-432	(−)	OK-432	(−)	OK-432	(−)	OK-432
		Autologous LN cells		K562		Patient's LN cell		K562	
12	Diffuse med. sized	0	8.2	10.3	51.1	9.8	4.1	36.2	57.2
13	" "	15.0	9.3	4.0	14.1	12.3	26.5	N.D.	N.D.
14	" large cell	2.7	17.1	9.8	22.1	10.7	15.8	16.4	37.0
15	" "	0	0	8.2	8.8	0	N.D.	25.3	N.D.
17	" small cell	0	11.1	69.0	78.5	0	5.6	12.7	25.1
18	Follicular med. sized	4.3*	22.6*	31.0*	66.6*	4.0*	6.3*	25.2*	37.4*
19	Hodgkin's disease	1.2	3.1	2.5	1.4	N.D.	N.D.	N.D.	N.D.
20	IBL or ch. lymphadenitis	0	2.9	17.2	26.5	0	9.8	35.5	43.6
21	Ch lymphadenitis	0	4.1	12.1	33.3	0	5.6	24.5	72.7

Fig. 16. Effect of *in vitro* treatment of effector cells with OK-432 on lymphocyte cytotoxicity against autologous lymph node (LN) cells of patients with malignant lymphoma and K562 (E:T = 25:1, *, E:T = 50:1). N.D., Not determined.

D. Other Immunological Functions of OK-432

Other than those described already, OK-432 is known to have many other important immunological functions. An adjuvant effect of OK-432 combined with lectin or vaccine was noted by Kataoka et al. (1979). Activation of the complement system by OK-432 with increasing levels of C4, C3, and factor B in serum and on the surface of malignant cells was discovered by Kondo et al. (1978). OK-432 was found to activate the hematopoietic microenvironment with increases of endogenous and exogenous hematopoietic spleen colony (CFU-S) formation (Hiraoka et al., 1981). Neutrophil-mediated tumor cell destruction was demonstrated after OK-432 injection into cancerous ascites, along with evidence of a cytostatic effect of ascitic and circulating neutrophils on self tumor cells (Katano and Torisu, 1982). It is certain that many other actions of OK-432 in modifying biological functions will be clarified with continued progress in immunological procedures.

IV. CONCLUSION

Immunotherapy with OK-432 is here considered from clinical and experimental points of view. Administration of OK-432 either alone or in combination with chemotherapy or radiotherapy has been confirmed to be effective at least in prolonging the survival of patients with cancer, even in advanced stages. Patients successfully treated with OK-432 clearly showed recovery from impaired immune response, especially in cell-mediated immunity, suggesting that the mechanism of action of OK-432 operates through activation of the host defense system. *In vivo* and *in vitro* immunological studies in humans and animals have demonstrated multiple and complicated functions of OK-432, including activation of T-cell-mediated cytotoxicity, modulation of regulatory T cells, activation of cytotoxic or cytostatic macrophages through increased target binding and phagocytosis, augmentation of NK-cell activity in accordance with production of γ-IFN, IL-1, and IL-2, elimination or impotence of NK-suppressor macrophages and probably additional NK-enhancing factors as well, and finally, augmentation of autologous cytotoxicity. Although clinical indications and optimal routes of administration of OK-432 are not conclusively defined yet, and there still remain many additional studies to be performed to clarify the effective mechanisms of OK-432, the preparation is believed to be hopeful for use in treatment of malignant diseases.

REFERENCES

Hiraoka, A., Yamagishi, M., Ohkubo, T., Kamamoto, T., Yoshida, Y., and Uchinoh, H. (1981). *Cancer Res. 41*, 2954-2958.
Hojo, H., and Hashimoto, Y. (1981). *Gann 72*, 692-699.
Ishida, N., Saito, M., Yamaguchi, T., Ebina, T., Koi, M., and Aonuma, E. (1982). *Cell. Immunol.*, in press.
Kai, S., Tanaka, K., Nomoto, K., and Torisu, M. (1979). *Clin. Exp. Immunol. 37*, 98-105.
Katano, M., and Torisu, M. (1982). *Cancer (Philadelphia) 50*, 62-68.
Kataoka, T., Oh-Hashi, F., and Sakurai, Y. (1979). *Cancer Res. 39*, 2807-2810.
Kimura, I., Ohnoshi, T., Yasuhara, S., Sugiyama, M., Urabe, Y. and Fujii, M. (1976). *Cancer (Philadelphia) 37*, 2201-2203.
Kondo, M., Kato, H., Takemura, S., Yoshikawa, T., Yokoo, N., Ikezaki, M., and Imanishi, H. (1978). *Jpn. J. Clin. Oncol. 8*, 27-30.
Mashiba, H., Matsunaga, K., and Gojobori, M. (1979). *Gann 70*, 687-692.
Matsunaga, K., Mashiba, H., and Gojobori, M. (1980). *Gann 71*, 73-79.

Micksche, M., Kokron, O., and Uchida, A. (1982). *In* "Current Concept in Human Immunology and Cancer Immunodulation" (B. Serrou, ed.), p. 639. Elsevier, Amsterdam.
Moriyasu, F., Miwa, H., and Orita, K. (1982). *In* Immunodulation by Microbial Products and Related Synthetic Compounds" (Y. Yamamura, ed.), p. 442. Excerpta Medica, Amsterdam.
Murayama, T. (1982). *Cancer Immunol. Immunother. 12*, 141-146.
Nakazato, H. (1976). *GAN-TO-KAGAKURYOHO 3*, 715-721.
Okamoto, H., Minami, M., and Shoin, S. (1967). *Jpn. J. Exp. Med. 36*, 175-186.
Oshimi, K., Wakasugi, H., Seki, H., and Kono, S. (1980a). *Cancer Immunol. Immunother. 9*, 187-192.
Oshimi, K., Kano, S., Takaku, F., and Okumura, Y. (1980b). *J. Natl. Cancer Inst. (US) 65*, 1265-1269.
Saito, H., and Tomioka, H. (1979). *Infect. Immun. 26*, 779-782.
Saito, M., Ebina, T., Koi, M., Yamaguchi, T., Kawade, Y., and Ishida, N. (1979). *Cell. Immunol. 68*, 187-192.
Shirakawa, S. (1982). *Proc. Int. Cancer Congr. 13th*, p. 412.
Suga, S., Tunekawa, H., Washino, M., Makino, N., Tamura, Z., and Goto, S. (1977). *Gastroenterol. Jpn. 12*, 20-25.
Takakura, K. (1982). *Proc. Int. Cancer Congr. 13th*, p. 165.
Torikai, T., Itoh, O., Satoh, M., and Osawa, T. (1980). *Gann 71*, 52-59.
Torikai, T., Itoh, O., Satoh, M., Okumurao, O., and Sawa, T. (1981). *Gann 72*, 92-97.
Uchida, A., and Hoshino, T. (1980a). *Cancer (Philadelphia) 45*, 476-483.
Uchida, A., and Hoshino, T. (1980b). *Cancer Immunol. Immunother. 9*, 153-158.
Uchida, A., and Hoshino, T. (1980c). *Int. J. Cancer 26*, 401-404.
Uchida, A., and Micksche, M. (1981). *Int. J. Immunopharmacol. 3*, 365-375.
Uchida, A., and Micksche, M. (1982a). *In* "Natural Killer Cell-mediated Immunity" (R. B. Herberman, ed.), Vol. 2, p. 431. Academic Press, New York.
Uchida, A., and Micksche, M. (1982b). *In* "Natural Killer Cell-Mediated Immunity" (R. B. Herberman, ed.), Vol. 2, p. 1303. Academic Press, New York.
Uchida, A., and Micksche, M. (1983). *J. Natl. Cancer Inst. (US) 71*, 673.
Uchida, A., Micksche, M., and Hoshino, T. (1982a). *In* "Immunodulation by Microbial Products and Related Synthetic Compounds" (Y. Yamaura, ed.), p. 446. Excerpta Medica, Amsterdam.
Uchida, A., Kolb, R., and Micksche, M. (1982b). *J. Natl. Cancer Inst. (US) 68*, 735-741.
Wakasugi, H. (1982). *J. Jpn. Surg. Soc. 83*, 38-52.
Wakasugi, H., Oshimi, K., Miyata, M., and Morioka, Y. (1981). *J. Clin. Immunol. 1*, 154-162.
Watanabe, Y., and Iwa, T. (1982). *Proc. Int. Cancer Congr. 13th*, p. 358.

Yagita, M., and Hoshino, T. (1983). *Clin. Hematol.* *24*, 368.
Yasue, M., Murakami, M., Suchi, Y., and Ohta, K. (1981). *Cancer Chemother. Pharmacol.* 7, 5-10.

DISCUSSION

MATHÉ: Have you investigated multiple sclerosis patients?

HOSHINO: My colleague, Dr. Uchida, extensively studied the depres-
            sion of NK activity in multiple sclerosis, but the
            presence of suppressor monocyte is not determined yet.

POSTE: The cytotoxicity values obtained with your "NK" prepara-
            tions are substantially higher than those published in
            the literature. Would you describe the criteria by which
            you identify the NK-cell preparations used in your
            studies?

HOSHINO: We use, for instance, lytic unit instead of percentage of
            cytolysis to express the NK values. However, since per-
            centage of cytolysis is more easily understandable, we
            expressed our figures as percentage of cytolysis. Our
            system of measuring NK activity is not different from the
            others.

YOSHIDA: How about the influence of OK-432 on specific T_s cell
            activity?

HOSHINO: OK-432 was found to suppress the action of suppressor T
            cells for mitotic responsiveness of T lymphocytes.

GOLUB: Do you have an explanation for the finding that the
            peripheral blood suppressor cell found postoperation was
            found only in the cancer patients?

HOSHINO: Now, the study is going to find out the reason of appear-
            ance of suppressor monocytes, but we suppose that tumor
            cell dissemination or escape from its cancer focus by
            operative procedure may concern this phenomenon, because
            no such suppressor monocytes is found in noncancerous
            patients who underwent major operation.

CHAPTER 34

SUCCESSFUL TREATMENT OF MALIGNANT ASCITES:
CLINICAL EVALUATION AND ROLE OF HOST'S INFLAMMATORY CELLS
IN TUMOR CELL DESTRUCTION IN ASCITES

Motomichi Torisu
Masaki Sakata
Takashi Fujimura
Hideaki Itoh

Department of Surgery
Kyushu University School of Medicine
Fukuoka, Japan

Yutaka Kimura
Masaharu Takesue

Kimura Surgical Hospital
Fukuoka, Japan

Takeshi Yoshida

Department of Pathology
University of Connecticut Health Center
Farmington, Connecticut

Mitsuo Katano

Division of Surgical Oncology
University of California at Los Angeles School of Medicine
Los Angeles, California

593

I. INTRODUCTION

In recent years, as a result of the medical progress in anti-cancer therapy, the prognosis of cancer patients has generally improved. However, most far advanced cancer patients who undergo noncurative surgery or inoperable patients still have poor prognoses despite the various therapies currently available, which involve immunochemotherapeutic agents, irradiation, or endocrine therapy. Often these patients tend to develop effusions in the abdominal cavity. Patients then have to struggle against such direct distress as dyspnea due to pressure on the thorax or anorexia that leads to hypoalbuminemia.

According to various references and our own experiences with these patients, the treatment for malignant ascites have been largely unsuccessful when various chemotherapeutic agents were used (Weisberger, 1958; Suhrland and Weisberger, 1965; Paladin *et al.*, 1976; Webb, 1978). Even immunotherapy is insufficient for managing this disease, because poor immune responses are well-known characteristics of malignant ascites, and most patients do not respond to general immunostimulants. Passive drainage of the effusion has only relieved the symptoms.

A streptococcal preparation called OK-432 has been produced (Koshimura *et al.*, 1964; Okamoto *et al.*, 1966; Sakurai *et al.*, 1972) and is now in clinical use as an immunomodulator in Japan (Kimura *et al.*, 1976; Uchida and Hoshino, 1980; Watanabe and Iwa, 1982). In 1976, we encountered a patient showing serious abdominal distension because of recurrent cancer, who was given this agent into his abdominal cavity for the purpose of treatment of ascites. We were surprised to see that his ascites completely vanished simultaneously with the disappearance of tumor cells in ascitic fluid in a short period. Moreover, his life span was considerably extended. We have performed the intraperitoneal injection of OK-432 on patients with malignant ascites routinely since that time. During our study, we accomplished wonderful results of this therapy as the fruit of our efforts. Furthermore, we found that host inflammatory cells induced by OK-432 destroyed tumor cells in ascites. Previously, we reported a part of our clinical trials and the role of host inflammatory cells in tumor cell destruction (Katano and Torisu, 1982, 1983; Torisu et al., 1983). In the present chapter, we describe all aspects of this study and show the mechanisms of host inflammatory cell-mediated tumor cell destruction.

II. CLINICAL TRIAL FOR MANAGEMENT OF MALIGNANT ASCITES

A. Management Protocol and Patients

1. Streptococcal Preparation, OK-432

The preparation of OK-432 (Chugai Pharmaceutical Co., Tokyo, Japan) has been described previously (Koshimura et al., 1964; Okamoto et al., 1966; Sakurai et al., 1972). OK-432 is produced by incubating the low-virulent SU strain of type III, group A Streptococcus hemolyticus of human origin in Bernheimer's basal medium with added penicillin G potassium followed by lyophilization of the incubation mixture. This lyophilized preparation is designated OK-432. A unit of KE (klinische Einheit) is used to express the strength of the preparation. One KE of OK-432 is equivalent to approximately 0.1 mg lyophilized preparation of heat-killed Streptococcus hemolyticus. This agent was shown to have not only stimulatory effects on cell-mediated immunity (Ishii et al., 1976; Sakai et al., 1976; Kai et al., 1979) but also direct cytotoxic activity on malignant cells (Sakurai et al., 1972; Ono et al., 1973). Biological activity of OK-432 remains stable for more than 2 years if stored dry at room temperature. The preparation is suspended in sterilized saline just before use.

2. Management Protocol

a. Intraperitoneal Injection of OK-432. Cytological examination was performed as ascitic fluid before treatment. Then, OK-432 was given intraperitoneally once a week at dosages ranging from 5 to 20 KE, suspended in 20 ml saline, until the fluid disappeared. If adhesions of the peritoneal cavity were remarkable and the ascitic cavity could not be confirmed clearly, the injection was carried out using echo-guide technique.

b. Intrapleural Injection of OK-432. OK-432 was given intrapleurally by the same schedule as the intraperitoneal injection.

c. Intradermal Injection of OK-432. OK-432 was given intradermally at dosages ranging from 1 to 2 KE, suspended in 1 ml
saline three times a week.

3. Patients

Two hundred patients with malignant ascites originating in
stomach and colorectal regions were divided into two groups,
called OK-432 therapy group and palliative therapy group. To
minimize bias in selection of patients, the selection was conducted in a blind manner. The selection ratio of OK-432 therapy
group to palliative therapy group was 3:1, 150 patients for OK-432
therapy and 50 for palliative treatment (Torisu *et al.*, 1983).
Thus, both groups were similar in terms of age, sex, performance
status, and type of disease (Table I). No patient in either group
was receiving chemotherapeutic agents at the time of this study.
Paracentesis was performed as required for patients' comfort.

4. Case Presentation

The patient is a 38-year-old man who had noticed heartburn
about 1 year previously. He came to the hospital because of a
sense of abdominal fullness, weight loss and anorexia. On examination, his abdomen was remarkably distended and measured
99-100 cm in girth. Cytological examination of the fluid
revealed numerous tumor cells in ascites. An upper GI series
showed a large mass in his stomach. Metastatic mass was suspected
in scintigram of the liver. According to these findings, the
disease was judged to be too advanced to benefit from any surgical
treatment.
Then, he was admitted to our hospital for treatment of
ascites. On Days 2 and 9 after admission, respectively, he was
given 10 and 15 KE of OK-432 intraperitoneally. In addition,
general management such as transfusion, correction of electrolytes,
and diuretics was started. During our treatment, ascitic fluid
began to decrease in volume and completely disappeared 15 days
after the first injection of OK-432. He left the hospital 1 month
after admission and was maintained by intradermal injection of
OK-432 three times a week.
Four months later, we decided to perform surgery, because his
general condition was remarkably improved, although tumor size
was unchanged according to an upper GI series. Laparotomy revealed no ascites, but the tumor had invaded the entire stomach,
transverse colon, small intestine, and distal pancreas. Total
gastrectomy and removal of involved organs were carried out. Nine
days after the operation, 10 mg of living BCG were injected intradermally for systemic immunotherapy (Torisu *et al.*, 1975). He
was discharged 3 months after the operation and had been maintained
by intradermal injection of OK-432 once a week.

TABLE I

Characteristics of Patients with Malignant Ascites
and Therapeutic Schedule

	OK-432 therapy group	Palliative therapy group
Number of patients	150	50
Male:female ratio	92:58	32:18
Age range (mean)	24-82 (57.4)	24-81 (55.6)
Gastric cancer	124	45
Colorectal cancer	26	5
Performance status		
Grade I	0	0
Grade II	0	0
Grade III	38	12
Grade IV	112	38
Therapeutic schedule	OK-432 ip, paracentesis, diuretics, blood transfusion	Paracentesis, diuretics, blood transfusion

Two years later, he was readmitted because of reaccumulation of ascites. Ten KE of OK-432 were given intraperitoneally once a week. On Day 14, ascitic fluid had again completely disappeared. He left the hospital 1 month after this admission, but he complained of dyspnea and weight loss 3 months after discharge. On examination, chest X-ray film showed right pleural effusion. Cytological examination of the fluid revealed many adenocarcinoma cells in the effusion. Ten KE of OK-432 were then given intrapleurally. On Day 4, pleural effusion had disappeared completely, and he left the hospital 20 days after admission. Currently, he is free from both ascites and pleural effusion. The clinical course of this patient is summarized in Fig. 1.

B. Clinical Evaluation of OK-432 Therapy

1. *Effect of Intraperitoneal Injection of OK-432*

The effect of intraperitoneal injection of OK-432 on malignant ascites of 150 patients was studied. After OK-432 therapy, 85 patients showed complete disappearance of ascites and 9 had a definite reduction of their ascites (Fig. 2). The two combined were classified as the responder group, which comprised more than 62% of the total number of patients. The mean period from the

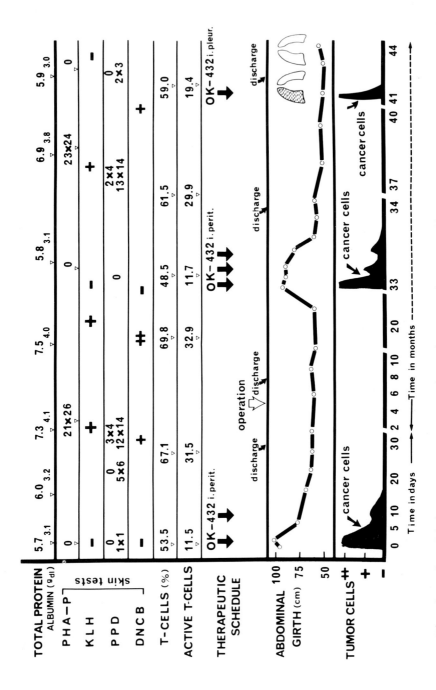

Fig. 1. The clinical course of a patient (see Section II,A,4) treated with intraperitoneal injection of OK-432.

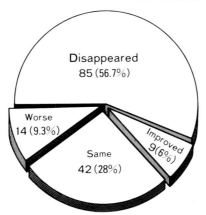

Fig. 2.   Effect of OK-432 therapy on 150 patients with malignant ascites. The effect was divided into four grades: disappeared, complete disappearance of ascites; improved, decrease in
abdominal girth by ≥ 10 cm; same, decrease in abdominal girth by
<9 cm or increase by <3 cm; worse, increase in abdominal girth by
>4 cm.

first disappearance of ascites to reaccumulation was 10.8 months,
ranging from 3.2 to over 38.6 months.
     The nonresponder group (56 patients) was composed of 42
patients who showed no significant change in volume of ascites
and 14 patients whose ascites increased despite the therapy. In
contrast, of 50 patients who received palliative therapy, only
12 had a very short transient decrease of ascites, ranging from
a few days to 1 month.
     In 85 patients who showed complete disappearance of ascites
after OK-432 therapy, the mean period from the first administration of OK-432 to its disappearance was 21.5 days, ranging from
9 to 48 days (Table II). Consequently, we consider that further
administration of OK-432 is not valid if a patient shows no significant reduction in ascitic fluid volume 2 months after the
first administration.

2. *Relationship between Disappearance of Ascites and Cytological
    Findings of Ascites*

     Cytological examinations were performed on ascitic fluid from
150 patients before therapy. Tumor cells were apparently detected
in samples from 85 patients. In our early experiences, we had
felt that this therapy was more effective in patients who were
positive for tumor cells in ascitic fluid prior to the therapy
than in negative cases. Consequently, we divided the patients
who received OK-432 therapy into two groups; one group contained
the patients who were positive for tumor cells in ascites (85),
and the other consisted of those who were negative (65).

600   MOTOMICHI TORISU ET AL.

TABLE II

Duration from OK-432 Injection to Disappearance of Ascites

Number of patients	Duration in days (mean ± SD)
85	9-48 (21.5 ± 6.9)

Interestingly, 68 of 85 patients (80%) with tumor cell-positive ascites had remarkable reductions in ascitic fluid volume after the therapy. In contrast, only 16 patients of 65 (24.6%) with undetectable tumor cells in ascites had seen improvement (Fig. 3). This difference is statistically significant ($p < .001$). These results strongly suggest that this therapy is more effective for patients with tumor cell-bearing ascites than for those who have only ascites.

The ascites of cancer patients appears to be caused by various mechanisms including portal or lymphatic obstruction by tumor mass, hypoproteinemia, complicated cirrhosis of the liver, and carcinomatous peritonitis. In particular, tumor cells usually do not appear in ascitic fluid caused by mechanical obstruction, hypoalbuminemia, or cirrhosis of the liver. Therefore, this therapy may be reasonable to perform only for patients with carcinomatous peritonitis.

3. Changes of Immunological Responses after OK-432 Therapy

It is well known that immune responses are markedly suppressed in advanced cancer patients, and that these suppressions are closely correlated to advances of disease despite primary lesions.

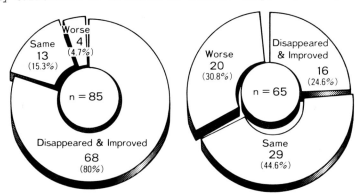

Positive for tumor cells   Negative for tumor cells

Fig. 3. Relationship between effects of OK-432 therapy and cytological findings as ascitic fluid before the injection.

TABLE III

Immune Responses in Patients with Malignant Ascites

Clinical parameters	Stage IV with ascites (n = 100)	Stage IV without ascites (n = 100)	Healthy (n = 100)
Skin test (% positive)			
PPD	12.3	21.6	92.6
PHA-P	20.5	33.8	97.3
DNCB	15.8	25.3	86.7
KLH	14.3	29.5	95.5
Cellular parameters[a]			
T cell (%)	40.3 ± 19.1	52.8 ± 11.3	64.5 ± 9.8
B cell (%)	48.6 ± 15.3	45.1 ± 9.8	35.1 ± 8.9
Active T cell (%)	19.8 ± 11.4	21.5 ± 10.3	39.8 ± 6.4
Random migration[b]	0.86 ± 0.54	1.92 ± 1.53	3.96 ± 1.13
Chemotactic activity (%)	26.4 ± 11.5	38.2 ± 19.3	99.7 ± 12.7

[a]Mean ± SD.
[b]Arbitrary unit in micrometer of microscope.

For example, the immunological potency of stage IV cancer patients
is more suppressed than that of stage III patients. Since the
early 1970s, we have conducted immunotherapy on advanced cancer
patients (Torisu *et al.*, 1975, 1977, 1978). Various skin tests,
such as PPD, DNCB, KLH, and PHA-P were employed. We also studied
circulating T-lymphocyte levels, active T-cell counts, random
migration tests, and chemotactic assays for the neutrophils.
Methodological details were described elsewhere (Boyden, 1951;
David *et al.*, 1964; Tachibana and Ishikawa, 1973; Torisu *et al.*,
1975, 1978).

To assess the immunological capability of patients with malignant ascites, immune responses of stage IV patients with ascites
were compared with those of stage IV patients without ascites
(Table III). All of these parameters were significantly suppressed
in patients at stage IV without ascites, but in particular, stage
IV patients with ascites were remarkably suppressed in these
parameters. Our previous experimences had shown that immune responses of stage IV patients with ascites were not improved despite inoculation of living BCG, which is one of the most powerful
immunopotentiators (Mathé *et al.*, 1969; Morton, 1970; Gutterman
et al., 1974). Therefore, the patients with malignant ascites are
thought to be in an immunologically deficient state.

Nevertheless, following our study, positive skin tests and
T-cell counts were significantly improved for responders (Fig. 4).
These improvements of various parameters usually appeared 1 month
after the first injection of OK-432. In addition, serum protein
levels of the responder group were gradually elevated after the
therapy. The elevation of serum protein level was closely associated with a decrease in protein level in ascites (Katano and
Torisu, 1983). Therefore, the immunological improvement could be
noted only after ascites became reduced. The improvement in general health certainly benefited the responder, because improvement
in the immunological parameters was not obtained if ascitic fluid
was merely removed by paracentesis.

In contrast, nonresponders had no significant changes despite
this therapy. For the patients who received palliative therapy,
none of these parameters changed.

4. Survival Time

On the results of intraperitoneal injection of OK-432, survival
time of the OK-432 therapy group was compared to that of the palliative therapy group. The mean survival time of the OK-432
therapy group was 10.2 months, ranging from 0.2 to 36.4 months;
that of the palliative therapy group was 2.9 months ranging from
0.2 to 10.3 months. This difference was statistically significant
($p < .05$). There were no significant differences in age, sex,
performance status, or stage or type of disease between the two
groups, retrospectively. When the responder group (85 patients)
was analyzed separately, the mean survival time was 15.3 months

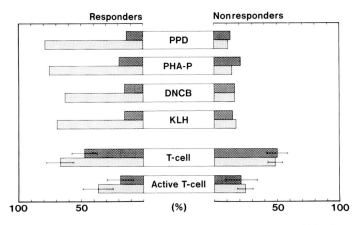

Fig. 4.   Changes in immune responses after OK-432 therapy. These parameters were measured before (dark shading) and 30 days after (light shading) the first injection.

($p < .001$), ranging from 2.9 to 36.4 months (Fig. 5) (Torisu *et al.*, 1983).   These results indicate that OK-432 therapy provides significant prolongation of survival time for patients with malignant ascites.

5. *Side Effects*

This therapy induced some side effects such as high fever, chills, nausea, and abdominal pain and distention.   High fever was experienced in 135 patients (90%) in the OK-432 therapy group; in 61 of these 135 patients, the high fever was accompanied by chills. Moreover, high fever generally continued for 2 to 3 days after each injection of OK-432, but it was easy to control with antifebrile medications.   Neutrophils increased in number not only in

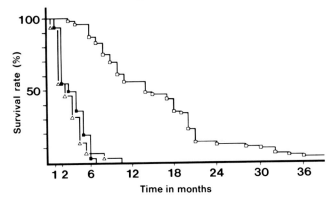

Fig. 5.   Comparison of survival rate between groups treated with and without OK-432.   □ Responders ($n = 85$); △ nonresponders ($n = 65$);   ■ , palliative therapy ($n = 50$).   (From Torisu *et al.*, 1983).

TABLE IV

Side Effects of OK-432 Therapy in 150 Patients

Clinical signs	Number of patients	Percentage
Fever	135	90.0
Chills	61	40.7
Nausea	43	28.7
Vomiting	8	5.3
Abdominal pain	33	22.0
Abdominal distension	37	24.7
Leukocytosis	138	92.0
Leukopenia	5	3.3

the abdominal cavity but also in the peripheral blood. The peripheral leukocytosis usually continued for 7 to 10 days and sometimes for more than a month without fever (Torisu *et al.*, 1983). This leukocytosis is a characteristic phenomenon of OK-432 therapy, unlike other chemotherapeutic agents, and it may be advantageous for cancer patients whose immune responses are generally depressed. Moreover, no other serious complication such as anaphylactic shock, liver dysfunction, renal failure, or ileus has been experienced throughout this study (Table IV).

III. INTERACTION BETWEEN HOST'S INFLAMMATORY CELLS AND TUMOR CELLS

During our clinical study, various inflammatory cells such as neutrophils, macrophages, and lymphocytes accumulated in the peritoneal cavity after the injection of OK-432. The inflammatory cells induced by OK-432 attached to tumor cells and finally destroyed them *in vivo*. In addition, inflammatory cells derived from ascites inhibited DNA synthesis of tumor cells *in vitro*. We previously reported preliminary data on our investigation and methodological details (Katano and Torisu, 1982, 1983; Torisu *et al.*, 1983).

After such preliminary study, we performed frequent examinations of ascitic fluid and study of DNA synthesis in tumor cells in additional patients. Details of cytological examinations are as follows. Ascitic fluid was obtained by paracentesis. Direct smear of fluid was made immediately before and 3, 6, and 12 hr after the injection of OK-432. Smears were then checked daily until the fluid had disappeared. Six cell types were identified by Giemsa and Papanicolaou stains: tumor cells, macrophages, lymphocytes, neutrophils, eosinophils, and mesothelial cells.

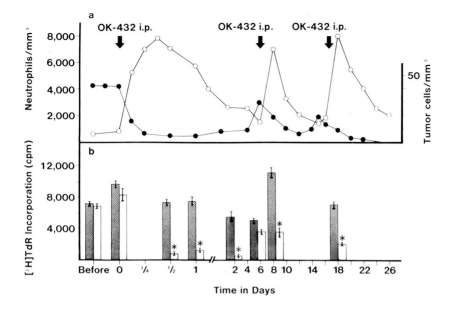

Fig. 6. Effect of neutrophils derived from ascitic fluid on
DNA synthesis of tumor cells. (a) Changes in number of neutrophils (○) and tumor cells (●) in ascites after OK-432 injection.
(b) Effects of neutrophils derived from ascitic fluid on DNA
synthesis of tumor cells. A neutrophil:tumor cell ratio of 100:1
was employed. Tumor cells (dark shading); tumor cells + PMNs
(light shading; * p < .001. (From Katano and Torisu, 1983.)

Careful cell counts were kept, and particular attention was paid
to the number of tumor cells and other inflammatory cells before
and after injection. In this section, we show the precise process
of interactions between various host's cells and tumor cells.
Moreover, we report that host's inflammatory cells that predominate
in killing tumor cells in ascites differ among patients.

A. Neutrophil-Mediated Tumor Cell Destruction

Numerous neutrophils usually accumulated in the peritoneal
cavity soon after the injection of OK-432. A typical example of
this process was observed between neutrophils and tumor cells in
ascites (Fig. 6). From 3 to 6 hr after the injection, neutrophils
strikingly increased in number in ascites. The neutrophils
reached their maximum number from 2 to 3 days after the injection,
then began to decrease in number. In contrast, tumor cells
rapidly decreased in number after the injection but began to increase in number on approximately Day 6 in this case. An
additional injection of OK-432 was performed in the same manner
as the first administration on Day 7. Neutrophils and tumor cells

showed a similar pattern in number in ascites. After the third
injection of OK-432, tumor cells completely disappeared from
ascites (Fig. 6a).

In order to examine whether disappearance of tumor cells
directly correlates with appearance of neutrophils derived from
ascites, the effect of neutrophils on the DNA synthesis of tumor
cells was studied by [^{3}H]thymidine incorporation. Tumor cell DNA
synthesis was significantly inhibited by neutrophils induced by
OK-432 but not by neutrophils before the injection (Fig. 6b).

Moreover, we could observe the morphological process of tumor
cell destruction on glass slides. After the injection, neutrophils surrounded clusters of tumor cells, attached tightly, and
infiltrated into the clusters in ascites. Finally, neutrophils
invaded the cytoplasm of tumor cells and destroyed them *in vivo*
(Fig. 7a-h). These results indicate that neutrophils induced by
OK-432 play a most important role in tumor cell destruction in
ascites.

B. Macrophage-Mediated Tumor Cell Destruction

Although neutrophils usually increased in number in ascites
after the injection, in some cases, macrophages greatly increased
in number. In these circumstances, we observed macrophages as
well as neutrophils surrounding, attaching to, and finally
destroying tumor cells on glass slides (Fig. 8a-d). In addition,
it was chiefly macrophages that destroyed tumor cells again after
the second injection. The macrophages induced by OK-432 were
thought to be in an activated state.

The effect of macrophages on DNA synthesis of tumor cells
was studied in eight patients with malignant ascites. Macrophages derived from ascitic fluid 4-6 days after the injection
significantly inhibited DNA synthesis in seven of the eight
patients (Fig. 9). However, macrophages obtained before the injection showed no significant inhibition of DNA synthesis of tumor
cells.

C. Lymphocyte-Mediated Tumor Cell Destruction

In other patients, lymphocytes played an important role in
tumor cell destruction in ascites. Lymphocytes induced by OK-432
dominantly attached and invaded the cytoplasm of tumor cells in
these cases (Fig. 10a and b). Previously we had identified the
lymphocytes as T-cell subpopulations (Katano and Torisu, 1983).
Moreover, lymphocytes obtained by paracentesis 4-6 days after the
injection were cultured with tumor cells. The lymphocytes strongly
inhibited DNA synthesis of tumor cells in four of seven patients
(Fig. 11).

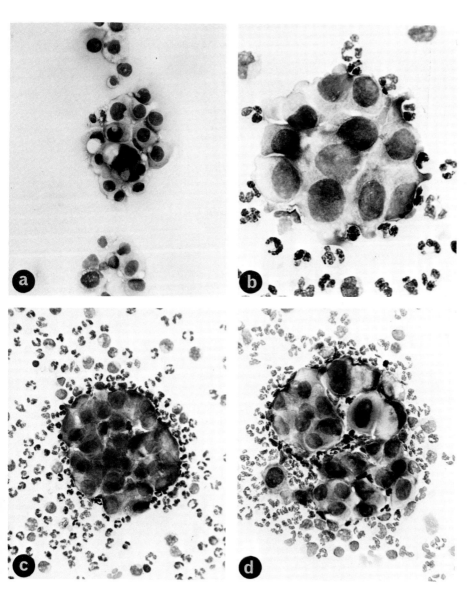

Fig. 7. Morphological interaction between neutrophils and
tumor cells in ascites after the injection of OK-432. (a) Tumor
cells are mainly found in ascites before therapy (×360). (b) Some
neutrophils start to associate closely with the cluster of tumor
cells, 3 hr after injection (×980). (c) Numerous neutrophils contact tightly with the cluster, 6 hr after injection (×360).
(d) Neutrophils begin to infiltrate the cluster, 12 hr after

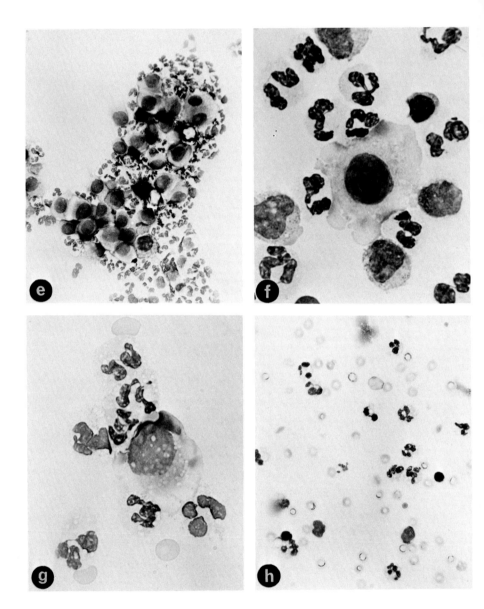

injection (×450). (e) Infiltrating neutrophils almost disconnect
the cluster, 24 hr after injection (×450). (f) Three neutrophils
invade the cytoplasm of tumor cell, 2 days after injection
(×1440). (g) Neutrophils have almost destroyed the tumor cell,
4 days after injection (×1440). (h) Tumor cells have completely
disappeared from ascites, 10 days after injection (×540).

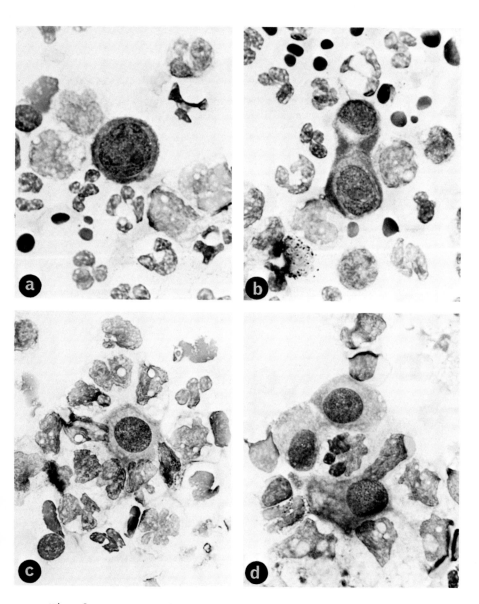

Fig. 8. Morphological interaction between macrophages and tumor cells in ascites after the injection of OK-432. (a) A tumor cell is surrounded by macrophages and neutrophils, 12 hr after injection (×1500). (b) Some macrophages attach to the tumor cells, 24 hr after injection (×1500). (c) Macrophages attach to the tumor cell more tightly, 2 days after injection (×1180). (d) Macrophages invade the cytoplasm of tumor cell, 3 days after injection (×1560).

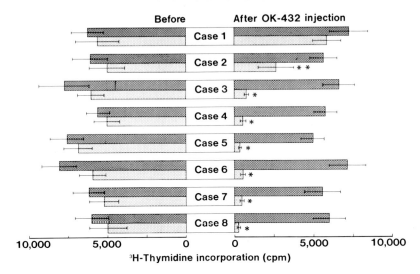

Fig. 9. Effect of macrophages derived from ascites on DNA synthesis of tumor cells. Macrophages were obtained 4-6 days after the injection of OK-432. A macrophage:tumor cell ratio of 10:1 was employed. Tumor cells (dark shading); tumor cells + macrophages (light shading); ** $p < .05$; * $p < .01$. (From Katano and Torisu, 1983.)

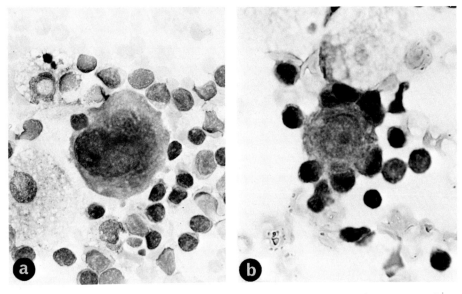

Fig. 10. Morphological interaction between lymphocytes and tumor cells in ascites after the injection of OK-432. (a) A tumor cell is surrounded by some lymphocytes, 4 days after injection (×1280). (b) Lymphocytes attach tightly and invade into the cytoplasm of tumor cell, 6 days after injection (×1440).

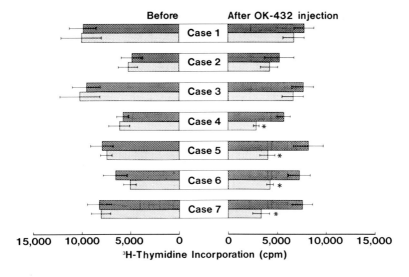

Before   **After OK-432 injection**

Case 1
Case 2
Case 3
Case 4
Case 5
Case 6
Case 7

15,000 10,000 5,000 0   0 5,000 10,000 15,000
³H-Thymidine Incorporation (cpm)

Fig. 11. Effect of lymphocytes derived from ascites on DNA synthesis of tumor cells. Lymphocytes were obtained 5-7 days after the injection of OK-432. A lymphocyte:tumor cell ratio of 20:1 was employed. Tumor cells (dark shading); tumor cells + lymphocytes (light shading); * *p* < .05. (From Katano and Torisu, 1983.)

IV. CONCLUSIONS

A total of 150 patients with malignant ascites caused by gastric or colorectal cancer were managed with the intraperitoneal injection of OK-432. In 85 patients (56.7%), ascites disappeared completely, and 9 (6%) had definite reduction in their ascites. Mean survival time of this therapy (10.2 months) was significantly prolonged over that of the palliative therapy group (2.9 months). In addition, an interesting characteristic of OK-432 therapy is an improvement of host's immune responses.

The effect of this therapy was closely correlated with cytological findings on effusions prior to the treatment. Namely, this therapy is more effective in patients who are positive for tumor cells in ascitic fluid than in negative patients. Therefore, OK-432 therapy may be the most effective in patients with carcinomatous peritonitis.

During our study, we were able to observe on glass slides that various inflammatory cells such as neutrophils, macrophages, and lymphocytes accumulated in the abdominal cavity after the injection of OK-432, attached to tumor cells, and finally destroyed them in ascites *in vivo*. Moreover, such inflammatory cells induced by OK-432 inhibited DNA synthesis of tumor cells *in vitro*. These results strongly suggest that host's inflammatory cells play an important role in tumor cell destruction in ascites.

Overall, we believe that the intraperitoneal injection of OK-432 is the most beneficial management of malignant ascites.

ACKNOWLEDGMENT

We express our thanks to Drs. F. Nakayama (First Department of Surgery, Kyushu University School of Medicine, Fukuoka, Japan) and T. Hirose (Hirose Surgical Hospital) for allowing us to study their patients.

The authors also thank T. Nishimura (Fukuoka University School of Medicine, Fukuoka, Japan), M. Ota (Central Laboratory, Kyushu University School of Medicine), and W. Goromaru (Kimura Surgical Hospital, Fukuoka, Japan) for their advice in preparing the cytological materials and photographs, and K. Matsui, Y. Horie, and K. Yasutake for their skillful technique.

REFERENCES

Boyden, S. W. (1951). *J. Exp. Med.* 93, 107-120.
David, J. R., Al-Askari, S., Lawrence, H. S., and Thomas, L. (1964). *J. Immunol.* 93, 264-273.
Gutterman, J. U., Mavlight, G., McBride, C. M., Frei III, E., and Hersh, E. M. (1974). *In* "Recent Results in Cancer Research" (G. Mathé and R. Weiner, eds.), Vol. 47, pp. 476-485. Springer-Verlag, Berlin.
Ishii, Y., Yamaoka, H., Toh, K., and Kikuchi, K. (1976). *Gann 67*, 115-119.
Kai, S., Tanaka, J., Nomoto, K., and Torisu, M. (1979). *Clin. Exp. Immunol.* 37, 98-105.
Katano, M., and Torisu, M. (1982). *Cancer 50*, 62-68.
Katano, M., and Torisu, M. (1983). *Surgery 93*, 365-373.
Kimura, I., Ohnishi, T., Yasuhara, S., Sugiyama, M., Urabe, Y., Fujii, M., and Machida, K. (1976). *Cancer 37*, 2201-2203.
Koshimura, S., Shimizu, R., Fujimura, A., and Okamoto, H. (1964). *Gann 55*, 233-236.
Mathé, G., Amiel, J. L., Schwarzenberg, L., Schneider, M., Cattan, A., Schlumberger, J. R., Hayat, M., and De Vassal, F. (1969). *Lancet 1*, 697-699.
Morton, D. L. (1970). *Surgery 68*, 158-164.
Okamoto, H., Minami, M., Shoin, S., Koshimura, S., and Shimizu, R. (1966). *Jap. J. Exp. Med.* 36, 175-186.
Ono, T., Kurata, S., Wakabayashi, K., Sugawara, Y., Saito, M., and Ogawa, H. (1973). *Gann 64*, 59-69.

Paladin, W., Gunningham, T. J., Sponzo, R., Donavan, M., Olson, K., and Horton, J. (1976). *Cancer 38*, 1903-1908.
Sakai, S. N., Ryoyama, K., Koshimura, S., and Migita, S. (1976). *Jap. J. Exp. Med. 46*, 123-133.
Sakurai, S., Tsukagoshi, S., Satoh, H., Akiba, T., Suzuki, S., and Takagaki, Y. (1972). *Cancer Chemother. Rep. 56*, 9-17.
Suhrland, L. G., and Weisberger, A. S. (1965). *Arch. Intern. Med. 116*, 431-433.
Tachibana, T., and Ishikawa, M. (1973). *Jap. J. Exp. Med. 43*, 227-230.
Torisu, M., Fukawa, M., Nishimura, M., Harasaki, H., Kai, S., and Tanaka, J. (1975). *In* "International Conference on Immunotherapy of Cancer" (C. H. Southman and H. Friedman, eds.), Vol. 277, pp. 160-186. *Ann. N.Y. Acad. Sci.*
Torisu, M., Miyahara, T., Fujiwara, H., Ohsato, K., Okano, H., and Tanaka, J. (1977). *In* "Immunotherapy of Malignant Disease" (H. Reiner, ed.), pp. 137-142. Schattauer Verlag, Stuttgart.
Torisu, M., Miyahara, T., Yamamoto, T., Harada, M., Fujiwara, H., Kitamura, Y., Jimi, M., Ohsato, K., Tanaka, J., and Fukawa, M. (1978). *Gann Monogr. 21*, 173-179.
Torisu, M., Katano, M., Kimura, M., Itoh, H., and Takesue, M. (1983). *Surgery 93*, 357-364.
Uchida, A., and Hoshino, T. (1980). *Cancer 45*, 476-483.
Watanabe, Y., and Iwa, T. (1982). *Proc. 13th Intern. Cancer Congr., Seattle 1982*, p. 358.
Webb, H. E. (1978). *Br. Med. J. 1*, 383-384.
Weisberger, A. S. (1958). *Ann. N.Y. Acad. Sci. 68*, 1091-1096.

DISCUSSION

COCHRAN: You show clear evidence of an acute inflammatory infiltrate followed by mononuclear cell accumulation. The slides showed tumor cells dying on contact with mononuclear cells. How strong is your evidence that polymorphs are the main tumor cell killers and in what proportion of patients are the polymorphs most important?

TORISU: Because of the relatively small number of patients we have examined, it is rather difficult to say the exact percentage. However, definitely more than 20% of cases have shown polymorphonuclear infiltrates predominantly throughout the treatment. As shown in my presentation, you can see tumor cells dying on contact with polys in such cases but not with mononuclear cells. I agree that sometimes polys infiltration is typically followed by mononuclear infiltration, although I wanted to stress the amazingly active participation of polys in destruction of tumor cells.

GOLUB: The neutrophils could mediate antibody-dependent cellular cytotoxicity via an Fc receptor. Do the ascites tumor cells have antibody on their membranes?

TORISU: That is a good question, but we have not looked at that yet.

COCHRAN: Is the leukocytosis due to polymorphs? Do patients who do not get a leukocytosis respond to therapy?

TORISU: Yes, it is due to polys. Those who do not get leukocytosis (about 10%) do not respond well to therapy.

COHEN: Is the pattern of inflammatory response constant in a given patient? In other words, if you find on one occasion neutrophils, are you more likely to find neutrophils than other inflammatory cells at the time of second treatment? Also, it may be better for the patient to have fever, as this could make the cells more active. Also, it may reflect interleukin-1 activity, which might activate lymphocytes.

TORISU: Yes, they usually follow the same pattern. It is possible that IL-1 activity is enhanced, although we have not examined this.

K. YOSHIDA: Is there any difference in drug sensitivity between a primary tumor and a recurring one?

TORISU: There is no difference.

MATHES: Do you get a similar result in other sites than the ascitic compartment?

TORISU: Not as dramatic as this with end-stage ascites tumor cells, but we do not have enough data to compare with other organs.

OKADA: You have clearly shown that in patients who have little or no tumor cells in ascites fluid, OK-432 administration affected them poorly. Does this mean that immunological unresponsiveness prevents, unexpectedly, invasion of tumor cells to the peritoneal cavity? Or, the absence of the tumor cells in the peritoneal cavity failed to stimulate immune response to tumor cells with the support of OK-432 administered intraperitoneally?

TORISU: I think you may have misunderstood our presentation.
            At the end stage of cancer, different factors may
            cause the accumulation of ascitic fluid. What I
            have shown in this presentation is that ascites
            caused by tumor cells disseminated into the peritoneal
            cavity could be remarkably cured by this treatment.
            However, the ascites fluid that might be caused by ob-
            struction of circulation, and so forth, by tumor mass
            in major organs such as liver and stomach, could not
            be affected by the treatment, since the treatment had
            only a minimal effect on the primary tumor lesion when
            injected intraperitoneally above.

CHAPTER 35

IMMUNOTHERAPY VERSUS CHEMOIMMUNOTHERAPY
AS ADJUVANT TREATMENT OF MALIGNANT MELANOMA

G. Mathé
J. L. Misset
B. Serrou
C. Jeanne
J. Guerrin
R. Plagne
M. Schneider
B. Le Mevel
R. Metz
Study analysis: M. Delgado and F. de Vassal
Statistical analysis: V. Morice

Institut de Cancérologie et d'Immunogénétique (INSERM, CNRS)
et Service des Maladies Sanguines et Tumorales
Groupe Hospitalier Paul-Brousse
Villejuif, France

BASIC MECHANISMS AND CLINICAL TREATMENT
OF TUMOR METASTASIS

I.   INTRODUCTION

     Satisfactory adjuvant treatment for melanoma is as yet un-
known. Preliminary reports were enthusiastic concerning
immunotherapy (Gutterman et al., 1973; Eilber et al., 1976), but
follow-up reports or final results of randomized trials have
been disappointing (Cunningham et al., 1979; Spitler and Sagebiel,
1980; Morton et al., 1982). However, most trials on immunotherapy of melanoma have shown, or still show, a transitory or
persisting beneficial effect (Eilber et al., 1976; Patterson et
al., 1979; Morton et al., 1982). Other trials have dealt with
adjuvant chemotherapy or chemoimmunotherapy (Banzet et al., 1978;
Beretta, 1982; Terry.et al., 1982; Wood et al., 1982). Although
here again the results arc not identical: several studies suggest
that any adjuvant treatment may be better than no adjuvant treatment at all (Beretta, 1982), or that chemoimmunotherapy may be
better than chemotherapy alone (Banzet et al., 1978; Wood et al.,
1982).
     In 1975, ONCOFRANCE Group (formerly Groupe Inter France of
GIF) initiated a trial on adjuvant treatment of melanoma. At
that time, reported results on immunotherapy (Gutterman et al.,
1973; Eilber et al., 1976) were considered quite convincing and
it seemed unethical to have a control group. Thus, GIF decided
to compare, in a randomized trial, adjuvant immunotherapy with
BCG for 2 years, with the same immunotherapy following 6 months
of adjuvant chemotherapy combining drugs active on melanoma:di-
ethyltriazenoimidazole carboxamide (DTIC) and 1-(2-chloroethyl)-3-
cyclohexyl-1-nitrosourea (CCNU) (Comis and Carter, 1974) and
epipodophyllotoxin (VM26), a spindle poison able to potentiate
the action of other cytotoxic drugs (Pouillart et al., 1975). A
total of 280 patients have entered the trial, and we present here
the results with a maximum follow-up time of 5 years and a median
follow-up time of slightly less than 3 years.

II.   PATIENTS AND METHODS

A.   Eligibility

     Conditions for eligibility for the trial were (a) histological-
ly confirmed malignant melanoma, either of Clark grade III, IV, or
V (McGovern et al., 1973), or with any Clark grade but with
positive regional lymph nodes, (b) surgical removal of all
detectable disease not more than 6 weeks before randomization
(lymph node dissection was mandatory only in case of suspicion of
lymph node involvement), (c) patients had to be under 70 years of
age, have no history of other malignant disease or of a disease

TABLE I

Stratification of Patients

Stratification criteria	Immunotherapy	Chemoimmunotherapy	p
Sex			
Males	61	74	.25
Females	72	73	.93
Stage			
I	120	130	.63
II	13	17	.44
Clark			
III	74	77	.80
IV	43	56	.19
V	11	12	.85
Unknown	5	2	--
Site of primary tumor			
Head and neck			
Stage I	15	20	.41
Stage II	2	1	--
Trunk			
Stage I	34	34	--
Stage II	6	2	--
Upper limb			
Stage I	13	20	.22
Stage II	2	3	--
Lower limb			
Stage I	58	56	.85
Stage II	4	10	--

contraindicating one of the treatment branches and (d) patients should not have previously received radio-, chemo-, or immunotherapy.

B. Stratification (Table I)

Patients were stratified according to lymph node status (stage I or II) and localization of the primary tumor (head and neck, trunk, upper limb (lower limb). At the time the trial was initiated, sex was not known to be a significant prognostic factor for melanoma and was not included as a stratification parameter. Fortunately, random allocation of patients in each treatment group was equalized as far as sex was concerned. The same applied to stratification according to Clark grade in Stage I patients, which happened to be equalized a posteriori.

C.   Treatment

Patients were allocated at random in each stratification
category mentioned, to receive either (group A) Immuno BCG
Pasteur, 75 mg on weekly scarification rotating on the four limbs
for 2 years, or (group B) the same immunotherapy following
6 months of chemotherapy as follows: VM26 60 mg/m^2 iv on Day 1
every 4 weeks, DTIC 150 mg/m^2 on Days 2, 3, 4, and 5 every 4 weeks,
CCNU 60 mg/m^2 on Days 2 and 3 orally every 8 weeks.

D.   Patients

Of the 280 patients who entered the trial between February
1975 and August 1980, 250 had stage I melanoma and 30 stage II.
A total of 151 had Clark III, 99 Clark IV, 23 Clark V, and 7 had
Clark level unknown but had stage II melanoma.   There were 135
males and 145 females.   Stage I primary tumors were located in
35 patients in the head and neck, in 68 patients in the trunk, 33
in the upper limb, and 114 in the lower limb.

III.   RESULTS

Tolerance of the regimen was good.   No major toxicity occurred,
and the chemotherapy as well as immunotherapy program could be
performed according to the protocol schedule in most cases.   Of
147 patients in the chemotherapy branch, 7 (5%) had to postpone
one or several cycles of chemotherapy or reduce the dosage of the
drugs because of hematological toxicity.   Sixteen patients (10.8%)
had their chemotherapy discontinued before completion of the
program because of hematological or gastrointestinal toxicity.
No complication of cytopenia was reported.   Of 280 patients receiving immunotherapy, 13 (4.5%) had to modify the schedule of
BCG (reduce the dosage or scarify only every other week) because
of local or general reactions (fever, malaise); 8 patients (2.8%)
refused continuation of the program because of these side effects.
Overall survival and disease-free survival curves are drawn
according to the Kaplan-Meier method (Peto, 1978) and comparison
of curves is made by the log-rank test.   At 5 years, 53.7% of the
patients are in first complete remission and 65.6% are alive.   At
median follow-up time of more than 2.5 years, 62% of the patients
were in first remission, and 76 were alive.
Prognostic factors were studied, and sex was significant in
favor of females for disease-free survival (p = .002) and for
survival (p = .008).   Clark level was significant in terms of
survival with a p value (test for trend) of .02.   No prognostic
value of the location of the primary tumor could be found (p = .9).

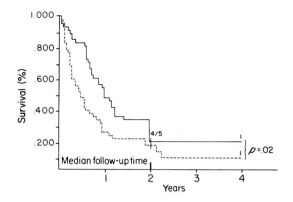

Fig. 1. Survival curve after relapse according to treatment
(*n* = 102). (———) Immunotherapy only (*n* = 47); (----) chemoimmunotherapy (*n* = 55).

According to the treatment arm, analysis performed in March
1982 with 6 years follow-up gives no difference between group A
and group B for disease-free survival, as for survival, but a significant difference (*p* = .02) (Fig. 1) in favor of immunotherapy
alone for survival after relapse, a difference that is not related
to the site of relapse or to the treatment of the relapse.

IV. DISCUSSION

We have no control group in this protocol and therefore can
therefore can draw no conclusion about BCG alone. However, it
can be noted that our survival curve is similar to that of
Spitler and Sagebiel (1980) (with or without levamisole); their
eligibility criteria were identical to ours, and our results with
immunotherapy alone are always better than chemotherapy followed
by immunotherapy. Therefore, immunotherapy by BCG might be better
than no adjuvant treatment. The difference, however, is not
likely to be major.
    Several authors (Banzet *et al.*, 1978; Beretta, 1982; Wood *et
al.*, 1982) have reported that chemoimmunotherapy is valuable as
adjuvant treatment for malignant melanoma. If we observe anything
in this trial, it is that chemoimmunotherapy may be less effective
than immunotherapy combined or interspersed with chemotherapy and
not, as in our study, following 6 months chemotherapy given alone.
If immunotherapy is of any value in melanoma, it may be very important to give it soon after (or even before) surgical removal of
the primary tumor and/or to avoid any immunosuppressive chemotherapy before immunotherapy.
    We conclude that chemotherapy followed by immunotherapy is
less effective than immunotherapy alone as adjuvant treatment for

malignant melanoma, but the difference is so far significant only for survival after relapse.

   This trial is now closed to patient accrual, but further analyses will be performed and reported. We are now conducting a new trial comparing, in a double-blind fashion, a control group with two immunoadjuvants acting selectively on T and NK cells, azimexon and bestatin.

REFERENCES

Banzet, P., Jacquillat, C., and Civatte, J. (1978). *Cancer 41*, 1240-1248.
Beretta, G. (1982). *In* "Immunotherapy of Human Cancer" (W. D. Terry and S. A. Rosenberg, eds.), pp. 259-263. Excerpta Medica, New York.
Comis, R. L., and Carter, S. K. (1974). *Cancer Treat. Rev. 1*, 285-304.
Cunningham, T. J., Schoenfeld, D., Nathanson, L., Wolter, J., Patterson, W., Cohen, M., Kuperminc, M., and Carbone, P. P. (1979). *In* "Adjuvant Therapy of Cancer" (S. E. Jones and S. E. Salmon, eds.), Vol. 2, pp. 507-517. Grune & Stratton, New York.
Eilber, F. R., Morton, D. L., Holmes, E. C., Sparks, F. C., and Ramming, K. P. (1976). *N. Engl. J. Med. 294*, 237-240.
Gutterman, J., Mavligit, G. M., McBride, C. M., Frei, E., Freireich, E. J., and Hersh, E. M. (1973). *Lancet 1*, 1208-1212.
McGovern, V. J., Mihm, M. C., Bailly, C., Booth, J. C., Clark, J., Clark, W. H., Cochron, A. J., Hardy, E. G., Micks, J. D., Levene, A., Lewis, M., Little, J. H., and Milton, G. (1973). *Cancer (Philadelphia) 32*, 1446-1457.
Morton, D. L., Holmes, E. C., Eilber, F. R., and Ramming, K. P. (1982). *In* "Immunotherapy of Human Cancer" (W. D. Terry and S. A. Rosenberg, eds.), pp. 245-249. Excerpta Medica, New York.
Patterson, A. H. G., Jerry, L. M., McClelland, A., McPherson, T. A., and Williams D. (1979). *Adjuvant Ther. Cancer 2*, 527-534.
Peto, R. (1978). *Biomedicine 28* (Special Issue), 24-36.
Pouillart, P., Schwarzenberg, L., Amiel, J. L., Mathé, G., Huguenin, P., Morin, P., Baron, A., Laparre, Ch., and Parrot, R. (1975). *Nouv. Presse Med. 4*, 721-724.
Spitler, L. E., and Sagebiel, R. (1980). *N. Engl. J. Med. 303*, 1143-1147.
Terry, W. D., Hodes, R. J., Rosenberg, S. A., Fisher, R. I., Makuch, R., Gordon, H. G., and Fisher, S. G. (1982). *In* "Immunotherapy of Human Cancer" (W. D. Terry and S. A. Rosenberg, eds.), pp. 251-257. Excerpta, New York.
Wood, W. C., Cosimi, A. B., Carey, R. W., and Kaufman, S. D. (1982). *In* "Immunotherapy of Human Cancer (W. D. Terry and S. A. Rosenberg, eds.). Excerpta Medica, New York.

CHAPTER 36

EVALUATION OF AN ANTICANCER ACTIVITY
OF A PROTEIN-BOUND POLYSACCHARIDE PS-K (KRESTIN)

Motoharu Kondo

Department of Medicine
Kyoto Prefectural University of Medicine
Kyoto, Japan

Motomichi Torisu

Department of Surgery
Kyushu University School of Medicine
Fukuoka, Japan

I. INTRODUCTION

Numerous investigations have demonstrated that a certain
species of bacteria or plant-derived polysaccharide exerts an
antitumor effect probably through potentiating host immune
responses. A protein-bound polysaccharide PS-K (Krestin) has

BASIC MECHANISMS AND CLINICAL TREATMENT
OF TUMOR METASTASIS
623

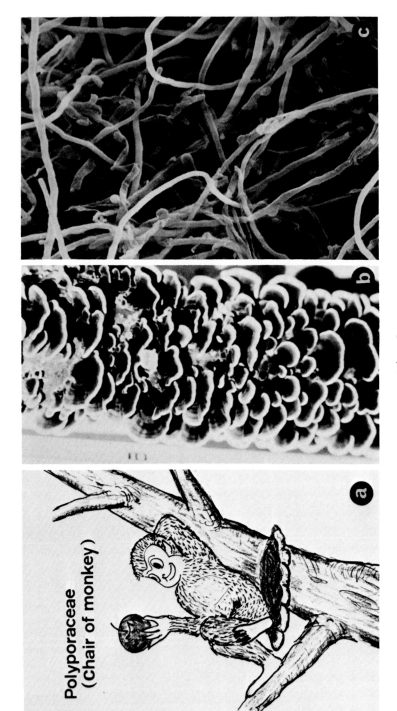

Fig. 1

been widely used for immunotherapy of cancer patients in Japan, and its efficacy in the clinical field has been evaluated in patients with advanced cancer in combination with either chemotherapy or radiotherapy (Itoh *et al.*, 1979; Hattori *et al.*, 1979; Tsukahara *et al.*, 1979). The present chapter examines the major function of PS-K and also presents a double-blind trial of PS-K on stage III gastric cancer patients.

II. PS-K

It is generally believed in Japan that a widely distributed Polyporaceae species has an antitumor effect in humans when its boiled extract is taken orally (Fig. 1a). Because it is difficult to cultivate the wild-growing Polyporaceae, *Coriolus versicolor* (strain 101), belonging to Basidiomycetes, as shown in Fig. 1b and c, was investigated for its antitumor effect. Heat extract of the cultured mycelia was precipitated by ammonium sulfate, and the desalted powder was designated as PS-K (protein-bound polysaccharide Kureha). This compound contains about 15% protein and its average molecular weight is approximately 100,000. The sugar protein consists of five kinds of sugar, mainly glucose, and the major protein has a straight-chain structure with β-(1→4)-glucan branching at the 6 or 3 position. The protein portion consists of 19 amino

Fig. 1. (a) Sarunokoshikake, a kind of mushroom that grows naturally on trees or in fields and has a shape like "the chair of a monkey," as it is called in Japan. By mycological definition, it belongs to the Polyporaceae of Basidiomycetes. For centuries it has been a tradition in Japan that the infusion of Sarunokoshikake was an effective therapy for malignant tumors. A researcher of Kureha Chemical Corporation (Tokyo, Japan) paid attention to this tradition and started the research. However, it was very difficult to obtain sufficient quantities of Sarunokoshikake for research development and commercial production. Finally, the company developed a procedure for obtaining large quantities of cultivated mycelia of *Coriolus versicolor* (Fr.) Quél. (Kawaratake) in Basidiomycetes. The characteristics of CM-101 fruit bodies (b) are compatible with those of *Coriolus versicolor*. The fungi grow on decayed trees, piling up fruit bodies in considerable numbers over a wide range of the world. The pileus is semicircular or fanshaped, 1-4 cm wide, and 0.5-1 mm thick. (c) The vegetative mycelium of CM-101 strain grows vigorously in natural media for fungal culture. A colony on agar plate is white and round, with a formation of aerial hyphae. The mycelium is 2-5 μm in width, showing branchings and septa. At the septal part, it forms clamp connections specific with Basidiomycetes.

acids, mainly aspartic acid, glutamic acid, and leucine. Since
Sephadex G-100 gel-filtered fractions of the preparation show
multiple peaks, it is obvious that PS-K is not composed of a
single substance. A brown, tasteless powder with a subtle odor,
PS-K dissolves easily in water. It is stable to temperature,
humidity, and light. When taken orally, the preparation has been
found to exert a suppressive effect on the growth of tumor.

III. ANTITUMOR EFFECT

Investigations of PS-K in animals bearing malignant tumors
have resulted in many reports demonstrating its effectiveness,
mainly in combination with chemotherapeutic agents (Tsukagoshi
and Ohashi, 1974; Yoshikumi et al., 1975; Ohno et al., 1975;
Usui et al., 1976; Akiyama et al., 1977; Ohashi et al., 1978;
Kataoka et al., 1979). The antitumor effect of PS-K is thought
to be caused mainly by the restoration of host-mediated immune
mechanism, and partly by its direct action on tumor cells, although the precise mechanism remains to be elucidated.

A. Direct Action on Tumor Cells

It has been shown that PS-K has an antitumor effect when it
is mixed with tumor cells in vitro (Katano et al., 1979). A
scanning electron micrograph of EL-4 cells incubated with
200 µg/ml of PS-K in RPMI 1640 medium at 37°C for 4 hr showed
shortening and bulging of microvilli on the cell surface, without
loss of viability. These workers also found that tumor cells incubated with PS-K lost their motility both in vitro and in vivo
using Ehrlich tumor cells and EL-4 lymphoma cells.

B. Host-Mediated Indirect Action of PS-K

It has been shown that PS-K has an antitumor effect against
Ehrlich ascites tumor cells and sarcoma 180 cells (Yoshikumi et
al., 1975), methylcholanthrene-induced sarcoma (Ohno et al.,
1975), and many other transplantable tumors. Although preliminary
experiments have been done by injecting PS-K into animals, it was
demonstrated by Tsukagoshi and Ohashi (1974) that PS-K was effective when administered orally. The mechanism of the antitumor
effect by orally administered PS-K is still obscure, but it is
speculated that PS-K restores the impaired immune response of the
tumor-bearing host.

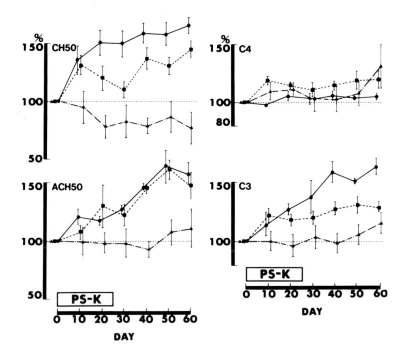

Fig. 2. Increase of serum complement levels in guinea pigs caused by oral PS-K administration. Dosages: (●, 2000 mg/kg (n = 4); ■ , 600 mg/kg (n = 5); ▲ , 60 mg/kg (n = 4).

1. Macrophage

The motility of macrophages was increased *in vitro* by PS-K. Peritoneal exudate cells obtained from guinea pigs were incubated with different concentrations of PS-K at 37°C for 24 hr, and their migration rates were investigated using the glass capillary method. The migration rate of macrophages was enhanced as the concentration of PS-K increased (Katano *et al.*, 1979). They also found that pretreatment with PS-K caused a significant increase in the number of macrophages, indicating that PS-K might have an enhancing effect on macrophage motility *in vivo* (Katano *et al.*, 1979). Since it was found that PS-K was not chemotactic for macrophages when examined using a Boyden chamber, it is obvious that PS-K enhanced macrophages *in vivo*.

2. Antibody Production

The ability to form antibodies in tumor-bearing mice was restored by the ip injection of PS-K, while no increase of antibody synthesis was observed when PS-K was given to normal mice (Nomoto *et al.*, 1975).

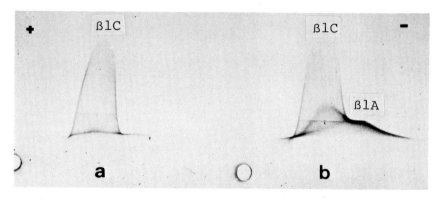

Fig. 3. Activation of complement component C3 by oral PS-K in humans as determined by conversion of β1C to β1A in cross-immunoelectrophoresis. Normal serum (a) and PS-K serum (b).

3. T-Cell Function

It is known that PS-K possesses a mitogenic effect on lymphocytes *in vitro* (Ohno *et al.*, 1975). It has also been shown that oral administration of PS-K results in an increase in the T:B ratio and blastoid transformation of lymphocytes, as well as enhancement of delayed hypersensitivity in humans as determined by PPD skin test (Yokoe *et al.*, 1979).

4. Complement

Activation of complement through the classic and the alternative pathways was observed when PS-K was incubated with normal human serum *in vitro* (Kondo *et al.*, 1978). Interestingly, oral administration of PS-K to guinea pigs enhanced serum complement level CH50 as determined by the lysis of sensitized sheep RBC, ACH50 by the lysis of unsensitized rabbit RBC, and also C4 and C3 protein (Fig. 2). Activation of complement was observed *in vivo*, when plasma of a patient, orally treated with 3 g/day of PS-K for 7 days, showed conversion of β1C to β1A, as determined by cross-immunoelectrophoresis (Fig. 3).

5. Other Actions

Administration of PS-K to normal mice increases serum interferon levels, which might enhance natural killer cell activity. An ability of mouse spleen cells to produce interferon is usually suppressed in tumor-bearing mice, whereas it is recovered by the use of PS-K.

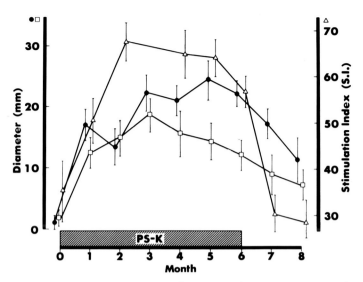

Fig. 4. Effects of PS-K on immunological parameters in aged immuno-deficient subjects without malignancy. ● , PHA; □ , PPD; △ , blastoid transformation. Vertical bars, mean ± SE (n = 10).

IV. APPLICATION OF PS-K TO AGED IMMUNE-DEFICIENT SUBJECTS

Results from various animal experiments suggested that PS-K might be useful in the treatment of human patients with malignant tumors by restoring their impaired immune response. However, since the immune response of the host-bearing malignancy is modified by the course of disease or by various forms of anticancer therapy, the effects of oral PS-K on immune responses in humans were first examined in aged individuals without malignancy who had decreased cellular immunity as determined by tuberculin (PPD) and phytohemagglutinin (PHA) skin tests as well as blastoid transformation of lymphocytes against PHA.

Ten aged individuals with decreased cellular immunity were selected from 290 subjects without malignancy, and they were treated with PS-K (3 g/day) for 6 months. It was found that the skin responses and the blastoid transformation of lymphocytes were significantly enhanced during the therapy, although their restored immune responses gradually decreased when PS-K was discontinued (Yokoe *et al.*, 1979), as shown in Fig. 4.

Thus, PS-K was found to enhance the previously impaired immune response in aged individuals during treatment with oral PS-K, suggesting that PS-K might be useful in the immunotherapy of human cancer patients. However, it is not known whether the amount of PS-K used in aged subjects without malignancy is sufficient to restore the impaired immune response in cancer patients, and further, it is not clear how long the preparation should be given to patients so as to keep potentiating their host immune response.

629

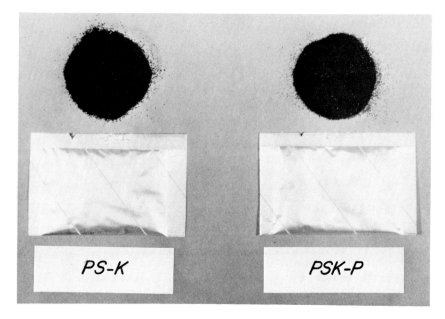

Fig. 5. This picture shows PS-K and PSK-P (placebo), which were used in our trial. By the external appearance of package and powder, PSK-P cannot be distinguished from PS-K.

Since immune response of the aged subjects decreased when the agent was discontinued, the ability of PS-K to restore host immune response seemed to be limited to the period during which it is given.

V. CLINICAL APPLICATION OF PS-K TO STAGE III GASTRIC CANCER PATIENTS

The anticancer effect of PS-K was next evaluated in patients with advanced gastric cancer by a double-blind trial. Placebo for PS-K (PSK-P) was prepared using a brown powder that resembled PS-K, as shown in Fig. 5. Placebo or PS-K was randomly given to two groups of patients who were matched for such factors as sex, age, surgical methods, histological findings, and performance status (Table I). The administration schedules of both PS-K and placebo are shown in Table II; these schedules were continued until distant metastasis or recurrence was found, at which time the patient received another operation and/or adjuvant immuno-chemotherapy. Various parameters were examined before the therapy, at 2 months, and at the time when recurrence was observed; however, no changes in serum protein, serum albumin, or red blood cell counts were seen (Fig. 6). The cellular parameters such as

TABLE I

Characterization of Patients with Gastric Cancer (Stage III)
and Therapeutic Schedule

	PS-K	PSK-P
Male:female ratio	48:24	42:30
Age (mean)	38-85 (51.4)	34-83 (52.3)
Therapeutic schedules		
Surgical method		
Partial gastrectomy	52	55
Total gastrectomy	20	17
Blood transfusion		
Yes	34	36
No	38	36
Histology		
Poorly differentiated adenocarcinoma	41	40
Moderately differentiated tubular adenocarcinoma	9	12
Well-differentiated tubular adenocarcinoma	8	9
Signet ring cell carcinoma	14	11
Performance status (group)		
I	25	24
II	30	31
III	17	15
IV	0	0

TABLE II

Administration Schedule

Administration period	PS-K (g/day)	PSK-P (g/day)
Before surgery	None	None
Surgery	None	None
After surgery[a]		
10-15 days to 2 months	3	3
2-14 months	2	1
Over 14 months	1	1

[a]When distant metastasis or recurrence was found during the
follow-up period, reoperation and/or adjuvant immunochemotherapy
was performed according to our original protocol.

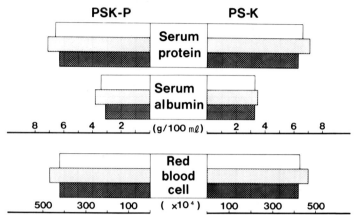

Fig. 6. Effects of PS-K and PSK-P on serum protein, serum albumin, and RBC counts in stage III gastric cancer patients. Pre-op (unshaded); 2 months post-op (light shading); recurrence (dark shading).

chemotactic activity and random migration of neutrophils were significantly enhanced in PS-K patients 2 months after the treatment, although there was no change in the number of T cells (Fig. 7). Among several skin tests for immunological parameters, only PPD was significantly increased in the PS-K group after the 2-month therapy (Fig. 8). Methodological details were described elsewhere (Boyden, 1951; David *et al.*, 1964; Tachibana and Ishikawa, 1973; Torisu *et al.*, 1975, 1978).

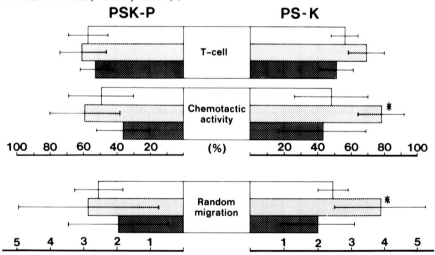

Fig. 7. Effects of PS-K and PSK-P on cellular parameters of stage III gastric cancer patients. Shading as in Fig. 6. (* $p < .05$). Horizontal bars for T cell and chemotactic activity represent percentage of mean control value from healthy volunteers, and random migration is expressed as an arbitrary unit from a micrometer in the microscope.

632

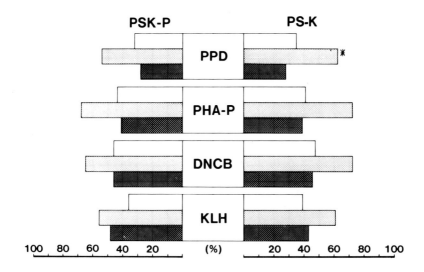

Fig. 8. Effects of PS-K and PSK-P on skin tests of stage III gastric cancer patients. Shading as in Fig. 6. (* $p < .05$).

The proportion of patients free of recurrence by the administration of PS-K and PSK-P is shown in Fig. 9, and it is clearly demonstrated that PS-K is effective in the stage III gastric cancer patients during the 80-month observation after their surgical treatments.

In the present investigation, all the patients received PS-K or placebo according to the administration schedule, and no chemotherapeutic agent was used. Although the disease-free period was significantly prolonged in the group treated with PS-K, whether the amount of PS-K used was adequate for the treatment of cancer patients should be further investigated.

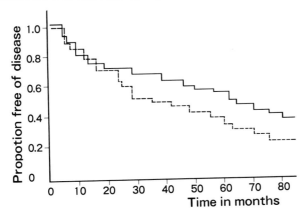

Fig. 9. Effects of PS-K (———) and PSK-P (----) on proportion of disease-free patients.

TABLE III

Side Effects of PS-K Administration

	Number of patients (%)	
Side effect	PS-K (n = 77)	PSK-P (n = 77)
Nausea	3 (3.9)	3 (3.9)
Vomiting	2 (2.6)	1 (1.3)
Appetite loss	5 (6.5)	2 (2.6)
Pigmentation of nail	4 (5.2)[a]	0
Diarrhea	4 (5.2)	1 (1.3)
Constipation	3 (3.9)	1 (1.3)
Cough on administration	7 (9.1)	2 (2.6)
Fever	0	0
Leukopenia	0	0

[a]Statistically significant (p = .001).

VI. SIDE EFFECTS

Complaints of patients during the administration of PS-K were compared with those of the patients receiving the placebo (Table III), although no specific side effects were seen in the PS-K group. Some patients complained of coughing due to the difficulty in taking the preparation in powder form, and this problem was resolved by dissolving PS-K in water before use.

VII. CONCLUSIONS

The present investigations demonstrated the usefulness of PS-K in the immunotherapy of cancer patients. Although there was a significant enhancement of disease-free period in stage III gastric cancer patients, the difference between the PS-K and placebo groups was not striking. Besides investigating optimum dosage of PS-K for the treatment of cancer patients, the preparation should be used in combination with chemotherapy or radiotherapy. The advantage of the preparation for clinical use is that it can be given to patients orally without disorder, since most of the bacterial or plant-derived so-called biological response modifiers are used in their injectable form. The duration of PS-K treatment must be as long as possible.

REFERENCES

Akiyama, J., Kawamura, T., Gotohda, E., Yamada, Y., Hosokawa, M., Kodama, T., and Kobayashi, H. (1977). *Cancer Res. 37*, 3042-3045.
Boyden, S. V. (1951). *J. Exp. Med. 93*, 107-120.
David, J. R., Al-Askari, S., Lawrence, H. S., and Thomas, L. (1964). *J. Immunol. 93*, 264-273.
Hattori, T., Niimoto, M., Koh, T., Nakano, A., Oride, M., Takiyama, W., and Nishimawari, K. (1979). *Jpn. J. Surg. 9*, 110-117.
Itoh, I., Sakai, T., and Mori, T. (1979). *Gan to Kagakuryoho 14*, 681-688.
Katano, M., Tanaka, M., Okano, H., and Torisu, M. (1979). *Proc. Jpn. Cancer Assoc. 38*, 299.
Kataoka, T., Oh-hashi, F., Tsukagoshi, S., and Sakurai, Y. (1977). *Cancer Res. 37*, 4416-4419.
Kondo, M., Kato, H., Yokoe, N., Matsumura, N., Hotta, T., and Masuda, M. (1978). *Gann 69*, 699-702.
Nomoto, K., Yoshikumi, C., Matsunaga, K., Fujii, T., and Takeya, K. (1975). *Gann 66*, 365-374.
Oh-hashi, F., Kataoka, T., and Tsukagoshi, S. (1978). *Gann 69*, 255-257.
Ohno, R., Imai, K., Yokomaku, S., and Yamada, K. (1975). *Gann 66*, 679-681.
Rinaldi, A., and Tyndalo, V. (1972). *In* "Mushrooms and Other Fungi" (A. Rinaldi and V. Tyndalo, eds.), p. 209. Hamlyn, London.
Tachibana, T., and Ishikawa, M. (1973). *Jpn. J. Exp. Med. 43*, 227-230.
Taguchi, T. (1979). *Recent Results Cancer Res. 68*, 236-240.
Torisu, M., Fukawa, M., Nishimura, M., Harasaki, H., Kai, S., and Tanaka, J. (1975). *Ann. N.Y. Acad. Sci. 277*, 160-186.
Torisu, M., Miyahara, T., Fujiwara, H., Ohsato, K., Okano, H., Fukawa, M., and Harada, M. (1977). *In* "Immunotherapy of Malignant Disease" (H. Reiner, ed.), pp. 137-142. Schattauer, Stuttgart.
Torisu, M., Miyahara, T., Yamamoto, T., Harada, M., Fujiwara, H., Kitamura, Y., Jimi, M., Ohsato, K., Tanaka, J., and Fukawa, M. (1978). *Gann Monogr. Cancer Res. 21*, 173-179.
Tsukagoshi, S., and Ohashi, F. (1974). *Gann 65*, 557-558.
Tsukahara, Y., Shiozawa, I., Noguchi, H., Iwai, S., and Fukuta, T. (1979). *Acta Obstet. Gyneol. Jpn. 31*, 889-893.
Usui, S., Urano, M., Koike, S., and Kobayashi, Y. (1976). *J. Natl. Cancer Inst. (US) 56*, 185-187.
Yokoe, N., Kato, H., Takemura, S., Yoshikawa, T., Kondo, M., Hosokawa, K., and Kodama, M. (1979). *Jpn. J. Clin. Oncol. 9*, 209-214.
Yoshikumi, C., Nomoto, K., Matsunaga, K., Fujii, T., and Takeya, K. (1975). *Gann 66*, 649-654.

DISCUSSION

COHEN: It was interesting that you could find PS-K-induced
            augmentation of macrophages in the abdominal cavity
            without effect on the tumor cells. This suggests that
            if you could combine PS-K with other therapy for
            macrophage activation, you might find good synergistic
            effects.

COLUB: Did you observe any immunological changes in the
            patients treated with PS-K placebo?

KONDO: No, there was no increase of immunity in the placebo
            group.

HOSHINO: What is the cause of the decline of PPD reaction after
            discontinuation of PS-K in elderly men? Is the PPD
            test a reaction of recalled antigen-sensitized lympho-
            cytes that are not decreased so fast?

KONDO: The reason is not known. But various kinds of skin
            tests are enhanced by the use of immunopotentiators
            other than BCG; therefore, the change of PPD skin test
            might reflect one, cellular immunity and the other,
            certain unknown mechanisms.

COHEN: There is another problem in skin testing. Cutaneous
            anergy can reflect either hyporeactivity or hyperreac-
            tivity. The latter occurs if the individual is mounting
            large-scale cellular immune responses elsewhere. This
            is the "mediator-excess" mechanism Dr. Yoshida and I
            described. Thus, to accurately assess delayed hyper-
            sensitivity, multiple parameters should be studied,
            including lymphokine production by isolated cells.

KONDO: I agree with you.

COCHRAN: What is the immunological significance of random migra-
            tion of neutrophils? What is the mechanism by which
            PS-K increases that migration?

KONDO: Since random migration of neutrophils corresponds to the
            stage of the patient, it seems to be useful to know
            nonspecific immune response of the host. The mechanism
            by which PS-K increases the migration is under investi-
            gation.

INDEX

A

N-Acetyl-D-galactosamine, inhibition of LIF, not of TMIF, 278
N-Acetyl-D-glucosamine, 105–106
Aclacinomycin, 484
Actinomycin D, 107–109
ADCC, see Antibody-dependent cellular cytotoxicity
Adhesion
  cell surface-associated molecules in receptor–ligand type interaction, 102
  intercellular, 102
  tumor cell *in vitro*, platelet-induced, 320–321
Adhesive factor
  cell surface-associated, 103–105
    characteristics of lectins, 110
    junction formation, 106–107
    release of macrophage-chemotactic factor from lymphocytes, 111
    and tumor cell adhesiveness, 118
  effect on mitosis, 110
  increase, of DNA synthesis, 110
    of protein synthesis, 110
  induction of blast transformation, 110
  mitogenic activity, 118
  regeneration, requiring protein synthesis, 108–109
  release by AH136B cells but not by AH109A cells, 111
  separation, 103–107, 109–112
    biochemical characterization, 103–106
    biological characterization, 106–107
    immunological characterization, 109–112
  serum-associated, 103–105
  stimulation of T lymphocytes, 110
  synthesis, biological characterization, 107–109
Adhesiveness
  cancer cells, 101–122
    adhesive factor separation, 103–107, 109–112
    adhesive factor synthesis, 107–109
    molecular mechanism, 101–122
    cell, three stages in process, 108–109

Adhesive substance and tumor cell differentiation, 102
Adjuvant treatment
  immunotherapy vs chemoimmunotherapy, 617–622
    eligibility, 618–619
    patients and methods, 618–620
    results, 620–621
    stratification, 619
    treatment, 620
  malignant melanoma, 617–622
Adrenal steroid hormones, 73
Adriamycin, *see* Doxorubicin
Albumin, serum, bovine, 195
Allogeneic tumor
  cells, immunostimulator, 224–225
  effect on lymph node metastasis, 228–229
  lentinan antitumor and tumor metastasis-inhibitory activities, 536–537
Alloimmunization and natural killer cytotoxicity augmentation, 135
ALS⁺, *see* Anti-lymphocyte serum
Alternative complement pathway (ACP), 256–259
  mechanism, 262–264
  in recognition of microorganisms, 262
Amnion
  human, histology, 211
    model for tumor invasion *in vitro*, 209–221
  invasion assay, 211–213
  preparation, 212–213
  polymorphonuclear leukocyte migration through, 214
  tumor cell, 214–217
    invasion, effect of chemoattractant and protease inhibitors, 216
    invasion, effect of inhibitors to protein and DNA synthesis, 216–217
    migration through, 214–215
ANA, *see* Antibody, antinuclear
Antibody, *see also* specific antibody
  adverse effect in tumor growth suppression, 255

Biology *(continued)*
  synthesis, 107–109
Blast transformation, and adhesive factor, 110
Blastogenesis, spleen cell, assay, 56
Bleomycin, 156–158
Bone marrow-derived cell
  in cancer tissues, 148–154
  pattern of accumulation: distance from
    cancer nests, 154
Breast
  cancer, adjuvant chemotherapy, 477–484
    biopsy and surgical specimens, 144
  carcinomas, mouse: resistance to metastasis
    from, 163–189
  tumor, 4–15
    cell heterogeneity, 4–8
    host cell heterogeneity of, 8–15
    macrophage and lymphocyte infiltration
      patterns in mouse, 8
    in mouse, model of tumor heterogeneity,
      4–5
    subpopulations, T cell content, 9, 10
BRM, *see* Biological response modifiers

C

CAC, *see* Complement-activating capacity
Calcium
  depletion, effect on cancer cell
    dissociation, 113–115
  ions, relationship with reduced
    adhesiveness of tumor cells for each
    other, 113
Cancer, *see also* specific cancer
  behavior, and lymphocyte and macrophage
    infiltration, 8
  biological significance of NK activity in
    human patients, 124–125
  human, and local T cell response, 143–161
    antigens defined with monoclonal
      antibodies, 145–148
    carcinogenic process and, 154–155
    clinical significance, 156–158
    functional role, 154
    patients and methods used, 144–145
    T and B cells in cancer tissues, 148–154
  immunotherapy, adoptive, 303
    tumoricidal macrophages in, 194–196
  invasion, biochemical and genetic
    mechanisms, 210
  invasive movements, active crawling of
    cells, 25–27
    due to growth, 25–26
  metastasis, 79–100
    cell biology, 96

  pathogenesis, and tumor cell
    heterogeneity, 79–100
  and research, 80
  neoplastic variability, 4
  patients, 385–404
    anti-osteogenic sarcoma monoclonal
      antibody in, 493–494, 496
    cell-mediated immunity regulatory
      mechanism, 289
    circulating immune complexes,
      386–387
    with IgG-rheumatoid factor and
      antinuclear antibody, 385–404
    immune complex of glomeruli, 385–404
    nephropathy, 387–388
    prognosis evaluation by measurement of
      immune complex, IgG ANA, and RF,
      402
    serum lymphokine activities in, 289
  therapy, subpopulation susceptibility to
    killing by, 86
  tissues, 148–154, 156–158
    thymus-derived and bone
      marrow-derived cells in, 148–154
    thymus-derived cell infiltration, clinical
      significance, 156–158
  treatment, clinical and experimental,
    447–636
Cancer cell
  adhesiveness, 101–122
    adhesive factor separation, 103–107,
      109–112
    adhesive factor synthesis, 107–109
    and dissociation, molecular mechanism,
      101–122
  autochthonous, T cell reaction to, 159
  autologous, specific killer T cell against,
    293–309
  capacity to grow in distant, heterotopic
    sites, 176
  and connective tissue barriers, 35–36
  dissociation, 112–117
    effect of calcium depletion, 113–115
    effect of intrinsic protease activation,
      115–117
  intravasation, 29
  target, T cell reaction directly to, 159
Carcinoembryonic antigen (CEA), 486
  and antibody system in cancer of
    gastrointestinal tract, 389
  in immune complexes, 387
Carcinogenesis
  immune response in, 155
  prevention by lentinan, 538–539
Carcinogenic process, and T cell response,
    154–155